Primary Care Orthopedics

Primary Care Orthopedics

Steven R. Brier, DC, ATC, CSCS

President, Island Medical Consultants
Freeport, Maine

Adjunct Associate Professor,
Department of Sports Medicine
College of Nursing
University of Southern Maine
Portland, Maine

with 382 illustrations

Mosby

A *Harcourt Health Sciences Company*
St. Louis   Philadelphia   London   Sydney   Toronto

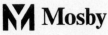

Publisher: John Schrefer
Executive Editor: Martha Sasser
Associate Developmental Editor: Christie M. Hart
Project Manager: Gayle Morris
Manufacturing Manager: Debbie LaRocca
Designer: Dana Peick
Cover Designer: Kathi Gosche

Printed in the United States of America

Mosby, Inc.
11830 Westline Industrial Drive
St. Louis, Missouri 63146

0-8016-6381-4

00 01 02 03 / 9 8 7 6 5 4 3 2

Contributors

Leo Varriala, M.D.,
Attending Physician,
Department of Orthopedic Surgery,
Mercy Hospital,
Rockville Centre, New York, and
Winthrop University Hospital,
Mineola, New York

Patrick J. DeRosa, M.D.,
Attending Physician,
Department of Orthopedic Surgery,
Mercy Hospital,
Rockville Centre, New York, and
Winthrop University Hospital,
Mineola, New York;
Team Physician,
Long Island University—C. W. Post College and Adelphi
   University

Forewords

Congratulations to Dr. Steve Brier on the publication of this superb volume. *Primary Care Orthopedics* is the best book of its kind I have seen in my 30 years in this field. I find it comprehensive, authoritative, and up-to-date. It is very well-organized, and his writing style is clear. You will find wonderful information about bone, joint, and muscle disorders in adults and children. He describes acute injuries, overuse syndromes, arthritic problems, neurovascular disorders, and infections.

This book correctly stresses the importance of an accurate diagnosis that leads to an intelligent treatment. You will improve diagnostic accuracy with the excellent chapters on orthopedic assessment and diagnostic imaging. The remaining chapters on specific joint and spinal areas instruct the reader about the structure, function, and problems that pertain to the specific body part discussed. It is here that you learn the best treatment options, which are multidisciplined in approach. Only someone with Dr. Brier's background and skill could have brought this information together in one volume. Each chapter has an extensive list of further references as well!

The text is richly enhanced by figures, photographs, line drawings, tables, algorithms, and decision-making flow charts. These make this book appropriate for students, practitioners, and the public. *Primary Care Orthopedics* definitely belongs on the bookshelf of anyone who is seriously interested in the diagnoses and treatments of a wide range of musculoskeletal ailments. I applaud Dr. Brier on this fantastic achievement.

William W. Southmayd, MD
Assistant Professor of Orthopaedics,
University of Massachusetts, Worcester, Massachusetts
Resident Training, New England Baptist Hospital,
Boston, Massachusetts
Medical Director, SportsMedicine Brookline,
Brookline, Massachusetts

Directed at the advanced student or clinician who wishes to gain a deeper understanding of the diagnoses and management of orthopedic conditions, *Primary Care Orthopedics* presents clinical information necessary to make an accurate diagnosis, integrate basic science principles with clinical management, and clearly illustrate conservative treatment protocols and guidelines. The text emphasizes early detection, appropriate referral, and sound, active conservative management of orthopedic injuries commonly encountered in an ambulatory care setting. Having known Steven Brier as a fellow chiropractic student, educator, and extremely competent and resourceful clinician, it was no surprise to read a well-organized, highly detailed textbook written in a clear concise style.

Each chapter opens with highlights and a brief description of the relevant anatomy and biomechanics, which clearly make up the basis for a scientific approach to assessment and conservative care of the locomotor system. Next, the author leads the reader through a logical sequence of examination procedures, which may include imaging and/or special studies, to aid the practitioner in making appropriate clinical decisions about evaluation and intervention strategies. Differential diagnostic lists are followed by comprehensive information about each selected disorder, including manual procedures and progressive exercise suggestions. The most helpful features of this text are the practical diagnostic and treatment algorithms and clinical pathways. Many algorithms in the clinical literature are cumbersome or difficult to follow and discourage clinicians from using them in everyday practice. Dr. Brier has organized numerous algorithms in a nonthreatening, easy-to-use style, which are valuable to the experienced practitioner, student, and those in the academic community.

Dr. Brier and his contributors are to be congratulated on their accomplishment of compiling a collection of valuable information in one comprehensive text. This book is a practical contribution to the management of musculoskeletal injuries and conditions commonly encountered by primary care–portal-of-entry providers. This is also an opportunity for me to thank Steven Brier for his contributions to the health sciences as a quality health care provider and consummate educator.

John G. Scaringe, DC, DACBSP, FICC
Clinical Professor
Los Angeles College of Chiropractic
Whittier, California

Preface

Target Audience

Primary Care Orthopedics is written for all providers of neuromusculoskeletal care that deliver conservative treatment. Some of us thrive as portal of entry physicians, while others specialize in various areas of musculoskeletal rehabilitation. It is imperative for all clinicians to strive to work in unison for a common goal—the well-being of the patient. As the new century arrives, there continues to be a great demand for the services of conservative, hands-on practitioners.

This text offers an appreciation for the various forms of treatment that are available for soft-tissue conditions: rehabilitation exercise, manipulation, clinical modalities, pharmaceuticals, and ergonomic and biomechanical alterations. I have presented to the reader other options for medical problems that do not respond to typical conservative methods and the more invasive procedures available to us at this point in time. Although all conservative health care providers strive to get each and every patient well, we all know that this is just not true in practice.

The key to successful intervention for orthopedic problems in a primary care practice is to know what conditions to refer and when and to whom to refer the refractory patient. Much depends on the primary or tentative diagnosis. Realizing that we all have significant limitations, we need to be aware of other disciplines and their penchant for results in treating soft-tissue injuries.

Chiropractors specialize in neuromusculoskeletal diagnosis and spinal manipulation, as do some osteopathic specialists. Physical therapists that specialize in orthopedic conditions use clinical modalities and rehabilitation exercise programs as the major course of treatment. Athletic trainers combine a keen knowledge of prevention and care of athletic injuries and are becoming increasingly more aware of hands-on active treatment for neuromuscular conditions. Strength and conditioning specialists use their advanced knowledge of training systems to enhance performance and prevent reinjury. Psychologists and naturopathic and homeopathic specialists are also finding their niche in the conservative treatment of soft-tissue conditions as well.

Tips for the Reader

Following the first two chapters that address orthopedic assessment and diagnostic imaging, we present a background on structure (applied anatomy) and function (clinical biomechanics) for each body part. Beginning with the upper limb and working through the axial skeleton and the lower limb, the reader will find common conditions that we meet each day in practice, as well as some not-so-common conditions. Each diagnosis comes with a table for physical examination findings, radiologic findings, and a treatment plan. Epidemiologic facts and differential diagnoses are also discussed. The generous use of clinical algorithms supports the didactic information, which allows the reader to get a "feel" for case management for various body parts at a glance. I have used highlight boxes for hot topics or controversial subjects, such as the anterior cruciate ligament–deficient knee dilemma.

Pedagogical Tips

For those students or instructors in the reading audience, you will find a series of clinical questions at the end of each chapter. These are topics of importance relevant to the chapter in which they appear. These self-help tests

will enable the student to assess his or her general knowledge of an orthopedic topic that is common in primary
care practice. Time should also be spent on the clinical
algorithms for each region, because they combine the sequencing of advanced imaging modalities, conservative
components for successful treatment, and clinical guidelines for referral of difficult cases. Key orthopedic terms
are found in the comprehensive glossary as a guide to
medical conditions and to increase understanding of the
diagnosis and management of soft-tissue injury.

Both the seasoned practitioner and the student or
intern engaged in neuromusculoskeletal education will
find it helpful to use this textbook to brush up on their
knowledge of clinical anatomy, to review biomechanical
principles for injury and disease, and to use this book as
a resource for multidisciplinary treatment options in
orthopedic care. We need to be cognizant of what other
providers may offer the patient and how we can better
coordinate successful, nonoperative care in the future.

Introduction

Primary care has become the mule of the health care professions. It has evolved into a complicated maze of provider networks, a switch board of clinical decisions and conclusions made by outside business professionals, and it continues to demand a balance between patient welfare and fiscal efficiency. What a task!

The facts in health care for the 21st century speak for themselves—roles are not so clear cut anymore. Too many hands are in the till; too many pairs of eyes are watching the statistical outcomes. Consequently, the patient—our reason for practicing our art in the first place—can get lost in the proverbial bureaucratic shuffle. Yet through this tumultuous time, some wonderful events are unfolding.

For one, the lines that once separated orthodox territories from alternative providers are fading. New and exciting research is uncovering promising therapies once discarded as the work of medical heretics. The dawning of a new age for the delivery of multidisciplinary health care is on our doorstep, and those that are entrusted with the public's welfare must heed the call.

Primary Care Orthopedics combines applied anatomy and biomechanics with clinical decision making for neuromusculoskeletal impairment. It presents true interdisciplinary models of treatment for common orthopedic maladies, along with a rationale of why they are effective. The text spends a great deal of time on sequencing advanced imaging modalities, as well as offers guidelines for specialty referral. It is precisely this micromanaging of each case that sets the effective provider apart from the crowd.

Basic tenets in musculoskeletal medicine are emphasized in the text: mechanical problems respond to graded therapeutic exercise; muscular impairment responds to motion; overuse syndromes require RICE before they are rehabilitated—beware of the diagnosis of a sprain in a young, active child, for example. There are also new conditions with which we are just beginning to grapple, such as CFIDS, fibromyalgia, and Lyme disease, as well as some old standbys, such as low back pain and anterior knee pain, presented from a slightly different perspective and stacked with some new ideas. Through it all, structure and function are entwined and co-dependent on one another. Bridging the gaps between allopathic, chiropractic, and osteopathic models of health care is a laudable goal—there are more similarities than differences.

Both portal-of-entry providers and allied health practitioners from varied disciplines will benefit from this text. It is my sincere hope that whichever initials follow your name—DC, DO, MD, ATC, PT, CSCS, or PhD—and from whatever educational background you may come, you will find clinical relevance and points of interest in the pages that follow. Our greatest challenge as providers of health care is to learn what works best, when it works best, and why it works best. This requires the almost Herculean task of checking your ego at the door, learning from your patients, and last, but not least, learning from each other.

Acknowledgments

Completing a project such as this is a good time to reflect on the past and pause to give thanks to the many individuals who have helped along the way. My deep gratitude to Charles R. Bianculli, DC, Patrick J. DeRosa, MD, and Richard Kroe, DC, who were wonderful mentors that always gave the time and effort to help me become a better clinician and person. I thank Robert Gariglio, ATC, MS, Avrum I. Musnick, DC, and Vincent Salamone, ATC, for teaching me humility and how to assess my limitations. I thank Robert Brier, PhD, and William F. Straub, PhD, who introduced me to academia and scholarship, to I. Edward Alcamo, PhD, who encouraged me to publish, and to Dennis Cardone, DO, and Eric Dorsky, JD, for 30 wonderful years of friendship.

Completing a book of this nature takes the methodical efforts of a team. My gratitude goes to Maxine Cappel Mayreis, DC, and to James Inzerillo, DC, for their moral support and hard work on the original manuscript. I thank John F. Clennan, Esq, medicolegal expert and magnificent writer of short stories, for his friendship and guidance. Special thanks go to my colleague and friend, Donald Holzer, MD, clinical assistant professor of neurology–Cornell University Medical College, for his assistance on electrodiagnostic medicine; to Richard Silvergleid, MD, and Manhasset Diagnostic Imaging, PC, to Robert Goodman, MD, and South Suffolk MRI, and to Douglas Obetz, DC, CCSP, for their work on the figures and technical aspects of this book; to Lisa Bloom, DC, for her medical illustrations; to Thomas M. Starace, DC, CSCS, for his help on the photographs of spinal and knee rehabilitation and for his continued support throughout my career; and to David G. Simmons, MD, and the late Janet G. Travell, MD, for their help and guidance on myofascial pain syndromes of the spine.

I would like to take this opportunity to thank Martha Sasser, Executive Editor at Mosby, for not giving up on this book as it made its way from Chicago to St. Louis. A special note of thanks goes to Gail Martin who completed the arduous task of taking the manuscript in midform and organizing and editing it to completion—what patience! Without Gail, this book would not have been published. I thank Kellie White at Mosby for holding down the fort during the middle relief innings, and to Dana Peick for her wonderful layout and art work in piecing it all together. Finally, I cannot thank enough Christie M. Hart, Associate Developmental Editor, for the amount of time and hard work she gave during the final 12 months to bring this book to fruition. Her keen eye and knack for content analysis is remarkable for a professional outside of the medical fields!

To all my former students at New York Chiropractic College, Long Island University–C.W. Post Campus, and The University of Southern Maine, thank you for the privilege of being a part of your education and for making me a better clinician.

Thank you to my wife, Dr. Kimberly Slade-Brier; your love and understanding is instrumental in every achievement in my life. I cannot begin to repay you for your kindness and devotion.

To my parents, Michael and Shelia, thank you for teaching me the value of education and of being a participant in life—not just a spectator; to my sister, Michelle, for her trust and the honor of confiding in me; and to Norma and Claire, the matriarchs of the family, for their endless strength and endurance.

Table of Contents

Primary Care
Orthopedics

Orthopedic Assessment

Basically a fact-finding mission, orthopedic assessment begins with the observation of patients as they enter the room. It may not end until the last diagnostic test is complete. The differential diagnosis of a patient's musculoskeletal malady requires (1) a thorough knowledge of anatomy and (2) the ability to listen carefully. The knowledge of anatomy is paramount; diagnosing a patient's condition involves primarily the application of anatomic knowledge. It is also necessary, however, to obtain an appropriate history by asking the right questions and listening carefully to the answers. Thus

applied anatomy + history = differential diagnosis

The key steps in drawing a tentative conclusion about a patient's complaint are (1) history taking, (2) observation, (3) palpation, (4) orthopedic testing, and (5) diagnostic procedures. Each constitutes a vital piece in the ever-challenging puzzle of the orthopedic diagnosis.

History Taking

A careful history is one of the most crucial elements of orthopedic assessment. An experienced diagnostician can form an idea of which structures are injured simply from the patient's history. Therefore listening is the key to history taking.

The questions should never steer the patient's answers unnaturally. Rather, they should provide the patient with options regarding the answers. For example, if the patient reports pain, the clinician may ask, "Does your pain stay at this spot, or does it travel somewhere else?" Open-ended questions (e.g., "Where do you feel the pain?") are more likely to elicit an accurate response than closed-ended questions (e.g., "Is this where your pain is?"), particularly from timid patients who may tell a clinician what they believe the clinician wants to hear. The phrasing is crucial; if the examiner does not give the patient an opportunity to describe the pain in detail, the examiner may miss a key piece of information for the differential diagnosis puzzle.

History Essentials

Every history of a musculoskeletal condition should cover certain key points. For example, were there any prior injuries to the joint in question or adjacent joints? History of trauma may help differentiate between inherent laxity (i.e., hypermobility of the ligaments and joint capsule) and past instability. It is also important to obtain a history of any trauma on the contralateral, or "good," side to permit comparison with the injured part for a true baseline measurement of joint stability.

What treatment was performed initially for the musculoskeletal problem? If an injury caused the problem, the clinician should determine whether the patient stopped the activity immediately, applied heat or ice packs, or administered any mode of self-treatment, such as bandage wrapping or immobilization. If the patient took any over-the-counter medications for the injury, the clinician needs to find out about their effect. Many times muscular problems do not improve with rest. The lack of external work or complete rest that occurs with immobilization can make the patient's condition worse in some cases. Injured joints and adjacent structures may be neglected, deconditioned, weakened, and atrophied from prolonged periods of protection, so it is important to inquire about the rest and activity of the injured area.

Did the patient consult any other clinician about the injury? It is important to learn the name and specialty of the practitioner who first examined the injury or the hospital where the patient visited the emergency room, the conclusion of the practitioner, and any treatment or rehabilitation recommended. If possible, it is wise to obtain the medical records.

What kind of trauma, if any, was sustained? What was the precise mechanism of injury? An accurate picture of the injury scenario, including the exact position of the injured area at the time of injury and the magnitude of stress and strain at the site, is essential. The extent of tissue damage produced through an overuse syndrome may differ greatly from that caused by a high-speed event. For example, repetitive microtears from overuse are not usually associated with gross joint instability, as is a high-acceleration skiing injury.

Did the patient hear a "pop" or feel a "snap?" A "pop" or "snap" may indicate an internal derangement of a joint, such as a subluxed glenohumeral joint or a torn meniscus in the knee. Stresses on articular structures (e.g., fibrocartilage and ligaments) may yield these noises.

On what type of surface did the injury occur? Injuries take place on surfaces as diverse as a snowy mountain top or synthetic turf for soccer, football, or baseball; different surfaces are known for different types of injuries. For example, synthetic turf may promote medial joint compartment injuries, such as cartilage or ligament tears from a fixed foot and knee rotation, whereas a slick and slippery playing surface may cause an athlete's legs to slide out from under him or her.

What were the impact forces of the injury? The speed of an automobile (e.g., 20 miles per hour versus 60 miles per hour) may affect the type of injury sustained in an automobile accident, for example. Similarly, an injury received as the patient is beginning to accelerate (e.g., running to first base after hitting a baseball) differs from an injury received as the patient is decelerating (e.g., preparing to round the bag).

Where is the pain? Does it move or radiate? It is best to ask the patient to point to the exact site of the pain. Patients may say that they have a pain in one location, such as the hip, but point somewhere else, such as the sacroiliac joint. The more distal the pain, the more accurately patients can determine its location because of increases in two-point discrimination, in sensory input, and in the population of pain receptors.

What provokes the pain or is palliative for it? Pain that arises with activity and decreases with rest is likely to have a mechanical cause. In addition, pain may vary during the course of the day. Morning pain and stiffness that ease during the day usually indicate a chronic inflammatory or arthritic cause. The pain may be positional; most cases of mechanical spinal pain have both a provocative and palliative arc of motion.

What are the patient's daily physical activities? Information about the patient's occupation can provide clues to the problem. For instance, because they spend significant amounts of time on a flexed knee, carpenters tend to have problems with their patellofemoral joints. Secretaries and hairdressers have postural myofascial disorders of the cervicodorsal and scapulothoracic regions. Thus the clinician should ask about the setup at work, the types of chairs that are used, the height of the display or computer terminal, and other ergonomic conditions. The patient's sleeping posture is also important.

How long has the patient had this pain? Many cases of myofascial pain, especially of the spine, are chronic in nature. Pain of this type may have developed during years of faulty posture.

What is the quality of the pain? Different types of pain are attributable to different types of tissue. Patients usually describe nerve pain, for example, as sharp or burning, with a specific distribution of a peripheral nerve. Bone pain is often deep, pinpointed, and boring. Muscular pain is dull, aching, and generally very diffuse. Sometimes, this kind of pain is referred to other areas and structures.

Pain Patterns

Because several patterns of pain that originate in the spine appear similar, spinal pain is one of the most difficult areas to diagnose differentially. There are three primary patterns: dermatogenous, myotogenous, and sclerotogenous (Figure 1-1).

A dermatome is the area of sensation attributed to a particular nerve root level; thus nerve root pain usually follows a specific dermatogenous pattern. Often described as sharp, stabbing, and well-demarcated, dermatogenous pain may result from herniated disks, stretch injuries, and tumors.

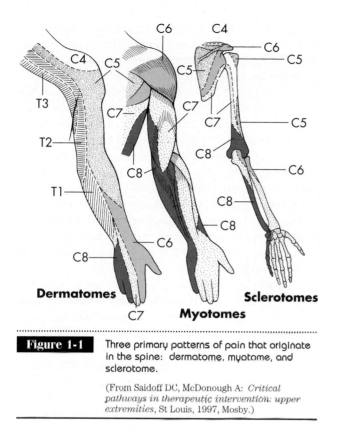

Dermatomes

Myotomes

Sclerotomes

Figure 1-1 Three primary patterns of pain that originate in the spine: dermatome, myotome, and sclerotome.

(From Saidoff DC, McDonough A: *Critical pathways in therapeutic intervention: upper extremities*, St Louis, 1997, Mosby.)

Pain referral with a muscular or fascial origin is called myotogenous pain. Areas known as trigger points refer pain to a distant site and are evident in patients with myofascial pain syndromes. Specific sites of tenderness that do not result from referred pain, termed tender points, develop in patients with varied soft-tissue, rheumatoid, and collagenic-vascular disorders, such as systemic lupus erythematous or fibromyalgia.[11,14] Information about inactivity or immobility is especially important for patients with chronic complaints, because a myotogenous or myofascial injury may indicate the need for extensive rehabilitation.

Pain referred from somatic structures, such as cartilage, ligament, joint capsule, or bone, may not follow a textbook dermatogenous pattern as does nerve root pain. Termed sclerotomes, these areas of common referral tend to show great variability among individuals, which makes somatically referred pain even more elusive in the differential diagnosis. Patients may describe this type of pain as dull, achy, diffuse, and difficult to pinpoint. They may point to a distribution area that involves several peripheral nerves. Scleratogenous-referred pain is one of the more common spinal pain patterns.

Some patients may not have a discriminating threshold of pain or may have little tolerance for pain. When these patients have a new complaint, it is easy to dismiss the new problem as "this week's pain." Such an attitude may cause the clinician to miss important information, however. It is essential to take a prudent history, including an outline of the details of the latest complaint.

Observation

The clinician begins to observe patients as soon as they enter the room and continues to make observations throughout the assessment. The clinician watches to see how patients rise from the reception room chairs, how and when they shift their postures, what their seated postures are, and whether they lean toward or away from the side of their chief complaints. Because the human frame is usually symmetric, it is essential to check for symmetry in muscle tone, laxity, motion, and shape. What is on the right should be on the left, although prior trauma and congenital defects can change the comparison value of a patient's contralateral side.

Palpation

Concentration and experience enhance the tactile art of evaluating human structures through palpation. The more sensitive sides of the fingers discriminate structures; the ends of the fingertips provide better sensory feedback when palpating a joint than do the pads of the fingers.

In an orthopedic assessment the clinician palpates for structural symmetry, resting muscle tone, periarticular myofascial tension, and jointlike pain. Supporting structures of ligament, tendon, muscle, and bone must be properly exposed for palpation. It is possible to detect joint effusions by meticulous palpation and to determine their origin, whether extraarticular or intraarticular (Figure 1-2). Any heat in a joint may indicate an inflammatory or infectious process.

Orthopedic Testing

Range-of-Motion Testing

Of all the orthopedic tests that a clinician performs on a patient, none is more crucial than the range-of-motion testing of the affected area. This testing provides information about the origin of the patient's pain, since movement reproduces the pain. The patient should be checked

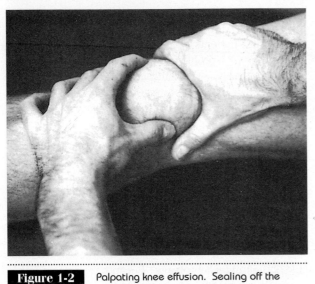

Figure 1-2   Palpating knee effusion. Sealing off the suprapatellar pouch enables the clinician to milk the fluid down into the joint cavity.

(From Mercier LR: *Practical Orthopedics,* ed 4, St Louis, 1995, Mosby.)

symmetrically for active motion of all articulations that may be involved in the dysfunction or injury. The examiner then takes the patient through the passive range of motion; in this process, the examiner evaluates the "end-feel" (i.e., springiness) of the joint in question.

The clinician must differentiate between a suspected spinal origin of pain (central) and an orthopedic condition that involves an extremity (peripheral). Range-of-motion tests reproduce spinal pain if it is mechanical in nature. In addition, the clinician evaluates joint stability during range-of-motion testing and later correlates the findings with stability test results.

Pinpointing the exact site of a soft-tissue lesion can be difficult. An important element of the physical examination process is identifying the site from which the pain or dysfunction is originating.

Local Versus Referred Pain

A simple yet complex procedure—putting joints and their juxtaarticular structures through their normal movements—yields invaluable information. Range-of-motion testing may be the only true clue to the etiology of nonmechanical back pain from a visceral origin, for example. Similarly, if a patient is complaining of a vague, dull elbow pain that emanates from the upper arm, the clinician puts the joints of the brachium through their

normal ranges of motion to rule out a local orthopedic lesion. If the result of testing is unremarkable, the clinician puts the cervical spine through its ranges of motion quite carefully; the patient's pain may be referred.

When asked to indicate the location of the pain, the patient with referred pain may point to a large generalized area; the patient can be more specific when the lesion is localized. If a patient complains of unrelenting spinal pain, yet has full, pain-free range of motion, a red warning light should go on in the examiner's head. Either the patient has an organic disease or the patient is not telling the truth. In the former scenario the patient probably has some viscerosomatic pain, perhaps ominous in reality, that mandates further diagnostic testing for a working diagnosis. In the latter case the pain may have a psychosocial cause.

If referred pain from a diseased organ system is mimicking a local orthopedic problem, the clinician should not hesitate to order appropriate tests and practice defensively. Determination of the erythrocyte sedimentation rate (ESR) is appropriate, for example, when the clinician suspects the presence of an inflammatory process. Patients with a history of malignancy should be handled carefully. Bone scanning to rule out skeletal metastasis and laboratory markers (e.g., measurement of serum calcium level) to investigate the possibility of a destructive bone tumor should be used at the earliest opportunity.[4] Certain types of cases should stand out further in the examiner's mind. Shoulder pain with no local orthopedic findings and full, painless range of motion in a patient who is over the age of 35 years and has a history of cigarette smoking may be a classic example of lung referral. A lordotic chest film of the lung apices should be taken to rule out a Pancoast's tumor. Visceral referral must be included in the differential list as well. In addition, the possibility of sympathetic nervous system involvement, as in Horner's syndrome, should be meticulously investigated.

Stability Testing

What radiology is to the diagnosis of fractures, stability testing is to the diagnosis of joint sprains. Stability testing indicates the extent of damage to a joint, the amount of instability present, and whether immobilization is necessary.

Because clinical examination reveals the degree of ligamentous or joint sprain (Table 1-1), the practitioner must be able to test accurately for joint instability. Stability testing is a series of stress tests that puts joint and

Table 1-1	Functional Capacity of Injured Ligaments						
Extent of Failure	**Sprain**	**Damage***	**Joint Motion, Subluxation**	**Residual Strength**	**Residual Functional Length**	**Residual Functional Capacity**
Minimal	First degree	Less than one third of fibers failed; includes most sprains with few to some fibers failed Microtears also exist	None	Retained or slightly decreased	Normal	Retained
Partial	Second degree	One-third to two-thirds ligament damage; significant damage, but parts of the ligament are still functional Microtears may exist	In general, minimal or no increased motion Remaining fibers in ligament resist opening	Marked decrease At risk for complete failure	Increased, still within functional range but may later act as a check rein rather than subtle control of joint motions	Marked compromise; requires healing to regain function
Complete	Third degree	Over two-thirds to complete failure; continuity remains in part	Depends on secondary restraints	Little to none	Lost	Severely compromised or lost
		Continuity lost and gross separation between fibers	Depends on secondary restraints	None	Lost	Lost

*Estimate of damage is often difficult; however, the different types listed can usually be differentiated. Anterior and posterior cruciate tears commonly exist with little to no abnormal laxity. The examination for medial and lateral ligamentous injury is usually more accurate.

(From Feagin JA, editor: *The crucial ligaments,* New York, 1988, Churchill Livingstone.)

periarticular structures through movements and end-range motions. It involves testing ligamentous tissues and joint capsules (Figure 1-3), since these important structures make it possible for the joint to withstand outside forces.

In view of the importance of symmetry, it is always wise to check both sides. Checking the uninjured side establishes a good, accurate baseline value of joint stability for comparison with that on the injured side. Bilateral ligamentous laxity shows that the patient's "instability" is normal, that laxity is inherent for this patient. It is not uncommon for patients with previously diagnosed sprains to exhibit the same amount of laxity on the contralateral side as patients with no history of trauma.

Joint Motion

It is a mistake to assume that the underlying cause of any movement restriction in a joint's passive range of motion is exclusively articular. Muscular hypertonicity can limit passive movement, for example, and often occurs in

Lachman Test

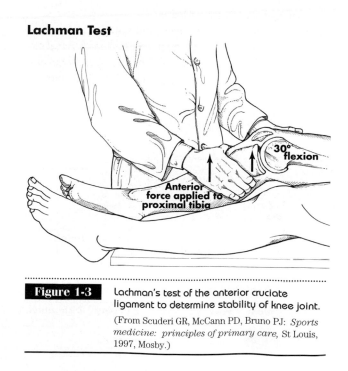

30° flexion

Anterior force applied to proximal tibia

Figure 1-3	Lachman's test of the anterior cruciate ligament to determine stability of knee joint.

(From Scuderi GR, McCann PD, Bruno PJ: *Sports medicine: principles of primary care,* St Louis, 1997, Mosby.)

association with articular lesions (joint dysfunction).[8] Chronic joint problems are also commonly associated with myofascitis. Distinguishing an articular from a muscular cause of movement restriction is not as clear-cut as once believed. Certain clinical findings in the skeletal system provide diagnostic clues, however.

Paraphysiologic Motion

To the examiner, the end of a joint's normal range of motion should feel palpable and springy. A hard and blocked sensation signifies an articular lesion or a pathologic articular physiology. It is possible to restore normal joint mobility by gapping (i.e., opening or overstretching) the joint beyond the normal physiologic range of motion without compromising the joint's integrity (e.g., causing a dislocation). Such manipulation, which takes place with a high-velocity, low-amplitude thrust, produces a characteristic cracking sound and moves the joint into the paraphysiologic range of movement (Figure 1-4).

If joint play (end-stage physiologic movement) is more affected than is normal active joint movement (before end stage), the cause of dysfunction is probably articular rather than muscular. Other signs of articular causes of dysfunction include the restoration of joint mobility through the manipulation of the affected joint in a neutral position and the observation of joint dysfunction after the administration of muscle relaxant medication.

Active and Passive Motion

Active or voluntary movement and passive or involuntary movement can reveal much during the physical examination. Although joint play is involuntary in nature, it does have a critical role in the normal health of synovial joints. Full, unrestricted passive movement is important for full, painless range of active motion. The term *joint dysfunction* signifies an aberration of passive joint movement.

Periarticular structures, such as muscles and tendons, are responsible for active movement. The synovial joint capsule and related structures are involved in passive movement. Thus a restriction on passive movement with joint blockage at end-feel suggests an articular cause for the dysfunction, with or without soft-tissue hypertonicity. If a painful arc of joint motion is seen when motion is induced, then the soft-tissue structures (i.e., muscle and tendon) are likely to be involved in pathomechanic motion.

At a gross kinetic level, active motion is essential for a healthy musculoskeletal system. The examiner should carry out manual muscle testing during the evaluation of active motion, first without examiner resistance and then with resistance. Strength is compared bilaterally and graded on a scale of 0 to 5. Passive joint dysfunction, although more subtle, may be responsible for many chronic syndromes of the synovial joint system. In most joints this passive movement is less than 4 mm.

Diagnostic Procedures

Practitioners use diagnostic testing not only to rule out a particular condition, but also to determine why a patient has not made the type of progress expected for the diagnosis or why a condition that had been under control has stopped improving or has become worse. A practitioner must always realize that when one type of therapeutic approach proves ineffective after a reasonable trial, it is necessary to try another approach or make a referral to another specialist. Also, appropriate testing may enable the clinician to reach a new, more accurate physical diagnosis (Table 1-2). A patient's pain level often prohibits full orthopedic testing on the first visit; follow-up testing allows a more accurate assessment of the condition.

For nontraumatic conditions, the first step is to determine whether there is an effusion. The presence of an effusion in association with a noneventful history suggests arthritides, infection, and neoplasm. Signs of sepsis in a joint include a hot, red, or swollen area; the joint's range of motion may be decreased if an infectious process is present. Swelling with no history of trauma tells the astute clinician to be quite suspicious. Radiologic studies, laboratory measurements, and further testing may be necessary to ensure an accurate diagnosis.

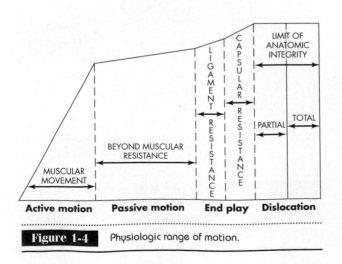

Figure 1-4 Physiologic range of motion.

Table 1-2	Indications for Diagnostic Procedures in Musculoskeletal Disease

Test	Indications
CT	Musculoskeletal trauma, particularly in the spine, acetabulum, and glenoid; back pain (e.g., herniation of nucleus pulposus, lumbar stenosis, facet joint arthritis); metabolic bone disease; tumor and congenital abnormalities (e.g., femoral anteversion, talocalcaneal coalition)
Conventional (contrast) arthrography	Tears of the rotator cuff, meniscal tears, adhesive capsulitis
Conventional tomography	Suspected occult fractures, delineation of fracture patterns in complex trauma, characterization of neoplastic and infectious processes
Electrodiagnostic tests	
EMG	Suspected denervating neuromuscular disease (e.g., nerve root lesions)
NCV	Suspected peripheral entrapment neuropathies
SSEP	Altered spinal cord function
Laboratory tests	Screening for malignancy, connective tissue disorders, infection, and general systemic illness
MRI	Spinal disk disease, radiculopathy, metastatic disease, avascular necrosis of the hip, meniscal tears, pathologic condition of the spinal cord, bone marrow disorders
Plain-film radiography	Initial workup for patients with musculoskeletal abnormalities, suspected fracture (minimum of two views), displacement of articular structures, arthritides, suspected pathologic condition of bone
Radionuclide scintigraphy (nuclear medicine)	Evaluation of bone pain when plain films are equivocal or normal; neoplastic disease, early diagnosis of stress fractures, avascular necrosis and osteomyelitis, evaluation of Paget's disease
US	Definition of soft-tissue anatomy, possibility of intraarticular and periarticular fluid (e.g., popliteal cysts, joint effusions), soft-tissue masses, pediatric hip pathology on a moving child

CT, Computed tomography; **EMG,** electromyography, **NCV,** nerve conduction velocity, **SSEP,** somatosensory-evoked potential, **MRI,** magnetic resonance imaging, **US,** ultrasonography.

For traumatic injuries, appropriate testing procedures include ordering plain films to rule out a fracture or dislocation or to diagnose subluxation or ligamentous instability.[2] A minimum of two views taken 90 degrees from each other is required. Computerized or conventional tomography may be necessary to diagnose accurately occult fractures or complex injuries that involve multiple sites.[1] Magnetic resonance imaging (MRI) is being used more for evaluating conditions of the central nervous system, the intervertebral disk, and the spinal cord itself.

Brand and associates reviewed and correlated clinical signs and symptoms of patients entering a busy emergency department after musculoskeletal trauma with the presence of fracture on subsequent radiographic films.[1] It was determined that the most accurate predictors for the presence of a fracture was bony deformity, instability, or crepitation at the fracture site. The next most accurate indicator was the presence of point tenderness.

Plain radiographic films have the advantage of ready availability; they can be obtained rapidly when it is necessary to rule out serious skeletal injury. They are also relatively inexpensive. Although clinical signs may cause the clinician to suspect a fracture, radiographic films are a definitive diagnostic procedure. In the spine, for example, plain films allow the clinician to visualize the bony elements clearly and to note degenerative changes (e.g., disk space narrowing). They provide little, if any, information concerning the contents of the spinal canal, however, and paraspinal information is minimal.[3] Moderate peripheral joint trauma may be an indication for a plain film series, primarily because of the vulnerability of the extremities. Their protective secondary restraints are not as powerful as those of the paraspinal structures.

Ancillary Procedure Protocol

Often, treatment or rehabilitation cannot begin the first day, because either the results of all diagnostic tests are not available or the patient's pain level does not permit the performance of all diagnostic tests. The sooner the patient's pain and swelling can be reduced, the sooner the clinician can complete the diagnostic work, reach a more accurate diagnosis, and begin rehabilitation. Thus it is essential to use ancillary procedure protocol if it is impossible to complete the assessment immediately.

The body's exaggerated inflammatory response to orthopedic trauma may cause not only pain but also a loss of joint mobility. The goal of preliminary treatment therefore is primarily to control pain and inflammation to facilitate joint function and permit completion of the assessment. The joint swelling caused by inflammation produces a painful response through the distention of the joint capsule and extravasation of intracellular fluid. Control of the swelling will help control the body's pain response. Indeed, control of pain and swelling permits early joint mobilization and an earlier return to homeostatic biomechanical function. Early intervention with rest, ice, compression, and elevation (RICE) is most effective in combating edema (Figure 1-5).[6,7,9,15]

Assessment in the Child

A child's anatomy, biomechanics, and skeletal physiology are very different from those of a fully grown adult. As a result, orthopedic trauma produces a different pattern of injury, and children may pose a diagnostic dilemma to the examiner. Trauma can have a drastic effect at the skeletal growth centers, for example, through widening of the epiphyseal plate or osseous displacement (Figure 1-6).[10] Thus when evaluating the condition of a youngster suffering from a traumatic injury, a practitioner must remember that an apparent ligamentous instability may in reality be a fracture to the growth plate.[5] Before diagnosing a "sprain" in preadolescents, it may be necessary to order radiographic studies to rule out a compromised epiphysis that will fail under external stress.

Since the periosteum is thicker and stronger in the young patient, it produces callus more quickly and in greater amounts than in adults. The osteoid of a child's bone is not significantly less calcified, but the density of a young bone is certainly less than that of an adult bone. Immature bone exhibits porosity with a pitted cortex, and the extensive haversian canals permit fracture easily.[5] Furthermore, the porous nature of a child's bone allows

RICE Regimen

Rest	Avoid activities that cause sharp pain. Ensure availability of crutches if patient cannot walk without a limp. Continue relative rest until pain and swelling are negligible on weight-bearing limb.
Ice	Ice provides local contraction of blood vessels so that blood flow is reduced to injured area. Reduction of swelling enhances healing. Ice provides some pain relief. Apply ice for 15 to 20 minutes initially every hour for 72 hours, then three to four times every 24 hours until pain, swelling, and inflammation dissipates.
Compression	Various compressive dressings combined with ice decrease swelling in acute inflammatory phase.
Elevation	Elevated limbs have a significant decrease in volumetric displacement because lymphatics have to work against decreased pressure to return excess fluid. As interstitial fluid and pressure increase past certain levels, a critical point is reached that causes collapse of lymphatic vessels.

Figure 1-5 Physiologic range of motion. RICE Regimen.
(Adapted from Brotzman S: *Clinical orthopaedic rehabilitation*, St Louis, 1996, Mosby.)

for failure in compression, as well as the failure in tension that occurs in the compact adult bone (Figure 1-7).[12,13]

In the spectrum of soft-tissue microtrauma, injury to an immature musculoskeletal system occurs most likely at the growth centers where tendons attach to puttylike structures called apophyses. The term *traction apophysitis* came about when tight muscle-tendon units, inflexible during adolescent spurts of growth, were found to cause types of traction insults at the growth centers responsible for growth (i.e., widening) of the long bones. Areas of tendinous insertion, such as the proximal tibia, proximal olecranon, and os calcis, are common sites of traction apophysitis. Whereas adults may develop muscle strains, tendonitis, and bursitis, the young patient (especially a physically active youngster) is more likely to develop a traction apophysitis and epiphysitis.

Conclusion

Sometimes, conditions with closely related symptoms require vastly different treatment schemes. For example,

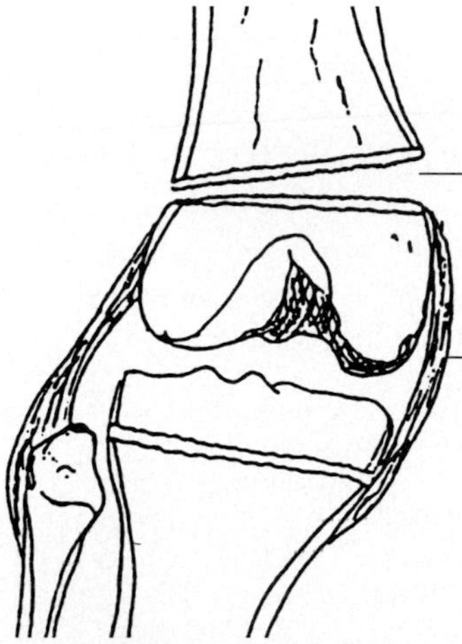
Epiphyseal plate
Medial collateral ligament

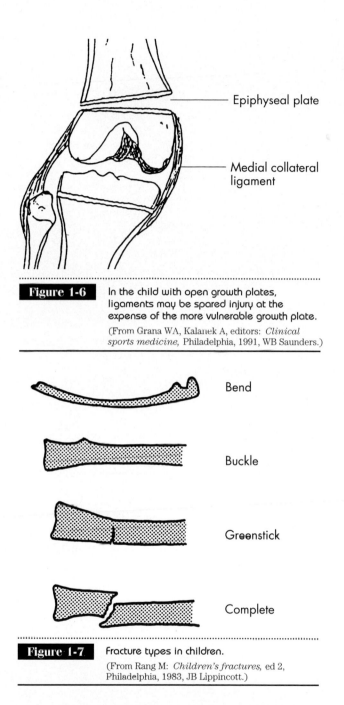

Figure 1-6 In the child with open growth plates, ligaments may be spared injury at the expense of the more vulnerable growth plate.

(From Grana WA, Kalanek A, editors: *Clinical sports medicine,* Philadelphia, 1991, WB Saunders.)

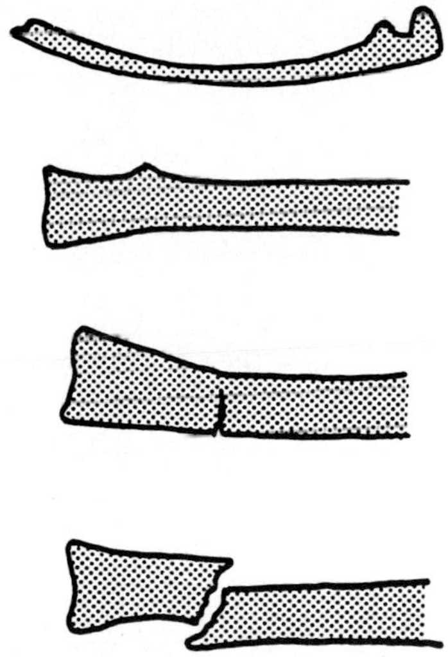
Bend
Buckle
Greenstick
Complete

Figure 1-7 Fracture types in children.

(From Rang M: *Children's fractures,* ed 2, Philadelphia, 1983, JB Lippincott.)

adhesive capsulitis of the shoulder requires immediate mobilization, whereas a dislocated shoulder requires immediate immobilization. Only with a thorough history, an appropriate assessment, and an accurate diagnosis can a proper treatment and rehabilitation program be prescribed. Prior experience usually allows the clinician to outline a treatment plan and estimate a time frame for patient recuperation and rehabilitation.

Review Questions

1. Hearing a "snap" or feeling a "pop" during an injury may indicate what type of trauma?
2. Morning stiffness is indicative of what ailment?
3. What is the usual origin of dull, achy, and diffuse pain?
4. Palpation is important in determining what clinical finding, indicating an internal derangement in a joint?
5. What may be the origin of unrelenting pain that cannot be reproduced on range-of-motion testing?
6. What are some of the clinical uses of plain x-ray films?
7. Describe the biologic differences between immature bone in the child and mature bone in the adult.

References

1. Brand DA et al: A protocol for selecting patients with injured extremities who need x-rays, *N Engl J Med* 306:333, 1982.
2. Bushong SC: *Radiologic science for technologists: physics, biology, and protection,* ed 5, St Louis, 1993, Mosby.
3. Deyo RA, Bigos SJ, Maravilla KR: Diagnostic imaging procedures for the lumbar spine, *Ann Intern Med* 111:865, 1989.
4. Gustillo RB, Kyle RF, Templemen D: *Fractures and dislocations,* vol 1, St Louis, 1993, Mosby.
5. Herndon WA: Acute and chronic injury: its effect on growth in the young athlete. In Grana WA et al, editors: *Advances in sports medicine fitness,* vol 3, Chicago, 1990, Year Book Medical Publishing.
6. Hocutt JE, Jaffe R, Rylander CR et al: Cryotherapy in ankle sprains, *Am J Sports Med* 10(5):316, 1982.
7. Knight KL, Londeree BR: Comparison of blood flow in the ankle of uninjured subjects during therapeutic applications of heat, cold, and exercise, *Med Sci Sports Exerc* 12:76, 1980.
8. Lewit K: The muscular and articular factor in movement restriction, *Manual Med* 1:83, 1985.
9. Meeusen R, Lievens P: The use of cryotherapy in sports injuries, *Sports Med* 3:398, 1986.
10. Micheli LJ: Overuse injuries in children's sports: the growth factor, *Orthop Clin North Am* 14:337, 1983.
11. Middleton GD, McFarlin JE, Lipsky PE: Prevalence and clinical impact of fibromyalgia in systemic lupus erythematous, *Arthritis Rheum* 8:1181, 1994.
12. Peterson MA, Burkhard SS: Compression injury of the epiphyseal growth plate: fact or fiction? *J Pediatr Orthop* 1:377, 1981.
13. Salter RB, Harris WR: Injuries involving the epiphyseal plate, *J Bone Joint Surg Am* 45A:587, 1963.
14. St. Claire SM: Diagnosis and treatment of fibromyalgia syndrome, *JNMS* 2:3, 1994.
15. Wilkerson GB: External compression for controlling traumatic edema, *Physiol Sports Med* 13:97, 1985.

Chapter Highlights

Conventional Radiography
Nuclear Medicine
Tomography
Discography
Magnetic Resonance Imaging
Contrast Arthrography
Diagnostic Ultrasonography
Myelography
Electrodiagnostic Testing
Thermography

Today's health care practitioner faces the enormous task of meticulously choosing for each patient the appropriate modality from the plethora of sophisticated imaging modalities available. It has become increasingly difficult to sequence the imaging procedures properly in the management of the patient with musculoskeletal problems. The difficulty of cost containment clouds the decision-making process, as the practitioner attempts to treat the patient appropriately in a well-defined, yet cost-effective, manner. Although the amount of information ultimately gathered through diagnostic imaging is enormous, the key to an efficient clinical practice is to know when, why, and where to use imaging techniques. Thus communication and cooperation between the primary care practitioner and the radiologist are imperative for efficient problem solving.

Conventional Radiography

Despite newer and more sophisticated imaging techniques, conventional radiography continues to provide a wide and diverse array of diagnostic data about musculoskeletal problems, such as soft-tissue injury, bony malalignment, loss of integrity of the osseous structures, and joint space abnormality.[2] It is usually the first step in identifying patients with osseous pathologic conditions. Other patients, who may need conventional radiography, are those who are over the age of 50 years and are experiencing new episodes of back pain, those who have a history of cancer or multiple traumatic episodes, those who have swollen joints, and those who have a history of recent infection.

Decisions regarding the need to expose the patient to ionizing radiation are complicated, as are the medicolegal issues involved. There are many gray areas in the decision to use plain-film radiography. For example, some practitioners believe that common muscle tension headaches are an indication for a plain-film series of the cervical spine; other practitioners disagree. It is essential for the clinician to base decisions to obtain radiographs on physical findings and patient history.

Proper Use of Plain-Film Radiography

The plain-film radiograph remains the most important method of imaging in musculoskeletal medicine. Although plain films often confirm what the astute practitioner already suspects from the findings of the physical examination, the number of abnormal findings may increase over the long run in both spinal and extraspinal cases. For example, small fractures in the extremities that are not immediately apparent after severe trauma may appear on a later radiographic film. The key to understanding and interpreting plain-film radiographs correctly is to learn normal radiographic anatomy and normal variants. Many spinal views, for example, contain normal variants, and the clinician must recognize them to avoid unnecessary further diagnostic studies.

Procedural Considerations

It is important to ensure that patients are exposed to a minimum amount of radiation (Table 2-1). Two films taken at 90 degrees to one another are sufficient for the diagnosis of most joint problems. Anteroposterior and lateral views may suffice for uncomplicated injuries in several regions of the body. Oblique projections and special views may be necessary to delineate more severe trauma and to rule out fractures and other pathologic abnormalities. A minimum of three films (i.e., oblique, lateral, and anteroposterior projections) are taken at joints with complex anatomic arrangements, such as the hand and wrist (i.e., carpus) and the foot and ankle (Figure 2-1 *A-C*). Sometimes an oblique projection is necessary to rule out trauma in other joints, such as the knee and elbow.

Because of the danger of secondary spinal cord compromise utmost care is essential in the treatment of injuries to the spine. A minimal initial radiologic examination of the cervical spine after trauma should include three views: lateral, anteroposterior, and odontoid (open mouth). If necessary, these cervical views can be taken while the patient is on a table in a non–weight-bearing position. If the clinician suspects instability or fracture and the initial films are unremarkable, a complete cervical series, including oblique, flexion, and extension views, may be necessary.[1] Oblique projections in the thoracic spine are rarely useful to the clinician, however.

Stress views can reveal more covert forms of instability, particularly when a patient has a history of multiepisodal trauma, such as work- or athletic-related injuries. In obtaining a stress view, the clinician places the joint at the point of greatest stress for the ligament or capsule involved, away from the stable closed-packed position to rule out occult instability that is not evident on a routine or neutral view (Figure 2-2). Stress views are quite useful in demonstrating acromioclavicular joint separation and sprains, as well as ligamentous instability at the ankle joint. They are less commonly ordered for the elbow, wrist, and knee.

Special precautions are warranted under certain circumstances. Because even small doses of ionizing radiation are damaging to a fetus during the first stages of development, it is essential to ask women of childbearing age if they are pregnant. It is safest to take plain films of women in this age group within 10 days of the first day of their last menstrual period, when they are almost certainly not pregnant. Other patients who require special consideration are those who have had large doses of radiation in the last 2 years (i.e., 12 to 16 x-ray films over the 2-year period) and those in the pediatric, prepubescent, or adolescent years. The relationship of the genital organs to the lumbar spine can make a plain film of this area genetically significant, and it is wise to reduce the gonadal dosage by (1) using a rare-earth screen with a green-sensitive film, (2) protecting the gonadal area with some type of shield, or (3) limiting the number of films taken. In the latter case, for example, the clinician may order two rather than five views for a standard lumbar examination and may reserve special projections

---

Table 2-1 Representative Radiation Quantities from Various Diagnostic X-Ray Procedures

Examination	Technique (kVp/mAs)	Skin Dose (mrad)	Mean Marrow Dose (mrad)	Gonad Dose (mrad)
Skull	76/50	200	10	<1
Chest	110/3	10	2	<1
Cervical spine	70/40	150	10	<1
Lumbar spine	72/60	300	60	225
Abdomen	74/60	400	30	125
Pelvis	70/50	150	20	150
Extremity	60/5	50	2	<1
CT (head)	125/300	3000	20	50
CT (pelvis)	124/400	4000	100	3000

CT, Computed tomography.

(From Bushong SC: *Radiologic sciences for technologists: physics, biology, and protection,* ed 5, St Louis, 1993, Mosby.)

for those cases in which they are essential for appropriate clinical diagnosis.[28]

Findings

Plain-film x-ray examination is an efficient way to discover dislocations, fractures, the static component of anatomic subluxations, certain types of stress injuries (e.g., stress fractures and tug lesions), metastatic disease, some types of primary tumors, metabolic disease (e.g., osteoporosis), degenerative arthropathic diseases (Table 2-2), and abnormalities in the growth plate. A plain-film x-ray examination is fast, since many primary care offices have x-ray equipment or are adjacent to facilities that do; it is relatively inexpensive for the patient and third-party payers and allows the clinician to rule out more severe injuries in patients who may need referral for care outside the primary care practice.

Dislocations, fractures, and anatomic subluxations require a minimum of two views for accurate diagnosis. Initial films of stress fractures are often equivocal. In this case, a follow-up x-ray series should be performed 10 to 21 days after the injury. Tug lesions are areas of calcification at muscle-tendon attachments to the periosteal bone interface (Figure 2-3 *A, B*). Common sites for tug lesions are the attachments of the deltoid muscle and latissimus dorsi muscle at the proximal humerus. Not

only do plain-film radiographs often reveal primary tumors, but also they are the first step in discovering metastatic disease. Similarly, a plain film is often part of the screening process for metabolic disorders, such as osteoporosis. However, approximately 30% of bone mass must be lost before these changes are visible on plain film. Osteopenia results from bone disorders in postmenopausal women who are not on estrogen replacement therapy, and it occurs in regions of the body that lose bone mineral content from disuse, such as a porous humerus in cases of adhesive capsulitis.

Table 2-2	Plain-Film Evaluation of Arthropathic Diseases
Diagnosis	**Site of Plain-Film Findings**
Psoriatic arthritis	Hand, sacroiliac joints (common); pubis symphysis, hip, knee (less common)
Rheumatoid arthritis	Wrist and hand, shoulder, knee, cervical spine, hip
Spondyloarthropathy	Sacroiliac joints, thoracolumbar spine
Osteoarthritis	Lumbosacral spine, hip, knee, foot and ankle, hand

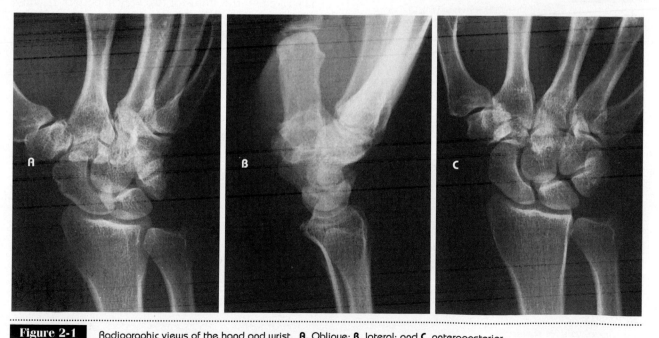

Figure 2-1   Radiographic views of the hand and wrist. **A,** Oblique; **B,** lateral; and **C,** anteroposterior

(From Scuderi GR, McCann PD, Bruno PJ: *Sports medicine: principles of primary care,* St Louis, 1997, Mosby.)

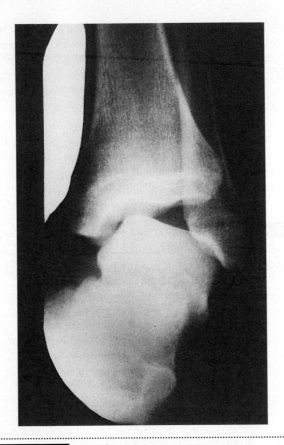

Figure 2-2   Inversion stress film showing talar tilt.

(From Nicholas JA, Hershman EB: *The lower extremity and spine in sports medicine*, ed 4, St Louis, 1995, Mosby.)

Soft-tissue structures require careful scrutiny on film because they may offer subtle clues to serious or underlying pathologic abnormalities. For example, signs of fat pad displacement at the elbow suggest the presence of a joint effusion.[1] Documentation of a joint effusion at a sprained ankle or knee may indicate that the injured ligamentous complex is intact. A severe ligamentous injury is more likely in the absence of a joint effusion, because capsular tears associated with a ruptured ligament allow extravasation of inflammatory fluid. If the patient has sustained a trauma, the examiner must rule out intra-articular fracture.[28] A lumbar film taken of a patient who is complaining of low back pain may reveal psoas spasm and hypertonicity.[27]

Plain-film analysis has its most clear and efficient use in detailing and documenting the effects of external stress on the musculoskeletal system. For such joint changes, plain-film radiography may provide better documentation than any other diagnostic test available (Table 2-3).

Skeletal-Age Determination

Plain-film radiography permits clinicians to distinguish skeletal maturity from chronologic age. During the physical examination, a prudent clinician assesses the level of skeletal maturity from the patient's appearance. Plain films confirm the status of two very important regions: the epiphyseal plate (Figure 2-4 *A, B*), which is responsible for the lengthwise growth of long bones, and the

Table 2-3   Clinical Conditions Diagnosed on Plain Films

Anteroposterior Lumbopelvic Projections	Lateral Lumbopelvic Projections	Oblique Projections	Flexion or Extension Projections
Facet tropism	Increased sacral base angle	Spondylolysis	Anterolisthesis, retrolisthesis
Asymmetric facet orientation	Degenerative disk disease	Visualized occult fracture or tumor	Ligamentous instability
Pelvic obliquity	Spondylolisthesis		
Transitional vertebrae	Swayback (i.e., hyperlordosis)		
Psoas hypertonicity or spasm	Hypolordosis		
Bertolotti's syndrome	Spondyloarthropathy		
Scoliosis			
Spondyloarthropathy			
Sacroiliitis			
Iliac apophysis for skeletal maturation			

apophyseal region (i.e., the interface between the growth cartilage and muscle-tendon unit), which is responsible for the widthwise growth of long bones.

Many children develop inflammation at the apophyseal region as a result of their rapid growth and the relative weakness of the cartilaginous growth center. Because the tractionlike pull of the muscle-tendon unit further reduces the flexibility of a joint that is tight as a result of growth, such an injury is called traction apophysitis. These lesions are self-limiting, but the clinician must investigate them and explain them in calming tones to anxious parents. Once the apophysis closes, the tendon-bone interface is more stable. Therefore it behooves the practitioner to take plain films on symptomatic children to obtain an accurate baseline record for future care and prognosis. Common areas of involvement include the os calcis, proximal tibia, olecranon, and anterior inferior and anterior superior iliac spines.

It is generally possible to determine skeletal maturity by examining the stages of growth-center ossification at two sites. First, a posteroanterior view of the wrist is compared with the standard in *Radiologic Atlas of Skeletal Maturity* to ascertain the relative osseous maturity.[12] Second, an anteroposterior lumbopelvic view

shows the iliac apophyseal ring, whose different stages of closure correlate with different degrees of skeletal maturity (i.e., Risser's sign). Because clinicians often use Risser's sign at the iliac apophysis to evaluate the growth stage of children with scoliosis, it is important to examine films of the lumbopelvic region in these children. Usually the orthopedic status of children with osseous abnormalities is more stable once their growth centers are fused. A closed growth plate may put the patient's parents and examining clinician at ease while the child undergoes treatment for the current symptomatology.

It is clear that plain films permit an expedient diagnosis that may rule out metabolic, physiologic, and oncologic disorders, as well as other types of serious pathologic conditions. Thus they help the practitioner decide whether to treat the patient in a primary care facility. The information from plain films is even more important when combined with proper clinical and laboratory procedures.

Traumatized Patient

Motorcycle or automobile accidents, construction or industrial site injuries, recreational or sporting mishaps, and household injuries are responsible for most multitrauma

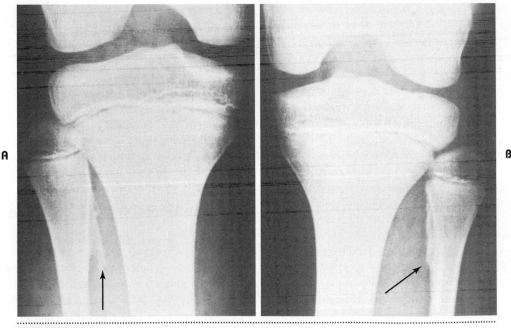

A   B

Figure 2-3 Examples of tug lesions. **A,** Cortical thickening; and **B,** irregularities as a result of muscle insertions. Tug lesions include the deltoid, latissimus dorsi, and margins of the fibula.

(From Keats TE: *Atlas of normal roentgen variants that may simulate disease,* ed 6, St Louis, 1996, Mosby.)

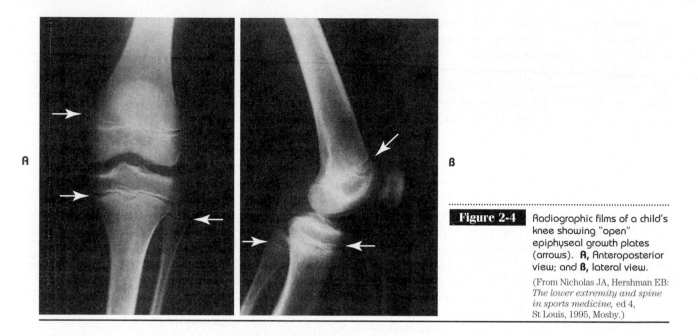

A

B

Figure 2-4 Radiographic films of a child's knee showing "open" epiphyseal growth plates (arrows). **A,** Anteroposterior view; and **B,** lateral view.

(From Nicholas JA, Hershman EB: *The lower extremity and spine in sports medicine,* ed 4, St Louis, 1995, Mosby.)

cases. After blunt or gross trauma, patients require special care to identify and treat a broad spectrum of potential injuries and complications. A fast, yet thorough, general body survey should begin once the patient recounts the events that led to injury. The clinician takes all vital signs, checks for displaced joints or gross deformity of bones, and searches for open or bleeding wounds that must have immediate attention. Once the patient's condition has been stabilized, a more thorough orthopedic and neurologic workup of the injury sites can be done.

A radiologic evaluation of the traumatized sites should include films of the adjacent joints. For instance, trauma to the soft tissues of the thigh should lead the clinician to order a radiographic examination of the hip, thigh, and knee joint in an effort to locate a fracture, displacement, or effusion. If there is a need for special films, such as oblique projections for suspected injury in the lumbar spine, or for films that are not musculoskeletal, such as chest or abdominal views, it may be necessary for the practitioner to refer the patient to a radiologist (Table 2-4). More advanced techniques may be used for diagnosing more severe bone and nerve injuries (Figure 2-5).

Care must be taken to investigate the possibility of associated injuries in trauma victims (Table 2-5). These patients may not mention secondary injuries to the examiner at first; in fact, they may not realize that such injuries have occurred. For example, patients who have been involved in an automobile accident or a contact sport trauma may initially sustain such debilitating shoulder or cervical spine injuries that they are not aware of secondary injuries (commonly to the sternoclavicular joint). Similarly, those who sustain severe internal derangements of the knee as a result of falls or skiing accidents may become symptomatic later because of an ankle or foot problem that stems from the same injury. Patients with whiplash injuries may develop low back pain after their debilitating neck pain has been resolved.

Blunt trauma and acceleration forces have the potential to cause internal organ pathologic conditions. Flank pain and hematuria in patients with a low back injury are indicative of kidney compromise, for example. Laboratory tests and radiologic procedures are helpful in confirming or ruling out a visceral disorder.

Nuclear Medicine

Examinations conducted with the use of nuclear medicine techniques, including bone scans, positron emission tomography (PET) scans, and single photon emission computed tomography (SPECT) scans, are valuable in diagnostic imaging because of their highly sensitive and fairly noninvasive nature. Whole-body scanning for metastatic and infectious diseases, as well as inflammatory and ischemic processes, is possible with scintigraphy. Furthermore, although radiographic films provide a static evaluation of an individual's anatomy,

Table 2-4 Preferred Radiographic Views for Evaluation of Skeletal Trauma*

Area	Specific Views	Area	Specific Views
Skull	Posteroanterior or anteroposterior Caldwell Townes Lateral (one lateral should be upright)	Sternum, sterno-clavicular joints	Posteroanterior Right and left anterior obliques with cephalad angle of tube Lateral
Facial bones	Waters Modified Waters Caldwell Lateral	Elbow	Anteroposterior Lateral Capitellum
Cervical spine	Anteroposterior Coned odontoid or orthopantogram Odontoid Lateral (cross-table or upright) Swimmer's lateral (cross-table) Both obliques, when possible	Radioulnar joints (forearm)	Anteroposterior or posteroanterior Lateral
		Wrist and hand	Posteroanterior Oblique internal, external, or both Lateral Navicular views, if needed
Thoracic spine	Anteroposterior Lateral (cross-table or routine) Swimmer's (coned to upper thoracic spine)	Pelvis, acetabulum	Anteroposterior Obliques (Judet)
		Hip, proximal part of femur	Anteroposterior pelvis Frog-leg or cross-table lateral Obliques
Lumbar spine	Anteroposterior Lateral (cross-table or upright) Lateral (coned to L5-S1)	Femur	Anteroposterior (to include hip and knee) Lateral (to include hip and knee)
Sacrum	Anteroposterior (tube-angled cephalad) Lateral	Distal part of femur and knee	Anteroposterior Lateral Tunnel Internal oblique
Chest	Posteroanterior or anteroposterior Left lateral (may not be possible in trauma) Lateral decubitus (pneumothorax, pleural fluid)	Tibia, fibula	Anteroposterior (to include ankle and knee) Lateral (to include both joints)
Ribs	Anteroposterior or posteroanterior Oblique	Ankle	Anteroposterior Oblique (mortise) Lateral
Shoulder	Anteroposterior (internal rotation) Anteroposterior (neutral) Transscapular lateral (Neer) Axillary	Calcaneus	Tangential Lateral
Humerus	Anteroposterior (to include elbow and shoulder) Lateral (to include both joints)	Foot	Lateral Anteroposterior Oblique Lateral
Clavicle	Anteroposterior or posteroanterior (to include both joints with and without weight bearing)		

*It is understood that most of the time the initial radiographic evaluation may have to be performed with a portable machine, and this may require modification of the positioning described in this table. This table also applies to pediatric trauma.

(From Gustilo RB, Kyle RF, Templeman DC: *Fractures and dislocations,* vol 1, St Louis, 1993, Mosby.)

bone scanning allows the evaluation of bone and joint physiology as well (Figure 2-6 *A, B*). A bone scan may permit the detection of bone changes days, weeks, or months before the changes become visible on plain x-ray films. Furthermore, it permits evaluation of multiple sites without added radiation exposure.[22]

Highly active individuals, such as competitive athletes, are prime candidates for bone scanning when the diagnosis is uncertain. For example, plain films may not reveal osseous pathologic conditions in a runner with lower leg pain that is recalcitrant to treatment, but a bone scan may show increased uptake of the radioactive

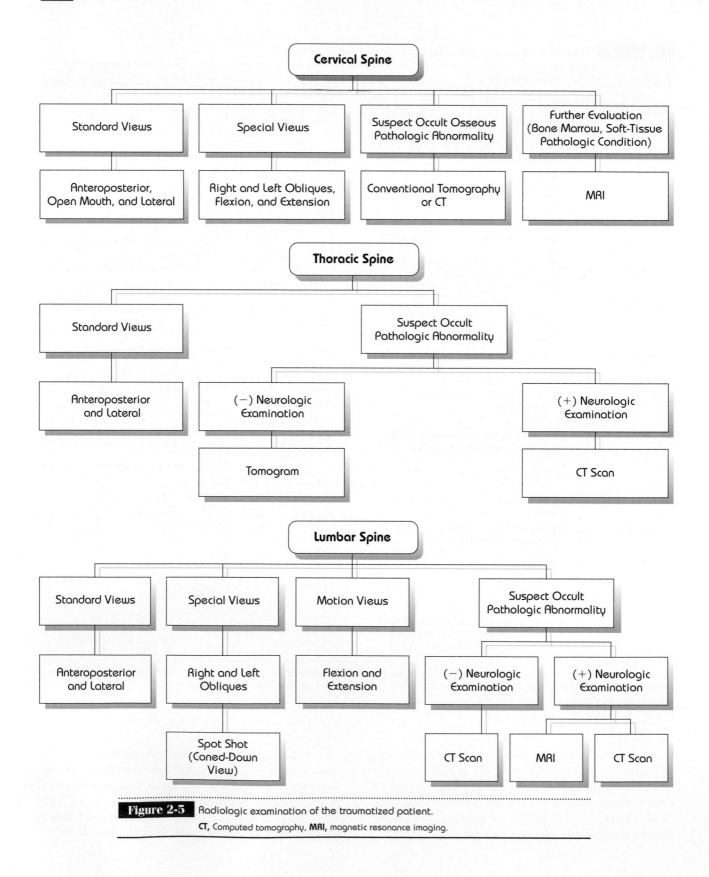

Figure 2-5 Radiologic examination of the traumatized patient.

CT, Computed tomography, **MRI,** magnetic resonance imaging.

Table 2-5	Clinical Dyads: Commonly Associated Injuries

Obvious Fracture	Associated Injury
Bone and bone	
Spine	Remote additional spinal fracture
Chest wall	Scapula fracture
Anterior pelvic arch	Sacrum fracture or dislocated sacroiliac joint
Femoral shaft	Fracture or fracture-dislocation of hip
Tibia (severe)	Dislocated hip
Calcaneus	Fractured thoracolumbar spine
Bone and viscera	
Chance fracture of spine	Ruptured mesentery or small bowel
Lower ribs	Laceration of liver, spleen, kidney, or diaphragm
Pelvis	Ruptured bladder or urethra
Pelvis	Ruptured diaphragm
Bone and vascular	
Ribs 1, 2, or 3	Ruptured aorta
Sternum	Myocardial contusion
Pelvis	Laceration of pelvic arterial tree
Distal third femur	Laceration of femoral artery
Knee dislocation	Popliteal artery laceration

(From Rogers LF, Hendrix RW: Evaluating the multiple injured patient radiographically, *Orthop Clin North Am* 21[3]:444, 1990.)

isotope consistent with a stress fracture (Figure 2-7 *A, B*). Although there may be a risk of more serious injury if these patients continue their normal activities with an injury that has not been identified and treated, they may be unwilling to temper their activities until conventional tests can provide an accurate diagnosis. The additional information provided by bone scanning becomes especially important in these cases.

Bone Scanning

The process of bone scanning (scintigraphy) involves the injection of an active agent, such as a technetium 99-labeled diphosphonate, that shows up on a special x-ray film to bring out covert pathologic conditions. Strontium 85 (^{85}Sr) was used in bone imaging at first, but it required a high radiation dose and a delayed time for processing.[6] Currently used compounds include condensed phosphates, diphosphonates, or imidodiphosphonate. Diphos-

phonates are not susceptible to enzyme breakdown in vivo and possess fewer plasma protein-binding properties, which enhance excretion.[6] Technetium 99m remains the most frequently used agent, however, because of its high avidity for bone localization and good renal excretion.

Bone Scanning Procedure

Although the nuclear medicine technologist performs the scan, a radiologist usually injects the isotope. The patient does not need to be prepared in any special way for a bone scan; however, all metallic jewelry and external prosthetic devices should be removed. The patient should be well-hydrated before the scan, but allowed to void before the procedure begins.

Bone imaging involves the use of a scintillation camera and a medium-high resolution, whole-body, low-energy collimator or single-pass diverging collimator. The patient lies under a gamma camera, which generally produces 3- × 5-inch Polaroid pictures. Normally, a whole-body scan includes both an anteroposterior and a posteroanterior view.

For most cases of musculoskeletal trauma and athletic stress injury, the primary procedure is a three-phase technetium bone scan:

1. *Dynamic or vascular phase.* Images of the area of clinical concern are obtained immediately and at intervals of 3 to 5 seconds for up to 1 minute after the intravenous bolus injection of technetium 99m. This type of examination is also called a flow study.[6]
2. *Soft-tissue or blood-pool phase.* Images are obtained 10 minutes after injection for approximately 500,000 counts.
3. *Delayed or osseous phase.* Images are obtained after waiting a minimum of 2 hours after injection. Longer delays tend to improve the target to background ratio. Multiple images are obtained over the skeleton. A 400,000 count is taken over the interior thorax. This procedure is also called a static image study.

A fourth stage may be useful when physical findings suggest the presence of an infection. A 100,000 count is taken over the area of interest; a similar count delayed for 24 hours may also be ordered. This kind of scan helps determine whether the injury involves soft tissue, bone, or both. It also indicates whether the injury is acute, subacute, or chronic, as well as the precise site of the injury. It is best used for differentiating between soft-tissue infection and osteomyelitis.

The images show areas in which the isotope has concentrated; the signal density may be either increased

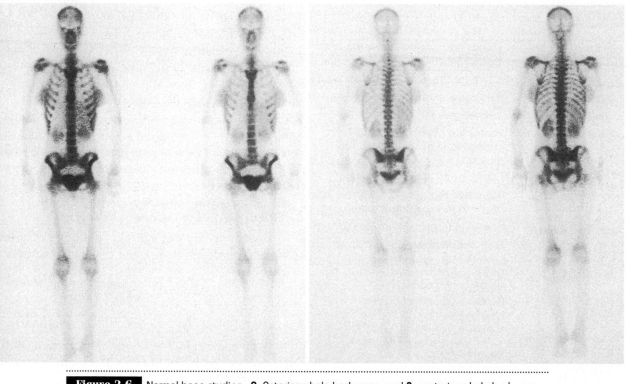

Figure 2-6 Normal bone studies. **A,** Anterior whole-body scan; and **B,** posterior whole-body scan.
(From Early PJ, Sodee DB: *Principles and practice of nuclear medicine,* St Louis, 1995, Mosby.)

or decreased, depending on the amount of tissue activity involved (e.g., blood flow and bone cell turnover). The normal areas of isotope concentration are the hematopoietic areas, such as the sternum, skull, acromioclavicular joint, sternoclavicular joint, costochondral junction, scapula tips, and pelvis. In a child, growth centers are also normal areas of concentration. An abnormal area of isotope concentration, sometimes called a "hot spot," indicates that a pathologic process has increased the focal metabolism normally present in the area under scrutiny. Blood flow increases with infection and tumors, for example, although not necessarily with trauma. The radiologist reads the scan, examining the symmetry of the isotope's uptake.

There should be at least a few days between scintigraphic examinations, even though the exposure to radiation for such an examination is usually minimal. In most patients the isotope is metabolized and cleared from the body within 1 or 2 days—definitely within 1 week. The kidneys excrete 50% of the technetium 99m diphosphonate injected into the body. The materials administered have a short, 6-hour half life. Thus total body radiation doses for bone scanning average 0.1 to 0.5 rad for the average 20m Ci adult dosage of the technetium 99m agent. The gonadal dose in a bone scan is similar to that received from either a barium enema study or a lumbar spine x-ray examination, which measures 0.2 to 0.5 rad.

Indications for Bone Scanning
Health care practitioners use bone scanning for a wide variety of purposes:
- Assessment of bone graft success
- Identification of early infections
- Evaluation of hip and knee prostheses
- Diagnosis of aseptic or avascular necrosis
- Management of Paget's disease
- Examination for bone tumors in patients with an increased alkaline phosphate level
- Assessment of bone tumors and biopsy sites
- Diagnosis of ankylosing spondylitis in sacroiliac joints
- Determination of the maturation or calcification of myositis ossificans
- Detection of reflex sympathetic dystrophy

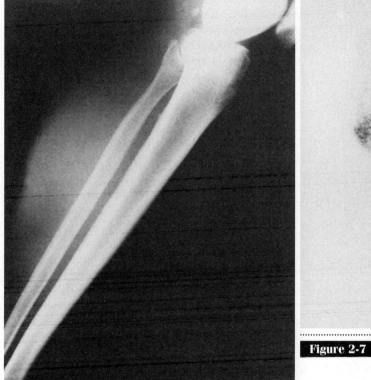

A
B

Figure 2-7 A, Normal radiographic film of runner with tibial pain. B, Bone scan of same patient demonstrating stress fracture.

(From Nicholas JA, Hershman EB: *The lower extremity and spine in sports medicine,* ed 4, St Louis, 1995, Mosby.)

- Diagnosis of discitis
- Assessment of posterior element pathologic condition of the spine (e.g., spondylosis, stress fracture)
- Determination of the status of spinal compression fractures
- Detection of primary tumors and metastatic disease
- Diagnosis of stress fracture of the extremity
- Diagnosis of occult fractures
- Confirmation of suspected osteomyelitis
- Information gathering in cases of suspected child abuse

Bone scanning has become common in the evaluation of child abuse. Very young children do not usually develop stress fractures of multiple fracture sites in normal living situations. A posterior rib fracture in a young child raises a high level of suspicion for child abuse. Generally a clinician first sees such a rib fracture on plain films in the office or emergency department before a bone scan.[18]

In chiropractic or medical practice, bone scanning is particularly helpful under two major circumstances. First, when the plain x-ray films are normal, but the patient continues to experience pain, follow-up bone scans may reveal an occult or stress fracture, or they may be normal. (Bone scanning can indicate not only the age of the fracture, but also, in a stress fracture, the stage of bone stress.) Second, when the x-ray films are abnormal, but the clinician is uncertain whether the findings are responsible for the acute complaint or are simply an incidental discovery, three-phase bone scanning can clarify the problem.

Although magnetic resonance imaging (MRI) has somewhat displaced bone scanning as the imaging technique of choice for avascular necrosis and for discitis, bone scintigraphy is still quite efficient and much less expensive than many other diagnostic modalities.

Positron Emission Tomography

PET is a very complex diagnostic imaging procedure that has been used experimentally since the 1950s; but only recently, with the advent of better instrumentation and computerization, has it become clinically useful. The basis of PET scan physiology is the positron, the positively charged data particle emitted from neutron-poor radionuclides. Conversion in the body is two gamma rays at 180 degrees from one another. There is no need for collimation.[7]

PET requires the interdisciplinary support of the physician, physicist, physiologist, chemist, and technologist. The procedure itself is noninvasive, but it involves the administration of a radioactive pharmaceutical substance in the creation of images of the brain, heart, lungs, and other organs. Radiotracers are used to "tag" organic molecules commonly found in the body. Specific diseased organs can be targeted; for example, glucose tagged with fluorine (^{18}F) can be used in imaging certain brain tumors, and ammonia tagged with nitrogen (^{13}N) can be used in imaging the heart.[7]

By means of PET, the investigator can peer into the working physiologic regions of the human brain and other organ systems to examine the nervous and biologic parameters without disturbing the normal homeostatic physiology. In the future, PET may be the diagnostic imaging of choice for certain central nervous system pathologic variations, because it may be able to demonstrate regional brain function that is not visible on an MRI or a computed tomography (CT) scan. Current PET studies are focusing on patients with epilepsy, Huntington's disease, stroke, Alzheimer's disease, and brain tumors, as well as spasmodic torticollis and other movement disorders.

Tomography

Conventional Tomography

Sometimes called routine tomography, conventional tomography differs from standard radiography in its ability to demonstrate anatomic structures precisely at specific levels. Conventional films (i.e., x-ray films) can mask the structure of interest by superimposing other structures on it, but tomography allows the technician to focus on a particular area. Through the synchronous motion of both film and x-ray tube, tomography produces images of the area that are sharp, whereas the anatomic structures away from that plane are blurry and poorly visible[29] (Figure 2-8 *A-C*).

The advent of CT and MRI has reduced the frequency with which practitioners order conventional tomograms. Currently, tomography is most often used in cases of orthopedic trauma when high-contrast images are needed to visualize a fracture.[5] Because of its ability to produce images in the sagittal and coronal planes, conventional tomography can also be a helpful adjunct in spinal imaging, for example, in the evaluation of nonunion defects. Occult fractures missed on plain x-ray films and only suggested by a technetium 99m bone scan may be confirmed by conventional tomography. In fact, conventional tomography demonstrates fine fracture lines that may not be apparent with CT. Tomograms are also helpful in assessing suspected osteochondral fractures in anatomically complex areas (e.g., the ankle), viewing alignment from a tibial plateau fracture, and confirming suspected cases of necrosis after fractures.[1]

Computed Tomography

The first CT scan was performed in 1970.[5] Since the early 1970s, CT scans have become an integral part of musculoskeletal diagnosis. The evolution of CT scanners has been impressive. First-generation scanners contained a slitlike beam that sliced through tissues 1 cm in width. Second-generation scanners had x-ray beams that were arranged in a fanlike configuration. Third- and fourth-generation scanners differ from their predecessors in that they permit the continuous, smooth motion of the x-ray tube around the patient in the gantry. Fourth-generation CT scanners are free of circular artifact. In addition, the use of a multicomputerized system accelerates the image reconstruction process. Multiplanar imaging is possible in these advanced computer systems, so reconstruction in the coronal and sagittal planes has become a reality.[23]

Modern CT scanners produce images with contrast resolutions far superior to those of plain radiographic films. Thus they provide better images not only of bony abnormalities, but also of soft-tissue structures. They offer the clinician a greater distinction between low-contrast objects, such as gray and white matter, than does conventional radiography. Moreover, CT has the potential for cross-sectional display and the reconstruction of the images in additional planes. On the other hand, the spatial resolution of CT is less than that of standard radiographic techniques, and the radiation dose is considerably higher. The level of radiation exposure for a single CT examination that does *not* scan an area more than once is intermediate between the level associated with radiographic films and the level associated with plain tomography.[13] Radiation exposure is inversely dependent on the thickness of the scan or tissue slice.

CT has been useful in a wide variety of musculoskeletal disorders, including those related to trauma (Figure 2-9 *A, B*), back pain (e.g., herniated nucleus pul-

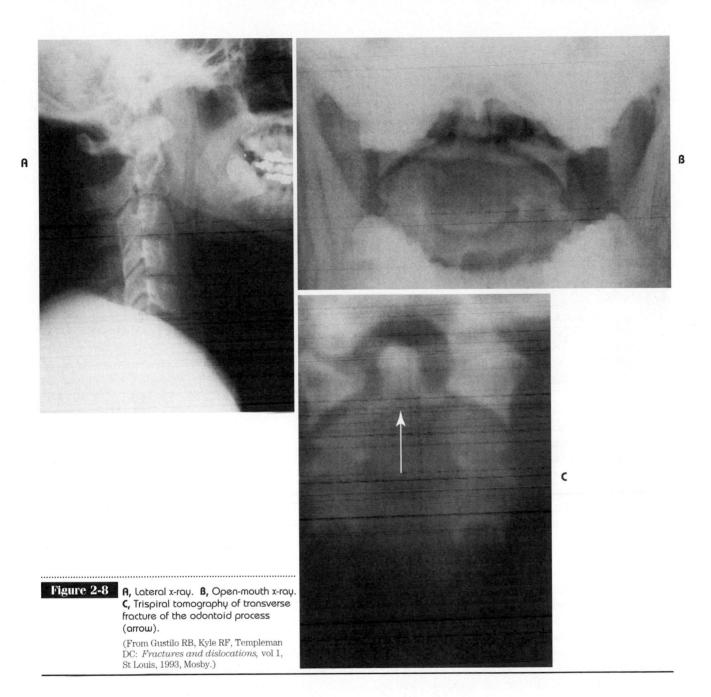

Figure 2-8 **A**, Lateral x-ray. **B**, Open-mouth x-ray. **C**, Trispiral tomography of transverse fracture of the odontoid process (arrow).

(From Gustilo RB, Kyle RF, Templeman DC: *Fractures and dislocations*, vol 1, St Louis, 1993, Mosby.)

posus, Figure 2-10), metabolic bone disease (e.g., osteoporosis), and tumor (e.g., soft-tissue masses).[29]

Quantitative Computed Tomography

Clinicians may use the noninvasive technique of quantitative CT to measure bone mineral density. Quantitative CT permits a determination of bone mineral content with three-dimensional localization. Furthermore, it allows separate measurements of cortical and trabecular bone.

Bone mass measurement at menopause can help identify women who are at greatest risk for osteoporosis. Thus quantitative CT can be an excellent screening tool to determine which patients will benefit from estrogen replacement therapy's ability to maintain bone mass.

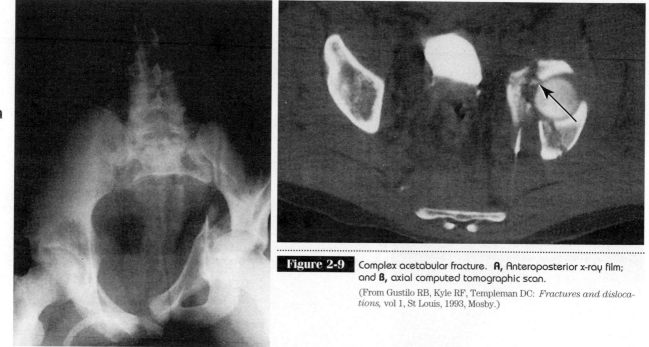

A

B

Figure 2-9 Complex acetabular fracture. **A,** Anteroposterior x-ray film; and **B,** axial computed tomographic scan.

(From Gustilo RB, Kyle RF, Templeman DC: *Fractures and dislocations,* vol 1, St Louis, 1993, Mosby.)

The use of quantitative CT has some drawbacks. It measures only the spine and may be subject to precision errors caused by variation in the fat content of bone marrow. Other practical techniques of bone mineral measurement include dual photon absorptometry and dual energy radiographic tomography.[15]

Discography

Although fairly effective, discography has been a controversial imaging modality for spinal disk disease. Clinicians still use discography for specific cases of spinal pain that are recalcitrant to conventional therapy, because discography provides information on spinal disorders that is unattainable by other imaging methods.

In a sterile environment the physician first administers a mild sedative and local anesthetic and then begins the injection of a water-soluble contrast dye. With fluoroscopy as a guide, the physician uses a double-needle technique (i.e., two probes), most often in an extradural fashion, to identify pain-site thresholds. Interpretation of results involves monitoring CT scans of the injected level and contrast volume, comparing pain pattern and neurologic distribution, and noting points of pain reproduction and thus resistance to injection.[17] (It

may also be possible to document the "chemistry" of pain at the intervertebral disk level by determining the levels of certain chemical compounds in the area that are known to be increased in patients with pain syndromes.)

Except for assessment of the conditions of a disk above a proposed spinal fusion, the indications for discography have been controversial in the past. In 1988 the North American Spine Society suggested that discography may be indicated in the evaluation of spinal pain that has continued for more than 4 months and is refractory to conservative care.[8] Current orthopedic and radiologic authorities offer the following guidelines pertaining to the indications for discography:

- To rule out disk involvement as a cause of postoperative pain
- To determine the appropriate level for spinal fusion
- To test the potential effectiveness of chemonucleolysis
- To visualize internal disk anatomy and to study the integrity of disk substructures

Of course, other diagnostic imaging modalities precede discography; the discogram seems to bridge the gap between the end of conservative care and the preparation for operative procedures.

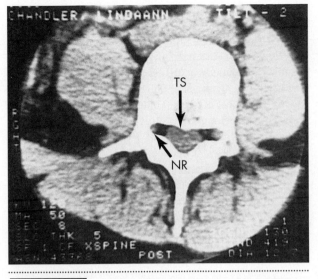

Figure 2-10 *Axial image showing a right paracentral herniation of the nucleus pulposus. Note the thecal sac (TS) insult and loss of fat signal around the displaced right nerve root (NR).*

Complications that have arisen with discography include nerve irritation, discitis, pain exacerbation, allergic reaction to the contrast dye, and subarachnoid puncture.[3]

Magnetic Resonance Imaging

The techniques of MRI are an extension of the techniques of nuclear magnetic resonance (NMR), which were discovered through physics and chemistry. The first human MRI scans were done in 1978.[5] In the space of a few short years, MRI has had a dramatic effect on the diagnosis and management of orthopedic problems. MRI has proven to be a valuable adjunct to CT and other imaging modalities; in some cases, it provides information on compromised anatomy that goes far beyond the capability of other imaging techniques, offering low-contrast resolution and direct multiplanar imaging, all without ionizing radiation.

MRI takes 40 minutes to 1 hour to complete. Claustrophobic patients may need a sedative before a scan by the older scanners, although open MRI scanners are now available. Some facilities have smaller, portable scanners for the assessment of peripheral, small joint injuries.

Techniques

Magnetic resonance involves the use of coils on the body surface and computer software to provide images with high-quality spatial resolution, tissue contrast, and anatomic detail. What appears to be an x-ray gantry contains not an x-ray tube and detectors, but a giant magnet, gradient coils, and a radiofrequency transceiver. More than 95% of all imagers are the superconducting type.[5] A radiofrequency pulse aligns protons in an electromagnetic field that uses no ionizing radiation. T1 and T2 proton densities provide the forum upon which clear images are submitted. Protons "flip" in an electromagnetic wave field. The T1 and T2 weights move in different planes. When computerized, they give different anatomic pictures.

Techniques of MRI vary, making it possible to show different types of anatomic or physiologic detail. Currently used in spinal imaging include dual echo and spin echo techniques, as well as imaging with various relaxation times. Not every MRI is both sensitive and specific, however. At the level of an intervertebral motor unit, for example, a desiccated disk may give the same signal as an osteophytic spur.

T1-weighted images involve short repetition and echo times, but provide great anatomic detail (Figure 2-11). The T1 relaxation time is the time required for the interactions between nuclear spins and tissues to return to normal after radiofrequency excitation.[5] T2-weighted images with prolonged relaxation time- and echo-time parameters afford great contrast resolution within hydrated tissues (Figure 2-12). On T2-weighted images, anatomic detail is sacrificed for the benefit of depicting the "path physiology" of the region. T2 relaxation time is the time required for the interaction between nuclear spins and adjacent activity to return to normal after radiofrequency excitation.

Cerebrospinal fluid gives a dark- or low-signal intensity; fat causes a bright- or high-signal intensity. The visibility of fat in MRI may enhance the contrast of normal anatomy, such as clearly visualizing the fat normally seen around the bone marrow. On the other hand, postdegenerative disk disease and herniated disks can obliterate the normal fat around nerve roots. As fat scatters radiation and obscures anatomic detail on a CT scan, the visibility of fat in MRI may, in fact, be one of MRI's advantages for obtaining useful images of the obese patient. Because of its water content, fat has a bright T2-weighted image on an MRI (Table 2-6).

Water and water absorption are very important in MRI. On a T1-weighted image for inflammatory discitis, hydration infiltrate is apparent on the image. Discitis on a T2-weighted image gives a bright-signal intensity, a larger signal than the normal disk.

Spinal Imaging with Magnetic Resonance

Several years ago, MRI of thick tissue areas, such as the lumbar spine, produced inadequate pictures, because the wave and spatial arrangement did not permit "photographs" of thin enough slices. With computer reformatting and the development of better magnets in recent years, the MRI pictures have become clearer and can now define the anatomy in these areas as accurately as a CT scan. It is still true, however, that a poor quality CT scan is better than a poor quality MRI picture. Of course, CT scanners are already in their fourth generation, and MRI is a relatively new modality.

T1-weighted images provide an excellent baseline for anatomic information. In a T2-weighted image the relaxation time is longer, and the cerebrospinal fluid in the canal appears white. Thus the fluid's appearance is similar to that obtained in a myelogram without the invasiveness of administering a contrast material.

It is sometimes difficult to differentiate between a disk bulge and a disk herniation on physical examination. An image obtained via MRI shows a disk bulge as a central or diffuse, symmetric bulging. The symmetry is the key to the report of a disk bulge. Disk herniations, however, are usually apparent on one side or the other.

A great disadvantage of MRI is that, unlike other imaging modalities, it cannot provide images of the cortices of bone. For pathologic abnormalities of the spinal cord, including that in the intradural space, MRI is the technique of choice, however. Thus MRI is preferred for detecting tumors, cord compression, and soft-tissue structures of the spine. It shows tissue contrast, blood flow in the veins, and direct imaging in all planes.

Table 2-6	Relative Values of SD, T1, and T2 Among Normal Tissues and Appearance of Each in an MRI (Value/Appearance)		
Tissue	**SD**	**T1**	**T2**
Fat and skin	High/white	Short/white	Long/white
Bone	Low/black	Very long/black	Very long/black
White matter	High/white	Short/white	Long/gray
Gray matter	High/white	Long/gray	Long/gray
CSF	Very high/white	Very long/gray	Very long/black

MRI, Magnetic resonance imaging; **SD,** spin density; **CSF,** cerebrospinal fluid.

(From Bushong SC: *Radiologic science for technologists: physics, biology, and protection,* ed 5, St Louis, 1993, Mosby.)

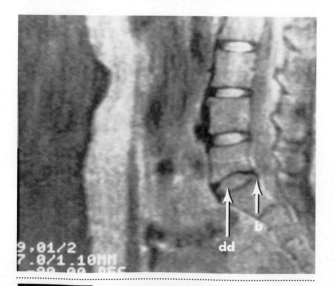

Figure 2-11 A mild decrease in signal intensity at the L5-S1 disk that indicates desiccation via the degeneration process (dd). There is also a small bulging (b) of the disk at this level.

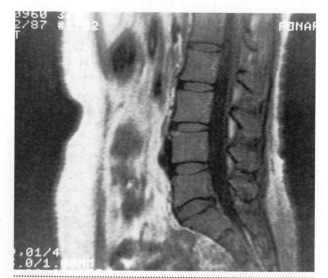

Figure 2-12 Sagittal T1-weighted image of the lumbar spine, showing normal spinal anatomy and healthy hydration of the intervertebral disks.

Imaging of the Knee Joint

The peripheral joint most extensively evaluated with MRI is the knee joint. Image quality has greatly improved since it has become possible to highlight the menisci and ligaments in a thin section, T1-weighted spin echo image (Figure 2-13 *A, B*).

MRI offers an excellent, noninvasive method of looking at osteochondral fractures and osteochondritis dissecans.[24] Furthermore, by virtue of its ability to provide images in multiple planes, MRI permits an examination of the entire medial and lateral meniscus, as well as the cruciate ligaments and the articular cartilage. Only the anterior cruciate ligament gives a mixed low-intermediate signal. Articular cartilage gives an intermediate signal intensity. T2-weighted images intensify the signal from edema within ligaments and tendons.

Indications

For certain pathologic conditions, MRI is the diagnostic procedure of choice:

- Spinal disk disease
- Medullary tumors
- Multiple sclerosis
- Cerebral edema
- Spinal stenosis
- Syringomyelia
- Metastatic disease
- Herniated disk
- Discitis (or infection)

- Avascular necrosis (especially of the femoral heads)
- Meniscal tears (fibrocartilage abnormalities)
- Central nervous system tumors
- Acoustic neuromas
- Soft-tissue tumors

In patients who have sustained head trauma with skull fractures either ruled out or confirmed on plain films, tomograms, or CT scans, MRI is an efficient way to identify the early signs of cerebral edema. It also generally detects any fluid or syrinx within the spinal canal.

MRI is more efficient than CT in detecting discitis, because this modality permits an earlier diagnosis. It may reveal discitis even before a bone scan can show it, since inflammation precedes osteoblastic activity. (Scintigraphy, of course, is very sensitive to osteoblastic activity.)

The test procedure of choice for diagnosing metastatic disease is an MRI scan. Metastatic disease gives a decreased signal intensity that appears dark. In contrast, benign tumors, such as hemangioma, may have an increased signal density.

When there is a question whether CT or MRI is the best modality for a particular patient, consultation with a radiologist is appropriate (Table 2-7).

Contraindications

The Food and Drug Administration (FDA) has not approved the use of MRI on pregnant women. In addition, patients who have a cardiac pacemaker, which may malfunction in the strong electromagnetic field needed for

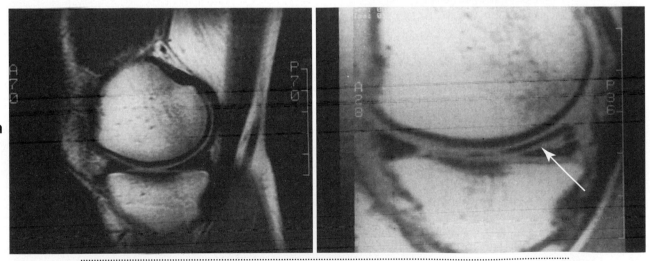

A   B

Figure 2-13 **A,** Magnetic resonance image of medial meniscus tear. **B,** Close-up of tear (arrow).

(From Gustilo RB, Kyle RF, Templeman DC: *Fractures and dislocations,* vol 1, St Louis, 1993, Mosby.)

Table 2-7 Magnetic Resonance Imaging versus Computed Tomography

Anatomic Area	Indications	Recommended Procedure	Anatomic Area	Indications	Recommended Procedure
Brain (including brain stem)	Initial evaluation (e.g., demyelination disease seizures)	MRI	Musculo-skeletal spine (cont'd)	Lower back or radicular pain in older person	MRI or CT*
	Previous normal CT	MRI		Cervical disk disease	MRI
	Previous abnormal CT	CT or MRI*		Spinal stenosis	
	Unchanged abnormal CT with increase in symptoms	MRI		Cervical	MRI
				Lumbar	CT or MRI*
	Contrast allergy	MRI		Tumors	MRI
	Acute trauma	CT		Metastatic disease	MRI
	Pituitary tumors	MRI	Hips	Early detection of aseptic necrosis	MRI
Ear, nose, throat, and eye	Neurosensory hearing loss (e.g., to rule out acoustic neuroma)	CT		Congenital hip dislocation or reduction	US
	Conductive hearing loss	CT	Extremities	Tumors, disease, or injury to muscle, ligaments, or cartilage	MRI
	Cancer staging (including laryngeal cancer)	MRI or CT*		Confirmation of calcification or fracture	CT
	Cholesteatoma of temporal bone	CT	Chest	Diseases of the hila	MRI
	Fractures of facial bones	CT		Diseases of the mediastinum	MRI or CT*
	Thyroid or parathyroid dysfunction (after US)	MRI		Lung disease	CT
	Sinus conditions	CT or MRI*	Abdomen and pelvis	General survey (e.g., to rule out tumor)	CT
	Orbital disease	MRI or CT*		Liver disease	CT or MRI*
	Disease of optic tracts and chiasm	MRI		Renal cell cancer staging	MRI
	Internal derangement of temporomandibular joint	MRI		Prostate disease	MRI, CT, or US
Musculo-skeletal spine	Lower back or radicular pain in younger person	MRI		Bladder disease	MRI or CT
				Abdominal aortic aneurysm	MRI
				Other	*

*Consult radiologist for imaging options.
CT, Computed tomography; **MRI,** magnetic resonance imaging; **US,** ultrasonography.
(Courtesy of Robert Goodman, MD, South Suffolk MRI, PC, Bayshore, New York.)

MRI; aneurysmal clips in the brain, which may torque from the electromagnetic field; cochlear implants that can be turned on and off by an electrofrequency pulse; or metallic foreign bodies within the eye should not undergo MRI.

Certain devices made from ferromagnetic materials, such as penile implants and shunt connections, may interfere with the signal detection and thus the usefulness of MRI. Orthopedic implants and pins usually have low ferromagnetic properties, however, and do not cause a noisy or distorted signal in MRI scanners.

Future

Despite the tremendous advances in other modalities of musculoskeletal imaging in the past decades, MRI has a promising future. Certain drawbacks and inconsistencies continue to be problematic in the use of MRI, however (Table 2-8). Also, other applications of MRI, such as its use with patients who have metabolic bone disease (e.g., osteoporosis), have yet to be thoroughly explored.

Research into the use of paramagnetic agents (e.g., gadolinium diethylenetriamine pentaacetic acid [gadolinium-DTPA]) as contrast agents in the examination of

Table 2-8	Shortcomings of Magnetic Resonance Imaging

Imaging Modality	Advantages over MRI
Conventional radiography	Increased spatial resolution of cortical and cancellous bone
Bone scanning	Full-body screening capability
CT	Increased spatial resolution of cortical and cancellous bone; cross-section depiction of calcified and osseous tissue; fracture detection
Contrast arthrography	Evaluation of intraarticular pathologic conditions

MRI, Magnetic resonance imaging; **CT,** computed tomography.

peripheral joints is needed as well. Such research could be accomplished via the intravenous or intraarticular administration of such materials.

Improvements in computer software and surface coil applications that are taking place in the field may permit the use of oblique planes of imaging and functional movement studies as a routine procedure.

Contrast Arthrography

The conventional use of arthrography in musculoskeletal disease involves the use of air to distend a synovial joint and a contrast agent (dye) to outline anatomic structures. The injection of iodinated contrast material into the joint space results in a clinical outline of the cartilage, menisci, ligaments, or synovium.[13] Arthrograms are most commonly ordered to identify tears in a joint capsule, fibrocartilage, and ligaments. Often this procedure can depict extravasation of synovial fluid through tears in the joint capsule or ligamentous structures.

Arthrography can be used with a contrast agent alone (i.e., conventional arthrography) or in conjunction with CT (i.e., computed arthrotomography). Conventional arthrography is used in orthopedic trauma to the shoulder, wrist, knee, and ankle (Table 2-9). Computed arthrotomography is most often used with rotator cuff disease of the shoulder joint.

The shoulder joint provides an excellent anatomic forum for both conventional arthrography and computed arthrotomography (Figure 2-14). Conventional arthrography is the gold imaging standard for adhesive capsulitis

of the shoulder joint, as well as for complete rotator cuff tears. Computed arthrotomography delineates the normal and pathologic variations of the joint capsules, as well as their muscular insertions. It maximizes visualization of the internal structures of the shoulder joint.

Tears of the glenoid labrum and partial thickness tears of the rotator cuff are most clearly visible on computed arthrotomograms. In fact, computed arthrotomography is particularly efficient in delineating and characterizing the glenoid labrum; also, this imaging technique is sensitive in exposing labrum lesions, such as detachments and attenuation. Because conventional arthrography is extremely accurate in the diagnosis of rotator cuff tears (99%), computed arthrography of the shoulder is not the procedure of choice for first documenting rotator cuff tears.[2] A computed arthrotomogram, however, detects subtle tears in the extreme anterior and posterior aspects of the rotator cuff and partial thickness tears that are not visible on a conventional arthrogram.

Arthrography was once the gold standard in diagnosing meniscus tears of the knee joint (Figure 2-15). Although arthrography remains an accurate imaging technique in this regard, most practitioners use MRI for this purpose.

Diagnostic Ultrasonography

For many years, ultrasonography (US) was the preferred musculoskeletal imaging modality for diagnosing tendon abnormalities and pediatric hip disease. Early scanners were high-contrast (bistable display mode) machines with only bright spots and no intermediate images. The later invention of gray-scale displays permitted intermediate densities.[5] Although the usefulness of this procedure is limited in diagnosing musculoskeletal disease because of the fact that the sound waves used in diagnostic ultrasound examinations cannot penetrate bone, US is a helpful procedure for diagnosing certain cases of soft-tissue pathologic variations.

US requires high-resolution equipment, including a high-frequency transducer. Furthermore, it is extremely operator dependent. It requires the ultrasonographer to be present at the time of the test. The ultrasonographer cannot come in at the end of the day and read all the studies at his or her leisure, which is a common procedure with MRI. If put on videotape, however, ultrasound images provide a dynamic picture of happenings within the tendinous structures, such as the rotator cuff mechanism.

Diagnostic US performs well in the detection of rotator cuff tears and other tendon abnormalities, as well as in the identification of some metabolic disease (e.g., Legg-Calvé-Perthes disease of the hip). The advantage

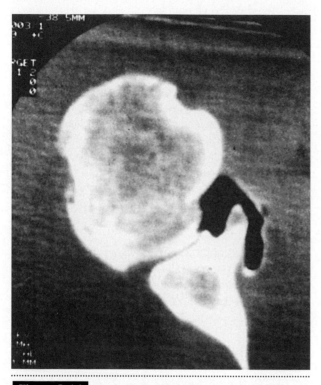

Figure 2-14 Computed arthrotomography of the shoulder.

(From Gustilo RB, Kyle RF, Templeman DC: *Fractures and dislocations*, vol 1, St Louis, 1993, Mosby.)

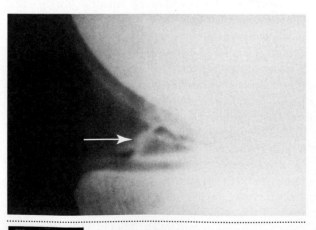

Figure 2-15 Arthrogram of medial meniscus tear.

(From Gustilo RB, Kyle RF, Templeman DC: *Fractures and dislocations*, vol 1, St Louis, 1993, Mosby.)

of US in the diagnosis of pediatric hip disease is that it can be performed on a moving child. In cases of suspected pediatric hip disease, such as congenital dysplasia or dislocation, US is the recommended primary imaging technique. It can be efficiently used in conjunction with conventional radiography.

Rotator cuff tears appear on the ultrasonogram as an absence of normal tendons on static and dynamic imaging. US usually demonstrates, in a rather reliable fashion, full thickness defects of 1 cm or greater in rotator cuff tears. It does not, however, demonstrate full thickness defects of less than 1 cm or partial thickness defects of any size.[4] Other pathologic conditions of the shoulder joint that are visible on an ultrasonogram include intraarticular bodies and various forms of tendonitis. Any narrowing of the subacromial space is also identifiable in most cases, suggesting that US may play a role in the diagnosis of impingement syndromes.[20,21] Finally, US has some limited value in the identification of fluid-filled cyst areas, such as the popliteal space of the knee.[14]

Although the indications for ultrasound examination may be more limited than are those for MRI or arthrography,[11] the primary care physician should keep in mind that US is quick, inexpensive, safe, and painless. Compared with the arthrographic examination, the ultrasonographic examination is substantially less expensive and less time consuming.[25]

Table 2-9 Joints Most Commonly Studied with Conventional Arthrography after Trauma

Joint	Purpose
Knee	Meniscus, cruciate and collateral ligaments, hyaline cartilage tears, osteochondral defects
Shoulder	Rotator cuff, glenoid labrum disruption
Hip	Hyaline cartilage integrity and tears, prosthetic joint loosening
Wrist	Triangular fibrocartilage, intercarpal ligament integrity
Elbow	Hyaline cartilage integrity, osteochondral defects
Ankle	Ligamentous tears, osteochondral defects
Temporomandibular	Disk and condylar integrity

(From Gustilo RB, Kyle RF, Templeman DC: *Fractures and dislocations*, vol 1, St Louis, 1993, Mosby.)

Myelography

Myelography, an invasive procedure, used to be the primary testing procedure for the diagnosis of spinal disk disease and pathologic variations of the spinal cord. With the advent of CT in the early 1970s and MRI in the 1980s, myelography has become an imaging technique of last resort in many cases of spinal pain when prior testing procedures of a noninvasive nature prove inconclusive.

Traditional myelographic techniques involve the introduction of small amounts of 170 to 300 mg percent water-soluble contrast medium into the subarachnoid space, either through a lumbar approach below the level of the conus medullaris or at the level of C1-C2 through a posterolateral approach.[13] Standard films of the spinal canal, including the nerve root and possibly the dural sleeve, are then taken to determine the presence or absence of a filling defect. The introduction of the contrast medium at the subarachnoid space of the lumbar spine may take place with or without the assistance and guidance of fluoroscopy. Some clinicians introduce the contrast material at the level of C1-C2 laterally.

In cases of acute spinal trauma, myelography may be used in conjunction with CT (Figure 2-16 *A, B*). The combination increases the sensitivity of the images, facilitating the detection of spinal cord or dural sac compression by small bone fragments or foreign bodies. Furthermore, when used in this combination the intrathecal administration of water-soluble contrast medium provides direct visualization of the spinal cord, nerve roots, and cauda equina. Thus it is possible to distinguish between intramedullary and extramedullary root or cord compression. The procedure demonstrates nerve root avulsion, the presence of a syrinx, and tears of the dura as well.[16] MRI is preferred for evaluating cord contusions, however, because of its ability to produce direct images of the spinal cord.

Myelography cannot thoroughly demonstrate neurogenic structure because the dura surrounds the nerve root only in a portion of the neurologic canal. The cerebral spinal fluid in the dura accepts the injected contrast medium; T2-weighted MRI displays this effect. Moreover, patients with failed back surgery and chronic low back pain secondary to infection or metabolic dis-

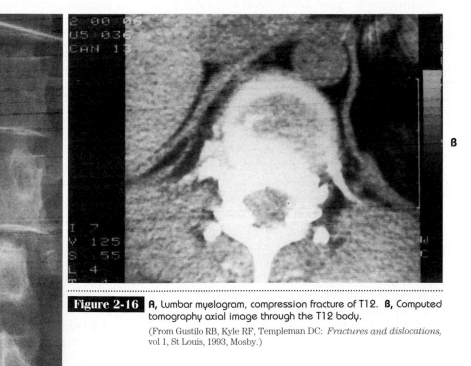

A   **B**

Figure 2-16   **A,** Lumbar myelogram, compression fracture of T12. **B,** Computed tomography axial image through the T12 body.

(From Gustilo RB, Kyle RF, Templeman DC: *Fractures and dislocations,* vol 1, St Louis, 1993, Mosby.)

ease can benefit from myelography. Spinal scans obtained by myelography, involving both intradural and extradural scans, are the best predictors of arachnoiditis. MRI with contrast is also effective.

Myelography remains valuable in the evaluation of intrinsic spinal cord and nerve root lesions, as well as dural tears associated with severe trauma. It is one of the rare imaging modalities that provides the clinician with dynamic information regarding flexion and extension positions in the spine (Table 2-10).

Electrodiagnostic Testing

Although electrodiagnostic testing can provide extremely valuable information, it does not stand alone as an accurate diagnostic entity (Table 2-11). Thus it is essential to correlate the data obtained with the physical examination findings and case history.[17] Two types of electrodes can be used in electrodiagnostic tests: needle electrodes and surface electrodes.

Motor Nerve Conduction Velocity

Measurement of motor nerve conduction velocity provides a valuable ancillary procedure in the diagnosis of various peripheral nerve lesions in both the upper and lower extremities. This form of testing involves stimulating a peripheral nerve at two separate positions along its course and recording the action potentials observed on an oscilloscopic screen. Stimulation occurs both distal and proximal to the testing site. The distance between stimulus points in millimeters divided by the latency times in milliseconds is equal to the nerve conduction velocity in meters per second. Because various delays occur at the myoneural junction, it is not possible to calculate conduction velocities of motor nerves from a single latency determination.[9]

Slow conduction times indicate nerve entrapment syndromes across the point at which the impulses are delayed (e.g., carpal tunnel). Routine nerve conduction velocity tests are not specific for conditions such as radiculopathy, but they may be helpful in cases of chronic pain that have a questionable spinal origin. Studies of nerve conduction velocity can rule out peripheral neuropathic conditions.

F Waves and H Reflex

When routine nerve conduction studies do not provide the necessary information about proximal nerve function

Table 2-10	Pros and Cons of Myelographic Studies
Pros	Cons
Studies of the subarachnoid space are possible.	Lesions removed from outside of the thecal sac can be missed.
Intraarachnoid lesions are shown.	Study variations are problematic.
Demarcation of multidisk levels is shown.	Poor detail in the dorsal spine is shown.
Information on surgical scars is provided.	Postoperative studies are impossible to read with accuracy.
Assessment of flexion and extension dynamics are possible.	Testing procedure is invasive.

and nerve root function, analysis of F and H waves is useful. The F wave results from an external stimulus applied to a myelinated nerve that conducts impulses both anterograde and retrograde. The anterograde impulse excites the nerve cell and produces an impulse that occurs slightly later than remaining impulses and is of lower amplitude. The length of time required to produce the F wave implies the state of proximal nerve root function.

The H reflex is dependent on a monosynaptic reflex arc. A mixed nerve (i.e., a nerve with both motor and sensory function, such as the posterior tibial nerve) is stimulated; the resulting sensory impulse is conducted into the dorsal root ganglion, which synapses with the anterior horn cell neuron, producing a contraction of the involved motor muscles (e.g., an ankle jerk). Practically, the H reflex can be obtained only from the posterior tibial nerve, and information about the ipsilateral S1 root can be inferred.

Sensory-Evoked Potentials

The electrical responses of nervous system sensory tracks are known as sensory-evoked potentials. A computer is used to average the repetitions of a large number of responses at different sites, and these averages are plotted on a graph in the form of a wave. Evoked potentials are most commonly recorded with surface electrodes, although needle electrodes may also be used.

Somatosensory-evoked potentials (SSEPs) are useful in the evaluation of various pathologic variations from the peripheral nerve through the spinal cord to the somatosensory region of the brain. Thus clinicians may use this test to assess diseases of the spinal cord, trauma to the spine, neuromuscular disease, and demyelinating disorders.

Spinal-evoked potentials reveal lesions at sites more proximal than the usual pathways studied by routine nerve conduction tests. After the stimulation of a peripheral nerve, these potentials are mapped out over the spinal cord or cauda equina.

Needle Electromyography

Widely used to diagnose nerve root lesions at the level of the spine and to differentiate a central spinal lesion from a peripheral neuropathic condition, needle electromyography (EMG) has the advantage of being an outpatient procedure that is relatively noninvasive and causes minimal morbidity. Results of the procedure are quite accurate in detecting disease of a neuromuscular origin.[10] For example, it is helpful in the diagnosis of myopathy, nerve root lesions, nerve root compression, and anterior horn pathologic abnormalities. The pattern of muscle innervation by the spinal root is the basis for the interpretation of needle EMG results.

Although needle EMG may detect the presence of root dysfunction and may possibly indicate the segmental level involved, it does not provide information as to the actual site of the lesion. Furthermore, it is not accurate during the first 3 weeks of a pain syndrome, since denervation potentials are generated after this time period.

EMG shows fibrillation potentials and possible motor unit changes in denervated muscles. Localization of this type of lesion may or may not be specific, depending on the anatomy of the patient and the distribution of abnormalities. Denervation of paraspinal muscle, for example, indicates that the individual patient has a lesion at the nerve root level. Findings of needle EMG in a patient who has dorsal root disease are normal, however.

Needle electrodes are fine wires that when placed intramuscularly stimulate the muscles around them. They are discomforting to the patient, since they can cause some local irritation. Surface electrodes are noninvasive and do not cause local irritation. These types of electrodes are only able to pick up muscular activity that is local and adjacent to the placed electrode.

In needle EMG, a thin wire needle electrode is placed intramuscularly at a specific site called the motor point. An oscilloscope is used to visualize the muscle ac-

---

Table 2-11 Pros and Cons of Electrodiagnostic Testing

Testing Modality	Pros	Cons
Nerve conduction velocity	Helpful in ruling out peripheral entrapment neuropathic conditions (e.g., prolonged latencies exhibited in carpal tunnel syndrome, tarsal tunnel syndrome), and ulnar neuropathic variations	Provides imperfect sensitivity; limited localization and determination of injury severity; timing of study is an important factor
F waves	Provides screening for late motor response with distal sweeps starting at the foot	Evaluates motor reflex only; possibly evaluates abnormal findings only in the presence of multiple-level injury
H reflex	Equivalent of ankle joint reflex; evaluates monosynaptic reflex with sensory and motor S1 function	Provides assessment of S1 nerve root only
SSEPs	Helpful in documenting sensory pathway disturbances in proximal neural injury and central conduction delays, as in myopathies and multiple sclerosis	Offers imperfect localization; findings are rarely abnormal if results of other electro-diagnostic tests are within normal limits
Needle EMG	Useful in assessing conductivity of neural tissues; helpful in determining site and severity of lesion; may be helpful in early assessment of recovery, screening for fibrillation potentials, and signs of denervation from nerve root compression disorders	Unable to detect denervation potentials for 14-28 days after injury; provides imperfect sensitivity; study timing is an important factor; proximal lesions are sometimes inaccessible anatomically; effectiveness is reduced after surgery

SSEPs, Somatosensory-evoked potentials; **EMG**, electromyography.

tivity. Motor unit potentials are taken first at rest and then during contraction, both minimal and maximal. The wave forms generated provide information on the type of injury (e.g., anterior horn versus muscle injury), time course (i.e., acute versus chronic), and degree of recovery (i.e., denervation versus reinnervation).

Surface EMG has been most widely used as a screening modality to infer muscle dysfunction in its broadest sense and as a monitoring device to assess response to therapy. It does not provide any information with respect to the locus of injury (i.e., root, nerve, and muscle) and, in fact, often reflects associated tissue injury rather than neurovascular dysfunction. Surface EMG is a vital component of biofeedback training paradigms that focus on the alleviation of chronic pain. On the other hand, needle EMG provides an accurate assessment of nerve root pathologic variations and is unaffected by associated soft-tissue injury.

Thermography

The premise that few of the imaging tests available depict the physiology of the body in a compromised state is the basis for thermography. Using temperature differentials in the body, thermography illustrates nerve fiber involvement in injury or disease. In fact, the word, *thermogram,* translates literally as "heat picture."

Among the major problems that arise in thermography are poor interexaminer reliability and poor reproducibility—possibly because the procedure requires proper cooling techniques, proper room situations, proper positioning, and proper room temperature ranges. Furthermore, thermograms do not provide specific information regarding the cause of nerve fiber irritation. They cannot differentiate between cervical causes of neural pain (e.g., herniated disk), scar tissue, and muscle spasm, for example. Also, thermography does not reveal the time of injury unless companion tests are taken in succession; temporary changes over a short time span may suggest the time of injury. Although thermograms do not show anatomic abnormalities as static radiographic films or CT scans do, thermograms do show what is happening physiologically to the muscles and nerves.[30]

Essentially two forms of thermographic imaging techniques are in use today: liquid-crystal and electronic infrared. Vascular heat patterns appear on the thermogram. Liquid-crystal thermography involves images that are both quantitative and qualitative. In electronic thermograms, data are gathered from the body by infrared detectors, processed via a signal onto a television screen, photographed from the screen, and put onto film. The color pattern scheme on the film reflects changes of temperature. A difference of 1° C causes a change in color on the film.

Thermography can be helpful in ruling out certain spinal conditions, such as myofascial pain syndromes and radiculitis, and in ruling out migraine and myofascial headaches. It may also help a clinician reach a definitive diagnosis of temporomandibular joint syndrome. Thermography can be particularly useful to document the need for ongoing medical care for patients with soft-tissue injury. Many times a patient whose diagnostic tests show no cause have a real pain syndrome that is responding to conservative care. In a number of whiplash cases involving the paraspinal soft-tissue structures of the cervical spine, for example, the thermogram was the only test on which the findings were abnormal.

With the exception of reflex sympathetic dystrophy,[26] thermography is specific for few clinical syndromes. Reflex sympathetic dystrophy is part of a spectrum of sympathetically mediated pain syndromes that usually occur in an extremity after a seemingly minor injury or a surgical procedure. During the course of follow-up care, when the affected area is normally healing, the patient begins to experience pain in that extremity. At times, autonomic dysfunction and loss of voluntary function accompany the pain. Common signs of this condition include coldness, blueness, sensitivity to touch or cold, and episodic mottling or cyanotic discoloration of the skin; however, the findings of electrodiagnostic studies are usually normal. Because the constriction of the blood vessels caused by the increased sympathetic signals typically reduces the blood supply to the involved extremity and makes it colder, thermography can aid in the diagnosis of reflex sympathetic dystrophy by confirming a temperature difference between extremities. Vasomotor abnormalities are quantified thermographically with asymmetries greater than 0.5° C.[19]

Conclusion

Diagnostic imaging and advanced testing procedures are always changing and leading the way to new technology. Certain procedures, such as the performance of a thorough physical examination and the correlation of the findings with a complete case history, remain standard protocols. After all, *practitioners* treat individuals with real musculoskeletal problems, not abnormal x-ray images or CT scans.

Results from diagnostic imaging procedures must be carefully correlated with clinical findings. Abnormal findings that are clinically significant must be painstakingly separated from incidental findings that bear little weight in the management of the case. Only extensive training and practice experience will make the clinician's decision-making process a smoother one regarding the sequencing and ordering of diagnostic tests.

Review Questions

1. (a) Name the most important and practical imaging technique in musculoskeletal medicine? (b) What is the minimum number of projections taken of a joint to be considered diagnostic for uncomplicated injuries? (c) Which articulations require three projections, and why?

2. Name three precautions that address the health hazards of ionizing radiation.

3. What anatomic sites are often used to clinically determine the skeletal age of children and adolescents?

4. Name four clinical uses for bone scanning.

5. (a) What are some advantages of CT scans compared with conventional plain-film radiography? (b) What are some advantages of CT scans compared with MRI?

6. What conditions suggest MRI as the modality of choice?

7. A patient with a history of cervical disk disease has signs and symptoms of carpal tunnel syndrome. What two electrophysiologic studies should be performed and why?

References

1. Becker E, Griffiths HJ: Radiological diagnosis of pain in the athlete, *Clin Sports Med* 6(4):699, 1987.
2. Belhobek GH, Richmond BJ, Piraino DW, et al: Special diagnostic procedures in sports medicine, *Clin Sports Med* 8(3):517, 1989.
3. Bogduk N, Aprill C, Derby R: Discography. In White AH, Schofferman JA: *Spine care,* vol I, St Louis, 1995, Mosby.
4. Burk DL, Karasick D, Kurtz AB et al: Rotator cuff tears: prospective comparison of MR imaging with arthrography, sonography, and surgery, *Am J Roentgenol* 153:87, 1989.
5. Bushong SC: *Radiologic science for technologists: physics, biology, and protection,* ed 5, St Louis, 1993, Mosby.
6. Datz FL: *Handbook of nuclear medicine,* ed 2, St Louis, 1993, Mosby.
7. Early PJ, Sodee DB: *Principles and practice of nuclear medicine,* St Louis, 1995, Mosby.
8. Executive Committee of the North American Spine Society: Position statement on discography, *Spine* 13:1343, 1988.
9. Feierstein MS: The performance and usefulness of nerve conduction studies in the orthopedic office, *Orthop Clin North Am* 19(4):859, 1988.
10. Getty CJ: "Bony sciatica"—the value of thermography, electromyography, and water-soluble myelography, *Clin Sports Med* 5(2):327, 1986.
11. Greenfield G, Stanish WD: Relieving shoulder pain without surgery, *PSM* 22(4):67, 1994.
12. Gruelich, Pyle: *Radiologic Atlas of Skeletal Maturity.*
13. Gustilo RB, Kyle RF, Templeman DC: *Fractures and dislocations,* vol 1, St Louis, 1993, Mosby.
14. Harcke HT, Grissom LE, Finkelstein MS: Evaluation of the musculoskeletal system with sonography, *Am J Roentgenol* 150:1253, 1988.
15. Harrington JT: Preventing osteoporosis in menopausal women, *J Musculoskel Med* 7:6, 1990.
16. Harris JH: Radiographic evaluation of spinal trauma, *Orthop Clin North Am* 17(1):88, 1986.
17. Kirkaldy-Willis WM, editor: *Managing low back pain,* ed 2, New York, 1988, Churchill Livingstone.
18. Kleinman PK et al: Factors affecting visualization of posterior rib fractures in abused infants, *Am J Radiology* 150:635, 1988.
19. Konowitz KB: Reflex sympathy dystrophy syndrome sometimes misdiagnosed, often misunderstood, JACA 35(6):58, 1998.
20. Mack LA et al: Sonographic evaluation of the rotator cuff: accuracy in patients without prior surgery, *Clinical Orthopedics,* 234, Year Book of Orthopedics, 1989.
21. Mack LA, Nyberg DA et al: Sonography of the post-operative shoulder, *Am J Roentgenol* 150:1089, 1988.
22. Martire JR: The role of nuclear medicine bone scans in evaluating pain in athletic injuries, *Clin Sports Med* 6(4):713, 1987.
23. Meschan I: *Roentgen signs in diagnostic imaging,* vol 2, Philadelphia, 1985, WB Saunders.
24. Mesgarzadeh M, Sapega AA, Banakdarpour A, et al: Osteochondritis dissecans: analysis of mechanical instability with radiography, scintigraphy, and MR imaging, *Radiology* 165:775, 1987.
25. Meyer SJ, Dalinka MK: Magnetic resonance imaging of the shoulder, *Orthop Clin North Am* 21(3):502, 1990.
26. Micheli LJ: Reflex sympathetic dystrophy may stem from sports (News Brief), *Physician Sports Med* 18(10):35, 1990.
27. Rogers LF, Hendrix RW: Evaluating the multiple injured patient radiographically, *Orthop Clin North Am* 21(3):437, 1990.
28. Thomas OC: Plain roentgenograms of the spine in the injured athlete, *Clin Sports Med* 5(2):353, 1986.
29. Weissman BNW, Sledge CB: *Orthopedic radiology,* Philadelphia, 1986, WB Saunders.
30. Wexler CE: *An overview of liquid crystal and electronic thermography,* Tarzana, Calif, 1983, Thermographic Services.

Chapter Highlights

Anatomy of the Shoulder
Examination of the Shoulder
Differential Diagnosis of Shoulder Pain
Disorders of the Glenohumeral Joint
Disorders of the Acromioclavicular Joint
Disorders of the Suprahumeral Space
Disorders of the Sternoclavicular Joint
Disorders of the Scapulothoracic Joint
Arthropathies of the Shoulder
A Word About Injections

A 45-year-old laborer with cervical disk disease, a 60-year-old smoker with lung cancer, and an 18-year-old baseball player may all have one thing in common: shoulder pain. The causes of shoulder pain are so diverse that such pain may be one of the most common ailments seen in a primary care practice. The cause of a patient's pain may be elusive, yet it may be as simple as an awkward sleeping posture. To add complications, the shoulder joint has the potential to mimic cervical pathologic abnormalities or refer pain to the spine.

Anatomy of the Shoulder

To accomplish an overhead movement or propel an object, there must be synchronous and painless shoulder motion. Thus the shoulder's capsule, surrounding muscles, nerves, blood vessels, and articulations make up quite a delicate and complex structure. The shoulder girdle, as it is generally known, encompasses four articulations that serve very different purposes and are vulnerable to vastly different problems:

1. The glenohumeral joint (Figure 3-1), often referred to simply as the shoulder joint, is highly functional, yet its tenuous bony restraints also make it highly unstable. Dislocations and subluxations are the result.
2. The acromioclavicular articulation (Figure 3-2) solidifies the portion of the posterior aspect of the shoulder girdle via the acromion process to the anterior bridge of the girdle at the clavicle. Chronic instability attributable to trauma, including occupational, recreational, and athletic injuries, earmark the typical history of acromioclavicular lesions.
3. The sternoclavicular articulation (Figure 3-3) joins the sternum, or breast bone, with the clavicle, or collar bone. Disorders of the sternoclavicular joint occur almost exclusively in association with athletic or motor vehicle trauma and with falls on an outstretched hand.
4. The scapulothoracic articulation joins the posterior shoulder region to the thoracic spine. It plays a major role in the normal excursion of the brachium (i.e., in the normal fluid motion of the arm from the side to an overhead position) and frequently suffers damage in gross blunt trauma from high-impact injuries and chronic postural syndromes.

The shoulder must rely on soft-tissue structures, rather than on osseous articulations, for its stability.

Examination of the Shoulder

History, observation, palpation, and orthopedic testing should reveal answers to the following questions about the mechanism and function of the shoulder:

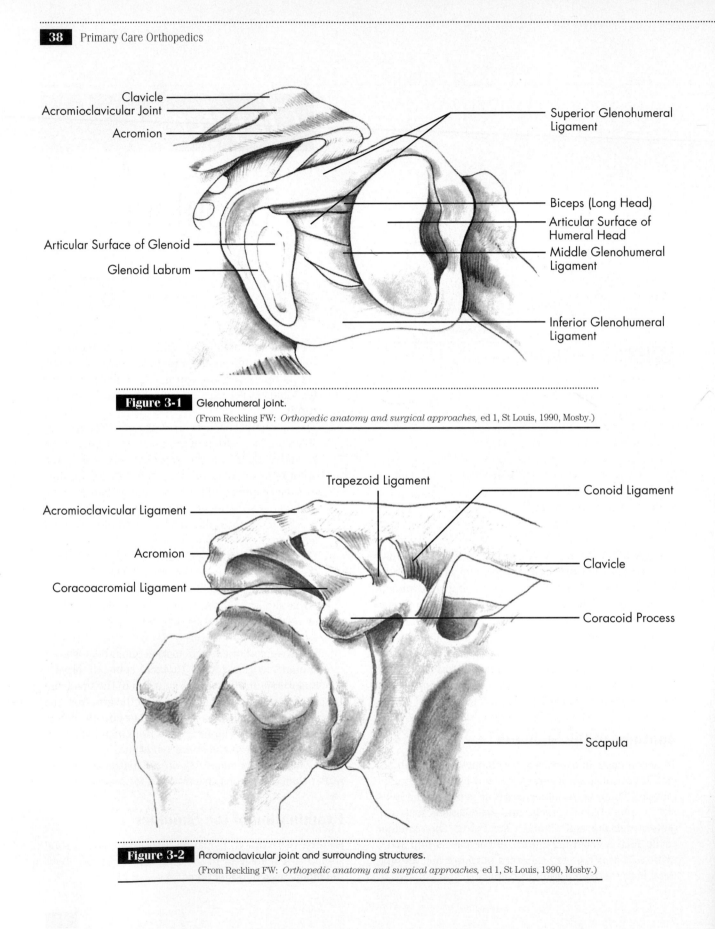

Figure 3-1   Glenohumeral joint.
(From Reckling FW: *Orthopedic anatomy and surgical approaches,* ed 1, St Louis, 1990, Mosby.)

Figure 3-2   Acromioclavicular joint and surrounding structures.
(From Reckling FW: *Orthopedic anatomy and surgical approaches,* ed 1, St Louis, 1990, Mosby.)

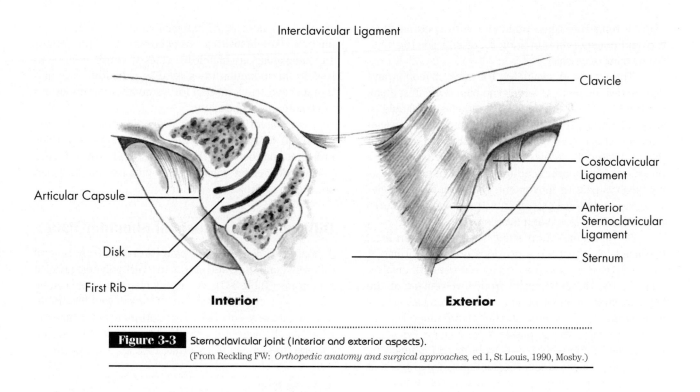

Interclavicular Ligament

Clavicle

Costoclavicular Ligament

Articular Capsule

Anterior Sternoclavicular Ligament

Disk

Sternum

First Rib

Interior

Exterior

Figure 3-3 Sternoclavicular joint (interior and exterior aspects).

(From Reckling FW: *Orthopedic anatomy and surgical approaches*, ed 1, St Louis, 1990, Mosby.)

- Is there a painful arc of movement associated with the patient's shoulder pain?
- If there is a painful abduction arc, where does it occur—at an angle of 0 degrees to 10, 45, 90 degrees or greater? (Different muscles exert their forces at various points along the arc.)
- Is there a history of trauma? If so, what are the results of stability testing?
- If there is no history of trauma, does the patient have a history of dermatologic conditions, poly-arthritis, or recurrent joint effusions?
- Is there any associated pain in the neck or elbow, or is there a relevant medical history of neck or elbow problems?
- Is there or has there been any swelling?
- What is the patient's position during sleep? Does he or she awaken with pain?
- Has there been any drastic change in workload in the patient's immediate past that could have contributed to the pain?
- Does the physical examination reveal any sign of glenohumeral instability? If so, is there an associated history of trauma? If not, the examiner should check other joints for inherent laxity (e.g., the metacarpophalangeal joints of the thumbs) and for subluxability (e.g., the patellofemoral joints).

- Was the arm forced into hyperabduction with external rotation, producing an occult glenohumeral subluxation?

Some practitioners mistakenly rush through the history-taking part of the shoulder examination. It is helpful to probe details, such as the sleeping postures of the patient and the time of day in which the shoulder is most troubling. In many adults, chronic pain stems from daily activities that they never associate with their problems.

If possible, the examiner should observe the patient taking off his or her outer garments to evaluate the shoulder's function and to note any grimace of pain. Some patients have had shoulder pain for so long that they have cleverly devised specific methods of disrobing without further aggravating their shoulder complaint.

Generally, the examiner begins with a bilateral inspection of the musculature at the anterior and posterior shoulder girdle. After looking for asymmetry, atrophy, and swelling, the examiner palpates the anterior capsule, biceps tendon, acromioclavicular joint, and anterior deltoid muscle to check for pain. Similarly, the examiner palpates the supraspinatus tendon and lateral deltoid muscle on the lateral aspect of the shoulder. Posteriorly, the examiner checks the scapula, rear deltoid muscle, and muscles of the rotator cuff for tenderness. A finding of palpable tenderness, in combination with a pertinent history and range-of-motion findings, often leads to an initial working diagnosis.

The examiner evaluates the arcs of motion and determines the point at which the pain is greatest along any troublesome arc. Range-of-motion testing should be active at first so that the examiner can assess muscle-tendon units. If testing reveals full and painless arcs of motion bilaterally, active testing with resistance is appropriate. The final procedure in range-of-motion testing involves passive movement, including shoulder elevation and rotational movements, to test inert structures (e.g., the joint capsule and ligaments).

It is extremely important to test abduction arcs, because such a test often provides precise information (Table 3-1). For example, it may differentiate involvement of the deltoid muscle from involvement of the supraspinatus or involvement of the acromioclavicular joint from involvement of the glenohumeral joint. Codman's drop-arm test makes it possible for the examiner to determine whether the rotator cuff is intact by testing the patient's ability to maintain arm abduction at 90 degrees. The apprehension sign is seen in patients with anterior glenohumeral instability. With the patient seated or supine, the examiner gently mobilizes the glenohumeral joint into external rotation and places one hand over the anterior capsule to feel for clicking or subluxing of the humeral head.

Hypomobility in a "capsular pattern" occurs in patients with adhesive capsulitis. These patients lose their capacity for internal or external rotation and hyperabduction. Patients with a loss of continuity of the rotator cuff mechanism are unable to achieve a continuous, painless arc of abduction; they tend to substitute scapulothoracic and trunk motion for a smooth, continuous arc of glenohumeral abduction.

An algorithm for clinical decision making for examination of the shoulder and management of various problems that occur in the shoulder is shown in Figure 3-4. Guidelines for diagnostic imaging for shoulder pain are shown in Table 3-2.

Differential Diagnosis of Shoulder Pain

As stated earlier, shoulder pain can result from several different conditions and can occur with a diverse array of symptoms (Table 3-3). A lengthy history of pain can be the result of chronic instability. If the relevant history reveals a traumatic episode, it is important to determine the exact mechanism of injury. If the arm was forced into hyperabduction with external rotation, for example,

---

Table 3-1 Pathologic Arcs of Abduction

Abduction Arc Affected	Possible Pathologic Conditions
0°-30°	Supraspinatus strain (tendonitis) Frozen shoulder
30°-90°	Deltoid strain, palsy Adhesive capsulitis Advanced rotator cuff disease
Greater than 90°	Acromioclavicular joint disease Trapezius strain Subacromial pathologic conditions • Biceps tendonitis • Subacromial bursitis • Rotator cuff strain • Impingement • Acromioclavicular arthritis Glenohumeral instability Scapulothoracic dysfunction

---

Table 3-2 Diagnostic Imaging for Shoulder Pain

Orthopedic Imaging	Clinical Indications
Computed arthrotomography	Partial thickness tear of rotator cuff, glenoid labrum tears or attenuation
CT	Infection, masses, metastatic lesions, abscesses, foreign bodies, complex fractures
Contrast arthrography	Adhesive capsulitis, complete tears of rotator cuff
Conventional tomography	Characterization of infectious and neoplastic processes
Fluoroscopy	Biopsies
MRI	Rotator cuff disease, capsular and tendon lesions, muscle tears, strains
Plain-film x-ray	Initial workup in all patients (frontal projections with arm in internal and external rotations)
Scintigraphy (bone scan)	Arthropathies (inflammatory), infection, neoplastic disease
US	Rotator cuff tear, tendonitis, intraarticular bodies

CT, Computed tomography; **MRI,** magnetic resonance imaging, **US,** ultrasonography.

Adapted from Resnick D: Diagnostic imaging for shoulder pain, *J Musculoskeletal Med,* 5(7):22, 1988.

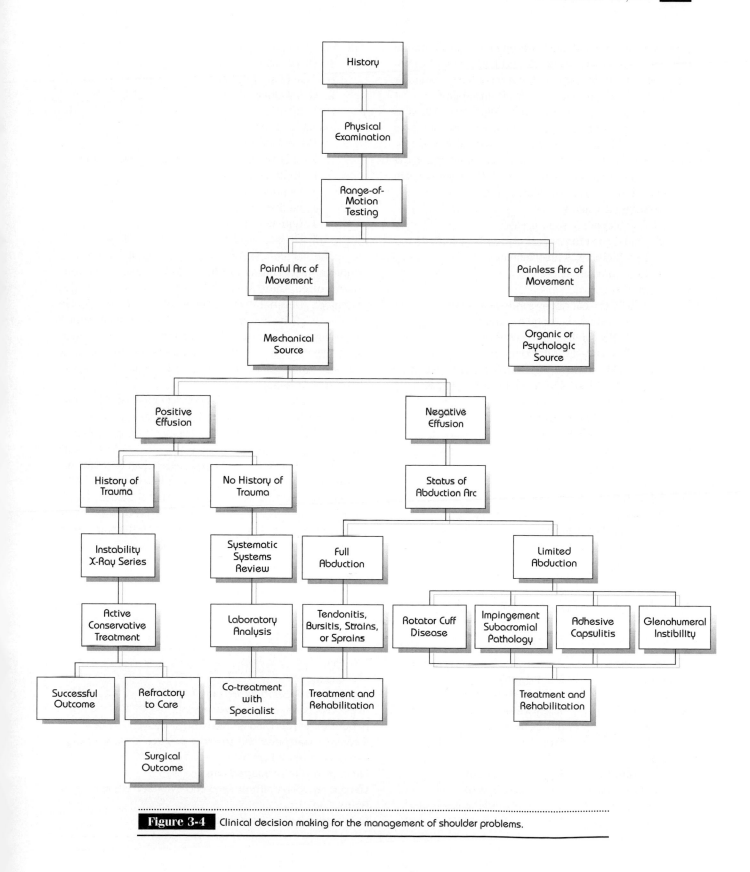

Figure 3-4 Clinical decision making for the management of shoulder problems.

there may be an occult subluxation in the glenohumeral joint. A delay in the diagnosis and treatment of glenohumeral instability may result in a second dislocation or subluxation with subsequent chronic instability.

Chronic soft-tissue overuse syndrome can also cause repeated episodes of shoulder pain. Subacromial and subdeltoid bursitis, as well as proximal biceps tendonitis, are common overuse syndromes involving the shoulder. The following is an outline of the origins of pain that may be referred to the shoulder:

I. Neurogenic origins
   A. Cervical nerve root disease
   B. Spinal cord tumors
   C. Brachial plexus involvement
      1. Traumatic
      2. Mechanical
         a. Cervical rib pressure on a nerve
         b. Anterior scalene syndrome
         c. Pectoralis minor syndrome
         d. Costoclavicular syndrome
         e. Malposition of first thoracic rib (e.g., as a result of sleeping in an awkward position)
   D. Scapulocostal syndrome
   E. Individual nerve trauma
      1. Suprascapular nerve
      2. Dorsal scapular nerve
      3. Long thoracic nerve
      4. Circumflex nerve
II. Sympathetic origins
   A. Causalgia
   B. Sympathetic dystrophy
   C. Shoulder-hand syndrome
III. Viscerogenic origins
   A. Diaphragm
   B. Pulmonary infarction
   C. Gallbladder
   D. Lung
IV. Hematologic origins
   A. Hemoglobinopathies
   B. Neoplastic disorders of hematopoietic tissue
      1. Multiple myeloma
      2. Lymphoma
      3. Leukemia
      4. Gaucher's disease
      5. Caisson disease

As people age, the acromioclavicular and glenohumeral mechanisms are likely to be involved in pain more often than are other articulations near the shoulder. Degenerative changes of the intraarticular meniscus of the acromioclavicular joint or subacromial spurring are the primary reasons for dysfunction, since they may lead to a painful arc of abduction with limited motion. Bony resorption, degenerative changes, and osteolysis can occur.[2]

Unless an individual is accustomed to working constantly with the arm abducted at an angle of 90 degrees or more, a sudden workload at the point of hyperabduction (e.g., painting or paper hanging) can produce a bout of subacromial pain. Individuals older than 35 years are more susceptible than younger people to acromioclavicular or subacromial pain from everyday activities. Some workers, such as insulators or house painters, may not experience these bouts of pain, however, because their shoulders are accustomed to this workload.

Table 3-3   Diversity of Shoulder Pathologic Conditions

Occupation or Activity	Site or Nature of Injury	Mechanism of Injury
Baseball pitcher	Rotator cuff strain or tendonitis	Throwing
Homemaker	Deltoid strain	Lifting groceries
Skier	Dislocated glenohumeral joint	Acute fall on hyperabducted arm
Weight lifter	Traumatic acromioclavicular arthritis	Repetitive bench pressing movements
Swimmer	Biceps tendonitis	Repetitive microtrauma of overhead swimming stroke
Student	Scapulothoracic dysfunction	Chronic forward head and shoulder position while studying
Elderly	Scapulothoracic dysfunction	Increased thoracic kyphosis
Football player	Sternoclavicular sprain	Arm tackling with abducted arm
Construction worker	Subacromial bursitis	Chronic, repetitive microtrauma and overhead lifting
Smoker	Vague, referred shoulder pain	Apical lung mass
Secretary	Adhesive capsulitis	Long-term guarding after shoulder strain

Disorders of the Glenohumeral Joint

Because the glenohumeral joint sacrifices bony stability for its exceedingly large range of motion, the glenohumeral articulation is the most commonly dislocated joint in the body.[10] The shoulder's modified ball-and-socket joint differs greatly from the deeply seated hip articulation. The glenoid portion of the scapula is small and flat. This shallow dish does not lend itself to stabilizing the humerus in dynamic movements of the brachium. The fibrocartilaginous glenoid labrum, which adds depth to the socket, is one source of stability for this articulation; the anterior glenohumeral ligament is another. Unfortunately, repetitive trauma causes microtears in the labrum that are associated with anterior glenohumeral instability (Figure 3-5 *A, B*).

Glenohumeral Dislocations

Shoulder dislocations can occur in a variety of ways and in several directions. It is of paramount importance to differentiate quickly between a dislocation that results from trauma and a dislocation that results from neuromuscular disease (e.g., muscular dystrophy), since the cause ultimately determines the appropriate management.

Most traumatic glenohumeral dislocations follow a forced or sudden hyperabduction and external rotation that has caused an anteroinferior translation of the humeral head. This is also known as a subcoracoid glenohumeral dislocation. High-impact trauma with a hyperabducted arm, as may occur in a skiing accident or fall, causes this type of injury. It is painful and disfiguring; moreover, the longer it takes to reduce the dislocation, the greater the muscle spasms and complications that can result. In some instances the arm and shoulder are so rigid that the practitioner must anesthetize the shoulder in the emergency room or office to achieve reduction. In other cases, reduction is possible immediately after the episode, even at the scene. It is always crucial to rule out an associated fracture and to check for neurovascular compromise distal to the site down the arm or in the hand.

More than 90% of traumatic glenohumeral dislocations are anterior.[75] One anatomic reason is that the shoulder capsule and glenoid are weakest at the antero-

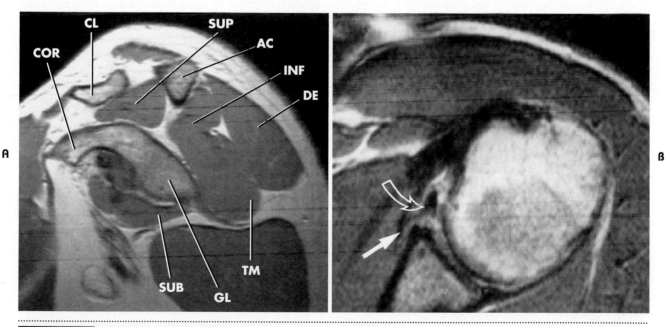

A

B

Figure 3-5 **A,** Sagittal oblique magnetic resonance image of shoulder. **B,** Instability. Labral detachments in a professional hockey player after acute injury. Note labral detachments from glenoid (open arrows) and capsular stripping from anterior glenoid neck (straight arrow).

AC, Acromion process; **CL,** clavicle; **COR,** coracoid process; **DE,** deltoid; **GL,** glenoid; **INF,** infraspinatus; **SUB,** subscapularis; **SUP,** supraspinatus; **TM,** teres minor.

(Part A from Kelley LL: *Sectional anatomy for imaging professionals,* ed 1, St Louis, 1997, Mosby. Part B from Nicholas JA, Hershman EB: *The upper extremity in sports medicine,* St Louis, 1995, Mosby.)

inferior point. Also, the position of the rotator cuff muscles places them at a disadvantage in their ability to stabilize and depress the head of the humerus during hyperabduction.

Radiographic Studies for Glenohumeral Dislocation

After a traumatic glenohumeral dislocation, plain films can help rule out gross deformity and associated fractures, such as an impact fracture of the head of the humerus. Standard x-ray films taken for a suspected dislocation include the two standard anatomic views (internal and external rotation) and an axillary view (Stryker notch).[58] If the examiner suspects other types of injuries, other approaches may also be necessary (Table 3-4).

A defect at the posterior aspect of the humeral head near the greater tuberosity can arise as a result of multiple dislocations or recurrent subluxations. This notch defect can also occur after a single dislocation, however.[23] With chronic anterior instability, the notch may enlarge at the posterolateral humerus, representing a stress reaction to a series of microfractures. This is termed a Hill-Sachs lesion and is seen with humeral head fractures on an axillary view (Figure 3-6 *A, B*). This view can best be obtained via the table-top method. The patient lies supine with an 8- × 10-inch plate behind the shoulder. The affected arm is put on top of the patient's head so that the axilla is exposed. Taken with the patient in this position, the film clearly shows the posterior aspect of the head of the humerus. This compression fracture defect of the posterolateral humeral head shows up as an indented "notch" on the x-ray film. The axillary or notch view accurately demonstrates the presence of a Hill-Sachs lesion. External rotation views obscure the lesion, although the

60-degree internal rotation view used by Adams, a researcher and clinician, brings the posterolateral surface into profile.[57] The axillary view continues to be a standard projection in confirming the diagnosis of previous traumatic anterior dislocations, however.

An anteroposterior projection affords another look at the glenohumeral joint. Many times the superior migration of the humeral head is evident in an anteroposterior projection. Attrition of the rotator cuff may cause this positional change of the humerus. The internal rotation sometimes makes it possible to visualize a Hill-Sachs lesion if it is of moderate magnitude. This view, however, is not a substitute for an axillary film of the posterolateral humeral head.[6]

Management of Glenohumeral Dislocation

First-time dislocations are often misdiagnosed. In addition, some patients do not see their physician when they first experience such an injury. The combination of these two factors can lead to an alarming recurrence rate in shoulder dislocations. The saying, "Once a dislocator, always a dislocator," does not hold true when the patient seeks treatment and carefully adheres to the proper treatment protocol from the beginning, however.

All first-time dislocations must be immobilized for a *minimum* of 3 weeks in the closed-packed position of arm adduction and internal rotation.[42] Pathologic changes, including Hill-Sachs lesions, are commonly associated with first-time, traumatic dislocations.[71] Careful testing of sensation around the shoulder is essential after a traumatic shoulder dislocation. Neuronal compression may lead to a weakness, numbness, or tingling, or a swelling into the hand.[63] Thus the practitioner should immediately rule out an axillary neurapraxia by neurologic testing of the C5 dermatome.[24]

It is necessary to immobilize the shoulder for as long as 4 to 6 weeks in some individuals. This lengthy period of immobilization allows the glenohumeral joint to form scar tissue, which, in effect, compensates for the loss of the stabilizing supports after the anterior capsule tears. The clinician must resist the temptation to permit early freedom of motion in the shoulder. In essence the clinician is caught in a dilemma. On the one hand is the need to stabilize a very unstable joint via adhesion formation; on the other hand is the worry about the need to reestablish the motion of what was once the most freely movable joint in the patient's body.

Adjunctive therapy measures can play an important role in the comfort and swelling reduction of a dislocated shoulder. Copious use of ice for controlling the

---

Table 3-4   Methods of Investigation for Suspected Injuries after Glenohumeral Traumatic Dislocation

Suspected Injury	Method of Investigation
Fracture of humeral head	Plain-film radiograph (axillary view)
Fracture of glenoid	Plain-film radiograph (AP view)
Axillary neurapraxia	Physical examination
Brachial plexopathy	Physical examination, needle EMG
Glenoid labrum tear	Arthrogram

AP, Anteroposterior; *EMG,* electromyography.

effusion in the shoulder is recommended, along with electrotherapy at a low-sensory stimulation level. When pain and swelling start to decrease, the patient can begin movement and isometrics for the rotator cuff.

Glenohumeral Subluxation

In a shoulder dislocation, the articulating surfaces are totally out of contact with one another, and there is a true gross deformity during the time that the joint is "out of its socket." In contrast, a subluxation of the glenohumeral joint encompasses a "shift" in the normal alignment of the articulation. Thus the symptoms and treatment of a glenohumeral subluxation differ from those of a dislocation (Table 3-5).

A subluxation can result from trauma similar to that involved in a shoulder dislocation, but the external forces are generally of less magnitude. In this case the patient feels the shoulder pop or shift out of place for a brief moment, then feels it spontaneously return to its normal position. This occurs secondary to muscle spasm. Similar to traumatic dislocation, traumatic subluxation is quite painful and causes mild-to-moderate swelling. Immobilization of the subluxed shoulder is necessary, but the patient may be able to start rehabilitation sooner than the patient with a dislocated shoulder.

Some patients who experience shoulder subluxation do not have a history of trauma; rather, they appear to have congenitally hypermobile joints (i.e., double jointed). The three most common lax joints are the patellofemoral joint, the first metacarpophalangeal joint of the hand, and the glenohumeral joint. These patients may relate a history of voluntary shoulder subluxation. In time their shoulder capsules are so stretched that the joint becomes painfully unstable. Because subluxation requires so little force in unstable shoulders, there is usually little or no swelling. Therefore these patients may require a sling or immobilization for only 1 or 2 days if they are experiencing pain. It is important for the practitioner to take a careful history and to check other peripheral articulations for hypermobility.

Subluxations of the glenohumeral joint without a history of trauma may also occur in patients with neuromuscular disorders. Muscular dystrophy is the most common cause of pathologic neuromuscular subluxations of the shoulder. Atrophy of the shoulder girdle may be severe, depending on the classification of the disorder. Careful laboratory studies are necessary to confirm the diagnosis. Electrodiagnostic studies are helpful in confirming a denervating neuromuscular disease.

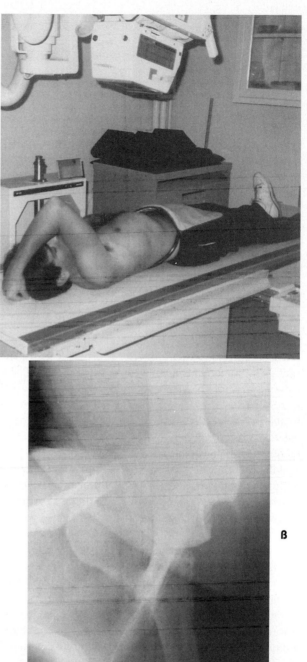

Figure 3-6 A, Patient positioning for the Stryker notch view. B, Stryker notch view demonstrating a Hills-Sachs lesion in a patient with anterior instability.

(From Nicholas JA, Hershman EB: *The upper extremity in sports medicine,* St Louis, 1995, Mosby.)

Table 3-5 Glenohumeral Dislocation versus Glenohumeral Subluxation

	Acute Glenohumeral Dislocation	Chronic Glenohumeral Subluxation
Physical examination findings	Effusion Inability to abduct or externally rotate shoulder Possible need for reduction Tenderness in rotator cuff muscles posteriorly Anterior capsule tenderness	Mild swelling possible Positive apprehension sign Hypermobility Tenderness at joint line
X-ray findings	Three views (internal, external, axillary) to rule out Hill-Sachs lesion and fracture of humerus	Three views (internal, external, axillary) to rule out Hill-Sachs (notch defect) and Bankart lesion (sclerosis of anteroinferior glenoid)
Treatment plan	Immobilization (3 weeks minimum) Ice Electrotherapy	Physical therapy, especially strengthening of periarticular structures

Recurrent Glenohumeral Instability

Patients with dynamic or transient recurrent anterior glenohumeral instability should undergo screening for (1) a Hill-Sachs lesion at the head of the humerus, posteromedially; (2) a Bankart lesion at the anteroinferior glenoid; and (3) a lax anterior capsule. If the recurrent glenohumeral instability results from multiple dislocations, axillary (Stryker notch) views generally reveal Hill-Sachs lesions. Chronically subluxed glenohumeral joints do not usually evidence the same degree of clinically significant radiographic findings, however. It is common to find a Bankart lesion that involves both the middle and inferior glenohumeral ligaments in patients with traumatic anterior glenohumeral instability. Diagnostic arthroscopy can be helpful in forming a definitive diagnosis and ascertaining the best treatment option.[19]

Factors That Contribute to Recurrent Instability

Although dislocations, subluxations, and glenoid labrum tears are responsible for the vast majority of shoulder instabilities, there are many patients with a subtle anterior glenohumeral instability that becomes apparent only through careful physical examination, radiographic examination, and history. The management of such a condition requires consideration of several factors (Figure 3-7).

Inherent laxity at the glenohumeral joint is more common in women, who may also experience knee and thumb hypermobility. Although laxity of articulations in the skeletal system differs from instability, the two seem to have a symbiotic relationship. Certainly, congenital laxity plays a role in the development of clinical musculoskeletal instability.

Repetitive microtraumatic overuse syndromes can also result in subtle glenohumeral laxity and anterior capsulitis. Often such overuse syndromes lead to labrum tears. Rotator cuff disease and impingement are frequently associated with anterior shoulder instability.[50] Occult tears of both the rotator cuff and biceps tendon can exert traction on the anterior capsule, thus increasing anterior glenohumeral instability. Repetitive stress at the extremes of motion can result in microtears at the anterior capsule and labrum. Recreational athletes who play overhead sports (e.g., tennis and racquetball) and competitive athletes who play throwing sports (e.g., baseball pitchers) can develop this condition because of their persistent, high-velocity overhead movements.[7,73] With the forceful contraction of the biceps muscle in the overhand movement, the upper portion of the glenoid rim may avulse as it separates from the labrum. The long head of the biceps causes this "bow-stringing," which can also subtly occur over time (microtrauma).

Treating shoulder pain in patients who compete in throwing sports can be unpredictable and somewhat perplexing. The correct diagnosis may be elusive. Two common causes of chronic anterior shoulder pain, subluxation and impingement, can be confused during the physical examination.[23]

Shoulder instability may be multidirectional in patients with hypermobility. Symptoms in these patients have varying degrees of severity. If persistent clicking and pain develop during the throwing motion and the patient does not respond to therapy, a radiographic or advanced imaging examination is necessary. Often these patients have labrum defects that may require an arthroscopic evaluation.[25] Labrum defects are commonly associated with shoulder instability and tears of the rotator cuff.[23] Competitive athletes in overhead sports who exhibit signs of anterior glenohumeral instability may be candidates for anterior capsulolabral reconstruction.[30]

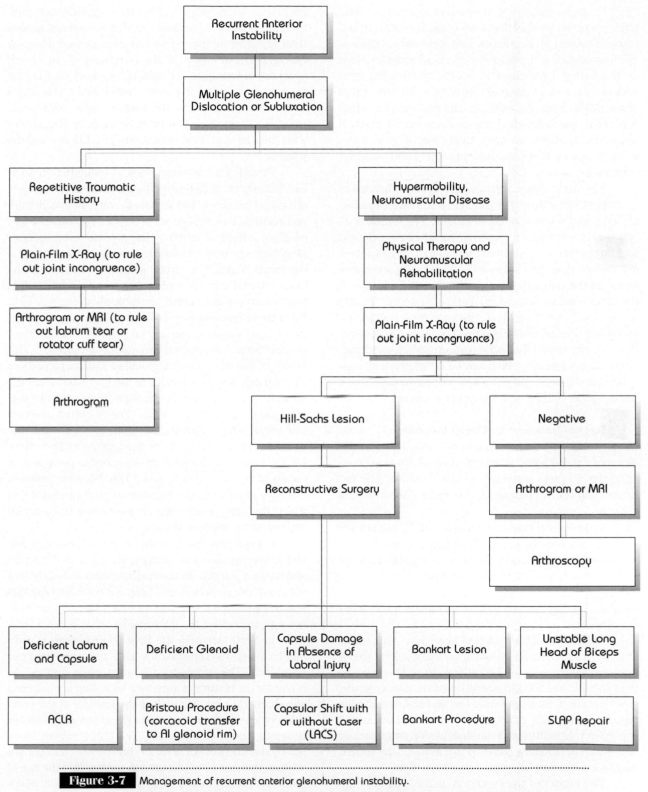

Figure 3-7 Management of recurrent anterior glenohumeral instability.

MRI, Magnetic resonance imaging; **AI,** anteroinferior; **ACLR,** anterior capsulolabral repair; **LACS,** laser-assisted capsular shift; **SLAP,** superior labrum anterior to posterior.

Posterior instability, as opposed to anterior instability, accounts for only 2% to 4% of patients with an unstable shoulder.[64] Recurrent posterior subluxation is often associated with high-force overhead activities, such as those that take place in sports. As the humerus adducts and rotates internally during the follow-through phase of throwing, for example, the periarticular structures (e.g., the deltoid and subscapularis muscles) reach maximum contraction force. Swimmers may also develop multidirectional shoulder instability and posterior subluxation.

The signs of recurrent anterior shoulder instability resulting from a defective glenoid labrum are catching, clicking, and popping of the shoulder. The "clunk test" can aid the examiner in determining whether a glenoid labrum tear is impinging in the shoulder. During the test the patient must be supine and relaxed. The examiner supports the patient's elbow with one hand and places the other hand behind the head of the humerus. Raising the patient's arm overhead, the examiner pushes the shoulder anteriorly while rotating the humerus. The result is positive when this manipulation produces a "clunk" or grinding sensation, which may be associated with capsular apprehension and glenohumeral pain as the head of the humerus collides with a tear of the labrum.

Surgical Treatment for Chronic Instability

Surgery is reserved as the last step to stabilize the condition of a patient who is experiencing constant pain attributable to gross instability of the shoulder. The patient's condition should meet one or more of the following criteria:

1. Patient has experienced multiple painful episodes of subluxing or dislocating glenohumeral joint.
2. Condition has been refractory to rehabilitation or physical therapy for 4 to 6 months.
3. Condition affects quality of life.
4. Joint incongruence is evident on radiographic examination.

Before opting for a surgical procedure, the patient must have experienced several episodes of painful glenohumeral subluxations or dislocations. In addition the patient should have tried to strengthen the shoulder girdle, including the rotator cuff muscles, and stabilize the lax glenohumeral joint during movement. If, however, a supervised physical therapy or rehabilitation program does not reduce or eliminate pain in 4 to 6 months, the patient may be a candidate for surgical reconstruction.

The impact of the condition on the quality of life is also a factor in determining whether surgery is appropriate. Many patients who have experienced multiple episodes of subluxation or dislocation can sublux their shoulder simply by rolling over in their sleep or reaching for an object in the back seat of the car. If everyday movements are difficult, surgery may be the treatment of choice. Similarly, if an individual is active in recreation and sports, the surgical option may be attractive. These decisions must be made by the patient with the advice of the primary care practitioner and the surgeon.[63]

Finally, joint incongruence as exhibited on an x-ray film may be an indication for surgery. Some types of structural damage to the glenohumeral joint may require reconstruction to restore some measure of stability. For example, a Bankart lesion, a defect of the anteroinferior glenohumeral ligament-labrum complex, appears as a calcification resulting from a stress fracture at the anteroinferior rim on a plain-film x-ray. This lesion is common in the chronically unstable shoulder.[75] A West Point view demonstrates the Bankart lesion by making it possible to evaluate the glenoid cavity without bony overlap from the coracoid process or acromion.[75] This view is sometimes called a modified axillary projection. The patient lies prone with a pillow underneath the shoulder to raise it, and the examiner places the film cassette superior to the shoulder. The resulting image of the relationship between the humeral head and the glenoid is similar to that obtained in the axillary view, but the anteroinferior glenoid rim is better visualized by means of the West Point view. This sclerotic defect is usually resolved via the Bankart surgical procedure, in which the orthopedic surgeon reattaches the anterior capsule to the anterior glenoid.

Capsulorrhaphy performed via arthroscopy has had its greatest success rates in patients with Hill-Sachs and Bankart lesions. In patients who have a detachment of the inferior glenohumeral ligament complex (Bankart lesion, Figure 3-8), the presence of a labrum tear does not appear to affect the outcome.[72]

In North America the Bristow procedure is commonly used to reconstruct the unstable anterior shoulder.[80] This procedure is most often applied directly for the recurrent anterior dislocating or subluxing glenohumeral joint. It involves the transfer of the coracoid process to the anterior margin of the glenoid fossa to create a bone block. It is hoped that this bony block will ultimately prevent another dislocation. A major advantage that has been documented regarding the use of a Bristow arthroplasty includes the avoidance of glenohumeral arthritis.[16]

A superior labrum anterior to posterior (SLAP) repair of the labrum is necessary if the long head of the biceps muscle is unstable.[34] An internal closure of the rotator cuff is indicated with concomitant cuff damage and instability, including minimal internal joint damage, hyperelasticity, or internal separation of the cuff. A capsular shift may be performed with or without laser assistance ([LACS] heat shrinkage), if there is no labral damage. As previously stated, an ACLR is performed when there is anterior instability with significant labral and capsular damage.[39]

Disorders of the Acromioclavicular Joint

Although there may be several reasons for acromioclavicular joint pain and dysfunction, generally they can be classified into two major groups: microtraumatic episodes or macrotraumatic episodes. Repetitive microtrauma can lead to arthritic changes at the acromioclavicular articulation, thereby leading to heterotopic bone formation that, in turn, leads to subacromial compromise. Repetitive overuse, such as in painting, throwing, and pressing motions in weight lifting, can result in subacromial spurring, degenerative arthritis of the acromioclavicular joint itself, or bony resorption of the distal clavicle. Over

time, for example, bench pressing movements can lead to microtears and degenerative changes at the acromioclavicular joint, along with meniscal damage, eventually leading to a condition often called weight lifter's shoulder (Table 3-6).

Macrotraumatic episodes, such as acute acromioclavicular sprains (separations), are quite common in recreational and competitive sports. There are two main mechanisms of acute acromioclavicular joint sprain. First, the patient may fall on the point of the shoulder with the arm in either the neutral or the adducted position. An ice hockey player, for example, usually hits the point of the shoulder into the boards or onto the ice, forcing the coracoid process and acromion downward; subsequent examination reveals point tenderness over the acromioclavicular joint, mild-to-moderate swelling, and a painful reduction in abduction and horizontal adduction. Second, the patient may fall on the hand of an outstretched arm. This second mechanism may, in fact,

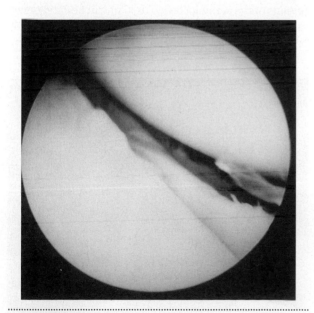

Figure 3-8 Arthroscopic view of the Bankart lesion with detachment of the anteroinferior labrum and capsule from the glenoid neck.

(From Nicholas JA, Hershman EB: *The upper extremity in sports medicine*, St Louis, 1995, Mosby.)

Table 3-6 Weight Lifter's Shoulder

Component	Description
History	Anterior shoulder pain with stress via chronic microtrauma to AC joint, chronic AC instability (individual often performs bench presses through pain)
Radiology	Studies to rule out traumatic AC arthritis, osteolysis of distal clavicle
Physical examination findings	Tenderness over AC joint, laxity of AC ligament, pain on hyperabduction, retrograde trapezius myospasm, meniscal damage, crepitus with degenerative arthritis
Secondary findings	Global weakness of shoulder girdle, suboccipital headaches, cervical joint dysfunction
Treatment plan	Rest, ice, electrotherapy, chiropractic manipulation of cervical spine, short-term immobilization for acute exacerbation of unstable AC joint
Follow-up care	Gradual strengthening program for shoulder girdle, including progression from isometrics to lightweight, short-arc isotonic movements; bench pressing maximum of two times per week with a light and heavy day followed by cryotherapy

AC, Acromioclavicular.

cause osseous injury to the distal forearm, wrist, or elbow joint, because the force of the fall is transmitted up through the acromioclavicular joint, which may bear the load of the person's body weight. The very young and the very old, because they are at special risk of falling, are particularly susceptible to upper limb fractures, such as a Colles' fracture. Participants in athletics, however, commonly injure their acromioclavicular joint.

The stability of the acromioclavicular joint depends on its ligamentous structures (see Figure 3-2). Together, the coracoclavicular and the acromioclavicular ligaments control the movements of the acromioclavicular joint. The coracoclavicular ligament is comprised of two bands, the conoid and the trapezoid, which anchor the lateral clavicle. The acromioclavicular joint allows a gliding motion of both the articular surface of the clavicle on the acromion and the rotation of the scapula on the clavicle during abduction of the arm. The joint itself contains a synovial membrane, and it may contain the anatomic variant of an articular disk.

Because the two ligaments of the joint lie in different planes, gross trauma is necessary to produce multidirectional instability. Usually these injuries result from a long, high-speed fall or from a motor vehicle or motorcycle accident. Total dissociation of the ligaments produces a complete rupture or dislocation of the joint. A concomitant fracture is also possible (Figure 3-9 *A, B*). Although these types of acromioclavicular sprains are not as common as mild or moderate sprains, they do occur in high-impact trauma and present problems for the primary care practitioner.

Orthopedic Evaluation of the Acromioclavicular Joint

Stress testing of the acromioclavicular complex is a primary component of the orthopedic evaluation for acromioclavicular joint stability. It is more efficient to test stability by placing two fingers over the anterior aspect of the clavicle while the other hand stabilizes the spine of the scapula. When pressing the two fingers down to "spring the clavicle" (i.e., push it up and down), the examiner can observe movement at the acromioclavicular joint. This applied stress causes a gliding motion through the acromioclavicular joint and may demonstrate abnormal laxity or produce pain. There may be a protective muscle spasm at the trapezius muscle of the side affected by a sprain. Mild swelling over the acromioclavicular joint may also be evident, along with a painful arc of abduction. Pain over 90 degrees of abduction almost always occurs, even in mild sprains.

Grading of Acromioclavicular Sprains

Sprains of the acromioclavicular joint can be categorized as mild (grade I), moderate (grade II), or severe (grade

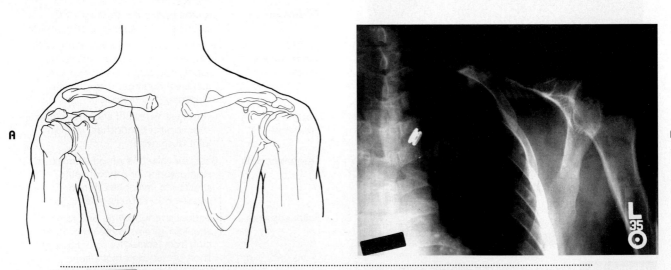

A   B

Figure 3-9 **A,** Grade III acromioclavicular separation with unilateral displacement of the distal clavicle superiorly. **B,** Plain radiographic film showing a grade III acromioclavicular separation with significant displacement of the distal clavicular head.

(From Ruiz E, Cicero JJ: *Emergency management of skeletal injuries,* ed 1, St Louis, 1995, Mosby.)

III). Traditional grading systems have used the first-, second-, and third-degree grades of injury.

- Grade I acromioclavicular sprains are mild in nature, with a minimal amount of pain, swelling, and ligamentous instability. They occur when a mild force causes tearing of only a few fibers of the acromioclavicular ligament and capsule. There is no gross instability of the joint.
- Grade II acromioclavicular sprains are moderate, but may cause marked pain, swelling, instability, and dysfunction. They occur when a moderate force tears the capsule and acromioclavicular ligament. Many times this injury leads to a subluxed acromioclavicular joint. The coracoclavicular ligament bands are intact.
- Grade III sprains are severe, caused by a large force that ruptures both the acromioclavicular and coracoclavicular ligaments. Grade III separations produce dislocations of the acromioclavicular joint and may, in fact, cause muscle avulsion and osseous fracture.

For the sake of flexibility in diagnosing acromioclavicular sprains, categories of disability may be added between the mild, moderate, and severe sprains. The system shown in Table 3-7 adds a plus (+) to cases that fall between the former broad categories of injury.

Table 3-7 Grades of Acromioclavicular Sprains

Grade	Physical Findings	X-Ray Findings	Grade	Physical Findings	X-Ray Findings
I	Palpable tenderness over AC ligament No gross instability Bogginess over AC joint Trapezius hypertonicity	No evidence of osseous deformity or gross instability	II+	Severe pain over AC ligament Pain over coracoclavicular ligament Pain in early abduction Inability to reach 90° 2+ laxity of AC joint testing Moderate elevation of clavicle Swelling over AC joint and supraclavicular area Moderate retrograde trapezius myospasm Cervical spine pain, hypomobility, and spasm	Evidence of moderate gapping on stress film Examination for associated fractures
I+	Palpable pain over AC ligament Pain over 90° of abduction No gross instability Minor swelling over AC joint Trapezius hypertonicity	No evidence of osseous deformity or gross instability			
II	Pain on palpation over AC ligament Tenderness over coracoclavicular ligament Painful arc of abduction to 90° Exquisite pain over 90° 1+ laxity of AC joint on stability testing (gapping) Swelling over AC joint Slight elevation of clavicle Mild retrograde trapezius myospasm Cervical discomfort and stiffness	No evidence of gross instability Slight increase in coracoclavicular interval in stress film with weights	III	Pain over AC joint and deltoid and trapezius muscles Pain (tearing) over AC and coracoclavicular ligaments 3+ laxity (dislocation) on stability testing Inability to place arm in neutral position Swelling over entire shoulder Elevation of clavicle (deformity) Cervical spine pain and spasm	Evidence of gross instability Examination to rule out associated fractures

AC, Acromioclavicular.

Treatment of Acromioclavicular Sprains

Mild acromioclavicular sprains require minimal treatment (Table 3-8). Recuperation from a moderate acromioclavicular sprain may take several weeks, and an integrated rehabilitation plan is necessary to return the patient to maximum function.

The use of an acromioclavicular splint or shoulder immobilizer is usually reserved for moderate separation or for more severe trauma to the shoulder. Essentially, if the individual does not feel pain while the arm is at his or her side, it is not necessary to immobilize the arm. If, however, the injured side is drooping and the patient is holding the arm in a position of protective adduction into the chest, immobilization for acromioclavicular in-

stability may be warranted. Once the patient shows signs of improvement, the immobilizer may be removed and rehabilitation can become more active.

Treatment of a grade III separation may be conservative or surgical. Post stated, "Often a grade III dislocation can be treated conservatively with results as good or better than those of operative methods."[56] When adopting a conservative care approach, the primary care practitioner generally recommends an aggressive program to control pain, swelling, and inflammation, as well as a lengthy immobilization period (i.e., 6 to 8 weeks). Some well-researched studies have provided evidence that favors the use of a conservative approach in treating displaced grade III acromioclavicular dislocations.[74,78] In fact, many orthopedic and sports medicine authorities believe that the nonsurgical approach is the treatment of choice for most patients with grade III acromioclavicular injuries.[4,17]

Table 3-8 Treatment for Acromioclavicular Sprains

Grade	Class	Treatment
I	Sprain	Ice Electrotherapy Examination to rule out cervical joint dysfunction CMT for cervical spine Progressive return to normal activity level after acute symptoms subside
I+		Ice Electrotherapy Examination to rule out cervical joint dysfunction CMT for cervical spine Use of sling for short time (1-3 days) Progressive return to normal activity level after acute symptoms subside
II	Subluxation	Ice Electrotherapy Immobilization for 7-14 days CMT for cervical spine
II+		Ice Electrotherapy Immobilization for 10-21 days CMT for cervical spine
III	Dislocation	Ice Electrotherapy Immobilization in Kenny-Howard AC splint for 6-8 weeks CMT of cervical spine Referral for pain medication

CMT, Chiropractic manipulative therapy; **AC**, acromioclavicular.

Conservative versus Surgical Treatment for Grade III Acromioclavicular Separation

Most current orthopedic literature suggests that surgical treatment has little advantage over conservative care for acromioclavicular disruptions. In addition, several of the surgical procedures that involve coracoclavicular screws or wires have been associated with a high complication rate. For example, there have been reports of superficial wound infections (i.e., any surgical procedure) and persistent loss of functional use. When Bargren, Erlanger, and Dick studied 63 grade III sprains treated by two operative methods, they found broken or bent Kirschner wires and osteolysis of the distal clavicle.[5] Eskola and associates reported similar problems.[22] Avikainen, Ranki, and colleagues studied 48 cases of complete acromioclavicular separations treated by Kirschner-wire fixation and reported their best surgical results in patients who were 30 years of age and younger; however, this age group reportedly did well with conservative treatment after traumatic separations.[3] Eidman, Siff, and Tullos, after studying 25 children with acromioclavicular dislocations, observed that, "...in children, conservative care should produce good or excellent results."[20] Similarly, a team of Norwegian orthopedic surgeons stated that, "...as long as nonoperative treatment gives *equal* or *better* long-term functional results, we do not recommend this operation in acute dislocations."[67]

In comparing the results of conservative treatment of grade III acromioclavicular sprains with the results of surgical treatment, MacDonald, Alexander, and colleagues found that outcomes in the nonsurgical group were statistically superior to outcomes in the surgical group.[38] Taft, Wilson, and Oglesby studied 127 patients who had an acute dislocation of the acromioclavicular joint and found that patients who underwent surgery had a higher rate of complications than did patients who chose conservative treatment. They concluded that the use of an immobilizer for 6 to 8 weeks, followed by a rehabilitation program, leads to acceptable clinical results without the risks of surgery.[70]

After studying 84 patients who had pronounced acromioclavicular dislocations that were treated by either a sling and bandage or an open-reduction operation with Kirschner wires, Larsen and associates strongly favored conservative care. They stated, "...they may make an exception for their patients with great prominence of the clavicle, but even in this group, an operation has little to commend it, since it creates a scar almost as disfiguring as the deformity."[35]

Only a small percentage of grade III injuries ever need surgical treatment. Surgery may be appropriate, however, for severe injuries in which the clavicle has come through its periosteal envelope (i.e., a buttonhole effect) or in which there is a disruption of the trapezius-deltoid mechanism or in which an avulsion fracture involves ruptured coracoclavicular ligaments. These types of injuries have sometimes been called grade IV dislocations and may prove to be exceptions to the general rule for conservative treatment.

In addition, there are a few scenarios in which a surgical procedure may be effective in relieving pain and dysfunction. For example, a chronic painful acromioclavicular joint in a failed dislocation treatment or subsequent acromioclavicular joint arthritis may respond to a distal clavicle excision (resection).[9] A surgical procedure usually alleviates the problem of a bony block (e.g., an irregular point of bone) that obstructs the arm's arc of abduction and prevents the patient from lifting the arm to the side without pain.

Disorders of the Suprahumeral Space

The shoulder complex plays a crucial role in an individual's everyday life. As such, movement of the arm in the frontal plane involves the structures of the suprahumeral space (also called the subacromial space). The bony architecture of this space is bordered by the acromion process superiorly (anteroinferior aspect), the coracoid process anteromedially, the acromioclavicular joint superiorly, and the tuberosity of the humeral head inferiorly. The coracoacromial ligament further compromises the subacromial space because of its relatively thick anatomic structure. This ligament runs from the coracoid process to the anteroinferior aspect of the acromion process. Several fibers also extend to the acromioclavicular joint. The anatomic function of this ligament is thought to center around controlling migration of the head of the humerus in a superior fashion.

Although it is most valuable for the evaluation of synovitis and occult rotator cuff disease, arthroscopy can be a helpful aid in diagnosing disorders of the subacromial area. Diagnostic arthroscopy permits visualization of the coracoacromial ligament and the underside of the anterior acromial surface, as well as debridement of the subacromial bursa. An orthopedic surgeon with experience in shoulder arthroscopy can evaluate the status of acromial erosion near the attachment of the coracoacromial ligament. The surgeon can also determine whether the patient needs an acromioplasty, since the extent of synovitis indicates the portion of acromion that requires removal or repair.[12]

Impingement Syndrome

Injuries to the subacromial bursa, acromioclavicular joint, supraspinatus tendon, and biceps tendon can cause the impingement syndrome. All these structures lie adjacent to the anterior acromion and coracoacromial ligament. Anterior impingement can result from biceps tendonitis, rotator cuff tendonitis, subacromial bursitis, or subacromial spurring.

Subacromial impingement prevents a comfortable range of motion in daily shoulder use because it compromises the soft tissue at the subacromial space. In vitro studies of the nature of impingement reveal that pressure is centered over the distal supraspinatus tendon.[45] The impingement syndrome causes wear and tear on the anterior one third of the acromion, anterior edge and undersurface of the acromion, coracoacromial ligament, and acromioclavicular joint itself at times.[27] As the individual raises the arm, the supraspinatus muscle passes under the acromial edge by the acromioclavicular joint, causing wear and tear of the supraspinatus tendon. Further anterior arc movement in overuse syndromes may also cause damage to the long head of the biceps tendon.

The supraspinatus muscle has an avascular zone that includes the region of its distal insertion.[60] It is believed that this avascularity may be attributable to the flat shape of the tendon, along with the common repetitive forces indicative of impingement syndrome. End-stage pathologic abnormalities, such as tendonitis, calcification, and frank rupture, tend to occur within this avascular region.[11] Such degeneration produces an inflammatory response that leads to the development of granulation tissue.

An impingement sign will appear during the examination of a patient with active symptoms. In the shoulder evaluation the examiner forcibly elevates the patient's arm in forward flexion, causing a "jamming" of the greater tuberosity against the surface of the anterior acromion.[40] The supraspinatus muscle can also be impinged during testing (Figure 3-10 *A, B*).

Since the impingement syndrome seems to be a continuous disease process, the goal of treatment is to arrest the inflammatory condition and prevent progressive degenerative changes.

Sports-Related Impingement Syndrome

Individuals who use their arms with an abduction arc greater than 90° (hyperabduction) are at risk for the impingement syndrome. Thus swimmers and throwing athletes are candidates for subacromial pathologic abnormalities.

Swimming. The average age at which swimmers begin their competitive careers is 10 years. Typically, impingement syndrome becomes evident in competitive swimmers at approximately the age of 18 years.[29] In one study, 92% of swimmers with shoulder pain swam freestyle, backstroke, or butterfly; 75% of these swimmers listed the freestyle or butterfly stroke as their best. Approximately 74% were sprint and middle distance swimmers, which relates to the explosive nature of sprinter and middle distance arm strokes.[29] A competitive swimmer who swims 10,000 yards per day, 5 days per week, 10 months per year, with 15 individual arm strokes for each length of a 25-yard pool, will log more than 1,200,000 arm movements per year.[13,61]

The underwater pull phase of the freestyle and butterfly strokes forces the humeral head up into the coracoacromial arch, causing microtrauma and irritation. At the point where the hand touches the water,

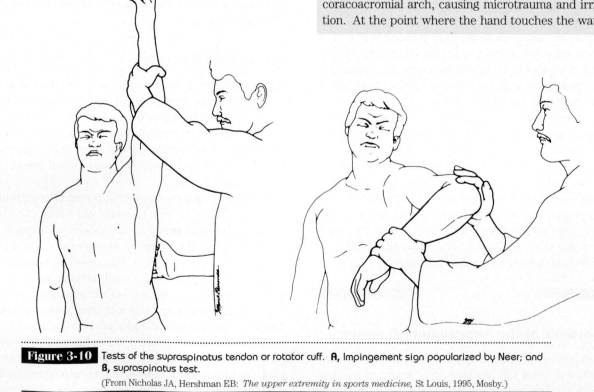

A   B

Figure 3-10 Tests of the supraspinatus tendon or rotator cuff. **A,** Impingement sign popularized by Neer; and **B,** supraspinatus test.

(From Nicholas JA, Hershman EB: *The upper extremity in sports medicine*, St Louis, 1995, Mosby.)

the supraspinatus insertion folds and compresses the midportion of the coracoacromial ligament; this repetitive microtrauma may lead to an impingement of the supraspinatus on the structures of the suprahumeral space, which is the primary cause of degeneration in the swimmer's shoulder.[14]

Tennis. Two movements that lead to the impingement syndrome are (1) the throwing motion required for the serve and (2) the overhead stroke. Of tennis players, 56% suffer shoulder symptoms.[36] Of these, 68% are anterior group problems; 13% are posterior group problems; and 11% involve parascapular pain, the symptoms of which are very similar to those of the impingement syndrome.

Baseball. The motion of pitching can be divided into four stages: (1) wind-up, (2) cocking, (3) acceleration, and (4) follow through. Because of the repetitive demands placed on baseball players, pitchers are most often affected by the impingement syndrome. In one study, 57% of professional pitchers who attended spring training experienced significant shoulder problems.[45] The injuries that professional pitchers experience are likely to arise from the fact that they throw at great velocities, since they use their muscles around the shoulder efficiently. The professionals use the subscapularis and latissimus dorsi muscles primarily, while using the supraspinatus, teres minor, and biceps brachii to a lesser degree.[31] Amateurs, however, continue to use all the rotator cuff muscles and biceps brachii through the acceleration stage of the pitch.[44]

Other Sports. Volleyball players and javelin throwers have a high incidence of shoulder problems. Approximately 44% of volleyball players and 29% of javelin throwers suffer shoulder problems. Of these, 90% are attributed to the explosive throwing motion required in these sports.[54]

Neer has classified three progressive stages of suprahumeral pathophysiology leading to the impingement syndrome[45]:

1. Edema and hemorrhage
2. Thickening and fibrosis
3. Rotator cuff tears, biceps tendon rupture, and osseous changes

The staging of pathologic abnormalities depends on a combination of clinical examination findings and radiographic evidence (Table 3-9).

Biceps Tendonitis

The role of the biceps tendon in the impingement syndrome may be vague or unclear. Symptoms of biceps involvement include anterior pain that can radiate distally toward the biceps muscle or anterior elbow. Forward flexion can cause pain, as can overhead motion.[47]

The long head of the biceps tendon is commonly involved not only in the impingement syndrome, but also in isolated bicipital tendonitis. Repetitive types of ballistic overhead movements involving hyperabduction and external rotation may lead to inflammation of the anterior shoulder capsule and the long head of the biceps tendon. The synovium of the shoulder capsule forms a common structure with the synovial lining of the bicipital tendon sheath; therefore anterior capsulitis and biceps tendonitis often occur simultaneously. Inflammation and swelling pose a major anatomic problem in this region because the injury is compounded as a result of the inability of the bicipital groove and the tight transverse humeral ligament to accommodate the tenosynovitis. Soon, the patient develops a chronic bicipital tendonitis that requires aggressive treatment.

Those who develop biceps tendonitis from macrotrauma include individuals whose upper extremity workload centering around the shoulder girdle suddenly increases. For example, an individual who must suddenly lift bulky, heavy boxes may develop this condition along with an anterior capsulitis. Common sporting activities, such as weight lifting, baseball, and softball, may cause anterior shoulder pain through repetitive microtrauma. In the case of weight lifting, excessive benchpressing movements without sufficient recuperation may lead to biceps tendonitis and anterior capsulitis. Baseball pitchers and softball players are also at risk for these conditions. Tennis players and others required to make frequent, repeated overhead arm movements may develop a case of tendonitis in the biceps concomitantly with strain or tendonitis in the rotator cuff. Once again, the cause is overuse.

Although the symptoms of biceps tendonitis can be vague, there is a simple test to identify any inflammation of this structure. The patient abducts his or her arm against resistance with the hand supinated. If the test produces pain over the biceps tendon and anterior capsular junction, the patient has biceps tendonitis. In Yergason's test for bicipital tendonitis, the examiner resists supination and flexion of the patient's arm (Figure 3-11 *A, B*). The clinical examination, tests, and history are of chief importance, because radiographic findings are usually normal (Table 3-10).

Table 3-9 Clinical Stages of the Impingement Syndrome

	Stage 1	Stage 2	Stage 3	Stage 4
Etiology	Commonly seen in people 25 years of age or younger Mild, reversible tendonitis of supraspinatus or biceps tendon Toothache-like discomfort that increases to pain on activity In some cases, consequence of trauma to AC joint	Patients usually 25-45 years of age Pain similar to stage 1, but more chronic and often worse at night Possible beginning of restricted movement Adhesive capsulitis or calcific tendonitis possible In some cases, irreversible lesion	Patients usually over 40 years of age Prolonged history of problem Refractory tendonitis, wearing, attrition of supraspinatus tendon and partial rotator cuff tears Possible prohibition of athletic endeavors	Full-thickness tear of rotator cuff
Physical examination findings	**Supraspinatus involvement** Point tenderness over greater tuberosity and usually anterior acromion Painful arc (maximum 90°) Positive impingement sign* Positive supraspinatus isolation muscle test** **Biceps lesion** Tenderness over the biceps tendon Positive Yergason's test Painful abduction with palm supinated against resistance	Similar to findings of stage 1, but more chronic and long-standing	Painful arc in early abduction Weakness; dependent on rotator cuff damage Adhesive capsulitis probable	Supraspinatus and infraspinatus wasting Tenderness over AC joint, greater tuberosity, anterior acromion Painful arc, inability to abduct arm fully Positive Codman's drop-arm test Decreased active, but full passive range of motion Adhesive capsulitis probable Weak abduction and external rotation
X-ray findings	Usually normal	Sclerosis of greater tuberosity possible Calcific tendonitis of supraspinatus or cystic changes (late)	Sclerosis of AC joint under anterior one third of acromion Greater tuberosity possible Irregular AC joint Cystic changes around greater tuberosity	Degenerative changes of AC joint (osteoarthritis) Narrowing of subacromial space
Treatment plan	Ice or ice massage Gentle stretching Isometrics graded to isotonics (short arcs) Pulsed ultrasound or electrotherapy	Ice or ice massage Mobilization for joint restrictions Isometrics graded to isotonics (short arcs) Ultrasound Change in work schedule Medical referral for antiinflammatory medication	Range-of-motion isometrics Medical referral for anti-inflammatory medication Trial of conservative treatment, followed by surgery, if necessary, to relieve pain Usually, inability to return to competitive activities	Conservative treatment to preserve strength Surgery to relieve pain Rarely returns to completely normal function

AC, Acromioclavicular.

*Patient expresses pain and facial grimace when arm is forcibly flexed forward, jamming the greater tuberosity against the anteroinferior surface on the acromion.

**With patient's arm 90° abducted, 30° flexed forward, and rotated fully internally, examiner exerts downward force; sign is positive if patient feels weakness and pain.

If isolated bicipital tendonitis has been so chronic that it is a factor in anterior impingement, an arthroscopic examination can confirm pathologic findings in the tendon sheath. Synovitis or fraying of the tendon within the shoulder joint is diagnostic and confirmatory. A tenosynovitis of the tendon sheath beneath the transverse humeral ligament may remain undetected at arthroscopy, however. Acromial arch decompression

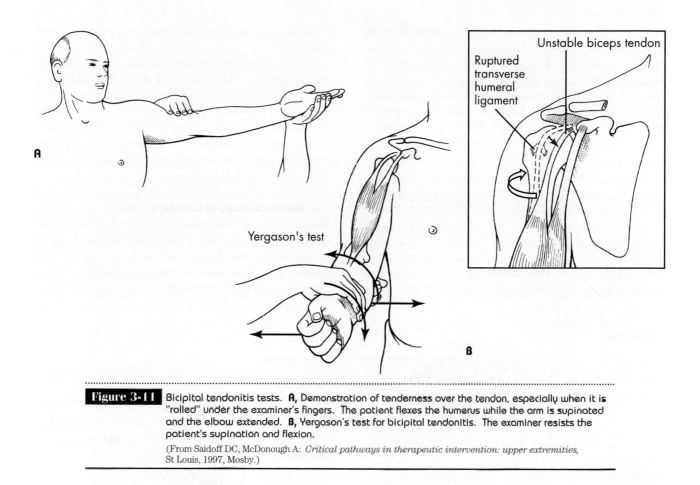

A

Yergason's test

B

Ruptured transverse humeral ligament

Unstable biceps tendon

Figure 3-11 Bicipital tendonitis tests. **A,** Demonstration of tenderness over the tendon, especially when it is "rolled" under the examiner's fingers. The patient flexes the humerus while the arm is supinated and the elbow extended. **B,** Yergason's test for bicipital tendonitis. The examiner resists the patient's supination and flexion.

(From Saidoff DC, McDonough A: *Critical pathways in therapeutic intervention: upper extremities,* St Louis, 1997, Mosby.)

may give the patient enough subacromial clearance to eliminate symptoms of biceps tendonitis; however, as a result of histopathologic changes in the tendon sheath, chronic tendonitis may remain symptomatic after surgical treatment for impingement.

Rotator Cuff Disease

Close to the arch of the acromion process of the scapula, the common rotator cuff tendon lies near the coraco-acromial ligament, subacromial bursa, and biceps tendon. This anatomic position makes the rotator cuff vulnerable to mechanical impingement.[60]

There are four muscles in the rotator cuff: (1) the supraspinatus superiorly, (2) the subscapularis anteriorly, (3) the teres minor posteriorly, and (4) the infraspinatus posteriorly. The rotator cuff muscles originate in the posterior shoulder girdle and hold the head of

most common

Table 3-10	Course of Biceps Tendonitis
Physical examination findings	Palpable tenderness along the anterior capsule of shoulder joint Discomfort on external rotation or resisted elbow flexion Positive supination-abduction test for pain at biceps tendon Boggy anterior aspect of glenohumeral joint
X-ray findings	Usually normal, but necessary to rule out calcific deposits in bicipital groove
Treatment plan	Ice massage Isometrics, then progression to short arcs Pulsed ultrasound Electrotherapy

the humerus in place anterolaterally (Figure 3-12). The muscles of the cuff end in flat, broad tendons that ultimately fuse with the fibrous capsule of the glenohumeral joint. Only the inferior portion of the joint does not possess this musculotendinous mass.[29] This anatomic fact, coupled with a weak anteroinferior capsule, creates an inherent weakness in human glenohumeral articulations.

Although the glenoid labrum and glenohumeral ligaments provide the glenohumeral joint's static stability, its dynamic stabilization revolves around the rotator cuff muscles. Along with the rotators of the scapula, the rotator cuff provides the biomechanical leverage necessary for producing a great deal of force while positioning the scapula for stability in the overhead position. In throwing sports, this leverage and strength become supremely important in the prevention of shoulder injuries, since the four muscles of the rotator cuff are responsible for suc-

cessfully and repetitively decelerating the arm in overhead motion.

Repetitive overhead activity may indeed compromise the anterior static restraints, thereby leading eventually to anterior instability.[8] Weakening of the scapula rotators and attenuation of the rotator cuff mechanism can lead to occult glenohumeral instability (subluxation) as a result of partial-thickness tears of the cuff, impingement of the rotator cuff mechanism, or concomitant anterior shoulder instability.[32]

Microvascularity of the Rotator Cuff

The circulation of the rotator cuff is unidirectional with poor flow at the insertion of the supraspinatus tendon.[60] Vessels within the tendon are sensitive to postural changes of the brachium. Decreased subacromial pressure associated with overhead activity may impede cir-

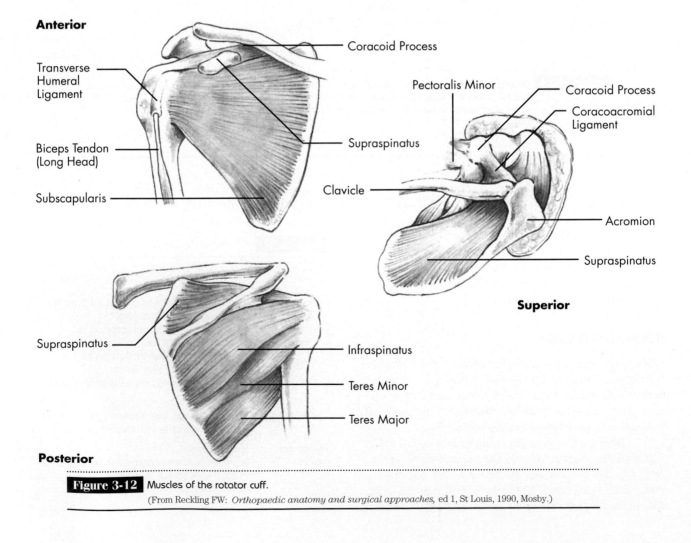

Figure 3-12 Muscles of the rotator cuff.
(From Reckling FW: *Orthopaedic anatomy and surgical approaches,* ed 1, St Louis, 1990, Mosby.)

culation. Furthermore, adduction of the arm decreases the perfusion of this area, whereas abduction leads to the filling of these vessels.[11]

Regarding the rotator cuff muscles, the subscapularis shows a coarse, railroad distribution of blood vessels. The teres minor shows a fine filigree pattern, and the infraspinatus has a pattern right between the two. The supraspinatus tendon has a zone of avascularity extending to within 1 cm of the point of insertion at the greater tuberosity.[11,60] It seems likely that this avascularity is attributable to the tendon's flat shape, as well as the compressive forces that are introduced on this portion of the tendon during adduction of the humerus. Compressive forces greater than 120 degrees against the coracoacromial ligament also play a role in relative avascularity. Breakdown changes, such as tendonitis, calcification, and rupture of the tendon, often occur in this area of avascularity. It can be theorized that, once a patient injures his or her rotator cuff mechanism and ceases to use the shoulder, this blood supply becomes even more tenuous because of the lack of a healthy abduction arc. After degeneration has begun, it begins to take on an accelerated inflammatory response that leads to the development of granulation tissue[60] (Figure 3-13).

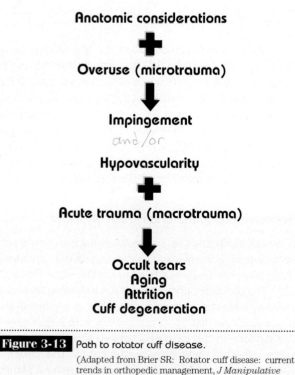

Figure 3-13 Path to rotator cuff disease.
(Adapted from Brier SR: Rotator cuff disease: current trends in orthopedic management, *J Manipulative Physiol Ther* 15(2):124, 1992.)

Etiology of Rotator Cuff Disease

Different authors offer different opinions concerning the mechanism of rotator cuff disease. Some focus on the effect of subacromial impingement on the rotator cuff tendons, primarily the supraspinatus, whereas others focus on the hypovascularity of the rotator cuff. Neer states that the functional arc of the shoulder occurs during forward flexion; therefore he concludes that mechanical impingement of the coracoacromial ligament and inferior aspect of the acromion process is the cause of injury to the rotator cuff.[41] Degeneration of the rotator cuff can and will come about with repetitive mechanical impingement and microtrauma.

Although repetitive microtrauma leading to an overuse injury can play a major role in cuff degeneration, an acute traumatic episode can start the degeneration process. Swelling and subsequent tenosynovitis occur in response to injury. Without careful attention and proper therapy, scarring and attrition of the tendon will occur (Figure 3-14). Victims of falls may land on a depressed shoulder with the arm in external rotation and abduction and strain the cuff. Wrestlers fall prey to these types of acute strains. In either case the arc of abduction and rotation are painful. The practitioner should immediately rule out rupture by diligently observing whether the patient can achieve an arc of abduction and maintain that abduction via a congruent motion.

Rothman and Parke stated that degeneration of the rotator cuff comes about secondary to hypovascularity.[62] Certainly, this fact seems to play a role in the etiology of supraspinatus injuries. De Palma concludes from his work on cadavers that the aging process plays a primary role in rotator cuff degeneration.[18]

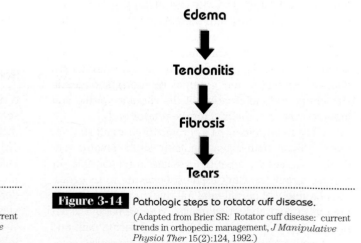

Figure 3-14 Pathologic steps to rotator cuff disease.
(Adapted from Brier SR: Rotator cuff disease: current trends in orthopedic management, *J Manipulative Physiol Ther* 15(2):124, 1992.)

Table 3-11 Management of Rotator Cuff Disease

	Supraspinatus Tendonitis	Chronic Rotator Cuff Strain	Advanced Rotator Cuff Disease
Physical examination findings	Painful abduction arc (0°-45°) Positive result on supraspinatus isolation test Palpable tenderness over lateral portion of greater tuberosity Discomfort at superior/lateral scapular spine Pain on initiation of abduction against resistance	Painful arc of early and late abduction (to 45° and over 90°) Painful arc of forward flexion (severely limited in impingement) Pain over supraspinatus muscle or tendon and possibly articular capsule Diffuse tenderness and myofascitis at posterior shoulder girdle	Incongruous motion of abduction Impingement sign Signs of adhesive capsulitis (multidirectional hypomobility) that is refractory to physical therapy Palpable tenderness over glenohumeral joint and posterior shoulder girdle Atrophy of rotator cuff Marked weakness of shoulder rotators Severe pain, dysfunction Tenderness over coracoacromial ligament
X-ray findings	Usually normal	Sclerosing at greater tuberosity Superior migration of humeral head	Marked decrease in suprahumeral space Superior migration of humeral head Sclerosing at greater tuberosity Heterotopic bone formation at glenohumeral joint
Treatment plan	Ice massage Electrotherapy Gentle stretching Isometrics	Ice massage Ultrasound Electrotherapy Mobilization Flexibility exercises and isometrics	Ice massage Arthrogram, either alone or with CT, to rule out rotator cuff tear MRI with or without contrast Medical referral for antiinflammatory medication Sometimes, orthopedic surgical consultation

CT, Computed tomography.

Clinical Management of Rotator Cuff Disease

The management of rotator cuff disease varies according to the location and severity of the condition (Table 3-11). Because superficial tendonitis responds to direct ice application, patients with this condition should use ice massage for 5 minutes per hour as often as possible. Acute tendonitis is best treated with cryotherapy, pulsed ultrasound, electrotherapy, and therapeutic exercise. Rehabilitation should center around the control the inflammatory process early, while maintaining neuromuscular health and flexibility. Isometric exercises performed in a doorway (internal and external rotation) and gentle stretching and mobilization of the shoulder girdle and humerus are often helpful for the rotator cuff.

The management of a chronic rotator cuff strain is more difficult than managing acute supraspinatus tendonitis. Generally, repetitive trauma is responsible for chronic strain; the clinician must be astute to recognize the possibility of partial- and full-thickness tears in a patient with poor abduction ability. When a patient is not progressing in treatment and is experiencing pain and shoulder dysfunction, such a tear is a likely cause.[1]

If the patient cannot abduct the arm and has a positive Codman's drop-arm test, an arthrogram is necessary to rule out a full-thickness tear of the rotator cuff. If the patient has difficulty abducting the arm, but can maintain the abducted position at 90 degrees, the clinician can order a computed tomography (CT) arthrogram instead to rule out a partial-thickness tear. Magnetic resonance imaging (MRI) may be appropriate if the results of other testing are equivocal or unsatisfactory (Figure 3-15).

Adhesive Capsulitis and Frozen Shoulder

Although similarities abound concerning the clinical presentation of adhesive capsulitis and frozen shoulder, these two orthopedic entities are not the same (Table 3-12). The parallels between them have clouded their definitions, however. Adhesive capsulitis is a clinical and histopathologic discovery in a patient with loss of shoulder motion. In the case of a "frozen shoulder," or end-stage adhesive capsulitis, movement of the patient's shoulder is usually severely restricted in several planes; in fact, almost no motion is possible.

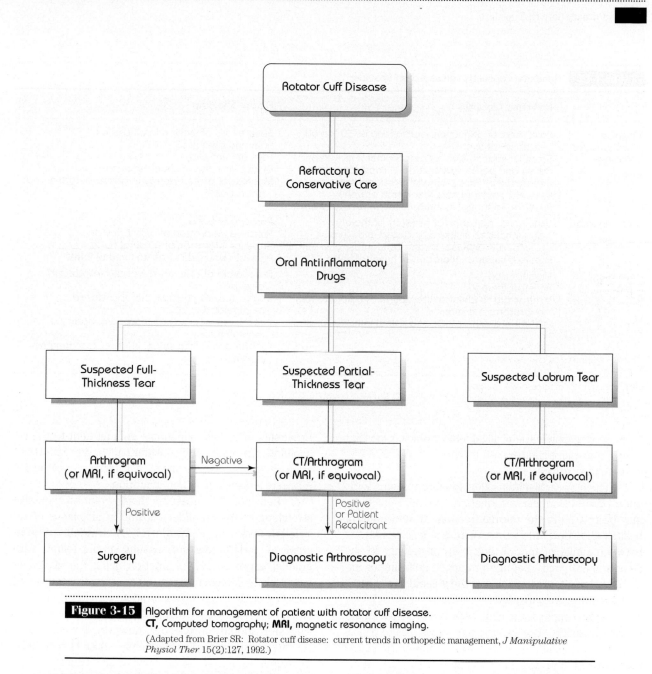

Figure 3-15 Algorithm for management of patient with rotator cuff disease. **CT,** Computed tomography; **MRI,** magnetic resonance imaging.

(Adapted from Brier SR: Rotator cuff disease: current trends in orthopedic management, *J Manipulative Physiol Ther* 15(2):127, 1992.)

Adhesive Capsulitis

In most instances the patient with adhesive capsulitis has some range of motion in the shoulder girdle, but the formation of dense fibrous adhesions combined with capsular contraction restricts mobility. The condition most often affects arcs of rotation and abduction. The onset may be insidious, and the patient will certainly experience increased pain as the restriction of motion increases. This close relationship between the amount of restricted movement and pain forms the basis for treatment protocol—mainly mobilization.[28]

The cause of adhesive capsulitis is obscure in many cases. For some reason, however, women between the ages of 35 and 55 years seem exceedingly prone to the condition.[77] There appear to be several possible contributing factors:

- Prolonged muscle guarding
- Prolonged disuse
- Prolonged immobilization
- Lack of complete rehabilitation after traumatic injury

| Table 3-12 | Adhesive Capsulitis versus Frozen Shoulder |

	Adhesive Capsulitis	**Frozen Shoulder**
Physical examination findings	Painful arc of abduction, particularly at 30° to 60°; external rotation Scapular substitution for glenohumeral movement Active and passive restriction in capsular pattern Restriction of joint play and functional movements Possible posterior shoulder girdle atrophy Possible joint hypomobility in lower cervical spine	Severe loss of motion in all planes Pain and disability Loss of joint play Disuse atrophy of shoulder girdle Myofascial trigger points in posterior girdle and rotator cuff
X-ray findings	Usually no indication of osseous pathologic abnormalities unless associated with chronic rotator cuff disease, chronic tendonitis, or arthritis Possible superior migration of humeral head	Porosity of bone Possible resorption of distal clavicle Superior migration of humeral head Possible sclerosis of glenohumeral joint
Treatment plan	Mobilization Physical therapy If refractory to physical therapy, arthrogram to rule out rotator cuff tear CMT for scapulothoracic and spinal joint dysfunction	Arthrogram to rule out advanced rotator cuff disease If refractory to physical therapy, closed manipulation If recalcitrant to closed procedure, open manipulation CMT for secondary spinal joint dysfunction and myofascitis

CMT, Chiropractic manipulative therapy.

- Poor scapulohumeral alignment (thoracic kyphosis)
- Progressive rotator cuff disease
- Arthropathies

The fibrocartilaginous glenoid labrum seems to be quite prone to adhesion formation, but this sensitivity may be related to the normal freedom of movement of healthy shoulders. Moreover, there is a delicate balance between range of motion and bony instability in the glenohumeral joint, and any prolonged guarding or immobilization after trauma makes the glenoid cavity more prone to adhesive capsulitis.

Arthrography is the diagnostic test of choice for adhesive capsulitis. The arthrogram shows loss of a normally loose, dependent fold of the glenohumeral joint and a decrease in contrast volume[46] (Figure 3-16 *A, B*). Many patients believed to have occult rotator cuff disease are found to have adhesive capsulitis when they undergo arthrography. Subacromial impingement can also mimic adhesive capsulitis.

A stiff and painful shoulder is not always adhesive capsulitis, but the best treatment of this condition is prevention. Therefore any suggestion of a loss of range of motion in a stiff and painful joint should be treated at once. Once the treatment has been selected, it must be pursued with vigor, aggressiveness, and determination. The patient must understand that the regimen and routine of exercises are time-consuming and discomforting.

He or she must make a genuine commitment to the rehabilitation program and consider pain or discomfort not as an enemy, but as a means of measuring success in the return to a normal freedom of motion.

Rehabilitative measures should emphasize passive stretching of the shoulder capsule in all planes of restricted movement (Figure 3-17 *A, B*). Gradual strengthening of periarticular soft tissues should follow, with gradual improvement of function being the clinician's yardstick for clinical progress. If conservative treatment fails, the patient may be a candidate for closed manipulation (i.e., noninvasive manipulation under anesthesia). This step should be reserved, however, for conditions that are refractory to physical therapy after 4 to 6 months in a supervised program of active range-of-motion exercises. If closed manipulation fails, the patient may undergo an open, surgical manipulation under anesthesia. Only patients whose function and pain are refractory to physical therapy and closed manipulation should undergo surgery (Figure 3-18).

Although adhesive capsulitis is considered a self-limited disease process, complete recovery without residual limitation and disability is neither assured nor common.[26] Conditions that will resolve do so within a 2-year period, and most people who elect to seek treatment do so because they are unwilling to accept this limited range of motion and incapacity.

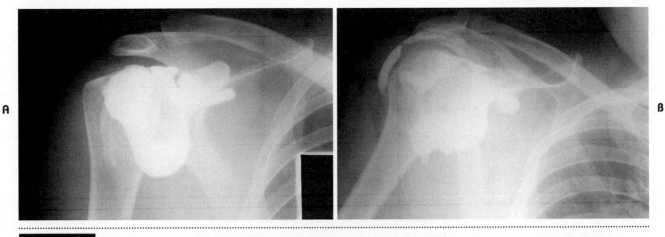

Figure 3-16 Arthrography of the shoulder. **A,** Normal. **B,** Classic subdeltoid and subacromial extravasation seen with complete rotator cuff tears. (Also noted are Hill-Sachs and Bankart lesions consistent with recurrent anterior dislocations.)

(From Ruiz E, Cicero JJ: *Emergency management of skeletal injuries,* ed 1, St Louis, 1995, Mosby.)

Frozen Shoulder

The patient with a frozen shoulder may seek treatment only after shoulder pain and motion restrictions have continued for several months and he or she can no longer compensate movement. The scapulothoracic joint may become tense or hypertonic as a result of overload from the anterior shoulder girdle. Because of the advanced shoulder dysfunction, the patient should undergo an arthrogram to rule out a concomitant rotator cuff tear.

Referral to a medical physician can be helpful for medication for pain and inflammation, as well as for a supervised physical therapy program. Many of these patients do not improve with this regimen, however, and such treatment can be terminated within 2 to 3 months if the range of motion does not increase. At that time, since everyday living is compromised, the patient is a candidate for a closed manipulation followed by physical therapy. Patients whose condition is refractory to a closed manipulative procedure may undergo an open manipulation, as illustrated in Figure 3-18.

Disorders of the Sternoclavicular Joint

Although the sternoclavicular joint does not provide the great excursion of motion of the glenohumeral joint, it does provide a fixed point of stability for humeral rotation. At 30 degrees of arm abduction, rotation of the clavicle and scapula takes place around the sternoclavicular line. At 100 degrees of elevation, the costoclavicular ligaments prevent further motion at the sternoclavicular joint.[51]

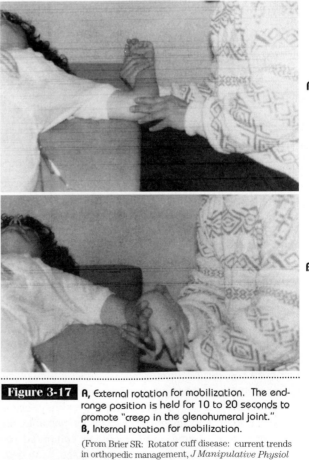

Figure 3-17 **A,** External rotation for mobilization. The end-range position is held for 10 to 20 seconds to promote "creep in the glenohumeral joint." **B,** Internal rotation for mobilization.

(From Brier SR: Rotator cuff disease: current trends in orthopedic management, *J Manipulative Physiol Ther* 15[2]:125, 1992.)

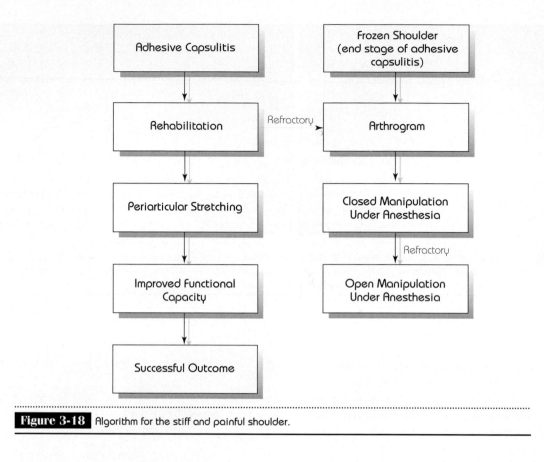

Figure 3-18 Algorithm for the stiff and painful shoulder.

The sternoclavicular joint also provides the only point of attachment of the upper extremity to the axial skeleton. The scapula and brachium hang at the lateral edge of the clavicle, but the sternoclavicular articulation serves as a stable anchor at the medial aspect of the shoulder girdle. Instabilities of this joint usually are the result of blunt trauma to the shoulder girdle, such as can occur in a motor vehicle accident or in contact sports or from an abrupt force on an extended arm in a posterior direction.

The humerus acts as a long lever and forces travel through the clavicle in a lateral to medial direction. Thus the clavicle can be displaced in varying degrees in an upward and forward fashion, as well as slightly anteriorly. Lines of force toward the sternal end of the clavicle place stress at the costoclavicular and sternoclavicular ligaments. In such an injury the tendons over the sternoclavicular joint and ligament are usually palpable. In cases of severe trauma, tomography, or computed tomography, is the imagery technique of choice.[79] A chest film may be warranted to exclude a pneumothorax.

Sternoclavicular Sprains

Like sprains of the acromioclavicular joint, sprains of the sternoclavicular joint are graded as first-, second-, or third-degree sprains (Table 3-13). In most cases of grade I or II sprains, treatment involves placing the arm in a simple sling in the closed-packed position of adduction and internal rotation until the patient no longer experiences pain. Ice applications are also palliative for pain and inflammation. Most patients have no pain after 2 or 3 weeks and experience no complications. A cosmetic deformity or bump at the sternoclavicular joint may be the only reminder of the episode. Alternative orthopedic procedures that involve open reduction with pinning are discouraged for anterior sternoclavicular dislocations and may produce subclavian vascular injury.[10] Posterior dislocation is a rare and potentially dangerous condition that can compromise anterior structures of the neck.

It may be necessary to immobilize third-degree sprains in a splint for 4 to 6 weeks with gradual restoration of arm motion. Chiropractic manipulative therapy (CMT) should be administered to the cervical spine be-

Table 3-13 Grades of Sternoclavicular Joint Sprains

	Grade I	Grade II	Grade III
Physical examination findings	Point tenderness over SC joint Discomfort with arm hyperabduction No gross laxity Usually no swelling	Palpable pain at SC joint Painful arm abduction Mild laxity with SC joint play Mild swelling Mild deformity at SC joint (anterior displacement)	Gross deformity at SC joint Anterior displacement of clavicle at sternum Moderate pain over SC joint Painful arm abduction Swelling, discoloration at SC joint Laxity of anterior SC joint
X-ray findings	Normal	Mild anterior displacement of clavicle	Displacement of clavicle at SC joint Examination to rule out associated fractures of sternum and clavicle
Treatment plan	Immobilization for pain relief Ice CMT for cervical spine	Immobilization for 2-3 weeks Ice CMT for cervical spine	Shoulder immobilization for 4-6 weeks Ice CMT for cervical spine

SC, Sternoclavicular; **CMT,** chiropractic manipulative therapy.

cause of shoulder girdle dyskinesia and the effects of the sling on the neck.

In many cases of trauma the multiplicity of injuries delays the diagnosis of sternoclavicular sprain or dislocation. The patient may not even complain of shoulder girdle pain until days later. Furthermore, conventional radiography is not always helpful in aiding the diagnosis, except when the clavicle is frankly dislocated.[52] Because multitrauma patients with a sternoclavicular injury may have occult injuries at a distal site, it is important to scan the appendicular skeleton when examining these patients.

Fractures of the Clavicle

The first long bone to ossify in the developing skeleton is the clavicle, and fracture of this bone is the most common fracture during birth and childhood.[79] Clavicular fractures often follow blunt trauma from an external blow or from a fall on the upper extremity. Most often, a force applied to the distal end of the clavicle produces shear at the middle third, resulting in a fracture of the clavicle at that site[79] (Figure 3-19) (Table 3-14). Most fractures heal uneventfully and rapidly under favorable conditions.

The patient exhibits point tenderness at the injury site and has a painful arc of shoulder abduction and scapulothoracic elevation and retraction. Radiographic films can confirm the diagnosis and rule out gross displacement. The primary care practitioner must make certain that there are no neurovascular or skin complications associated with the clavicular fracture. As long

Table 3-14 Fracture of the Clavicle

Physical examination findings	Local deformity at fracture site Painful abduction and forward flexion Painful scapulothoracic elevation or retraction History of external blow or fall on upper limb
X-ray findings	Fracture usually evident in middle third of clavicle
Treatment plan	Ice Immobilization for 4 weeks Range-of-motion movements in second or third week

as these criteria are met, the fracture can be treated conservatively with either a sling-and-swathe or a figure-8 bandage.[69] Gentle motion can be included in the home treatment program as early as the second week after injury, provided that the patient's pain is reduced.

Disorders of the Scapulothoracic Joint

The status of the scapulothoracic articulation as a true joint has been the subject of debate. Clearly, however, this region plays a major role in both primary and secondary function of the shoulder. In fact, shoulder movement, stability, and integrity require a healthy scapulo-

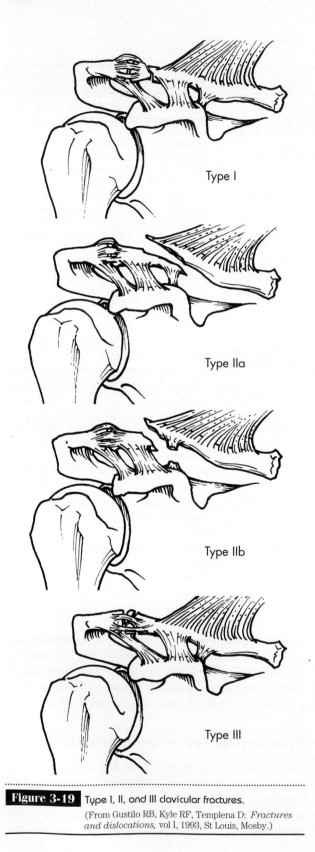

Type I

Type IIa

Type IIb

Type III

Figure 3-19   Type I, II, and III clavicular fractures.

(From Gustilo RB, Kyle RF, Templena D: *Fractures and dislocations,* vol I, 1993, St Louis, Mosby.)

thoracic mechanism. With the initiation of abduction, scapulothoracic motion involves a ratio of 1.25:1 between glenohumeral and scapulothoracic components.[55] After the first 20 degrees of abduction, the scapula contributes 1 degree of rotation for every 2 degrees of glenohumeral motion.[66]

The soft-tissue integrity and strategic positioning of the scapula stabilize the shoulder. The scapulothoracic joint allows the scapula to form a stable platform against which the humerus can move. Optimal functioning of the shoulder girdle rotators provides stability as the scapula moves with precision under the humeral head. The trapezius, rhomboid, and serratus anterior muscles, together with the spine, provide the scapulothoracic joint with both dynamic and static support.[33]

Movements of the scapulothoracic joint closely resemble those of the sternoclavicular and acromioclavicular joints. With the retroscapular musculature and anterior shoulder articulations, the thoracic spine forms a kinetic chain in which motion at one joint causes movement in another. This is one reason the examiner stabilizes the scapula posteriorly when examining the acromioclavicular joint for stability. The axis of the sternoclavicular, acromioclavicular, and scapulothoracic joints in the closed-packed position is at an angle of 50 degrees in protraction; in the loose-packed position, it is at an angle of 70 degrees.[28]

When examining this articulation of the shoulder girdle, the practitioner needs to rule out gross or postural deformation, such as posterior protrusion of the scapula (i.e., "winging"), scoliosis, Sprengel's deformity, or Klippel-Feil syndrome. These kinds of conditions can lead to mechanical dysfunction of the shoulder girdle, cervicodorsal spine, and brachium. For the examination the patient performs a push-up against the wall as the examiner determines whether the medial border of the scapula moves away from the chest wall and protrudes posteriorly. Winging can be an indication of serratus anterior weakness or long thoracic nerve palsy. It is also necessary to check the posterior shoulder girdle for atrophy to rule out suprascapular nerve damage. If such damage exists, the supraspinatus and infraspinatus muscles will be weak or atrophied.

Scapulothoracic Myofascitis, Dysfunction, and Dyskinesia

Many patients who have had anterior shoulder trauma and cervical whiplash find that, after their primary traumatic episode has been treated, they have tender areas in the posterior shoulder girdle near the shoulder blade. Furthermore, prolonged immobilization, rotator cuff disease, and adhesive capsulitis each can cause scapulothoracic problems.

Scapulothoracic myofascitis and dysfunction can have several presentations. One is an altered scapulohumeral rhythm. The scapulothoracic joint has an important role in a sound, healthy scapulohumeral rhythm. Normally, there is a 3:2 ratio between the range of the glenohumeral joint movement and the range of the scapulothoracic joint movement throughout the full abduction arc. Patients with a pathologic arc of abduction secondary to adhesive capsulitis or rotator cuff disease usually "scapula substitute," trying to shrug their arm up into abduction or to use their trunk. Reverse scapulohumeral rhythm is another name for this form of scapula substitution, in which movement originates at the scapulothoracic joint instead of at the glenohumeral joint.

In another possible scenario, a motor vehicle accident may cause the cervical spine to experience a hyperflexion-hyperextension sprain or strain, also known as whiplash. Once the joint dysfunction, the paracervical soft-tissue inflammation, and the loss of articular mobility have been treated, many patients begin to feel the effects of secondary scapulothoracic dysfunction.[49] Tender points along the levator scapula, trapezius, and rhomboid muscles become evident (Table 3-15). The scapulothoracic myofascial syndrome can actually cause pain referred up toward the insertion of many muscles at the level of the occiput.

Although scapulothoracic dyskinesia secondary to chronic glenohumeral instability is biomechanically understood, the condition per se is rarely treated. Despite the major focus on the clinical, physical, and radiographic elements of the primary pathologic condition, however, the secondary complaint of subscapular pain may be quite alarming and disabling to the patient. Hypertonicity, stiffness, and lack of scapula and humeral excursion can compound the problem of a painful arc of shoulder abduction. Mobilization and manipulation of the scapulothoracic joint can often alleviate many of the secondary complaints of glenohumeral instability (Figure 3-20).

Of course, any prolonged immobilization of the glenohumeral joint can cause stiffness of the entire shoulder girdle and scapulothoracic articulation. Frequently, chronic subacromial impingement and rotator cuff disease lead to scapulothoracic dyskinesia over time. If paraspinal myofascitis is present, a combined treatment protocol of ultrasound and electrical stimulation

Table 3-15	Scapulothoracic Myofascitis, Dysfunction, and Dyskinesia
Physical examination findings	Palpable tender points at vertebral border of the scapula
	Active trigger points at origin of levator scapulae
	Middle trapezius hypertonicity
	Possible suboccipital cephalgia
	Myofascitis of scapula musculature with arm, shoulder, and hand referral
	Crepitus or fixation of scapulothoracic articulation
X-ray findings	No evidence of osseous pathologic variations
	Superior migration of humeral head on anteroposterior shoulder film as a result of posterior shoulder girdle hypertonicity
Treatment plan	CMT for cervical spine, scapulothoracic joint
	Identification and adjustment of extension fixations in thoracic spine
	Scapula mobilization
	Isometric scapula retraction exercises
	Correction and rehabilitation of postural faults
	Ultrasound and electrical stimulation combination therapy for myofascial trigger points

CMT, Chiropractic manipulative therapy.

with scapula mobilization and manipulation helps ease the patient's pain and dysfunction.[43]

Scapulothoracic Postural Faults

With or without external loading, postural faults are the primary cause of posterior shoulder girdle and scapula pain. Medial and retroscapular pain has a direct link to head and arm positioning in relation to the upper torso. Workplace trauma and muscle fatigue can originate in muscle weakness and awkward shoulder and arm postures. Workers should be able to position their hands near waist level and near the body when they are working. The repetitive lifting of objects and the constant performance of fine manual assembly tasks can prove quite debilitating to the upper back region. Many workers who suffer from shoulder pain state that they have been working with their hands primarily at or above the level of the

Table 3-17	Psoriatic Arthritis versus Rheumatoid Arthritis	
Clinical Characteristics	Psoriatic Arthritis	Rheumatoid Arthritis
Onset	Insidious or acute	Insidious
Pattern	Asymmetric	Symmetric
Sex predominance	No difference	Female
Distal interphalangeal disease	Yes	Rarely
Nail involvement	Yes	No
Shoulder involvement	30%	57%-62%*
Rheumatoid arthritis factor in blood	Not often present	Often, especially with family history

*Sartoris DJ, Resnick D: Target area approach to arthritis of the small articulations, *Contemp Diagn Radiol*, 8:1, 1985.

the first joint affected, however. Patients with psoriatic arthritis and spondylitis may have a higher incidence of shoulder disease. Bilateral shoulder involvement is not uncommon.

A Word About Injections

Patients with tendonitis, capsulitis, or exacerbations of chronic arthritis may discuss with their physician the possibility of administering an injection to ease the painful inflammation. It is best to keep treatments as noninvasive and conservative as possible. If adjunctive therapies, such as ice, exercise, electrotherapy, or ultrasound treatments, do not improve a patient's condition and the pain is severely affecting the patient's life style or sleep, the next progressive step is to prescribe an oral, nonsteroidal antiinflammatory drug (NSAID). Medications such as indomethacin (Indocin), sulindac (Clinoril), ibuprofen (Motrin, Advil, Nuprin), naproxen (Naprosyn), tolmetin sodium (Tolectin), and diclofenac sodium (Voltaren) are as effective as aspirin in inhibiting prostaglandin synthesis and are less irritating to the gastrointestinal tract.

If the oral administration of NSAIDs does not rid the patient of pain, an injection may be helpful. Intraarticular corticosteroids may help relieve inflammation and night pain in shoulder arthritis. If the patient has pinpoint tenderness (i.e., pain that is localized rather than diffuse), the injection provides a more favorable result.

study

Review Questions

1. Name the four major articulations that comprise the shoulder girdle and the orthopedic conditions that are common to each.
2. Match the best imaging procedure with its clinical indication.
   A. Computed tomography   1. glenoid labrum tears
   B. Contrast arthrography   2. degenerative arthritis
   C. Computed arthrotomography   3. adhesive capsulitis
                                          4. complex fractures
   D. Conventional radiography
3. (a) What is the most common type of glenohumeral dislocation? (b) What is the mechanism of injury? (c) What are two important steps during initial care that will reduce future morbidity?
4. (a) Name some clinical signs and symptoms of an acute traumatic shoulder separation (acromioclavicular sprain)? (b) What are some high-risk sports for acromioclavicular trauma?
5. What anatomic structures occupy the suprahumeral space?
6. A 50-year-old woman complains of generalized stiffness and pain in the shoulder for 2 months duration; she recalls no prior trauma. On examination, she exhibits severe loss of external rotation and abduction of the arm. (a) What is your tentative diagnosis? (b) What is your diagnostic imaging test of choice? (c) What is your primary treatment?
7. A 60-year-old man complains of shoulder pain for a 4-week duration that becomes worse at night. He has had no prior trauma, is afebrile, and is a two pack-a-day cigarette smoker for 40 years. Orthopedic examination findings are unremarkable with full range of motion. (a) What diagnosis should be ruled out? (b) What tests should be ordered?

References

1. Andrews JR: *Management of rotator cuff injuries in the throwing athlete*, Baltimore, 1998, NATA 49th Annual Meeting and Clinical Symposium.
2. Andrews JR, Whiteside JA, Wilk KE: Rehabilitation of throwing and racquet sport injuries. In Buschbacher RM, Braddom RL, editors: *Sports medicine and rehabilitation: a sport-specific approach*, St Louis, 1994, Mosby.
3. Avikainen V, Ranki P et al: Acromioclavicular complete dislocation: analysis of the results in 48 patients, *Ann Chir Gynaecol* 68(4):117, 1979.
4. Bach BR: Commentary on acromioclavicular research, *Adv Orthop Surg* 16(5):327, 1993.

5. Bargren JH, Erlanger S, Dick HM: Biomechanics and comparison of two operative methods of treatment of complete acromioclavicular separation, *Clin Orthop* 130:267, 1978.

6. Barth E, Berg E: Practical pointers for common shoulder pain complaints, *J Musculoskel Med* 6(6):38, 1989.

7. Bigliani LU, Codd TP, Connor PM, Levine WN, Littlefield MA, Hershon SJ: Shoulder motion and laxity in the professional baseball player, *Am J Sports Med* 25:609, 1997.

8. Bigilimi LU, Kimmel J, McCoon PD: Repair of rotator cuff tears in tennis players, *Am J Sports Med* 20:112, 1992.

9. Bigilimi LU, Nicholson GP, Flatow EL: Arthroscopic resection of the distal clavicle, *Orthop Clin North Am* 24(1):133, 1993.

10. Booher JM, Thibodeau GA: *Athletic injury assessment,* ed 3, St Louis, 1994, Mosby.

11. Brier SR: Rotator cuff disease: current trends in orthopedic management, *J Manipulative Physiol Ther* 15(2):123, 1992.

12. Caspari RB, Savoie FH: Shoulder arthroscopy: present status of a promising technique, *J Musculoskel Med* 6(1):39, 1989.

13. Ciullo J: Swimmer's shoulder, *Clin Sports Med* 5(1):1, 1986.

14. Ciullo J, Stevens G: The prevention of injuries to the shoulder in swimming, *Sports Med* 7:182, 1989.

15. Cofield RM: Degenerative and arthritic problems of the glenohumeral joint. In Rockwood C, Matsen F, editors: *The shoulder,* Philadelphia, 1990, WB Saunders.

16. Cofield RM, Irving JF: Evolution and classification of shoulder instability, *Clin Orthop* 223:32, 1987.

17. Cox JS: Acromioclavicular joint injuries and their management principles, *Ann Chir Gynaecol* 80:155, 1991.

18. De Palma AF: *Surgery of the shoulder,* ed 3, Philadelphia, 1983, JB Lippincott.

19. Detrisac DA, Johnson LL: Arthroscopic shoulder capsulorrhaphy using metal staples, *Orthop Clin North Am* 24(1):71, 1993.

20. Eidman DK, Siff SJ, Tullos HS: Acromioclavicular lesions in children, *Am J Sports Med* 9(3):150, 1981.

21. Ellison AI: *Athletic training and sports medicine,* Chicago, 1984, American Academy of Orthopedic Surgeons, National Athletic Trainers' Association.

22. Eskola A et al: Acute complete acromioclavicular dislocation: a prospective randomized trial of fixation with smooth or threaded Kirschner wires or cortical screw, *Ann Chir Gynaecol* 76(6):323, 1987.

23. Glousman RE: Instability versus impingement syndrome in the throwing athlete, *Orthop Clin North Am* 24(1):89, 1993.

24. Goldberg TI, Boone RS: Brachial plexus lesions associated with dislocated shoulder, *Adv Orthop Surg* 16(2):139, 1992.

25. Gross TP: Anterior glenohumeral instability, *Orthopaedics* 11(1):3, 1988.

26. Harding WG: Keep your shoulders in the "safe zone," *Phys Sports Med* 21(12):93, 1993.

27. Hawkins RJ, Abrams JS: Impingement syndrome in the absence of rotator cuff tear, *Orthop Clin North Am* 18:373, 1987.

28. Hertling D, Kessler R: *Management of common musculoskeletal disorders,* ed 2, Philadelphia, 1990, JB Lippincott.

29. Hill JA: Epidemiologic perspective on shoulder injuries, *Clin Sports Med* 2(2):241, 1983.

30. Jobe FW, Giangarre CE, Kuitne RS, Glousman RE: Anterior capsulolabral reconstruction of the shoulder in athletes in overhead sports, *Adv Orthoped Surg* 16(5):332, 1993.

31. Jobe FW, Gowan I: A comparative electromyographic analysis of the shoulder during pitching, *Am J Sports Med* 15(6):586, 1988.

32. Jobe FW, Kvitne RS: Shoulder pain in the overhand or throwing athlete: the relationship of anterior instability and rotator cuff impingement, *Orthop Rev* 18(9):963, 1989.

33. Jobe FW, Moynes DR, Brewster CE: Rehabilitation of shoulder joint instabilities, *Orthop Clin North Am* 18(3):473, 1987.

34. Jobe FW, Screnar PM, Brewster CE: *Management of shoulder instability in throwing athletics,* Baltimore, 1998, NATA 49th Annual Meeting and Clinical Symposium.

35. Larsen B, Berg/Nielsen A, Christensen P: Conservative or surgical treatment of acromioclavicular dislocation: a prospective, controlled, randomized study, *J Bone Joint Surg* 68A:552, 1986.

36. Lehman R: Shoulder pain in the competitive tennis player, *Clin Sports Med* 7(2):304, 1988.

37. Lewit K: Relationship of faulty respiration to posture, with clinical implications, *J Am Osteopath Assoc* 79(8):525, 1980.

38. MacDonald PB, Alexander MJ et al: Comprehensive functional analysis of shoulders following complete acromioclavicular separation, *Am J Sports Med* 16(5):475, 1988.

39. McFarland EG, Shaffer B, Glousman RE, Conway JE, Jobe FW: Clinical and diagnostic evaluation. In Jobe FW, editor: *Operative techniques in upper extremity sports injuries,* St Louis, 1996, Mosby.

40. Magee DJ: *Orthopedic physical assessment,* ed 3, Philadelphia, 1992, WB Saunders.

41. Marone PJ: *Postgraduate advances in sports medicine,* vols II-IX, Berryville, Vir, 1987, Forum Medicum.

42. Meyers JF: Injuries to the shoulder girdle and elbow. In Sullivan JA, Grana WA, editors: *The pediatric athlete,* Park Ridge, Ill, 1990, AAOS.

43. Micheli L: Scapulothoracic motion in shoulders with glenohumeral instability syndrome: investigation (abstract), *Med Sci Sports Exerc Suppl* 22(2):104, 1990.

44. Miniaci A, Fowler PJ: Impingement in the athlete, *Clin Sports Med* 12(1):91, 1993.

45. Neer CS: Impingement lesions, *Clin Orthop* 173:70, 1983.

46. Neviaser TJ: Adhesive capsulitis, *Orthop Clin North Am* 18(3):439, 1989.

47. Neviaser TJ: The role of the biceps tendon in the impingement syndrome, *Orthop Clin North Am* 18(3):383, 1987.

48. Neviaser RJ, Eisenfeld LS, Wiesel SW et al: *Emergency orthopaedic radiology,* New York, 1988, Churchill Livingstone.

49. Norlander S, Gustavsson BA: Reduced mobility in the cervicothoracic motion segment: risk factor for musculoskeletal pain: a two-year prospective follow-up study, *Scand J Rehab Med* 29:167, 1997.

50. O'Brien SJ, Warren RF, Schwartz E: Anterior shoulder instability, *Orthop Clin North Am* 18(3):395, 1987.

51. Peat M: Functional anatomy of the shoulder complex, *Phys Ther* 6(12):1861, 1986.

52. Percy A et al: Dislocation of the sternoclavicular joint: a review of 49 cases, *Int Orthop* 12:187, 1988.

53. Percy EC, Birbrager D, Pitt MJ: Snapping scapula: a review of the literature and presentation of 14 patients, *Can J Surg* 31:248, 1988.

54. Peterson L, Renstrom P: *Sports injuries: their prevention and treatment,* Chicago, 1983, Year Book Medical Publishers.

55. Plancher KD, McGillicuddy: *Clavicle fractures in cyclists*, San Francisco, 1997, AAOS.
56. Popper NK, Walker PS: Normal and abnormal motion of the shoulder, *J Bone Joint Surg* 58:195, 1976.
57. Pring DJ, Constant O, Bayley JI et al: Radiology of the humeral head in recurrent anterior shoulder dislocations: brief report, *J Bone Joint Surg* 71B(1):141, 1989.
58. Protzman RR: Anterior instability of the shoulder, *J Bone Joint Surg* 62:909, 1980.
59. Rames RD, Karzel RP: Injuries to the glenoid labrum, including SLAP lesions, *Orthop Clin North Am*, 24(1):45, 1993.
60. Rathburn JB, MacNab I: The microvascular pattern of the rotator cuff, *J Bone Joint Surg* 52B:540, 1970.
61. Roodman W: Etiologies of shoulder impingement syndrome in competitive swimmers, *Chiropractic Sports Med* 3(2):27, 1989.
62. Rothman R, Parke W: Vascular anatomy of the rotator cuff, *Clin Orthop* 41:176, 1965.
63. Rowe CR: Recurrent anterior transient subluxation of the shoulder: the "dead arm" syndrome, *Orthop Clin North Am* 19(4):767, 1988.
64. Rowe CR, editor: *The shoulder*, New York, 1988, Churchill Livingstone.
65. Sartoris DJ, Resnick D: Target area approach to arthritis of the small articulations, *Contemp Diagn Radiology* 8:1, 1985.
66. Shrode LW: Treating shoulder impingement using the supraspinatus synchronized exercise, *J Manipulative Physiol Ther* 17(1):43, 1994.
67. Skjeldal S, Lundblad R, Dullerud R: Coracoid process transfer for acromioclavicular dislocation, *Act Orthop Scand* 59(2):180, 1988.
68. Smith AN: Scapular fracture in a collegiate football player, *J Athletic Training* 33(2):5-30, 1998.
69. Stanley D, Morris SH et al: Recovery following fractures of the clavicle treated conservatively, 19:162, 1988, *Yearbook of Orthopaedics 1989,* Chicago, Yearbook Medical Publishers.
70. Taft TN, Wilson FC, Oglesby JW: Dislocation of the acromioclavicular joint: an end-result study, *J Bone Joint Surg* 69A(7): 1045, 1987.
71. Taylor DC, Arciero RA: Pathologic changes associated with shoulder dislocations: arthroscopic and physical examination findings in first-time traumatic anterior dislocations, *Am J Sports Med* 25:306,1997.
72. Tensor R, Uribe J, Shildkrout K: Selections of patients for arthroscopic shoulder capsulorrhaphy, *Medicine and Science in Sports and Exercise* (abstract suppl), 22(2):103, 1990.
73. Thomas J, Matsen F: An approach to the repair of avulsion of the glenohumeral ligaments, *J Bone Joint Surg* 71A(4):506, 1989.
74. Tibone J, Sellers R, Torino P: Strength testing after third-degree acromioclavicular dislocation, *Am J Sports Med* 20(3):328, 1992.
75. Weissman BN, Sledge CB: *Orthoped radiology,* Philadelphia, 1986, WB Saunders.
76. Wiker SW: Shoulder posture and localized muscle fatigue and discomfort, *Ergonomics* 32(2):211, 1989.
77. Wiley AM: Diagnostic arthroscopy and adhesive capsulitis, *Arthroscopy* 7(2):138, 1991.
78. Wojtys EM, Nelson G: Conservative treatment of grade 3 acromioclavicular dislocations, *Clin Orthop* 268:112, 1991.
79. Yocum TR, Rowe LJ: *Essentials of skeletal radiology,* vol I, Baltimore, 1987, Williams & Wilkins.
80. Young DC, Rockwood CA: Complications of failed Bristow procedures and their management, *Adv Orthop Surg* 16(1):41, 1992.

A functional hinge joint, the elbow provides approximately 140 degrees of flexion and allows for terminal extension in the closed-packed position. The humeroulnar articulation determines the anatomic angle (i.e., carrying angle) of the elbow. In the extended or supinated position, the forearm has an outward (valgus) carrying angle of up to 15 degrees. Full elbow flexion brings about an inward (varus) angle of approximately 10 degrees.[34]

Biomechanics of the Elbow

Unlike the shoulder, the elbow possesses great bony stability. It is normally a well-aligned joint with a tight bony articulation; an alteration in this structure, such as by a traumatic event, frequently causes a loss of motion. The anterior and posterior bundles of the medial (ulnar) collateral ligament contribute significantly to the medial stability of the joint. Likewise, the lateral (radial) collateral ligament and annular ligament provide stability for the lateral portion of the elbow (Figures 4-1 *A, B*). The radial collateral ligament plays a small role in tensile strength, however.

The soft-tissue structures of the wrist, such as the flexors and extensors, add to the stability of the elbow. In fact, the elbow can retain its stability in spite of the loss of some of its bone stock as long as the radial head remains unaffected. In addition, the loss of some range of motion in the elbow does not destroy its functional usefulness for common daily needs. For instance, only approximately 50 degrees of supination and pronation and 30 to 100 degrees of flexion are necessary for everyday motions. This narrow range of movement, of course, may not be acceptable to a baseball pitcher or tennis player.

The elbow rotates by means of the proximal radioulnar joint. It has approximately 90 degrees of supination and pronation, provided that there is no compromise of the radial head. Injuries to the radial head generally result in radioulnar dysfunction and subsequent loss of rotation.

The anterior capsule provides stability in extension through valgus and varus joint loading. It is quite sensitive even to mild trauma, however, which can lead to the common flexion contracture. Compressive loads are greatest through the radial side of the elbow. Approximately 60% of axial compression forces are distributed via the lateral portion of the elbow joint.

Pathologic valgus loading of the lateral side of the elbow may result from repetitive overhead activities, such as throwing a baseball or playing tennis. Constant valgus stresses may cause such orthopedic conditions as osteochondral fractures of the capitellum, osteochondritis dissecans, and radial head injuries.

Tensile loads across the medial portion of the elbow increase the tension of the soft-tissue structures. Medial shear forces produce tensile loading of the wrist flexor and forearm pronator group, stretching of the medial collateral ligament, and ultimately spurring of the coronoid process and medial collateral ligament. Through medial stresses, these inflammatory conditions may adversely affect the ulnar nerve at the cubital tunnel or the two heads of the flexor carpi ulnaris.[22]

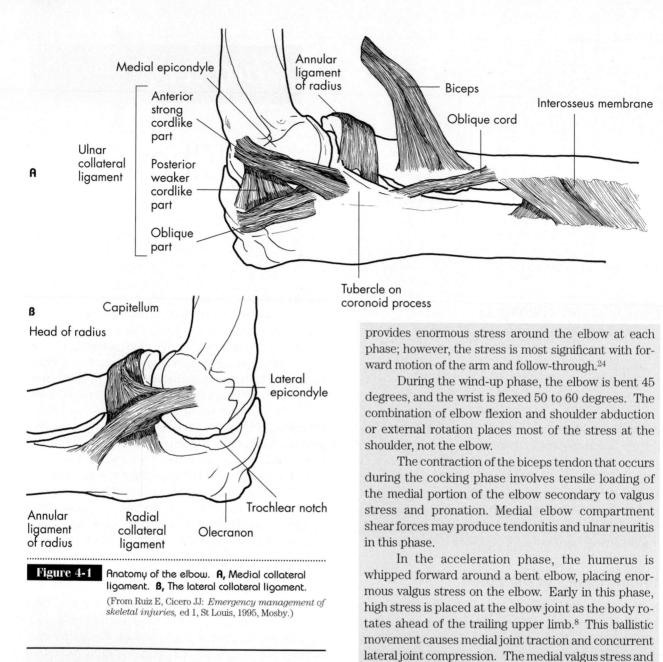

A

Medial epicondyle

Annular ligament of radius

Biceps

Interosseus membrane

Oblique cord

Ulnar collateral ligament

Anterior strong cordlike part

Posterior weaker cordlike part

Oblique part

Tubercle on coronoid process

B

Capitellum

Head of radius

Lateral epicondyle

Annular ligament of radius

Radial collateral ligament

Olecranon

Trochlear notch

Figure 4-1 Anatomy of the elbow. **A,** Medial collateral ligament. **B,** The lateral collateral ligament.

(From Ruiz E, Cicero JJ: *Emergency management of skeletal injuries,* ed 1, St Louis, 1995, Mosby.)

Biomechanics of the Throwing Motion

In recreation and sport, only the act of running is more common than the act of throwing. An understanding of the mechanisms of action in throwing is crucial to an understanding of pathologic makeup of the elbow. The pitching motion in baseball, for example, has five phases: (1) wind-up, (2) cocking, (3) acceleration, (4) release, and (5) follow-through. Valgus strain provides enormous stress around the elbow at each phase; however, the stress is most significant with forward motion of the arm and follow-through.[24]

During the wind-up phase, the elbow is bent 45 degrees, and the wrist is flexed 50 to 60 degrees. The combination of elbow flexion and shoulder abduction or external rotation places most of the stress at the shoulder, not the elbow.

The contraction of the biceps tendon that occurs during the cocking phase involves tensile loading of the medial portion of the elbow secondary to valgus stress and pronation. Medial elbow compartment shear forces may produce tendonitis and ulnar neuritis in this phase.

In the acceleration phase, the humerus is whipped forward around a bent elbow, placing enormous valgus stress on the elbow. Early in this phase, high stress is placed at the elbow joint as the body rotates ahead of the trailing upper limb.[8] This ballistic movement causes medial joint traction and concurrent lateral joint compression. The medial valgus stress and the radiohumeral compression are greatest during this stage. If stresses are repetitive through the acceleration phase, medial ligament or flexor and pronator muscle strain may occur. Also, lateral compartment osteochondrosis and degenerative changes may take place (Table 4-1). If the throwing motion is more sidearm than directly overhead, elbow stress appears to increase during throwing.

The usual position of the elbow during the release phase is extension, with the upper arm abducted 90 degrees from the upper trunk.

In the follow-through phase of throwing, proximal radioulnar motion controls the ball. As the elbow rapidly extends, stress occurs along the triceps muscle to the olecranon process. Not only can the compressive forces of the capitellum and radial head injure the posterior compartment of the elbow, but the hyperextension may also.

Faulty mechanics may originate in the person who uses poor segmental progression of large muscle groups (e.g., not effectively using the legs and hips to dissipate force)—extending the lead arm (glove hand), lifting the back foot from the ground too soon, and opening the lead shoulder too soon. As a result, the power of the torso and legs is lost, and the throw must be made with the arm alone. Anatomic factors include leg length discrepancy, scoliosis, dorsal kyphosis, and leg paresis.

Examination of the Elbow

The clinical examination and subsequent decision making on the appropriate treatment for a patient with elbow dysfunction begins with the history (Figure 4-2). When there is a history of macrotrauma, the clinical suggestion of internal structural damage to the elbow

joint may be strong. Certain microtraumatic events, such as the high velocity and repetitive trauma of pitching, can also result in an internal derangement of the elbow, however.

It is essential that the examiner compare the size, contour, and attitude of the injured elbow with the same characteristics of the elbow on the "good" side. The examiner should also palpate for effusion, symmetry, and tenderness of the underlying anatomy and order x-ray films when a traumatic episode brings the patient to the office or if the history indicates repetitive microtrauma or multiple painful episodes. If the patient fell on an outstretched hand, for example, the practitioner should examine the wrist, proximal radioulnar joint, and shoulder (especially the acromioclavicular joint). Inspection for full pronation and supination is necessary to rule out damage to the radial head.

Symptomatology in the Elbow

Pain in the medial compartment of the elbow is usually located at the medial collateral ligament, ulnar nerve, or flexor or pronator muscle-tendon unit. Overuse, especially in racquet sports and baseball, can damage any or all of these structures. A single traumatic episode is more likely to cause a medial collateral ligament sprain than an ulnar neuritis or flexor strain, however (Table 4-2). Chronic flexor strains can cause fibrosis and adhesions

Table 4-1 Sports-Related Elbow Injuries and Precipitating Stresses

| | Resulting Injuries | |
Type of Stress	Adult	Child
Diffuse	Humeral hypertrophy; radial head coronoid process hypertrophy; olecranon process hypertrophy	Hypertrophy and hypermaturity radial head, capitellar, trochlear epiphyses; hypertrophy and hypermaturity medial epicondylar apophysis
Humeral shaft	Spiral fracture humeral shaft	Same as adult
Medial tension	**Acute:** avulsion fracture medial epicondyle; fracture ulnar spur **Chronic:** ulnar traction spur; hyperostosis ulnar groove; loose bodies	**Acute:** avulsion medial epicondylar apophysis; **Chronic:** traction apophysitis medial epicondylar apophysis
Lateral compression	**Acute:** osteochondral fracture **Chronic:** loose bodies	**Acute:** osteochondritis dissecans **Chronic:** aseptic necrosis radial head; anterior angulation deformity radial head; loose bodies
Extension	**Acute:** avulsion olecranon process **Chronic:** osteochondral loose bodies	**Acute:** avulsion olecranon apophysitis **Chronic:** traction apophysitis medial epicondylar apophysis

(From Gore RM, Rogers LF, Bowerman J et al: Osseous manifestations of elbow stress associated with sports activities, *AJR* 134:971, 1980. Reproduced by permission.)

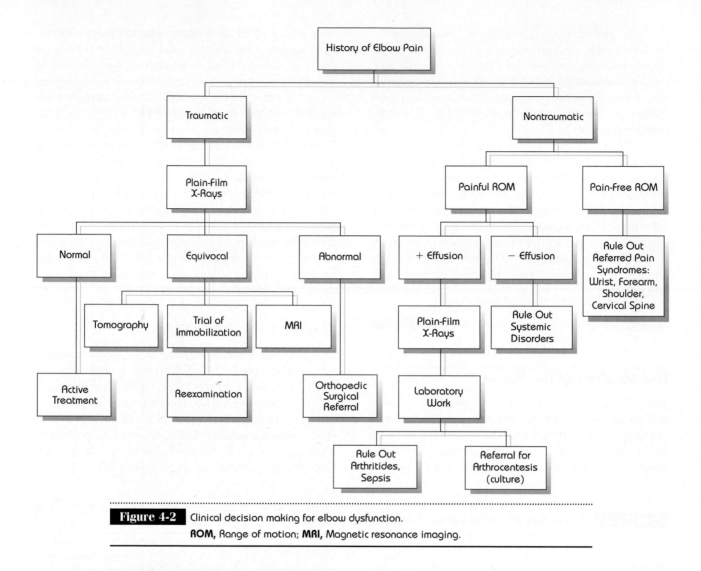

Figure 4-2 Clinical decision making for elbow dysfunction.
ROM, Range of motion; **MRI,** Magnetic resonance imaging.

that, in time, can affect the ulnar nerve because of its anatomic proximity to the muscle-tendon unit.

Lateral elbow symptomatology can center around the extensor compartment, such as in tennis elbow. In adolescents, compression of the radiohumeral joint may cause osteochondritis dissecans, bony overgrowth, or, ultimately, loose bodies (i.e., bone fragments).

Structures that may be damaged in the anterior compartment of the elbow include the joint capsule, biceps tendon, and median nerve. Soft-tissue bogginess and palpable tenderness occur in cases of capsulitis and bicipital tendonitis. Usually, participation in athletics suggests a history of heavy lifting or exertion. Pronator teres syndrome is a peripheral entrapment neuropathy of the median nerve just distal to the elbow, where it

splits the pronator teres muscle. Numbness, tingling, and pain along the distal course of the median nerve, as well as night pain, are telltale signs of this syndrome. Anterior forearm compartment myofascitis may also accompany this exertional injury.

Diagnostic Studies

Routine radiographic films of the elbow include tripositional views. An anteroposterior view is taken with the elbow in full extension, a lateral view with the elbow flexed to 90 degrees; and either an oblique or axial view with the elbow joint flexed to 110 degrees and the tube angled at 45 degrees to profile the olecranon and trochlea of the humerus. Stress views taken with the elbow in

Table 4-2	Medial Compartment Localization of Pathologic Conditions	
Patient Group	**Site or Structure Involved**	**Examination Finding**
Children	Trochlea	Changes in ossification patterns
Adolescents	Trochlea	Heterotopic bone in competitive athletic populations
Chronic overusers	Ulnar nerve Medial collateral ligament	Laxity, neuropathy, chronic strain Heterotopic bone, fibrosis, and flexor mass scarring

valgus may be warranted, especially in athletes, to determine the extent of medial joint opening. These films stress the integrity of the medial collateral ligament. Computed tomograms or arthrograms may aid in diagnosing capsule and cartilage tears in the elbow joint.

Hemarthrosis commonly accompanies fractures of the elbow. On plain films it may initially appear as the elevation of the anterior and posterior fat pads, otherwise known as the positive fat pad sign. The effusion in the joint displaces these fat pads. Because ulnar neuritis is also common in the traumatically injured elbow, electromyographic and nerve conduction studies can be quite helpful in differentiating elbow abnormalities from cervical radiculopathy or more distal neuropathies.

Acute Traumatic Injuries

Dislocation of the Elbow

In adults the elbow is the third most commonly dislocated joint (the shoulder and the interphalangeal joints being first and second, respectively). In children, the elbow is the most commonly dislocated joint. Approximately 80% to 90% of all elbow dislocations are posterior or posterolateral in nature[6]; (Figure 4-3 *A, B*) the ulna and radius are displaced posteriorly in relation to the humerus (Table 4-3).

Indirect force from a fall on an outstretched upper limb accounts for the vast majority of these injuries. Hyperextension of the joint may occur, or a direct posterior force applied while the elbow is in mild flexion can cause the injury.[10] Contact sports such as football and wrestling are major contributors to the incidence of this injury.

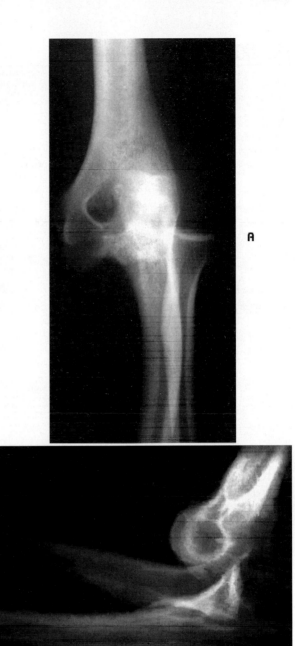

A

B

Figure 4-3 Posterolateral elbow dislocation. **A,** Anteroposterior view. **B,** Lateral view.

(From Ruiz E, Cicero JJ: *Emergency management of skeletal injuries*, ed 1, St Louis, 1995, Mosby.)

The flexor mass of the elbow is usually sufficient to maintain the functional ability of the arm, even though the elbow joint may be unstable medially. It is necessary to take radiographic films, however, to rule out associ-

Table 4-3 Traumatic Elbow Injuries

| | Posterolateral Dislocation | Fractures | |
		Medial Epicondyle	Radial Head
Physical examination findings	Effusion and deformity Flexion contracture Radial head tenderness Loss of pronation and supination	Effusion Palpable pain over medial epicondyle Lack of elbow motion	Effusion Palpable tenderness at radial head Limited, painful pronation; supination Restricted flexion and extension
X-ray findings	Standard three-view series (i.e., anteroposterior, lateral, oblique) Visualization of posterior dislocation of radius and ulna Associated humeral fracture ruled out	Standard three-view series (i.e., anteroposterior, lateral, oblique [medial]) Visualization of fracture at medial epicondyle of humerus Displaced fragment ruled out	Standard three-view series (i.e., anteroposterior, lateral, oblique) plus other oblique films Visualization of vertically oriented fracture of radial head's lateral aspect
Treatment plan	Referral to orthopedic surgeon Immobilization for 4-8 weeks Treatment of any associated fractures Early limited mobilization Monitoring of shoulder and cervical spine on involved side	Referral to orthopedic surgeon Immobilization for a minimum of 3-4 weeks Monitoring of shoulder and cervical spine on involved side	Referral to orthopedic surgeon Cast immobilization for 4-6 weeks Monitoring of shoulder and cervical spine on involved side

ated fractures and to confirm bony alignment. Complications that may result from a dislocated elbow include the following:

- Malalignment of bony fragments
- Brachialis contusion at the distal humerus
- Fracture of the medial epicondyle
- Myositis ossificans, secondary to immobilization
- Postimmobilization capsular tightness

Dislocations of the elbow are usually reducible via closed methods. Nonsurgical treatment with cast immobilization, usually for 4 to 8 weeks, is preferable to primary ligamentous repair, because traumatized elbows generally exhibit less motion loss and fewer continuing symptoms after conservative treatment.[13] Rehabilitation centers around the control of the swelling and inflammation, as well as the use of gentle active ranges of motion to regain mobility. Passive stretch should be avoided, since it can cause a myositis injury to the elbow flexors. Because early limited mobilization is the key to future success, initiation of motion at some point within the first 2 weeks is normal treatment for simple elbow dislocation.[1,17] Persistent displacement or deformity that can be visualized radiographically requires operative treatment.

Elbow Fractures

Medial Epicondyle Fractures

Both medial and lateral epicondyles project from the distal humerus proximal to its articular surfaces. The medial epicondyle is the larger and more prominent of the two and thus the more often injured (Figure 4-4). It is also the site of origin of the common flexor mass of the forearm and the medial collateral ligament.

Avulsion fractures of the medial epicondyle of the humerus may accompany direct trauma, such as the following:

- Posterior or posterolateral elbow dislocation
- Acute medial collateral ligament (rupture) sprain
- Osteochondral fracture or loose fragment (primarily in adolescents)

As muscle mass and strength increase in adolescence and young adulthood, these injuries occur with increasing frequency. They are more common among participants in the throwing sports. Such sports as baseball and wrestling, for example, are notorious for acute and chronic medial compartment trauma. These types of fractures may also accompany posterolateral dislocations of the elbow. Not uncommonly, these injuries can be associated with impacted fractures of the radial head.[25] In some cases the forearm flexors may pull a bone fragment distally toward the anterior.

The treatment parallels that of an elbow dislocation. It centers on early motion after immobilization for a minimum of 3 to 4 weeks to promote collagenous healing of the medial epicondylar physis. Open treatment is necessary if there is severe soft-tissue damage at or around the ulnar nerve, or if bony displacement has occurred.

Radial Head Fractures

Most cases of radial head fracture, an injury quite common in adults, result from a fall on an outstretched arm. There may be a concomitant medial elbow soft-tissue injury as a result of valgus stress placed at the elbow, along with ligamentous disruption.

The injury compromises proximal radioulnar joint movement and causes effusion. Swelling may make flexion and extension of the elbow joint painful. The radial head is quite tender to palpation. Special films may be necessary for patients with a history of trauma, compromised proximal radioulnar motion, or an elevated fat pad sign, since some fractures may go unnoticed on a particular projection[27] (Figure 4-5). In addition to the standard anteroposterior, lateral, and supination anteroposterior (oblique) views, the clinician may order other oblique films to document fully a fracture line. Similar to medial epicondyle fractures, radial head fractures may be associated with dislocations of the elbow.[33]

Fractures of the radial neck are uncommon in adults, although they may occur with other, more substantial injuries resulting from multiple trauma. Many times these injuries appear on the lateral film as a "step-off" (i.e., a disruption in the line of bone) between the radial head and neck. The fracture heals in 2 to 3 weeks, with early mobilization the usual rule.

Mechanical Syndromes of the Elbow

The elbow is a commonly afflicted joint in overuse syndromes, such as throwing injuries and "tennis elbow." Repetitive movements that irritate the musculoskeletal system cause microtearing at the soft-tissue level. In essence, the body's physiologic ability to heal wounded tissues cannot keep up with the repetitive nature of microtrauma. Hence, progressive changes in soft-tissue structures take place.[2]

Soft-tissue syndromes around the elbow may be classified into three broad categories according to their functional anatomy: (1) medial compartment syndrome,

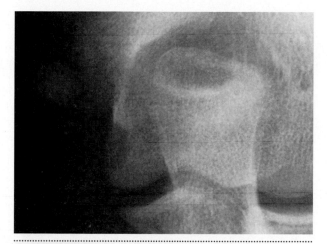

Figure 4-4 Severely displaced fracture of medial epicondyle.

(From Canale ST, editor: *Campbell's operative orthopaedics*, ed 9, vol 3, St Louis, 1998, Mosby.)

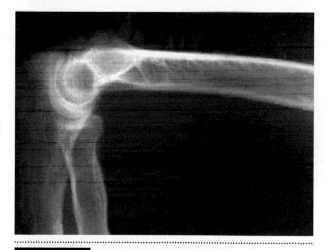

Figure 4-5 Lateral view of the elbow with a radial head fracture. The anterior fat pad is elevated. The posterior fat pad has become discernable. The supinator line is obscured.

(From Ruiz E, Cicero JJ: *Emergency management of skeletal injuries*, ed 1, St Louis, 1995, Mosby.)

(2) lateral compartment syndrome, and (3) posterior compartment syndrome. The chief mechanism of elbow trauma is a valgus stress injury with forced extension. Angular velocity produces a shearing force medially and a compressive force laterally. Medial elbow injuries are caused by constant distraction of the soft-tissue structures and large valgus forces; in contrast, lateral elbow injuries are the result of an overload of compressive forces.[9]

Repetitive loads into extension can promote chronic injuries to the posterior compartment of the elbow, as well as injuries to the olecranon and osteoarthritis.

Medial Compartment: Shear and Stress Injuries

Medial Sprains

Most elbow sprains result from a valgus stress overload with forced extension. Avulsion of a ligament from its bony attachment or a secondary ulnar nerve injury mandates surgical exploration and repair. Elbow sprains usually involve the medial collateral ligament. Sprains at grade II or higher involve the posteromedial joint capsule and, possibly, the capsular ligament. Effusion, posterior instability, and a painful arc of elbow flexion are significant findings (Table 4-4). Radiographic films are essential to exclude fracture. The clinician also checks pronation and supination for possible radial head damage. Laxity of the medial collateral ligament leads to joint instability from 30 to 90 degrees of elbow flexion. Swelling, however, may prevent the patient from achieving flexion in the acute stage of injury.

Table 4-4 Shear and Stress Injuries to the Elbow

	Medial Elbow Sprain	Chronic Medial Collateral Ligament Sprain	Ulnar Neuritis	Medial Epicondylitis
Physical examination findings	Effusion Palpable tenderness over MCL Partial arc of elbow flexion Capsular or radial head tenderness	Pain and tenderness over medial epicondyle Palpable discomfort 0.5" below medial epicondyle Tenderness over anterior aspect of elbow joint Gapping (laxity) on valgus stability testing of ligaments (see Chapter 1) Pain on valgus stress No terminal extension Possible signs of ulnar neuritis (e.g., presence of Tinel's sign, compression pain, referral to hand)	Dysesthesia and paresthesia distal to elbow in ulnar nerve distribution, especially fourth and fifth digits Presence of Tinel's sign Painful repetitive elbow flexion Weakness in hand interossei, grip, or pinch (Froment's sign)	Palpable tenderness at medial humeral epicondyle Pain on resistive wrist flexion Tenderness at common flexor or pronator muscle group Discomfort on forearm pronation
X-ray findings	Effusion Need to rule out separation or fracture of medial epicondyle	Possible heterotopic bone formation evident on plain films Possible calcific spurring at ulnar coronoid process (MCL attachment) Need to rule out separation of medial epicondyle Abduction stress testing (gravity testing) at 15°-20° of flexion to detect medial compartment instability	Three views (anteroposterior, lateral, axial) Need to rule out degenerative changes at coronoid of ulna and medial epicondylar changes	Usually normal Need to rule out chronic medial elbow instability
Treatment plan	Ice and immobilization Electrotherapy Referral to orthopedic surgeon in presence of fracture or advanced joint instability	Ice and rest Evaluation of stability for rehabilitative prognosis or surgery Consultation with orthopedic surgeon	Ice massage Pulsed ultrasound Gentle stretching of flexor mass Surgical referral if ulnar nerve is subluxing	Ice massage Pulsed ultrasound or electrotherapy Strengthening and stretching exercises

MCL, Medial collateral ligament.

If there is any question regarding medial joint instability or a medial collateral ligament tear, a gravity stress film taken with the patient supine is helpful. The arm is abducted to 90 degrees to the side, and the shoulder is externally rotated. After the elbow is flexed to 20 degrees to clear the olecranon from the olecranon fossa, gravity is allowed to impose a valgus stress at the elbow. An anteroposterior projection indicates the degree of medial joint opening. The patient may have to be anesthetized for this study.

An acute tear of the medial collateral ligament may be splinted for 3 to 6 weeks, after which the patient begins rehabilitation.

Chronic Medial Compartment Laxity

Repetitive trauma associated with excessive overhead arm motions, such as those required in baseball and tennis, may result in chronic tearing of the medial collateral ligament. An increased carrying angle may also play a role in medial compartment syndrome. In the adult, chronic medial stress can cause small traction spurs at the attachment site of the medial collateral ligament to the coronoid process of the ulna.

Chronic laxity of the medial compartment of the elbow joint brings about a host of secondary neurologic problems that can be quite debilitating. Ulnar neuropathy can occur secondary to stretching or rupture of the unstable medial collateral ligament over the ulnar groove. Also, a peripheral entrapment neuropathy secondary to either chronic ligament sprain or chronic flexor strain can affect the ulnar nerve because of the close proximity of the ulnar groove to the scar tissue that forms at the medial joint. In some athletes whose sport requires a great deal of throwing, the presence of scar tissue makes surgical transposition of the ulnar nerve necessary.[8]

Ulnar Neuritis

There are many causes of ulnar nerve pain at the elbow joint: nerve subluxation during overhead movements, cubital tunnel scarring secondary to chronic flexor mass strains, and intraneural fibrosis as a result of repetitive mechanical trauma. Repetitive stress to the medial compartment of the elbow, as occurs with baseball pitching, is the most common cause of the problem.

Ulnar neuritis, or cubital tunnel syndrome as it is commonly called, is the second most common peripheral entrapment neuropathy of the upper extremity—second only to carpal tunnel syndrome.[9] Conditions associated with ulnar neuritis include the following:

Tardy ulnar N, palsy: sxcoms laiter

- Chronic medial epicondylitis or tendonitis
- Chronic flexor strains (repetitive microtrauma to the flexed elbow)
- Ulnar nerve contusion
- Bony compression because of an old fracture, loose body, or osteophyte (seen in chronic medial stress syndrome)
- Ulnar nerve subluxation behind the medial epicondyle

Patients with ulnar neuritis develop numbness and paresthesia in the hand along the ulnar nerve distribution. As in angina pectoris, pain may radiate down the medial arm into the fourth or fifth digits in ulnar neuritis. Repetitive elbow flexion and a tap at the cubital tunnel often provoke a dysthetic response distal to the elbow (i.e., Tinel's sign). Weakness in pinch or grip, as well as a subtle difficulty in handwriting, may also be present. Late motor changes in the disease include atrophy of the hand (i.e., in the first dorsal interossei) and Froment's paper sign (i.e., weakness in thumb interphalangeal joint flexion with attempted pinch).

Nerve conduction velocity studies can pinpoint the area of entrapment and dysfunction, as can sensory studies of the ulnar nerve's dorsal cutaneous branch to the hand. Electrophysiologic studies may reveal a nerve entrapment syndrome at the elbow or above. These studies are also useful in differentiating between a central (cervical spine) and peripheral (e.g., elbow, wrist, hand) nerve lesion.

Medial Epicondylitis

The pain associated with tendonitis of the common flexor mass usually arises at the tendinous attachment of the flexors at the medial humeral epicondyle. Inflammation and scarring around the medial compartment of the elbow can cause localized pain and tenderness at the flexor-pronator mass. Although there is usually no distal referral of the flexor strain itself, the accumulation of scar tissue near the ulnar nerve as a result of chronic strains and tendonitis may irritate the nerve, and there may be transient pain on wrist flexion. Resisted pronation also causes pain because the pronator muscle arises in part with the common flexor tendons. Provocation of pain with resisted wrist flexion and with the elbow in extension is a standard test finding in patients with medial epicondylitis.

Although termed *golfer's elbow*, many other social and athletic activities can cause flexor tendonitis around the elbow. If these activities overload the flexor-pronator muscle group and it is not strong enough to dissipate the overload, tendonitis and pain can develop. For example, repetitive hard throwing in track and field events such as the javelin and baseball often result in symptoms of medial epicondylitis. Thus repetitive mechanical strain, rather than macrotrauma, is usually responsible for medial epicondylitis.

Treatment centers on correcting the faulty forearm biomechanics and building up the strength of the forearm and wrist flexors.[15] Ice, pulsed ultrasound treatment, electrotherapy, and muscle rehabilitation are important features of treatment. Stretching the flexor-pronator mass in elbow and wrist extension is also helpful. Neither bracing nor the injection of steroids and antiinflammatory medications is usually necessary for this injury, however. Poor body mechanics and failure to rest aggravate the situation; thus chronic problems of the medial compartment can persist.

Lateral Compartment: Compression Injuries

Osteochondral Lesions of the Radial Head

The combination of repeated compression and valgus stresses may lead to osteochondral defects at the lateral elbow. As a result, loose bodies may form at the radial head; ultimately, these loose bodies can migrate toward the posterior compartment of the joint. Deformity, decreased range of motion, pain, and swelling are all common findings in patients with such lesions. Terminal extension is usually lost, as well as the final 20 to 30 degrees of elbow flexion.

Occasionally, loose bodies appear in the lateral compartment secondary to osteochondral chip fractures of the radial head. Arthrotomography and MRI are helpful procedures for the identification of such lesions. Although there is a much higher rate of complication from elbow arthroscopy than with either knee or shoulder arthroscopy, this procedure proves most beneficial in patients who have loose bodies removed.[21]

rule out 1st ⟹ Radial (subl

Lateral Epicondylitis (Tennis Elbow)

Best known by the general term *tennis elbow,* an overuse soft-tissue lesion to the extensor-supinator group on the lateral portion of the elbow can affect one or more areas. For example, involvement of the tendon-bone interface at the lateral epicondyle of the humerus affects the extensor carpi radialis longus muscle. Inflammation of the periosteum may be an aggravating factor, along with tendonitis of the musculotendinous junction. A lesion at the attachment of the extensor carpi radialis brevis tendon sometimes causes pain in the posterior olecranon area. Orthopedic maneuvers, such as Mills' test and Cozen's test, cause pain during physical examination

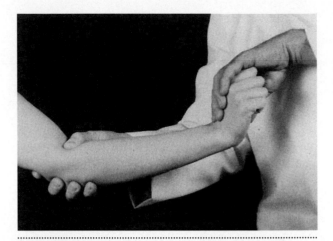

Figure 4-6 Cozen's test. With the affected elbow slightly flexed and pronated, the patient actively dorsiflexes the hand and wrist. The examiner applies pressure against the dorsum of the patient's hand as the patient resists flexion. Pain elicited at or near the lateral epicondyle suggests epicondylitis.

(From Evans RC: *Illustrated essentials in orthopedic physical assessment,* St Louis, 1994, Mosby.)

(Figure 4-6).[7] Concomitant myofascitis of the extensor group as a whole is not uncommon and is usually found several inches distal to the elbow joint at the forearm.

Most adults with tennis elbow are between the ages of 30 and 55 years. The rate of recurrence is higher in tennis players who are over the age of 40 and have a prior history of pain.[12]

Etiology of Lateral Epicondylitis. Etiologic factors of this ailment range from a varus stress on the elbow in the follow-through phase of racquet sports to improper backhand technique in tennis as follows:
- Poor choice of tennis racquet (e.g., graphite is a better choice than aluminum)
- Use of racquet that is too heavy
- Inappropriate grip (hand) measurement
- Excessive tension on strings
- Poor technique in one-handed backhand
- Improper biomechanics of hitting (e.g., failure to use the whole body, use of only the arm)
- Carrying heavy bags with a straight arm
- Overuse in weight training (e.g., repetitive arm extension)
- Excessive hammering (e.g., by carpenters)
- Use of a hard and "fast" surface by a novice tennis player

Incorrect technique in tennis increases the stress on the extensors of the forearm. One of the best ways to decrease stress on the arms is to use the legs to get into the proper position to hit the ball.

An improper grip, such as one that is too small or too large, can cause muscle fatigue that can lead to tendon injury. A racket that is strung at a tension that is too high increases the stresses on the muscles of the forearm and the structures of the elbow joint because it absorbs too little shock at impact. Similarly, hard surfaces such as cement courts can be deleterious to the soft-tissue structures of the upper extremity because they increase the speed at which the tennis ball moves, thus increasing the force transmitted to the tennis racket and, ultimately, to the elbow joint.

Treatment of Lateral Epicondylitis. Most patients with lateral epicondylitis respond to conservative measures.[5] Many patients find the following strengthening exercises extremely beneficial:

- Putty exercises
- Wrist curls (flexion)
- Reverse wrist curls (extension)
- Pronation and supination with dumbbell

For those whose condition is refractory, it may be necessary to employ more aggressive, more advanced stages of treatment along the following continua:

- Rest (active), transverse friction massage, ice, pulsed ultrasound, electrotherapy, putty exercises (e.g., squeezing Play-Doh), and counterforce brace, when active
- Rest, ice, pulsed ultrasound, electrotherapy; use of nonsteroidal antiinflammatory drugs; putty exercises and counterforce brace, if tolerated
- Rest, ice; use of nonsteroidal antiinflammatory drugs; manipulation; phonophoresis
- Rest, ice; corticosteroid injection; immobilization
- Surgical decompression (lateral release)

Patients should allow each stage of treatment a fair trial before proceeding to the next stage (Table 4-5). At least 95% of individuals recover with ice, rest, and electrotherapy, or, in advanced cases, with these treatment components and antiinflammatory agents.[20]

On resistant cases, elbow manipulation may have fair to good results. The hand and wrist are put into a flexed position with the forearm pronated. Using one hand at the patient's wrist to bring the elbow into terminal extension, the practitioner grasps the radial head with the other (Figure 4-7). The thrust into extension should produce an audible release that may indicate a breakdown of adhesions that have formed at the common extensor origin.

Although several authors have described this procedure as one to be performed while the patient is under

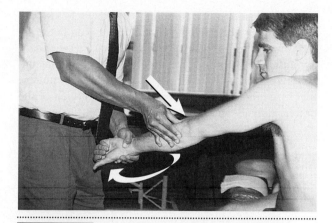

Figure 4-7 Manipulation of the elbow consisting of pronation and extension. Contact is on the radial head proximally and on the long lever of the forearm distally.

anesthesia,[30] as well as after surgery has failed, manipulation is best used as a last step in conservative care—without the administration of anesthesia. If the patient does not feel improvement after the first two or three manipulations, the treatment is usually not going to be effective. The patient may be more likely to benefit from another corticosteroid injection. Such an injection is most helpful for the patient who has a somewhat narrowly pinpointed area of tenderness and has not responded well to physiotherapy, exercise, and oral nonsteroidal antiinflammatory medication.[30]

Nirschl and Sobel and other investigators have advocated for several years the use of a counterforce brace in treating tennis elbow.[20,28] The brace is a wide, nonelastic support that is curved to fit the conical shape of the forearm (Figure 4-8). Usually the brace has dual tension straps that extend its width for adjustment purposes. The use of such a brace prevents full muscle expansion, thereby decreasing the working force of the tendon sheath. Rigid immobilization of the elbow reduces pain, but at the price of muscle atrophy and deconditioning. Therefore such a brace is not recommended for routine use. Patients with resistant conditions whose daily activities may exacerbate the injury, however, may benefit from the use of a counterforce brace.

Only those patients with conditions that have been recalcitrant to all attempts at conservative care, with symptoms of more than 6 months' duration and continual pain without aggravating activity, should undergo surgical debridement. Failure of a series of three corticosteroid injections is a sufficient trial for the efficacy of nonoperative treatment before surgery.

Myofascitis of the Forearm

Lateral epicondylitis does not only refer pain both distally and posteriorly, but also it can lead to a secondary myofascial syndrome of the forearm. Trigger points emanating from the common exterior mass at the muscle belly are common, as are focal areas of irritation of the brachioradialis and supinator muscles. Swelling is infrequent, but a generalized weakness in grip and a loss of functional capacity are common. Combination therapy (ultrasound with electrical muscle stimulation), manual ischemic compression, stretching of the wrist flexors and extensors, and full range-of-motion wrist isotonic exercises are helpful in regaining full capacity of the forearm.

Refractory Pain in the Lateral Elbow

Clinicians should closely evaluate lateral elbow pain that is especially resistant to prudent, systematic care for the possibility of posterior interosseous nerve syndrome. A branch of the radial nerve, the posterior interosseous nerve splits into sensory and motor branches at the elbow, and the short radial extensor muscle of the wrist receives its innervation from both branches. The nerve is susceptible to compression at the level of the two heads of the supinator muscle. Anatomically, this area is referred to as the Arcade of Frohse. If the compression affects the sensory branch, the patient may experience lateral elbow pain; if it affects the motor portion, weak wrist extension and a lack of finger extension may result. Nerve conduction studies will show retardation of nerve impulses across the Arcade of Frohse.[9]

Posterior Compartment: Forced Extension Injuries

Repetitive extension may result from either force or high-velocity movements. The concavity of the olecranon fossa of the humerus facilitates elbow extension to 0 de-

---

Table 4-5 Compression Injuries to the Elbow

	Lateral Epicondylitis	Myofascitis of Forearm
Physical examination findings	Palpable tenderness anterior and distal to lateral epicondyle at extensor carpi radialis brevis Sometimes direct tenderness at lateral epicondyle Pain on active extension, with or without resistance Bogginess or thickening over common extensor aponeurosis Weakness in grip Positive Mills' and Cozen's tests	Pain on wrist extension Palpable tender points (trigger points) in extensors of forearm Hypertonicity of wrist extensors Weak grip
X-ray findings	Usually normal Necessary to rule out soft-tissue calcification around lateral epicondyle	Normal
Treatment plan	Active rest, transverse friction massage, ice, electrotherapy, putty exercise Counterforce brace for heavy activity Strengthening exercises for forearm Rest, ice, electrotherapy, or pulsed ultrasound Counterforce brace Oral NSAIDs If refractory, rest, ice, injections (limited to series of three), manipulation Surgical debridement as last resort	Ice massage, ultrasound, soft-tissue stretching Acupressure, isotonic exercise

NSAIDs, Nonsteroidal antiinflammatory drugs.

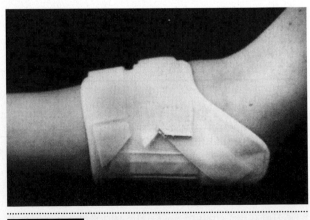

Figure 4-8 Use of a counterforce brace, the Nirschl tennis elbow support, to immobilize and compress the injured tendon.

(From Torg JS, Shephard RJ: *Current therapy in sports medicine,* ed 3, St Louis, 1995, Mosby.)

grees (i.e., terminal extension). The fossa itself, together with the anterior capsule and biceps muscle,[29] checks any extension past the terminal point. Continuous impaction of the olecranon process into the olecranon fossa causes arthritic bone build-up and a flexion deformity at the joint.

Variations in the elbow's normal terminally extended position can occur in a congenital or an acquired scenario. The individual who can actively hyperextend the elbow usually has a generalized ligamentous and capsular laxity. On the other hand, an individual may develop a flexion contracture as a result of extension overload and posterior abutment that causes recurrent anterior capsular sprains. Degenerative changes at the olecranon fossa may also alter an individual's terminally extended position. Some patients may be unable to flex their elbow actively because of posterior capsule sprains, triceps tendonitis, or intraarticular loose bodies.[32]

Triceps Strain and Tendonitis

The primary means of controlling elbow extension is the triceps muscle; the anconeus muscle participates in extension control to only a small degree. The act of throwing may cause pain in the triceps muscle, since both the valgus extension overload during the early acceleration phase and rapid deceleration phase of throwing can cause pain.

Rapid acceleration may cause a wedging of the olecranon in the olecranon fossa. Rapid deceleration in the throwing motion not only causes severe tension in the triceps mechanism, but it also creates traction on the anterior capsule. At this point in the throwing movement the rotator cuff and triceps must decelerate the upper limb in motion, and the triceps must strongly and efficiently complete an eccentric contraction. Posterior impingement may result in further degenerative changes at the posterior compartment of the elbow joint.

Carpenters, baseball players, and weight lifters who repeatedly subject their elbows to resisted extension are likely candidates for the familiar flexion contracture and posterior elbow tenderness (Table 4-6). Often, degenerative changes in the olecranon fossa impede terminal extension in these individuals.

When attempting to help patients with internal derangements of the elbow regain complete extension postimmobilization, the clinician must proceed with caution. It is essential to avoid passive forced extension; otherwise, the development of a myositis of the anterior brachial musculature may further complicate matters. Gentle, gradual active mobilization exercise is a wiser choice.

Degenerative Arthritis of the Posterior Compartment

The actual mechanism of injury in the patient with degenerative arthritis of the elbow is similar to that in the patient with posterior muscle strain. Because the history of dysfunction and pain is usually a lengthy one in degenerative arthritis, the periarticular soft-tissue structures can no longer absorb the forces placed on the elbow, and therefore the osseous structures must bear the stress at the posterior compartment.

Traumatic Olecranon Bursitis

Although not an extension injury by nature, traumatic bursitis of the elbow involves the olecranon bursa and posterior aspect of the elbow. The patient either accidentally bangs the point of the elbow down on a hard surface or sustains a contusion through an external moving force. In either case the elbow swells posteriorly as the bursa sac fills with a combination of synovial fluid and blood (Figure 4-9). Just as there is no true effusion in a prepatellar bursitis at the knee, there is no true effusion in traumatic bursitis of the elbow.

Because of the extraarticular soft-tissue swelling, flexion is painful for patients with traumatic olecranon bursitis. The amount of trauma endured at the elbow joint determines the need for radiographic studies and the type that should be taken. Treatment consists of the application of ice and compression, protection of the bursa from further insult, and further investigation to rule out concomitant traumatic injuries. Only in isolated, stubborn cases should the blood be drained from the bursa, and only as a last stage procedure, when pain and swelling are recurrent, should a bursectomy be performed. In the latter case the body may form another synovial sac to replace the old bursa.

Athletic individuals who continue to participate in contact sports (e.g., wrestling, hockey, football) should wear protective padding over the affected posterior elbow. This will help discourage the development of chronic traumatic changes, such as coagulation of blood ("rice-body" formation). Once such changes take place, the bursa is usually chronically tender to external pressure.

Pediatric Elbow Injuries

Throwing sports and gymnastics are responsible for a large portion of pediatric elbow injuries.[18] Repetitive activities such as overhead throwing make particularly imposing demands on the skeletally immature elbow. Injuries from such athletic endeavors as baseball pitching

Table 4-6 Injuries to the Posterior Compartment of the Elbow

	Triceps Strain and Tendonitis	**Degenerative Arthritis**	**Traumatic Olecranon Bursitis**
Physical examination findings	Posterior elbow tenderness Discomfort at proximal olecranon Painful forced extension with resistance Possible pain on full elbow flexion	Flexion contracture Joint stiffness and lack of functional mobility History of painful extension	Swelling No true joint effusion Painful flexion Point tenderness over olecranon fossa
X-ray findings	Usually normal after acute injury	Posterior osteophytes Traction spurs at olecranon process Joint space narrowing	Usually normal Need to rule out olecranon fracture in advanced trauma
Treatment plan	Ice massage Rest Underwater ultrasound Graded exercise	Continuous ultrasound Maintenance of remaining range of motion Strengthening through functional pain-free arcs	Application of ice and compression Protective padding for athletics Need to rule out concomitant injury

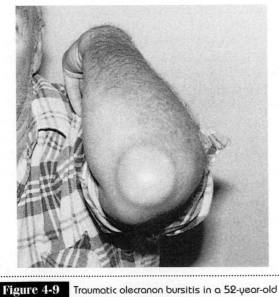

Figure 4-9 Traumatic olecranon bursitis in a 52-year-old laborer.

may potentially damage a youngster's epiphyseal plate, muscle-tendon units, and articular cartilage.[16] It is actually possible to begin to predict subsequent orthopedic problems in child athletes, for example, depending on the specific biomechanical demands of the sport and age of the patient.

Although the mechanisms of injury are similar in children and adults, the pathologic effect of injury in the immature recreational athlete is directly correlated to bone age. Bones are stronger when they have matured and when the growth plate has closed (Table 4-7). During periods of rapid growth, a child's joints are quite susceptible to muscle-tendon imbalance, and they lack flexibility. Furthermore, growth cartilage is less resistant to repetitive loads. As a result, youngsters tend to have overuse injuries near or at the epiphyseal plate or the tendon attachment at the apophysis. Thus skeletal maturity and time of fusion of the secondary ossification centers play a role in the type of injury sustained and the prognosis for complete recovery.

Osteochondritis Dissecans

Typically occurring in the skeletally immature patient, osteochondritis dissecans is a disease of the articular cartilage and bone at the capitellum. It has been postulated that the cause of this disorder is either trauma or a vascular aberration, but the true cause probably lies somewhere in between. Repeated athletic movements such as those required in baseball or racquet sports usually bring about the typical symptomatology: intermittent effusions, locking, limited extension, lateral joint line pain, and stiffness (Table 4-8).[35]

The compressive forces placed on the lateral side of the elbow by throwing activities can lead to articular cartilage damage in the distal humerus, either alone or concomitantly with osteocartilaginous lesions of the radial head (Figure 4-10).[26] During the follow-through phase of throwing a baseball, for example, the elbow pushes through extension with forearm pronation causing a valgus thrust and shearing stress of the radio-

Table 4-7	Secondary Centers of Ossification in the Pediatric Elbow	
		Age (years)
Capitellum		2
Medial epicondyle		4
Radial head		5
Trochlea		8
Olecranon		9
Lateral epicondyle		10

capitellar joint. Anterolateral elbow pain is a clinical sign of lateral compartment incongruence. The practitioner should check the motions of the proximal radioulnar joint to make certain that the patient with anterolateral elbow pain does not have a fractured radial head.

Loose bodies do not form in the beginning stage of osteochondritis dissecans. At this point the clinical picture is similar to that of Panner's disease—an osteochondrosis of the capitellum that may or may not be related to trauma and affects primarily boys between the ages of 5 and 10 years. Usually, Panner's disease involves the entire capitellum, but it runs a benign course. Both osteochondritis dissecans and Panner's disease may be the result of lateral elbow compression that can lead to vascular insult and bony fragmentation. If there is no loose body formation, children who develop osteochondritis dissecans when younger than the age of 13 years generally recover uneventfully with rest and physiotherapy to reduce pain and swelling.

Adolescents and young adults must be treated according to the amount of dysfunction and joint incongruence, loose body formation, and pain. Competitive pitchers in baseball are frequently treated surgically, if they do not respond to conservative care. In the presence of advanced articular cartilage destruction and loose fragments, surgery may enable them to continue their athletic careers.

Osteochondritis dissecans is seldom seen in an adult thrower, because it usually forces an adolescent with the condition to curtail his or her career. In essence, the adolescent's throwing arm never reaches the active competitive stage in early adulthood.

Little League Elbow

Although the overuse syndrome sometimes called *Little League elbow* is found mostly in young baseball players, any skeletally immature person may suffer the conse-

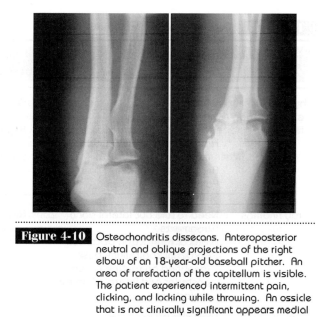

Figure 4-10 Osteochondritis dissecans. Anteroposterior neutral and oblique projections of the right elbow of an 18-year-old baseball pitcher. An area of rarefaction of the capitellum is visible. The patient experienced intermittent pain, clicking, and locking while throwing. An ossicle that is not clinically significant appears medial to the trochlea of the humerus.

quences of soft-tissue microtrauma at the elbow. Thus the syndrome includes a number of orthopedic disorders that result from repetitive valgus stress to the young elbow joint.

Many young athletes must throw hard continuously. There are more than 2 million participants in Little League baseball alone. Young pitchers, especially those under 15 years of age, usually lack the control and accuracy of older, more highly skilled pitchers; as a result, the youngsters throw more balls than strikes and must throw more pitches per inning. In these young pitchers the repeated valgus stress of pitching applies traction forces to the medial growth center of the elbow. Tensile forces in the acceleration phase of throwing can create stresses that lead to medial traction apophysitis, as well as flexor strain associated with medial epicondylitis. Throwing sidearm or "leading" with the elbow and slinging the ball appears to increase these shear forces and exposes the youngster to an even higher risk of injury.

Compressive forces affect the lateral portion of the elbow joint. This pathomechanical situation leads to radiocapitellar disease with or without loose body formation. Osteochondritis of the capitellum can lead to loose body formation. The distal epiphyseal plate is the weak link in the adolescent radius,[14] and osteochondral defects at the radial head can destroy articular surfaces, leading to lateral compartment incongruence.

Youngsters aged 9 to 12 years are most affected by Little League elbow. However, older adolescent throwers

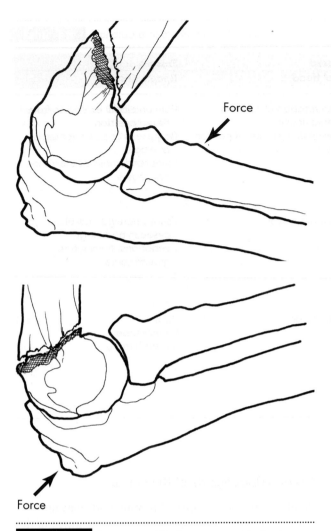

Force

Force

Figure 4-11 Extension and flexion supracondylar fractures.
(From Ruiz E, Cicero JJ: *Emergency management of skeletal injuries*, ed 1, St Louis, 1995, Mosby.)

Case Study

A 20-year-old pitcher from a college baseball team had a 6-month history of elbow pain, medial joint tenderness, and intermittent swelling. Valgus stress tests resulted in medial elbow pain; wrist flexion and forearm pronation were painful to the patient.

A standard three-view x-ray film series of the dominant right elbow was taken. A chip fracture of the medial epicondyle was clear in the anteroposterior projection, but displacement was minimal. Because

the patient had not responded to rehabilitation (at his college's athletic training facility) consisting of ice, ultrasound treatment, and exercises, the clinician ordered an arthrogram of the affected elbow to rule out the presence of an intraarticular loose body. The arthrogram was normal.

Although the diagnostic study had ruled out a loose body in the elbow joint, the fact that the condition had been refractory to conservative care measures remained a matter of concern. The patient was a throwing athlete who required a significant amount of strength, function, and mobility at the elbow. In addition, the chip fracture was most likely larger than had been visualized on the plain x-ray film, because the fracture had also broken off a dime-sized cartilage cap that did not appear on the film.

The orthopedic surgeon felt that an arthroscopy would not be appropriate because the fragment was not within the articulation; the chip and cap were in the flexor mass off the medial epicondyle. An arthrotomy was scheduled, and the patient made a complete recovery following the procedure.

In summary:

Physical examination findings	• Intermittent swelling of right elbow • Painful flexion, pronation • Palpable tenderness of medial epicondyle
X-ray findings	• Chip fracture of medial epicondyle, right elbow
Diagnosis	• Fracture of medial epicondyle with osteochondral fragment
Treatment plan	• Arthrogram to rule out loose body • Excision • Postsurgical splinting for 7 to 10 days, then follow-up physical therapy

Review Questions

1. (a) State the biomechanical forces at the elbow joint that produce structural tensile loads? (b) What is the chief mechanical stress to the elbow during the throwing motion?

2. (a) What structures may cause pain in the medial compartment of the elbow? (b) What structures may

cause pain in the lateral compartment? (c) What structures may cause pain in the anterior compartment? (d) What structures may cause pain in the posterior compartment? (e) What is indicated in a patient with a hemarthrosis and an elevated fat pad sign on x-ray films?

→ 3. (a) A patient that complains of pain over the extensor mass at the lateral elbow with positive Mills' and Cozen's tests most likely has what condition? (b) Name a minimum of three etiologic factors. (c) Conservative treatment includes what therapies? *a) Lat. epi.*

4. (a) Chronic injury to the medial compartment, including repetitive stress from pitching, often leads to what type of peripheral entrapment neuropathy? (b) What are the signs and symptoms of this condition?

5. (a) Describe Little League Elbow. (b) List ways to prevent this condition.

References

1. Blackard D, Sampson JA: Management of an uncomplicated posterior elbow dislocation, *J Athletic Training* 32(1):63, 1997.
2. Buschbacher RM, Braddon RL: *Sports medicine and rehabilitation: a sport specific approach,* Philadelphia, 1994, Hanley & Blefs.
3. Ciccartelli P: Avoiding elbow pain: tips for young pitchers, *Phys Sports Med* 22(3):65, 1994.
4. Congeni J: Treating and preventing Little League elbow, *Physician Sports Med* 22(3):54, 1994.
5. Drechsler WI, Knarr JF, Snyder-Mackler L: A comparison of two treatment regimens for lateral epicondylitis: a randomized trial of clinical intervention, *J Sports Rehabil* 6:226, 1997.
6. Eppright RH, Wilkins KE: Fractures and dislocations of the elbow. In Rockward CA Jr, Green DP, editors: *Fractures,* Philadelphia, 1975, JB Lippincott.
7. Evans RC: *Illustrated essentials in orthopedic physical assessment,* St Louis, 1994, Mosby.
8. Fox GM, Jebson PL, Orwin JF: Overuse injuries of the elbow, Phys Sports Med 23(8):58, 1995.
9. Gerstner DL, Omer GE: Peripheral entrapment neuropathies in the upper extremity, *Clin Sports Med* 5(4):37, 1988.
10. Gustilo RB, Kyle RF, Templeman DC: *Fractures and dislocations,* vol I, St Louis, 1993, Mosby.
11. Ireland ML, Andrews JB: Shoulder and elbow injuries in the young athlete, *Clin Sports Med* 7(3):473, 1988.
12. Jobe FW, Nuber G: Throwing injuries of the elbow, *Clin Sports Med* 5(4):621, 1986.
13. Joseffson PO et al: Surgery versus non-surgical treatment of ligamentous injuries following dislocation of the elbow, *Clin Orthop* 212:163, 1987.
14. Keats TE: *Radiology of musculoskeletal stress injury,* St Louis , 1990, Mosby.
15. Lachowetz T, Drury D, Elliot R, Evon J, Pastiglione J: The effect of an intercollegiate baseball strength program on the reduction of shoulder and elbow pain, *J of Strength Conditioning Res* 12(1):46, 1998.
16. Maffuli, N, Chan D, Aldridge MJ: Derangement of the articular surfaces of the elbow in young gymnasts, *J Pediatr Orthop* 12(3):344, 1992.
17. Mehlhoff TL, Noble PC, Bennet JB, Tullos HS: Simple dislocation of the elbow in the adult: results after closed treatment, *J Bone Joint Surg [Am]* 70:244, 1988.
18. Meyers JF: Injuries to the shoulder girdle and elbow. In Grana WA, Sullivan JA, editors: *The pediatric athlete,* Park Ridge, Ill., 1990, American Academy of Orthopedic Surgeons.
19. Morrey BF: *The elbow and its disorders,* Philadelphia, 1985, WB Saunders.
20. Nirschl RP: Elbow tendinosis/tennis elbow, *Clinics in Sports Med* 11(4):851, 1992.
21. O'Driscoll SW, Morrey BF: Arthroscopy of the elbow: diagnostic and therapeutic benefits and hazards, *Adv Orthrop Surg* 16(5):285, 1993.
22. Post M: *Physical examination of the musculoskeletal system,* Chicago, 1987, Yearbook Publishers.
23. Rang M: Children's fractures, *Pediatr Clin North Am* 37(6):1523, 1986.
24. Russotti GM, Cooney WP: *Advances in orthopaedic surgery,* Baltimore, 1987, Williams & Wilkins.
25. Russotti GM, Cooney WP: Throwing injuries in baseball pitchers: a review, *Adv Orthop Surg* 11(4):247, 1987.
26. Stanitski CL: Combating overuse injuries: a focus on children and adolescents, *Phys Sports Med* 21(1):87, 1993.
27. Suzuki K, Minami A, Svenaga N, Kondoh M: Oblique stress fracture of the olecranon in baseball pitchers, *J Shoulder Elbow Surg* 6:491, 1997.
28. Torg JS, Shephard RJ: *Current therapy in sports medicine,* ed 3, St Louis, 1995, Mosby.
29. Tullos H, Bennett JB: Ligamentous and articular injuries in the athlete. In Morrey BF, editor: *The elbow and its disorders,* Philadelphia, 1985, WB Saunders.
30. Wadsworth TG: Tennis elbow: conservative, surgical and manipulative treatment, *Br Med J* 294(6572):621, 1987.
31. Wadsworth TG: *The elbow,* New York, 1982, Churchill Livingstone.
32. Warhold LG, Osterman AL, Skirven T: Lateral epicondylitis: how to treat it and prevent recurrence, *J Musculoskeletal Med* 10(6):55, 1993.
33. Weissman B, Sledge C: *Orthopaedic radiology,* Philadelphia, 1986, WB Saunders.
34. Whiteside JA, Andrews JR: Common elbow problems in the recreational athlete, *Clin Sports Med,* 6(2):17, 1989.
35. Williamson LR, Albright JP: Bilateral osteochondritis dissecans of the elbow in a female pitcher, *J Fam Pract* 43:489, 1996.

Chapter 5

Wrist and Hand

PART ONE: THE WRIST

The wrist is made up of an intricate network of complex joints. Because it is so complex, many problems may occur with the wrist, and the condition of a patient with wrist pain is frequently misdiagnosed or undertreated.

Wrist pain often poses a diagnostic dilemma to the examining physician. The physician must be quite meticulous in taking a case history and, as such, ascertain whether the patient's pain has a traumatic or nontraumatic origin. In addition, the location of the pain and its quality and alleviation are important components of the physician's history taking process. Knowledge of surface anatomy is paramount.

Both young and old persons can sustain acute wrist injuries from a fall. Often these injuries occur with an extended wrist and result in significant injuries such as fractures and sprains. Inflammatory conditions evolving from repetitive stress syndromes, either from work-related activities or fitness routines, can cause wrist pain as well.

Anatomy and Function of the Wrist

Not only is the anatomy of the wrist complex (Figure 5-1), but its functions are diverse. Thus the wrist is a network of bones and joints that must be both mobile and stable. No muscles insert directly into the wrist; muscle-tendon units outside the wrist at the forearm control wrist motion, while a network of strong ligaments across the carpus provides stability (Figure 5-2). Therefore the wrist is inherently a weak joint and vulnerable to several types of injuries.

Evaluation of the Wrist

Because of its complex anatomy, a thorough evaluation of a wrist problem includes a complete history and a meticulous physical and radiographic examination. The history is crucial in evaluating wrist pain (Figure 5-3). Acute pain at the wrist generally is the result of trauma or overuse. Sports injuries that involve throwing, twisting, impact, or weight bearing can lead to wrist pain and disability.[63] Chronic pain at the wrist can be mysterious, often with few clinical signs during the examination. It may result from rheumatic, osseous, or metabolic disease:

- Arthritis
- Osteonecrosis (seen in fracture of scaphoid)
- Peripheral neuropathies (e.g., carpal tunnel syndrome, ulnar neuritis)
- Posttraumatic carpal instability
- Malunion of fractures
- Collagen-vascular disease

Radiographic evaluation, laboratory work, and specialist referral may be necessary to determine the cause of chronic wrist dysfunction in difficult cases.

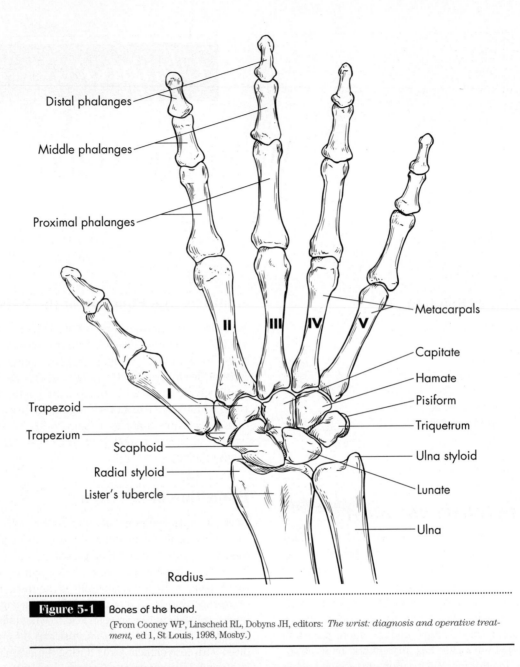

Distal phalanges

Middle phalanges

Proximal phalanges

II III IV V

Metacarpals

Capitate

Hamate

Pisiform

Trapezoid

Triquetrum

Trapezium

Ulna styloid

Scaphoid

Radial styloid

Lunate

Lister's tubercle

Ulna

Radius

Figure 5-1 Bones of the hand.

(From Cooney WP, Linscheid RL, Dobyns JH, editors: *The wrist: diagnosis and operative treatment,* ed 1, St Louis, 1998, Mosby.)

Physical Examination

A history of trauma suggests the possibility of fracture, osteonecrosis, carpal instability, or secondary neurovascular compromise. Pain without a preceding event may be from rheumatoid disorders, an infectious process, or a systemic illness. X-ray films should be scrutinized for ligamentous instability, bony union, and alignment and joint integrity. Stress fractures must be ruled out in athletes who participate in contact sports, such as football and karate (Figure 5-4 *A, B*), or activities that involve repetitive loading of the upper limb, such as gymnastics.

In the physical examination the practitioner asks the patient to perform functional tasks such as wrist movements, thumb opposition, and grip. A bilateral comparison for deformity, swelling, and strength follows. After palpating the carpus and distal forearm to distinguish any unilateral point tenderness, the examiner evaluates the radial aspect of the wrist over the first extensor compartment, thumb, and distal radius on both the dorsal and palmar surfaces. The examiner then palpates the floor of

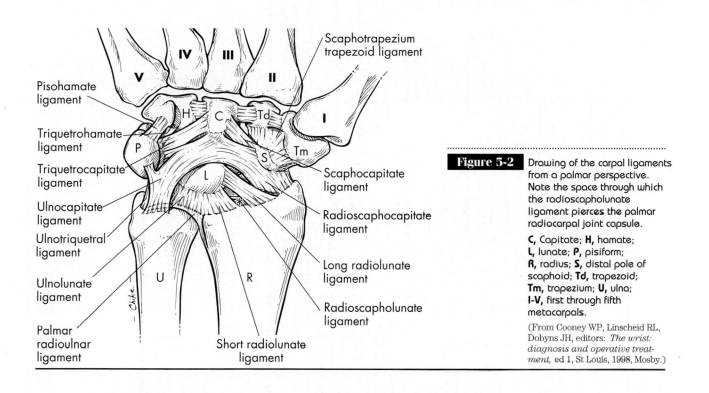

Figure 5-2 Drawing of the carpal ligaments from a palmar perspective. Note the space through which the radioscapholunate ligament pierces the palmar radiocarpal joint capsule.

C, Capitate; **H**, hamate; **L**, lunate; **P**, pisiform; **R**, radius; **S**, distal pole of scaphoid; **Td**, trapezoid; **Tm**, trapezium; **U**, ulna; **I-V**, first through fifth metacarpals.

(From Cooney WP, Linscheid RL, Dobyns JH, editors: *The wrist: diagnosis and operative treatment*, ed 1, St Louis, 1998, Mosby.)

Figure labels:
Scaphotrapezium trapezoid ligament
Pisohamate ligament
Triquetrohamate ligament
Triquetrocapitate ligament
Ulnocapitate ligament
Ulnotriquetral ligament
Ulnolunate ligament
Palmar radioulnar ligament
Short radiolunate ligament
Scaphocapitate ligament
Radioscaphocapitate ligament
Long radiolunate ligament
Radioscapholunate ligament

the anatomic snuffbox for scaphoid tenderness. In addition, the examiner performs the following:

- Exerts digital pressure over the lunate to check the central carpus
- Palpates the ulnar aspect of the wrist over the distal styloid at the triangular fibrocartilage complex and Guyon's canal to investigate the possibility of ulnar nerve referral
- Palpates the tendon sheaths for point tenderness, the presence of ganglion cysts, and generalized swelling
- Tests the motor strength of the wrist flexors (median nerve), wrist extensors (radial nerve), and intrinsic muscles of the hand (ulnar nerve)
- Performs Tinel's tap over the palmar carpal ligament-flexor retinaculum and Phalen's test on wrist flexion to reproduce median nerve symptomatology (Figure 5-5 *A, B*)
- Tests opposition strength of the thumb and thenar musculature to rule out median nerve entrapment at the carpal tunnel

Additional tests may include orthopedic examination of the elbow to rule out more proximal entrapment neuropathies or examination of the cervical spine to exclude radiculopathy secondary to a cervical disk syndrome or spondylosis.[60] Electrodiagnostic studies can be ordered to complement the physical examination and to differentiate between a peripheral (i.e., arm, wrist, hand) and a central (i.e., spine) lesion.[75] Helpful electrophysiologic studies may include somatosensory-evoked potential (SSEP) and dermatomal-evoked potential (DEP) determinations, nerve conduction velocity (NCV) tests, electromyography (EMG), and F wave tests.

Radiographic Examination

The standard radiographic projections needed to investigate a wrist problem include a minimum of three views: (1) posteroanterior, (2) posteroanterior oblique, and (3) lateral. Posteroanterior ulnar deviation films are a key component of routine imaging in patients with a suspected scaphoid fracture.[52] Carpal tunnel views with the wrist in flexion can aid in the diagnosis of hamate fractures.

It is wise to inspect the posteroanterior view for three normal arcs at the wrist, as well as to examine the spacing of the intercarpal joints. Angles between the individual carpals become significant in screening for carpal instability. The scapholunate angle should come under particular scrutiny in any patient who complains of wrist

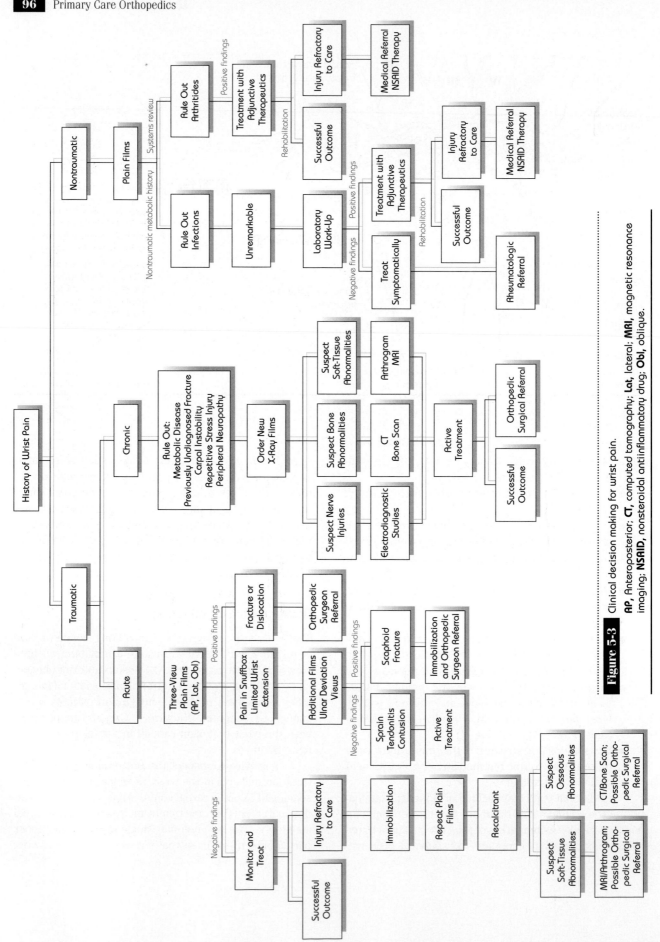

Figure 5-3   Clinical decision making for wrist pain.

AP, Anteroposterior; **CT,** computed tomography; **Lat,** lateral; **MRI,** magnetic resonance imaging; **NSAID,** nonsteroidal antiinflammatory drug; **Obl,** oblique.

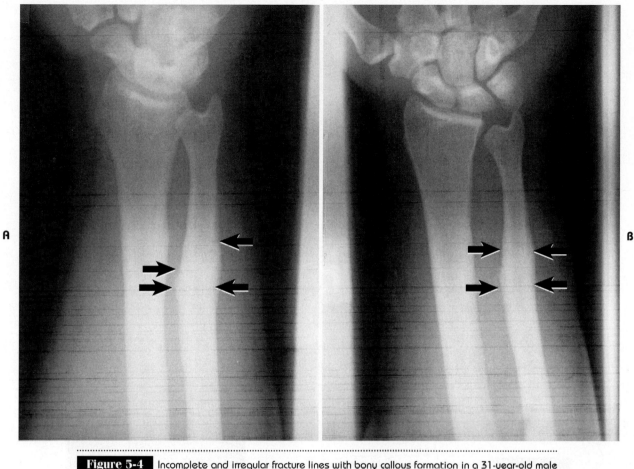

Figure 5-4 Incomplete and irregular fracture lines with bony callous formation in a 31-year-old male martial arts participant. History of forearm pain over the ulna for the previous 1½ years suggested multiepisodal stress fractures with incomplete bony healing. **A,** Oblique projection. **B,** Anteroposterior projection.

pain of unknown origin (Figure 5-6 *A, B*).[66] The presence of a Terry Thomas sign (i.e., a gap more than 2 mm on the posteroanterior film) suggests a scapholunate dissociation.

The lateral projection provides an easy window to observe the scapholunate angle, which should be approximately 60 degrees. This view also illustrates the position of the lunate distal to the radius.

The practitioner may order supplemental films, depending on the type and amount of past trauma or the strength of a clinical suspicion of underlying carpal instability. In some cases, advanced imaging modalities may be necessary to reach an accurate diagnosis. Conventional and computed tomography (CT) are helpful in the diagnosis of occult fractures, metabolic osseous disorders (e.g., osteochondrosis), and stress reactions of

bone.[74] Nuclear scintigraphy can be helpful in assessing stress fractures at the wrist and localizing metabolic bone lesions.[77]

Magnetic resonance imaging (MRI) is an effective technique in the evaluation of wrist disease and dysfunction.[52] It is useful in identifying soft-tissue lesions at the wrist, such as tendonitis,[52] and investigating the cause of chronic nonspecific wrist pain (Figure 5-7).[99] Arthrography and MRI at the wrist facilitate the evaluation of the triangular fibrocartilage complex. Special films can rule out ligamentous or capsular instability.

Disorders of the Wrist

For simplicity, the causes of wrist dysfunction can be divided into three categories:

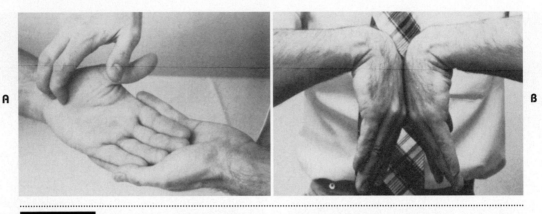

A

B

Figure 5-5 **A,** Tinel's tap. Percussion of the median nerve at the carpal tunnel may reproduce pain and tingling along the median nerve distribution. **B,** Phalen's test. The symptoms may also be reproduced after 1 minute of acute wrist flexion against resistance.

(From Mercier LR: *Practical Orthopedics,* ed 4, St Louis, 1995, Mosby.)

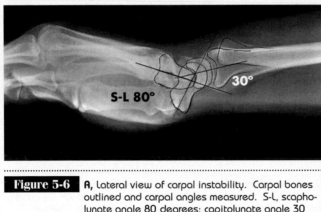

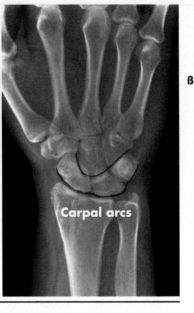

A

B

Figure 5-6 **A,** Lateral view of carpal instability. Carpal bones outlined and carpal angles measured. S-L, scapholunate angle 80 degrees; capitolunate angle 30 degrees. **B,** Posteroanterior view of the wrist demonstrates carpal arcs of the proximal carpal row (scaphoid, lunate, and triquetrum) and distal carpal row (capitate and hamate).

(From Cooney WP, Linscheid RL, Dobyns JH, editors: *The wrist: diagnosis and operative treatment,* ed 1, St Louis, 1998, Mosby.)

1. Inflammatory conditions, including De Quervain's tenosynovitis, tendonitis of the wrist, intersegmental carpal dysfunction, and synovitis
2. Traumatic conditions, such as scaphoid fractures, hook of the hamate fractures, Colles' fractures, post-traumatic carpal instability, Kienböck's disease, ganglion cysts, triangular fibrocartilage tears, and extensor carpi ulnaris subluxation
3. Neurovascular injuries, including carpal tunnel syndrome and Guyon's tunnel syndrome or ulnar neuritis

Inflammatory Conditions

De Quervain's Disease

Described as an inflammation of the first extensor compartment (Table 5-1), De Quervain's disease is a tenosynovitis of two specific tendons: the abductor pollicis longus and the extensor pollicis brevis. These two tendons can become inflamed as they pass through the first dorsal extensor compartment of the wrist at approximately the level of the radial styloid. Progression of the inflammation leads to swelling of the tendons, thickening of the sheaths, and, ultimately, fibroses.[27] The patient may per-

Table 5-1   Inflammatory Conditions of the Wrist

	De Quervain's Disease	Tendonitis	Intersegmental Carpal Dysfunction	Synovitis
Physical examination findings	Swelling over first extensor compartment Palpable tenderness over radial styloid Painful ulnar deviation (Finkelstein's test)	Possibly some localized swelling or bogginess over extensor hood, near retinaculum or more distal along each particular extensor tendon sheath Painful passive stretch and active resistance Flexor inflammation, palpable tenderness along flexor tendon sheath or near volar carpal ligament Need to rule out carpal tunnel syndrome	History of previous trauma, immobilization, or arthritide Negative effusion Unremarkable neurovascular examination findings Weakness in functional tasks Painful to pressure or extremes of joint motion	Effusion Often limited and painful range of motion Evaluation of neurovascular status Possible fever and lymphadenopathy Need to rule out systemic and osseous pathologic conditions
X-ray findings	Normal	Usually normal	Usually not taken unless underlying arthritide or bony instability from trauma is suspected	Important to rule out arthritide, infection, or carpal instability Minimum of three views
Treatment plan	Ice and electrotherapy Immobilization, if necessary Medical referral for medication or injection in cases of advanced disease	Ice and electrotherapy in cool water or pulsed ultrasound underwater Immobilization, if necessary Gradual strengthening exercises	Ice Careful evaluation of lunate Protection of dysfunctional segment Mobilization or manipulation to hypomobile and fixated carpal segments	Ice and electrical stimulation Possible need for laboratory evaluation Medical referral sometimes needed for infection or advanced rheumatoid disease

ceive pain as distal as the first metacarpophalangeal joint and as proximal as the distal one third of the forearm.

De Quervain's disease is more common in women, occurring at a ratio of 4 to 1.[78] It frequently occurs in recreational athletes (e.g., participants in racquet sports), schoolteachers, machinists, typists, and printers —those who engage in constant, repetitive motions that require ulnar deviation of the wrist. In addition, the number of women who develop De Quervain's disease during pregnancy and in the postpartum period has increased, suggesting an association between the disease and the levels of estrogen. In the past, hormonal influx has been shown to cause peripheral neuropathies, such as carpal tunnel syndrome.[82,83]

Diagnosis of De Quervain's Disease. Physical examination of the patient with De Quervain's disease usually reveals a local tenderness and bogginess at the wrist, often associated with soft-tissue swelling at the level of the radial styloid; this area is usually quite tender to palpation. Extension of the thumb brings out the contour of the painful tendons.

It has been said that tenderness on thumb flexion to the palm and ulnar deviation (Finkelstein's test) is a pathognomonic sign of first extensor compartment tenosynovitis (Figure 5-8 *A, B*). Usually, pain is exquisite in the region of the radial styloid. There should be a bilateral comparison if Finkelstein's test reveals tenderness, however, since the test can cause some discomfort

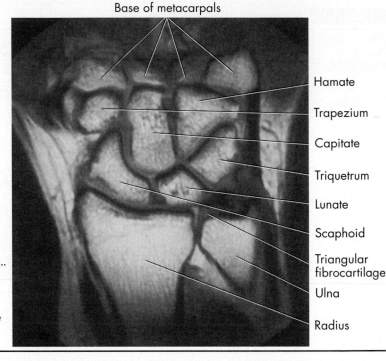

Base of metacarpals

Hamate

Trapezium

Capitate

Triquetrum

Lunate

Scaphoid

Triangular fibrocartilage

Ulna

Radius

Figure 5-7 Magnetic resonance image showing the soft tissues, bony detail, and cartilage structures of the wrist.

(From Bushong SC: *Magnetic resonance imaging: physical and biological principles,* ed 2, St Louis, 1996, Mosby.)

either to the average patient who has first extensor compartment tendonitis without the clinical signs or to the patient who has basal-thumb arthritis. If the first metacarpophalangeal joint is compromised in any way, either via osteoarthritis or rheumatoid arthritis, a plain x-ray film should help the practitioner differentiate between the two clinical entities.

Treatment of De Quervain's Disease. The stage of the disease determines the appropriate treatment for De Quervain's disease, and the length of time that the patient delays before seeking care may determine the stage of the disease. An individual with De Quervain's tendonitis may wait 6 days, 6 weeks, or 6 months to seek treatment after the onset of pain. To complicate matters further, De Quervain's disease can be very resistant to treatment.

In the early stages of De Quervain's disease, when the inflammatory process seems to be limited to some synovial irritation of the tendon sheath, the patient's symptoms may resolve with the use of aggressive cryotherapy and electrotherapy. In the latter stages of the disease, when the condition is refractory to all channels of care, thickening of the roof of the first dorsal extensor compartment can actually lead to stenosis of the canal through which the tendons pass. When this occurs, conservative treatment may be ineffective. Sometimes the patient needs a medical referral for medication, injection, and in rare instances decompression surgery.

Many patients use their hands even when their hands are injured. It may be easy to rest a knee or an ankle by not walking, but many basic daily activities, such as eating and dressing, involve the thumb and wrist. It is imperative to prevent further injury by changing the mechanics in the patient's workplace early in treatment and to stabilize the injury initially with the use of ice, electrotherapy, and a brace, if needed. When ordering this treatment, the primary care provider should explain that the condition is often highly resistant to treatment; therefore it is very important for the patient to follow the instructions carefully.

There are five stages of care, ranging from the most conservative to the most invasive. The first stage of care involves the use of electrotherapy in the office of the primary care provider and the application of ice at home for 10 to 15 minutes of every hour possible to reduce inflammation and swelling. Obviously, any activity that requires ulnar deviation should be curtailed. At this stage it is not usually necessary for the patient to stay out of work, although he or she should try to work around the injury. Active treatment with underwater electrotherapy, cryotherapy, and words of caution until the symptoms abate are usually sufficient at this stage.

The second stage of care is necessary when symptoms are more severe. In addition to the components of the first stage of care, the patient may need a thumb spica brace to immobilize the wrist during the performance of some mechanical tasks. This brace helps alleviate some of the tenderness in the first extensor compartment when the patient must constantly use the hands. Braces that only go around the wrist are ineffective; simultaneous immobilization of both the first extensor compartment and the thumb is essential.

The patient who does not seek care for several weeks, who has not followed the provider's instructions, or who reinjures the wrist needs the third stage of care. Treatment at this time involves continued electrotherapy and cryotherapy, as well as the continued use of the thumb spica brace, but the patient's pain and discomfort may also require time off from work and the oral administration of antiinflammatory medication. Usually the patient should begin drug therapy by taking an over-the-counter drug, such as ibuprofen or naproxen sodium, particularly if the patient has had any previous gastric sensitivity to prescription-strength nonsteriodal antiinflammatory drugs. If the patient's condition does not respond, a referral to a medical physician is often helpful to obtain a prescription for a stronger antiinflammatory medication.

When the condition is not responding to medication and conservative treatment, care moves into the fourth stage. At this point, continued pinpoint tenderness may warrant referral for an injection of an anesthetic and a steroid to alleviate the patient's severe discomfort and pain. Usually a combination of the anesthetic lidocaine (Xylocaine) with the steroid methylprednisolone (Depo-Medrol) is helpful. The patient should continue to ice the area aggressively at home; in addition, he or she should stay out of work and continue to use the immobilizer.

Fortunately, few cases of this tenosynovitis require the fifth stage of care and only if the condition has been recalcitrant to all other levels of care. A patient with such advanced disease has so much fibrosis and chronic adhesion formation in the first extensor compartment that a stenotic situation develops over the radial styloid. A true stenosing tenosynovitis that has resisted all types of conservative and nonconservative care requires surgical decompression in which the surgeon splays open the tendon sheaths. Although its location (hand and thumb) makes this tenosynovitis a difficult clinical entity to treat, most patients do not have to resort to surgical decompression.

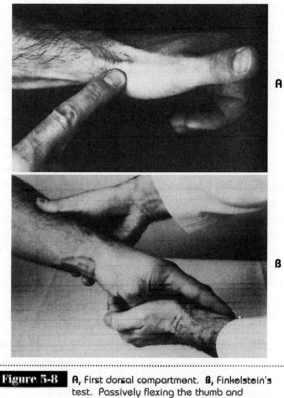

Figure 5-8 A, First dorsal compartment. B, Finkelstein's test. Passively flexing the thumb and adducting the wrist reproduces pain in the first dorsal compartment.

(From Mercier LR: *Practical Orthopedics*, ed 4, St Louis, 1995, Mosby.)

Tendonitis of the Wrist

People who are physically active are more likely to develop tendonitis of the wrist. They may complain of pain over the common extensor tendon hood or over the wrist retinaculum, or they may have flexor tendonitis over the flexor tendon sheath.

Clinical examination reveals a well-localized tenderness over the involved tendons. Passive stretching generally accentuates the pain. The practitioner should also make the patient actively contract the associated muscle against resistance. Plain x-ray films are usually normal. If the patient's pain has persisted for some time or if initial treatment has failed, radiographic studies are helpful in ruling out any underlying osseous abnormality. In the older patient the plain films may reveal calcific flecks within the affected tendon sheath.

Most cases of tendonitis in the wrist are associated with overuse. The history often uncovers subtle changes in activity levels. The individual may have suddenly begun to carry out new tasks at work or to participate in new physical activities. The patient with tendonitis of the wrist usually has a point tenderness localized over the tendon sheath or the retinaculum, as well as stiffness and a deep dull ache that is aggravated by activity. Often, patients seek treatment only because a recent event has caused them exquisite pain; they may have experienced discomfort for several months or even years without seeking treatment.

Treatment should center on the use of ice, electrotherapy, or pulsed ultrasound performed under water, along with the avoidance of any aggravating activity for several days. If the tendonitis is especially resistant to treatment, it may be necessary for the patient to place the wrist in an immobilizer during the period of aggressive treatment. Workers or athletes who may have to participate in activities that compromise the wrist may need the wrist taped in a thumb spica.

Most cases of extensor or flexor tendonitis of the wrist are not as difficult to treat as cases of De Quervain's disease. In general, tendonitis of the wrist can be treated conservatively, without medication, and in a steplike manner. A graduated exercise program involving grip, extension and flexion of the wrist, and flexibility training frequently hastens the patient's recovery.

Intersegmental Carpal (Wrist) Dysfunction

Among the conditions that commonly lead to joint dysfunction at the wrist are osteoarthritis, early- to middle-stage rheumatoid arthritis, and postimmobilization intercarpal dyskinesia. Usually, intersegmental dysfunction of the wrist centers around the intercarpal joints or the radiocarpal articulation. Patients with this condition may have had a prior traumatic episode or a moderate soft-tissue injury that was never fully rehabilitated. A physical examination reveals few neurovascular findings, no effusion, pain with wrist pressure or extreme joint movement, and weakness in functional tasks.

Several joint play movements can be performed at the wrist: (1) long-axis traction, (2) anteroposterior glide, (3) side-to-side glide, and (4) side tilt. Candidates for such manipulations must meet the following orthopedic criteria:

- No recent history of a macrotraumatic episode
- No effusion
- No radiographic evidence of carpal instability at the site of the proposed manipulation
- No physical or clinical evidence of intersegmental hypermobility at the site of the proposed manipulation

Each carpal bone can be mobilized individually in the stabilization of the adjacent carpal bone during each of the four joint play movements listed. For example, the practitioner can check the scaphoid for anteroposterior glide by fixating the radius with the proximal hand. The thumb is then in a semiopposition posture, as in a modified Finkelstein's maneuver (see Figure 5-8).

Long-Axis Traction. At the distal radioulnar joint, the convex head of the ulna articulates with the concave ulna notch of the distal radius. The radiocarpal joint involves the convex surfaces of the scaphoid, lunate, and triquetrum, articulating with the concave surface of the radius.[20] Both of these regions are included in long-axis traction mobilization. First, the clinician performs a bilateral comparison of the patient's joint movement to determine the inherent motion and laxity of the joint. The practitioner then uses one hand to stabilize the long bone of the patient's forearm. This hand will grip the distal radioulnar joint proximal to the patient's wrist. The practitioner places the other hand just distal to the carpus and provides a gentle yet firm distractive force at the wrist-carpus interface. This movement places long-axis traction on the wrist.

Anteroposterior Glide. During an anteroposterior glide, the practitioner checks both the proximal and distal rows of carpal bones. First, the practitioner places the stabilizing hand just proximal to the radiocarpal joint, in a position similar to that used in long-axis traction. The distal hand is around the proximal row of the carpal bones. The two hands should be next to each other.[38] The force of the distal hand applied through the proximal row of carpals creates the anteroposterior sliding motion as the proximal hand stabilizes the radiocarpal joint.

Next, the mobilizing hand moves down to the distal carpus to produce movement in the carpal bones. At this point the stabilizing hand should firmly grasp the proximal row of carpals. The mobilizing hand exerts a gliding force through the distal row of carpal bones.

The lunate warrants careful attention during these manipulations, because it is frequently the culprit for carpal dysfunction. Many times it is painfully fixated, but it usually responds to manipulation and short-term inactivity or protection.

Side-to-Side Glide. There is less gross joint play of the carpus in the side-to-side glide than in the previous two movements. It is always important to check for symmetry of movement at the opposite wrist. The actual technique of the side-to-side glide is similar to that of the anteroposterior glide; the practitioner follows the procedure described earlier for each row of carpal bones.

Side Tilt. In a side tilt of the carpals, the practitioner stabilizes the distal radiocarpal joint with the stabilizing hand while providing ulnar and radial deviation of the carpus with the mobilizing hand.[56]

Synovitis of the Wrist

Nonspecific inflammation and swelling of the wrist may be a sign of metabolic or osseous pathologic variations. A complete history is imperative in determining the primary cause of pain and dysfunction. It is necessary to evaluate the range of motion, neurovascular status, and strength of the hand and wrist. Rheumatoid arthritis, Kienböck's osteonecrosis, posttraumatic carpal instability, and collagen-vascular disorders can all cause a synovitis of the wrist. Cuts, bites, and puncture wounds suggest infection. In addition to an examination for lymphadenopathy and fever, laboratory tests and cultures may be necessary to rule out infection. The practitioner who suspects a bony pathologic abnormality or an osseous deformity as a result of rheumatoid arthritis should order x-ray films.

Treatment generally involves the application of ice and electrical stimulation to relieve pain and swelling. Immobilization for a short period of time may help alleviate pain and protect the injury site. Strengthening exercises with putty or rubber bands may help the patient return to full activity. A program of functional, task-oriented exercise is best for these individuals. Referral to a medical physician may become necessary should the patient require antiinflammatory medication. Patients with advanced rheumatoid disorders may best be co-treated with a rheumatologist.

Traumatic Conditions

Scaphoid Fractures

The scaphoid bone plays a crucial role in carpal stability by acting as a scaffold (hence, the name scaphoid) between the two rows of carpal bones. The anatomic linkage of the proximal and distal rows of carpal bones provided by the scaphoid and its associated ligaments prevents collapse and deformity in the healthy wrist.

Diagnosis of a Scaphoid Fracture. The examiner can assess the contributing role of the scaphoid in any posttraumatic carpal instability by measuring the angle between the scaphoid and adjacent bones. For example, the scapholunate angle should be approximately 60 degrees on a routine lateral plain x-ray film. In addition, the proximal margins of the scaphoid, lunate, and triquetrum should line up on a posteroanterior projection of a healthy wrist. A dissociation between the scaphoid and the lunate of more than 2 mm is a pathologic sign frequently cited in cases of posttraumatic carpal instability (i.e., Terry Thomas sign). It appears on the posteroanterior wrist projection and is diagnostic of ligamentous instability at the wrist.[95]

The scaphoid is the most commonly injured carpal bone.[14] A prompt, accurate diagnosis of a fracture is of paramount importance. The typical presentation of a scaphoid fracture includes a history of a blunt blow to the wrist or a fall on an outstretched hand and wrist (Table 5-2). In a fall, scaphoid injury usually occurs when the wrist is dorsiflexed and radially deviated; distal radial fractures can occur when the wrist is only slightly dorsiflexed.[32] For any patient with such a history and wrist pain, the practitioner should check for the following:

- Limited and painful dorsiflexion
- Palpable tenderness in the floor of the anatomic snuffbox
- Swelling

Patients who exhibit any two of these findings should immobilize the wrist and have another x-ray film taken in 7 to 10 days if the first films are equivocal.

Multiple radiographic views are strongly recommended for patients who may have a scaphoid fracture. In addition to the three standard wrist views (i.e., anteroposterior, lateral, and oblique), the clinician should obtain an ulnar deviation projection. The latter projection sometimes demonstrates a subtle fracture line. More advanced imaging such as magnetic resonance is often helpful after fracture to detect avascular necrosis.[92]

Treatment of a Scaphoid Fracture. The primary reason for the high nonunion rate of a scaphoid fracture is a delay in diagnosis and inadequate immobilization.[47] Therefore treatment should be quite aggressive. As noted earlier, immobilization should begin with suggestive symptomatology, even in the absence of radiographic signs of fracture. Sometimes, 7 to 14 days must pass before there is sufficient resorption along the fracture line to make the injury clear on a radiographic film.

Fractures to the scaphoid make up more than 60% of all carpal fractures.[95] Of these, 70% occur in the middle third of the bone (waist).[47] Because the scaphoid's blood supply enters distally, fractures to the distal and middle third tend to heal at a faster rate than fractures of the proximal pole. The latter may require periods of immobilization as long as 12 to 16 weeks, whereas the former may require immobilization for 8 to 12 weeks.

Distal, horizontal-oriented fractures are usually treated successfully with a short-arm thumb spica cast.

Table 5-2 Fractures of the Wrist

	Scaphoid Fracture	Hook of the Hamate Fracture	Colles' Fracture
Physical examination findings	Limited and painful dorsiflexion Palpable tenderness in anatomic snuffbox History of trauma Swelling	Palpable tenderness over hook of hamate Weakness in grip strength Ulnar nerve paresthesia Tenosynovitis of ulnar aspect of wrist	Dorsal swelling, deformity of distal radius (e.g., abnormal contour of bone, bumps, angles) Lack of distal radioulnar joint motion Traumatic fall on outstretched hand Point tenderness over distal fracture site Need to rule out carpal tunnel syndrome
X-ray findings	Minimum of four views: postero-anterior, lateral, oblique, and ulnar deviation Fracture line most likely visible on oblique or ulnar deviation projection*	Four views: carpal tunnel, antero-posterior, lateral, and oblique Lateral trispiral tomography at 1-mm to 2-mm increments, if diagnosis is in doubt	Forearm films, including wrist and elbow "Silver fork" deformity in distal fracture of radius
Treatment plan	Immobilization Ice and electrical stimulation Referral to orthopedic surgeon	Referral to orthopedic surgeon Immobilization, if diagnosed early Excision of fracture fragment, if conservative care is ineffective	Referral to orthopedic surgeon for cast immobilization Evaluation for concomitant injuries to ipsilateral shoulder and cervical spine

*If the physical examination findings suggest scaphoid fracture, but the x-ray findings are normal or equivocal, the clinician immobilizes the wrist as if it were fractured and reorders x-ray films in 10 to 14 days.

Proximal, vertical-oriented fractures exhibit the greatest mobility.[36] In these cases the orthopedic surgeon may consider open reduction with fixation.

Immobilization usually continues until there is radiographic evidence of healing. Follow-up films reveal trabecular continuity if the fracture is healing properly. Bone resorption along the margins of the fracture with the typical formation of cystlike areas of radiolucency is an indication of inadequate healing (Figure 5-9). Electrical stimulation of bone and nerve cells may be a beneficial adjunct in treatment.

Traditionally, the treatment of a nonunited scaphoid fracture centers around either iliac bone grafting and internal fixation with Kirschner wires (K wires) or, when CT or MRI shows avascular necrosis (i.e., death of bone), an arthrodesis.[22] The purpose of these procedures is to stabilize the wrist and relieve pain, however, not to correct the problem in its entirety. Thus it is not assumed that aggressive treatment at this point will increase the patient's range of motion or grip strength.[87]

The most important considerations in selecting the appropriate treatment for a patient with a scaphoid fracture are the amount of pain and the extent of disability the patient is experiencing. Unless the patient has multiple cysts, is experiencing posttraumatic carpal instability, and has markedly lost wrist function, the primary care practitioner and a conservatively minded surgeon may take a "wait and see" approach.

Hook of the Hamate Fracture

In general, a hamate fracture is the result of a direct blow to the carpal region or chronic repetitive strain at the wrist, as may occur in racquet sports or baseball. Diagnosis is usually delayed within the spectrum of primary care, because routine radiographic studies rarely demonstrate the fracture.[23] If there is a high enough level of clinical suspicion, an immediate referral to an orthopedic surgeon may be in order.

There is a tenderness over the hook of the hamate and a weakness in grip strength. Carpal tunnel views or trispiral tomography may be necessary to diagnose this type of fracture (Figure 5-10). Scintigraphy is helpful in cases in which imaging is equivocal, but the level of suspicion is high.[69] The consequences of late diagnosis include tenosynovitis and ulnar nerve injury.[10] Sometimes, excision of the fragment is necessary.

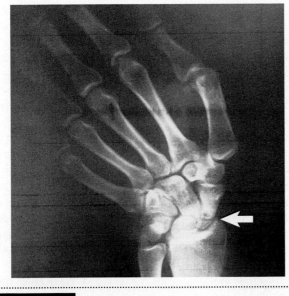

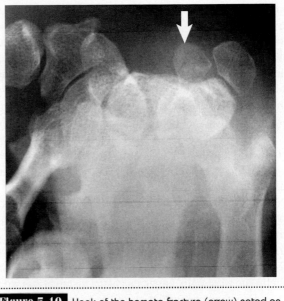

Figure 5-10 Hook of the hamate fracture (arrow) noted on carpal tunnel view.

(From Cooney WP, Linscheid RL, Dobyns JH, editors: *The wrist: diagnosis and operative treatment,* ed 1, St Louis, 1998, Mosby.)

Colles' Fracture

Representing one of the most common ailments of the traumatized wrist-forearm complex, Colles' fracture occurs most often in the young, the old, and anyone else who is subject to falls. The weight of the body as it falls on an outstretched hand produces the fracture force, while displacing the distal radius fragment into the typical "silver fork" position (Figure 5-11 *A, B*). Associated injuries to the ulnar styloid or ulnar collateral ligament of the wrist are also common. It is important to rule out carpal tunnel syndrome through both neurologic examination and physical examination after a trauma. Once again, anatomic derangements, whether severe or minute, can potentially impair local neurophysiology. Referral to an orthopedic specialist should be prompt to reduce the deformity as much as possible.

Colles' fracture has traditionally been treated conservatively with closed reduction and cast immobilization. Countertraction helps reduce the typical radial and dorsal displacement of the fracture. Follow-up x-ray films, sometimes at intervals of several weeks, are very helpful.[12] An anteroposterior film allows the clinician to inspect the degree of comminution and the radial angle, as well as to determine whether there is any radial displacement or radial shortening. Dorsal compression and displacement are clear on a lateral projection. Surgical

correction may be necessary for some of these types of problems.[86] The surgeon may prescribe an external fixator over cast immobilization if there is radiologic evidence of radial shortening of 4 mm or greater.[1]

The problem of posttraumatic compressive neuropathies has come under a great deal of discussion in the past decade. It may be more common than was once thought.[3] Late compressive neuropathy involves the median nerve most frequently, but it may also involve the ulnar nerve. The relationship between malunions and compressive neuropathies also needs a more thorough investigation.

Posttraumatic Carpal Instability

Chronic wrist pain and loss of hand function may result from carpal instability. The disruption of dynamic ligamentous integrity and normal bony alignment because of a traumatic event (e.g., perilunate dislocation, recurrent lunate subluxation, scaphoid malunion, multiple carpal fractures) or cumulative overload (e.g., repetitive strain injuries) is termed posttraumatic carpal instability.

Ligament instability at the wrist adversely affects the proximal row of carpal bones primarily, leading to longitudinal collapse and articular dissociation. Scapholunate dissociation, the most common form of carpal instability, may be the result of repetitive trauma to the wrist or a combination of injuries, such as carpal fracture and dislocation.[19,64] For example, a force to the hypothenar region with the wrist dorsiflexed and the ulna deviated can cause scaphoid dorsiflexion, placing the volar side of the scapholunate interosseous ligament under failure load and leading to scapholunate dissociation.[31,62] Depending on the articular surface of the lunate in its orientation in a dorsiflexed or palmar-flexed axis, the instability can occur in a dorsal or palmar fashion.[95] Sometimes the terms *dorsiflexed intercalated segment instability* or *palmar-flexed intercalated instability* are used.

The clinical signs and symptoms of posttraumatic carpal instability include pain, intermittent disability, crepitus, and carpal hypermobility (Table 5-3). Loss of grip strength on the dynamometer or manual testing may also occur. Antecedent trauma, combined with a history of chronic wrist pain, suggests carpal instability as well.

Radiologic examination of the wrist for carpal instability generally includes the standard posteroanterior, lateral, and oblique projections, plus optional ulnar-radial deviation views and, possibly, stress films with the fist in a clenched position (i.e., compression posteroanterior film).[6] Some authorities advocate the use of additional lateral films with the wrist in dynamic positions.[34] CT or MRI are helpful in the diagnosis of osteonecrosis and malunion.

There are several types of carpal instability patterns. For example, carpal shifts to the anterior or posterior can reduce the capitate-lunate angle, which is normally 30 degrees. A lateral projection that reveals an abnormal or increased scapholunate angle (i.e., larger than its normal 30 to 60 degrees) may result from a scaphoid fracture, lunate subluxation or dislocation, or palmar flexion sprains.[34,79] The interval between the scaphoid and the lunate may increase from its normal spacing of 2 mm or less. As noted earlier, a scapholunate distance of greater than 2 mm (i.e., Terry Thomas sign) is suggestive of ligamentous disruption, and a distance of 4 mm is confirmatory; it is evident on the posteroanterior standard wrist projection (Figure 5-12). An abnormal scaphoid rotation visible on the neutral posteroanterior and the ulnar deviation stress film(s) together are called the "ring sign" (Figure 5-13).

After immobilization or surgical treatment for carpal instability, the wrist and hand may become stiff. Physical therapy not only can improve the range of motion in the joint, both actively and passively, but it can help prevent the tendonitis that can occur secondary to prolonged immobilization.[97] Strengthening exercises can be gently and slowly intensified in the patient's rehabilitation schedule. Possible long-term results of scapholunate instability include irregularity of the scaphoid fossa of the radius, spur formation, and loss of joint

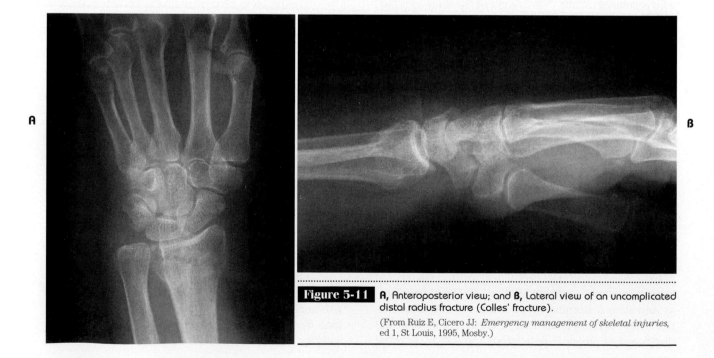

A

B

Figure 5-11 **A,** Anteroposterior view; and **B,** Lateral view of an uncomplicated distal radius fracture (Colles' fracture).

(From Ruiz E, Cicero JJ: *Emergency management of skeletal injuries,* ed 1, St Louis, 1995, Mosby.)

| **Table 5-3** | Traumatic Conditions of the Wrist |

	Posttraumatic Carpal Instability	Kienböck's Disease	Ganglion Cyst	Triangular Fibrocartilage Tear	Extensor Carpi Ulnaris Tendonitis or Subluxation
Physical examination findings	Limited and painful motion Scapholunate tenderness upon palpation Possible synovitis Loss or decrease in grip strength History of trauma	Usually a history of trauma Progressive dysfunction and chronic pain Limited dorsiflexion of wrist Palpable tenderness at central carpus Swelling in dorsum of wrist	Soft-tissue mass on dorsum of wrist Freely movable cyst in extensor tendon sheath Prominence in wrist flexion Palpable tenderness	Dorsal-ulnar pain Crepitus and clicking Bogginess and swelling at wrist	Reproduction of symptoms or sub-luxation of tendon on hypersupina-tion or flexion Crepitus or clicking on repetitive forearm rotation History of acute or repetitive mechanical move-ment of wrist
X-ray findings	Three standard views, plus scaphoid projec-tion at a minimum Evaluation for altered scapho-lunate angle Evaluation for Terry Thomas sign (i.e., scapholunate dissociation or subluxation) Evaluation for osteonecrosis of posttraumatic bony changes	Minimum of three views Initial films often normal Dense, sclerotic lunate visible on follow-up projection	Not applicable	Three-view series to rule out fracture Arthrogram or MRI to confirm diagnosis	Normal
Treatment plan	Rehabilitation, ice, electrotherapy Need to rule out rheumatoid disease in selected patients Referral to ortho-pedic or hand surgeon, if gross instability is seen on radiographic films or if function is lost Possibly bracing for work tasks or acute exacerbations CT or MRI to evaluate post-traumatic bony pathologic variations	Immobilization, ice, electrical stimulation Gradual exercise program Referral to ortho-pedic or hand surgeon for advanced pathologic abnormalities or protracted pain in spite of treatment Exercises with therapeutic putty	Rest, activity modification, ice, underwater ultrasound Referral to ortho-pedic surgeon, if condition remains refractory to care	Ice, immobilization Referral to ortho-pedic surgeon, if condition is refractory to conservative care	Ice, electrotherapy Trial of immobili-zation, manipu-lation in chronic cases Referral to ortho-pedic surgeon for refractory or grossly unstable cases

CT, Computed tomography; **MRI,** Magnetic resonance imaging.

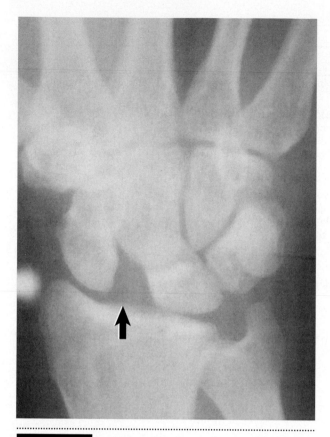

Figure 5-12 Terry Thomas sign.

(From Deltoff MN, Kogon PL: *The portable skeletal x-ray library,* ed 1, St. Louis, 1998, Mosby.)

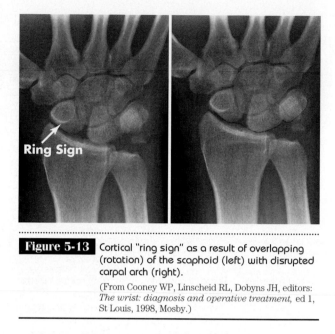

Figure 5-13 Cortical "ring sign" as a result of overlapping (rotation) of the scaphoid (left) with disrupted carpal arch (right).

(From Cooney WP, Linscheid RL, Dobyns JH, editors: *The wrist: diagnosis and operative treatment,* ed 1, St Louis, 1998, Mosby.)

space.[33] Radioscapholunate osteoarthritis is common in untreated injuries.[93]

Kienböck's Disease

The cause of Kienböck's disease is largely unknown. Described as an avascular necrosis of the lunate bone, it generally follows repetitive microtrauma or an acute traumatic injury to the wrist that goes undiagnosed.[67] Rarely an individual develops this condition without antecedent trauma.

Patients with Kienböck's disease usually experience progressive wrist pain, loss of motion, and weakness on job-task completion. They often ignore the chronic pain until they can no longer work around the problem. There is palpable tenderness at the central carpus, with limited extension. The application of direct pressure by clamping the lunate between thumb and forefinger causes pain.[78] Swelling occurs on the dorsum of the central carpus.

X-ray films taken shortly after the initial injury may be normal. Only when a second set of films is taken months later does the clinician see the vascular changes caused by Kienböck's disease. At first, change appears as a chalky whiteness of bone at the lunate (Figure 5-14); this dense and sclerotic appearance may later degenerate into carpal collapse or fragmentation.[60] Degenerative arthritis and carpal instability commonly follow.

Treatment includes early immobilization of the wrist, preferably in a thumb spica splint. Ice, electrical stimulation, or antiinflammatory medication can help reduce swelling and pain. Gentle range-of-motion movements and exercises with therapeutic putty help restore wrist and hand function. Later stages of Kienböck's disease may require referral to a hand surgeon, since an arthrodesis (fusion) may become necessary.

Ganglion Cyst

Accounting for 50% to 70% of all tumors in the wrist and hand region, ganglion cysts are fairly common, benign soft-tissue lesions. They are more common in women (43 per 10,000) than in men (25 per 10,000).[46] This type of cyst is a mucinous mass found in a tendon sheath, most frequently on the dorsum of the wrist (Figure 5-15), and is sometimes the result of trauma. The size of the cyst may change according to the activity level of the patient, and the mass is freely movable. It becomes painful in some individuals, especially if it increases in size.

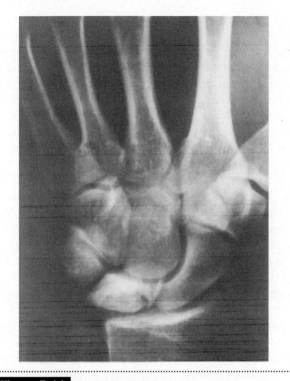

Figure 5-14 Kienböck's disease.

(From Deltoff MN, Kogon PL: *The portable skeletal x-ray library,* ed 1, St Louis, 1998, Mosby.)

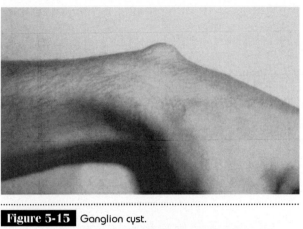

Figure 5-15 Ganglion cyst.

(From Mercier LR: *Practical orthopedics,* ed 4, St Louis, 1995, Mosby.)

Conservative treatment includes rest, avoidance of any repetitive mechanical use of the wrist and hand, application of ice, and underwater ultrasound. Should the cyst be painful or progressive, a referral to an orthopedic surgeon may be necessary. Care at this point can be either aspiration of the cyst or injection of a steroid compound into the cyst to reduce swelling and inflammation. Should these remedies prove ineffective, surgical excision may be indicated. Surgery should be viewed as a last resort, however, because ganglion cysts can recur after treatment.

Triangular Fibrocartilage Tears

Practitioners whose patients include a large percentage of athletes frequently encounter individuals with dorsal-ulnar wrist pain. When a triangular fibrocartilage tear is the cause of the pain, symptoms include clicking, crepitus, and swelling at the dorsal-ulnar aspect of the wrist. Blunt trauma (e.g., from a blow that forces the wrist into dorsiflexion and pronation) and repetitive trauma (e.g., from a sport such as gymnastics) are the most common causes of such injuries to the triangular fibrocartilage

complex.[47] Gymnasts are particularly vulnerable to debilitating wrist injury because of the frequency with which their sport requires them to place their weight on their arms; weight bearing unique to the upper limbs of gymnasts places large compressive forces at the distal forearm and wrist.

Anatomically, the triangular fibrocartilage complex lies between the articular lip of the radius and the styloid process of the ulna (Figure 5-16). The complex not only serves as the articular surface for the triquetrum and lunate, but it also provides a surface for weight bearing. When intact, the fibrocartilage absorbs approximately 40% of the distal load, and the radius absorbs about 60% of the weight-bearing load transmitted across the wrist. The triangular fibrocartilage also aids in the maintenance of the distal radioulnar joint by increasing its congruency (e.g., fit, stability).[26] Individuals with a positive ulnar variance are more likely to experience triangular fibrocartilage tears.[17,25]

The differential diagnosis of dorsal-ulnar pain at the wrist includes a variety of conditions (Table 5-4). The first step is to order a routine, three-view plain x-ray film series of the wrist to rule out fracture or metabolic bone disease. Arthrograms or MRI studies show the amount of fibrocartilage damage (Figures 5-17 *A, B*). Special instability series views can rule out ligamentous capsular instability at the wrist.

The condition is usually refractory to conservative care of ice application, splinting, and active rest. Failure of the triangular fibrocartilage under compressive loads over time may lead to chondromalacia of the articular surface of the ulna, ulnocarpal impingement, and degenerative joint disease.[25] Arthroscopic debridement of the triangular fibrocartilage and the tear itself may be necessary in some patients.

Extensor Carpi Ulnaris Tendonitis or Subluxation

Although there are still occasional clinical references to it, subluxation of the extensor carpi ulnaris tendon is largely a forgotten entity in orthopedic practices.[2,39,71] Other forms of tendonitis seem to occur more often.

The extensor carpi ulnaris tendon lies in a shallow groove at the medial border of the distal ulna and depends on stability of the distal radioulnar joint. There are several possible causes of tendonitis or subluxation. For example, a sudden, forceful supination with ulnar deviation and a palmar (volar) flexor force can rupture the fibro-osseous tunnel that contains the extensor carpi ulnaris tendon at the distal radioulnar joint.[71] This injury can occur from a forceful follow-through at the end of a baseball swing[44] or a forceful forehand stroke in tennis.[80] Other potential causes include chronic overstretching of the tendon sheath, overuse, and repetitive participation in racquet sports.

Hypersupination via a laborious or athletic endeavor can cause a mechanical subluxation of the extensor carpi ulnaris. In this instance the tendon slips as the forearm goes through rotary movement; the patient feels pain at the distal forearm or wrist. Pronation may cause a spontaneous reduction of the tendon back into place.

Both the severity of the injury and the length of time between the injury and the initiation of treatment determine the appropriate treatment of extensor carpi ulnaris subluxation. X-ray films are usually normal. Acute subluxation may need a period of 4 to 6 weeks of immobilization with the arm in pronation and radial deviation and dorsiflexion to allow the ruptured membrane to heal.[90] In more chronic cases, immobilization is less effective.[80] A trial of strengthening and manipulation may alleviate some of the symptoms. Conditions that are refractory to conservative care may need reconstructive surgery that creates a new tunnel from the slip of the extensor retinaculum.[15,81,90]

Table 5-4 Differential Diagnosis of Dorsal-Ulnar Wrist Pain

Diagnosis	Diagnostic Studies	Signs and Symptoms
Triangular fibro-cartilage tear	Arthrogram or MRI Plain films often not helpful	Pain in dorsal ulnar aspect of wrist Crepitus Greatest pain on compression
Avascular necrosis of lunate (Kienböck's disease)	Plain x-ray films CT or MRI	Synovitis of wrist Joint line pain with referral Limited volar and dorsiflexion
Guyon's canal syndrome (ulnar nerve compression)	Electrodiagnostic studies (nerve conduction velocity, electromyography)	Interossei weakness Dysthesia or paresthesia in 4th or 5th digits
Tendonitis	X-ray films normal	Pain on active motion with resistance Discomfort with passive stretching
Hook of hamate fracture	Plain x-ray films (including tunnel view) CT or scan, if plain films equivocal	Point tenderness over hamate Ulnar neuropathy with familiar referral
Extensor carpi ulnaris subluxation	Plain films unremarkable	Pain on hyper-supination or flexion Crepitus or clicking with forearm rotation Palpable tenderness over tendon at ulnar styloid

MRI, Magnetic resonance imaging; *CT,* computed tomography.

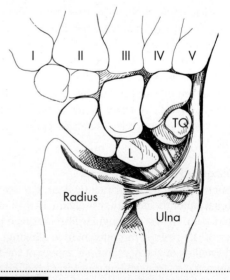

Figure 5-16 Triangular fibrocartilage complex.

(From Nicholas JA, Hershman EB: *The upper extremity in sports medicine,* St Louis, 1995, Mosby.)

Neurovascular Conditions

The median nerve is commonly affected in neurovascular conditions of the wrist. The most common compressive neuropathy of the wrist is carpal tunnel syndrome. Many injuries or illnesses have been associated with carpal tunnel syndrome, including blunt trauma, overuse, nutritional deficiencies, pregnancy, and diabetes.

After it runs by the flexor digitorum superficialis in the middle of the palm, the median nerve passes below the flexor retinaculum. It comes down into the hand and gives off common palmar digital nerves (Figure 5-18). These divide into the digital nerves and supply cutaneous innervation to the three and one-half radial digits. (The median nerve does not provide cutaneous innervation to the one and one-half digits on the ulnar side, however, because the superficial branch of the ulnar nerve innervates these digits.[96]) The median nerve also has motor branches and a recurrent branch to the thenar musculature.

The flexor retinaculum helps form the carpal tunnel. It also bridges the gap along the carpal bones and forms a fibrous and osseous canal. The tendons from the flexor digitorum superficialis and flexor digitorum profundus pass under the flexor retinaculum, which, along with the palmar aponeurosis and the fibrous flexor sheath that extends over the digits, form portions of the deep fascia in the palmar portion of the hand. The palmar carpal ligament is the lower part of the antebrachial fascia, and it continues into the deep fascia of the hand. The median nerve transverses this carpal tunnel; and the fascia, ligaments, and retinaculum add to the tightly wound compartment of connective tissue. This arrangement is the anatomic reason that soft-tissue swelling, inflammation, and fibrosis can impinge on the median nerve in the carpal tunnel.

Carpal Tunnel Syndrome

As noted earlier, the most common peripheral entrapment neuropathy of the upper extremity is carpal tunnel syndrome. This condition has gained widespread attention in recent years because of a clinical entity known as repetitive stress injury (RSI), which frequently occurs among industrial workers (e.g., packers) and civil service individuals (e.g., postal workers).

The cause of carpal tunnel syndrome may be repetitive mechanical motion in the workplace, as well as isolated traumatic episodes of stress and strain on the hand and wrist. It can also result from retention of water, par-

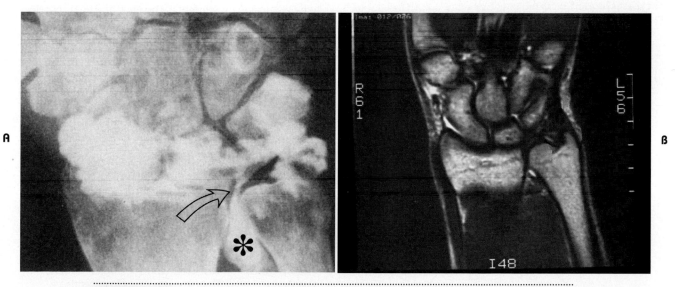

A   **B**

Figure 5-17   **A,** Wrist arthrogram demonstrating a tear within the triangular fibrocartilage (TFC) (open curved black arrow), allowing communication between the radiocarpal compartment and the distal radioulnar joint (asterisk). **B,** Magnetic resonance image of complete tear of the central portion of the TFC.

(Part A from Jobe F, editor: *Operative techniques in upper extremity sports injuries*, ed 1, St Louis, 1996, Mosby. Part B from Cooney WP, Linscheid RL, Dobyns JH, editors: *The wrist: diagnosis and operative treatment*, ed 1, St Louis, 1998, Mosby.)

ticularly in pregnant women; osteoarthritis or degenerative changes in older individuals; metabolic disorders, such as diabetes mellitus and alcoholism; and secondarily from trauma that injures the flexor compartment (e.g., Colles' fracture).

The clinical features of carpal tunnel syndrome are fairly well-known (Table 5-5); they become evident during neurologic testing of the upper extremity. Paresthesia or dysesthesia of the three and one-half fingers on the radial (thumb) side of the hand occurs frequently. The most common symptom is pain that grows worse at night, with numbness and tingling into the thumb and first and second digits. Water retention, such as that experienced by women at certain points in the menstrual cycle, can place pressure on the median nerve in the carpal tunnel. Any type of swelling underneath the flexor retinaculum or palmar carpal ligament can cause symptoms. The presence of Tinel's sign over the palmar carpal ligament and the reproduction of symptoms in Phalen's wrist flexion test indicate the common pathways of pain. X-ray films are not usually helpful in identifying carpal tunnel syndrome, but electrodiagnostic studies are useful in distinguishing this syndrome from cervical radiculopathy.[45]

Differential diagnosis includes median nerve entrapment at the pronator teres musculature at the forearm. If the results of Phalen's test are normal, but passive supination to stretch the swollen pronator teres reproduces symptoms, the condition may involve a forearm lesion rather than carpal tunnel syndrome. A trigger point on the flexor carpi radialis muscle can also refer pain to the palm and wrist and mimic carpal tunnel syndrome.[5] There are three stages of carpal tunnel syndrome: mild, moderate, and severe (Table 5-6). One of the biggest problems in treating the condition is in preventing any irritation of the wrist and hand, such as hyperflexion, that compromises the carpal tunnel. Conservative care is indicated initially, yet a prolonged delay before surgical intervention may reduce the chance of success with operative intervention.

Mild Carpal Tunnel Syndrome. In the mild stage of carpal tunnel syndrome, a careful case history should reveal whether the problem arises from the patient's sleeping posture (e.g., with the wrist in flexion) or from irritating the wrist in some kind of recreational activity (e.g., riding a bicycle that is not the proper size for the rider's stature).

Nerve root compression or stretching may occur concomitantly with wrist trauma or motor vehicle accidents. In the latter case, some patients have cervical radiculopathy, as well as peripheral entrapment neuropathy. The wrist injury may go unnoticed at first. Because it usually occurs in association with a hyperflexion-hyperextension movement of the head and neck, cervical acceleration-deceleration (CAD) injuries initially occupy the examiner's attention. Such a "double crush" injury is often disabling.[89] Electrodiagnostic studies may be helpful in determining whether the patient has a central lesion that affects the nerve root or a peripheral lesion that involves irritation at the carpal tunnel.

The chiropractic physician can treat the peripheral entrapment neuropathy by means of underwater ultra-

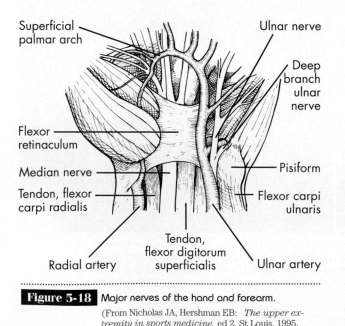

Figure 5-18 Major nerves of the hand and forearm.

(From Nicholas JA, Hershman EB: *The upper extremity in sports medicine,* ed 2, St Louis, 1995, Mosby.)

Table 5-5 Clinical Features of Carpal Tunnel Syndrome

Factors	Symptoms	Signs
Female gender	Nocturnal pains	Thenar atrophy
Pregnancy	Paresthesia	Tinel's sign
Diabetes mellitus	Weakness	Reduced two-point
Rheumatoid	Clumsiness	discrimination
arthritis	Activity-induced	Phalen's test (15,
Stenosing flexor	symptomatology	30, or 60 sec)
tenosynovitis	Numbness	Loss of grip
Colles' fracture		strength

sound, vitamin B6 therapy in a dosage of 50 mg three times a day, and an examination of the cervical spine for any dyskinetic or neurologic problems.[58] Most mild cases respond to conservative therapy in 3 to 6 weeks. If the clinician believes that the patient has not improved, is experiencing worse paresthesias or a dysesthetic response, shows any signs of a loss of grip strength, a weakness in wrist flexion, or thenar atrophy, the clinician should order electrodiagnostic tests immediately. Motor changes and a constant symptomatology suggest that conservative management is unlikely to be successful.[43]

Moderate Carpal Tunnel Syndrome. One of the most difficult clinical challenges for the primary care physician is moderate carpal tunnel syndrome. If the condition does not respond to conservative treatment, the practitioner must begin an aggressive treatment regimen with ancillary therapeutic care and must allow a finite period of time for improvement. Moderate carpal tunnel syndrome does not respond to ancillary proce-

dures carried out once or twice each week; there must be at least three treatment sessions per week. The patient may use either a splint that keeps the thumb and wrist in the neutral position or a cock-up splint that helps prevent night pain. In addition, the patient should avoid all activities that aggravate the wrist. The administration of vitamin B6 and antiinflammatory medication may reduce swelling inside the carpal tunnel, thereby reducing pain and paresthesia.[85]

It is important to follow the patient closely to ensure that he or she is adhering to the treatment program and that the condition is improving. For example, the practitioner should check periodically for sensorimotor changes and atrophy of the thenar eminence. Careful monitoring of the cervical spine for concomitant radiculopathy is also necessary. Weakness may occur in pinch strength and, possibly, wrist flexion.

The results can be disastrous if the patient undergoes several months of ineffective treatment, since the

Table 5-6   Stages of Carpal Tunnel Syndrome

	Mild	Moderate	Severe
Physical examination findings	Tenderness at flexor retinaculum Palpable tenderness over volar carpal ligament Positive Tinel's sign History of dysesthesia or paresthesia in thumb and first two digits No motor changes No atrophy	Pain, paresthesia, and dysesthesia in thumb and first two fingers Positive Phalen's test Positive Tinel's sign Possible swelling and thickening over volar carpal ligament and flexor retinaculum Weakness in grip, pinch strength, and wrist flexion Possible early thenar atrophy	Thenar atrophy and weakness Provocative orthopedic tests Pain worse at night Progressive motor changes
X-ray findings	Normal Electrodiagnostic study, if no abatement of symptoms in 3-6 weeks	Usually normal	Usually normal Possible porosity of bone attributable to disuse
Treatment plan	Underwater ultrasound in pulsed mode CMT to cervical spine Vitamin B6 (50 mg tid) Cock-up splint at night, if pain occurs only at night or patient has postural problem during sleep	Underwater ultrasound Antiinflammatory medication Vitamin B6 (50 mg tid) Cock-up splint, especially at night Monitoring of cervical spine Intensive care for 2 weeks Referral for EMG and NCV studies and orthopedic evaluation, if condition fails to improve	Electrodiagnostic studies (EMG and NCV) Surgical referral Immobilization Physical therapy and rehabilitation

CMT, Chiropractic manipulative therapy; **EMG,** electromyography; **NCV,** nerve conduction velocity.

nerve compression continues during this period. Therefore the patient should undergo an intensive regimen of ancillary therapeutics for 2 weeks. If six treatment sessions fail to produce any reduction in pain or other improvement, the practitioner should order an EMG series. Once again, it is essential to rule out proximal compressive neuropathies.[30,70] Consultation with an orthopedic surgeon is appropriate at this time to determine whether the patient is a candidate for surgical decompression.[70] An accurate diagnosis that isolates the neuropathy to the carpal tunnel is imperative to avoid poor surgical outcome in patients with ongoing hand and wrist pain.

Severe Carpal Tunnel Syndrome. Signs of severe carpal tunnel syndrome include motor changes, constant numbness in the hand, and tingling with night pain. Severe compression of the median nerve, which provides motor branches to the thenar muscles (except one of the heads of the flexor pollicis brevis and the radial two lumbrical muscles), results in total loss of hand function. Thus holding a pencil or a coffee cup becomes difficult. Sensation to the palmar thumb, index finger, and middle finger is compromised, as it is in other stages of carpal tunnel syndrome. Wrist flexion, opposition, and thumb adduction are usually weak. The space in the canal is compressed, and fibrosis may be advanced. There may be evidence of atrophy in the first radial interossei muscle, as well as atrophy and flattening of the thenar eminence.

The patient may not be able to localize the symptoms. At times, the patient may awaken because of the numbness and tingling and may have to relieve the pain and paresthesia by shaking and massaging the hand. Sometimes, the symptoms do not abate even with these actions.

Phalen's test and Tinel's sign are both provocative tests. Nerve conduction velocity tests reveal pathologic changes at the carpal tunnel and thenar muscles. In fact, the sensitivity of nerve conduction studies is approximately 85% to 90%.[40,54,57] Typical electrodiagnostic findings in patients with severe carpal tunnel syndrome are distal wrist latency delay in nerve conduction velocities, loss of amplitude, or conduction slowing at the median nerve. Cervical nerve root involvement appears as denervation potentials on EMG testing with normal distal nerve conduction.[29] Electrodiagnostic evidence of advanced disease (e.g., delay of terminal sensory or motor latencies) and delayed diagnosis reduce the likelihood of success of a surgical procedure. To further complicate matters, electrodiagnostic tests frequently show not only median nerve involvement, but also ulnar nerve neuropathy.

Nonsurgical treatment may offer relief of symptoms in some patients with severe carpal tunnel syndrome. Patients who exhibit severe sensory loss, thenar muscular atrophy, or symptoms for a prolonged period are unlikely to respond well to nonoperative care, however. Any motor change is a particular cause for concern. At this late stage the administration of vitamin B6 and cervical spine care are not helpful unless the patient also shows signs of a cervical radiculopathy. If splinting the wrist in a neutral position of dorsiflexion, prescribing antiinflammatory medication, or administering underwater ultrasound treatment does not help, the practitioner should refer the patient to an orthopedic surgeon for consultation. Injection of a corticosteroid into the carpal tunnel may be the last resort in the effort to avoid a surgical procedure. Axonal loss and persistent symptoms usually necessitate surgical intervention, however.

Patients who are older than 50 years of age, whose symptoms have persisted for longer than 6 months, who experience constant numbness or tingling, or whose condition has progressed from the mild or moderate level to the severe level in a period of 8 to 12 weeks should probably undergo surgical decompression of the carpal tunnel. The basic goal of surgery is to relieve the mechanical compression on the median nerve by dividing the transverse carpal ligament and opening up the flexor retinaculum. If the surgery does not relieve the patient's symptoms, the reason may be an incomplete sectioning of the transverse carpal ligament, inadequate removal of the hypertrophied flexor tendon synovium, or the presence of a more proximal or coexistent site of entrapment.[94]

Postoperative care generally includes wrist immobilization in the neutral position for a minimum of 2 to 3 weeks. Postsurgical rehabilitation may span several months to ensure the restoration of the patient's hand function and ability to complete everyday tasks. Occupational and physical therapy may be necessary. The patient must work on grip strength, thumb opposition, and finger flexion through the use of putty or a clothes pin or various grip-enhancing devices. After surgical rehabilitation, the results of static and two-point discrimination tests, as well as the patient's ability to perform fine manipulation tasks, should improve.[51]

Surgery for severe carpal tunnel syndrome is not always successful. Failure does not necessarily reflect inadequate surgical techniques, but it may be the result of an inaccurate diagnosis; the presence of other, previously unrecognized neurologic injuries at the wrist level or more proximal locations (e.g., thoracic outlet syndrome);

radiculopathy or radiculitis; or tumor. Metabolic disorders such as diabetes mellitus and alcoholism may also affect surgical results.

Guyon's Canal Syndrome and Ulnar Neuritis

Peripheral entrapment of the ulnar nerve can occur both at the wrist and at the cubital tunnel of the elbow. The nerve passes through the tunnel of Guyon between the pisiform bone and the hook of the hamate bone. Among the potential causes of ulnar nerve entrapment are pisiform fracture; hook of the hamate trauma, including acute fracture and stress fracture; distal radius fracture; posttraumatic carpal instability; or tumor.[9] Hypothenar atrophy and intrinsic weakness of the hand muscles may occur concomitantly with ulnar neuritis. Pain may refer distally to the fourth and fifth digits of the hand.

The clinician can palpate the tunnel of Guyon region by placing the thumb on the palmar surface of the patient's wrist at the ulnar side, pointing the thumb at the patient's index finger, and pressing down. Routine wrist films are taken with carpal tunnel projections to rule out a hook of the hamate fracture. Nerve conduction velocities may be slowed and should be correlated with clinical findings.

Rest and immobilization are the primary components of the initial treatment (Table 5-7). Referral to an orthopedic surgeon is indicated for fracture care. Those who participate in sports such as baseball and tennis may require extensive rehabilitative therapy to regain the functional hand and wrist strength that they need for their sports.

Table 5-7 Guyon's Canal Syndrome and Ulnar Neuritis

Physical examination findings	Pain at Guyon's canal
History of trauma or carpal fracture
Distal referral to 4th and 5th digits
Palpable tenderness over hook of hamate or distal ulnar-pisiform interface
Intrinsic hand weakness
X-ray findings	Standard films, plus special projection, such as carpal tunnel view sometimes required for fracture
Treatment plan	Rest and immobilization
Referral for fracture care
Rehabilitative therapy

PART TWO: THE HAND

Mechanically, the hand is a delicately balanced system of bones, ligaments, tendons, and small muscles. It is a sophisticated instrument used to manipulate and feel the environment. Sometimes, minor changes in the hand's function as a result of disability or injury can cause major changes in an individual's daily life. Rheumatoid arthritis in the hand, for example, can make brushing the teeth or holding a fork a major task.

Anatomy and Function of the Hand

The back of the hand is the dorsal aspect; the front of the hand is the palmar or volar aspect (Figure 5-19). The digits are referred to as the thumb and the index, long (middle), ring, and little fingers. (Referring to the digits by the numbered system, such as first or second finger, is confusing in persons who are missing a digit.) Any point on the thumb side of the finger is referred to as the radial aspect of the finger, and any point on the little finger side is referred to as the ulnar aspect of the finger.

The bones of the hand include five metacarpals, one for each digit. The distal aspect of each is called the head, and it has a significantly peculiar anatomy in the fingers; it is bulbous on its palmar aspect, compared with its distal aspect.

The fingers each have three phalanges, called proximal, middle, and distal phalanges. The thumb has two phalanges, proximal and distal. In addition to the metacarpophalangeal joints, the fingers have a proximal interphalangeal joint and a distal interphalangeal joint; these joints are the articulations of the proximal and middle phalanges and of the middle and distal phalanges, respectively. Because the thumb has only two phalanges, it has only one joint, called the interphalangeal joint.

Each finger and thumb joint has radial and ulnar collateral ligaments that prevent excessive lateral motion. The normal ranges of motion of the finger and thumb joints are the following:

1. Metacarpophalangeal joints: minus 30 degrees (extension) to 95 degrees (flexion)
2. Proximal interphalangeal joint: minus 5 degrees (extension) to approximately 110 degrees (flexion)
3. Distal interphalangeal joint: minus 5 degrees (extension) to approximately 100 degrees (flexion)
4. Metacarpophalangeal joint of the thumb: 0 degrees (extension) to approximately 80 degrees (flexion)
5. Interphalangeal joint of the thumb: minus 5 degrees (extension) to approximately 90 degrees (flexion)

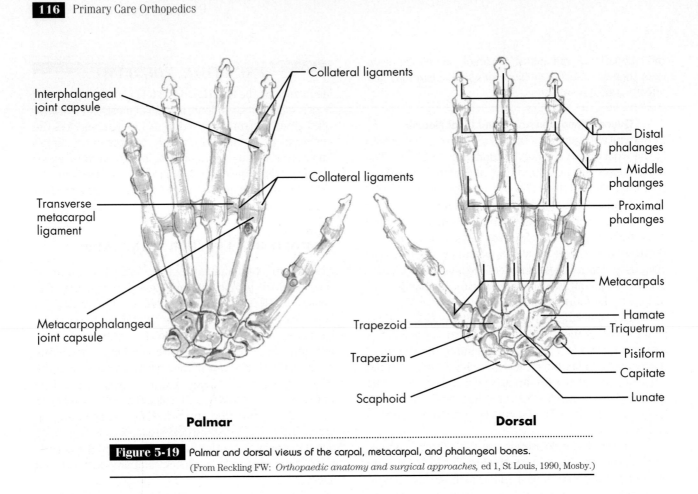

Palmar view labels: Interphalangeal joint capsule, Collateral ligaments, Transverse metacarpal ligament, Collateral ligaments, Metacarpophalangeal joint capsule

Dorsal view labels: Distal phalanges, Middle phalanges, Proximal phalanges, Metacarpals, Hamate, Triquetrum, Pisiform, Capitate, Lunate, Trapezoid, Trapezium, Scaphoid

Palmar   **Dorsal**

Figure 5-19 Palmar and dorsal views of the carpal, metacarpal, and phalangeal bones.
(From Reckling FW: *Orthopaedic anatomy and surgical approaches*, ed 1, St Louis, 1990, Mosby.)

The muscles that control the movements of the hand are divided into two groups: extrinsic or intrinsic muscles. In the extrinsic groups involved in hand function, the muscle bellies originate in the forearm and elbow area.

The long (extrinsic) muscles that control the hand have lubricating and protecting synovial sheaths. On the dorsal side of the hand, the synovial sheaths are located primarily in the wrist, under a fascial band called the extensor retinaculum (Figure 5-20). On the palmar aspect of the hand, each finger has its own synovial sheath from the midpalm area to the end of the digitorum profundus tendon. The thenar (thumb) and hypothenar (little finger) synovial sheaths extend proximally to the wrist, where they communicate with each other.[65] The flexor tendons to the fingers are also encased in fibrous tendon sheaths that facilitate their mechanical action by keeping them close to the bones and joints during flexion and extension of the fingers. Without their sheaths, for example, the tendons would bow during flexion and thus be unable to function properly.

The small (intrinsic) muscles of the hand are divided into the thenar, hypothenar, and interosseous and lumbrical groups (Figure 5-21). The thenar muscles control several of the motions of the thumb, such as adduction and opposition. Muscles of the forearm, however, are responsible for other thumb movements (Table 5-8). For example, the abductor pollicis longus abducts and extends the thumb at the carpometacarpal joint, whereas the extensor pollicis brevis extends the thumb at the carpometacarpal and metacarpophalangeal joints.[65] Actions of the thumb include the following:

- Abduction (i.e., laying the back of the hand flat on a table and pointing the thumb upward)
- Extension (i.e., laying the palm flat on a table and attempting to point the thumb toward the ceiling)
- Adduction (i.e., sliding the thumb across the palm)
- Opposition (i.e., bringing the thumb over to touch the little finger)

The interosseous and lumbrical muscles of the hand originate from the metacarpals and insert into the extensor hood, where the extensor communis digitorum

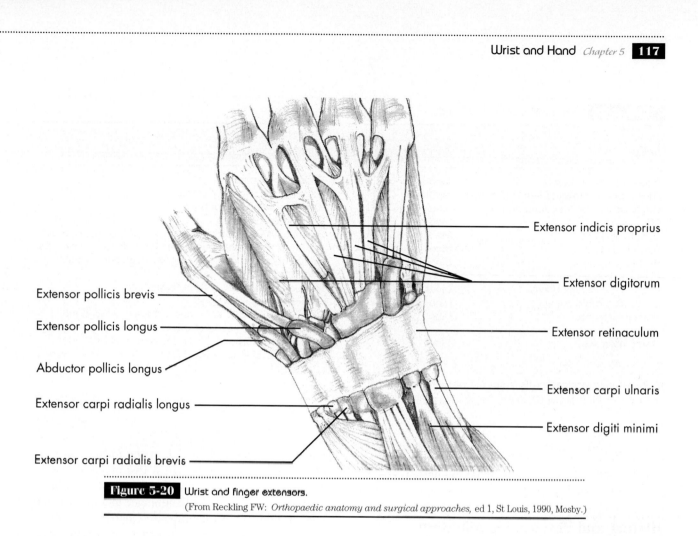

Extensor indicis proprius

Extensor pollicis brevis

Extensor digitorum

Extensor pollicis longus

Extensor retinaculum

Abductor pollicis longus

Extensor carpi radialis longus

Extensor carpi ulnaris

Extensor digiti minimi

Extensor carpi radialis brevis

Figure 5-20 Wrist and finger extensors.
(From Reckling FW: *Orthopaedic anatomy and surgical approaches,* ed 1, St Louis, 1990, Mosby.)

tendon joins the tendons of the interossei and lumbrical muscle tendons.[65] These muscles flex the metacarpophalangeal joints and help extend the interphalangeal joints. They also abduct and adduct the fingers. Moving the index, ring, and little fingers away from the long finger is abduction, for example; moving these fingers back toward the long finger is adduction.

The skin and subcutaneous tissues of the dorsal and palmar aspects of the hand have different characteristics. On the dorsal side of the hand, the epidermis and dermis are thinner than on the palmar aspect. The dorsal skin is also less firmly adherent to the deeper tissues to allow for more excursion during the flexion of the fingers. On the palmar side of the hand, the epidermis and dermis are more tightly affixed to the deeper structures, including the tendon sheath and bone, to provide a firmer grasp of objects. Deep to the epidermis, dermis, and subcutaneous fat in the palm, there is a layer of fibrous tissue called the palmar fascia. The tendons and the neurovascular structures lie beneath this fascia.

The nails grow from a nailbed. As it grows from proximal to distal, the hard nail grows over an area known as the nail matrix. The epidermis that grows over the proximal and lateral edges of the nail is known as the perionychium.

The arterial supply to the hand is from the radial and ulnar arteries, which branch into the hand and form the deep and superficial arterial arches of the hand. From the superficial arch, the digital arteries arise to supply the fingers. Each finger has a radial and an ulnar artery that lie on the palmar-lateral aspect of the finger.[18] Digital veins and nerves accompany these arteries in the finger.

The innervation of the hand comes from the ulnar, median, and radial nerves. The ulnar nerve provides the motor supply to the intrinsic muscles of the hand, with the exception of the two radial lumbricals and the thenar muscles.[60] It also innervates the little finger and one half of the ring finger. The median nerve supplies the thenar muscles and two radial lumbrical muscles. The median nerve provides sensory supply to the palmar aspect of the

Table 5-8 Intrinsic Muscles of the Hand

Muscle	Nerve	Segmental Innervation	Primary actions
Abductor pollicis brevis	Median	C8, T1	Abduction of thumb
Flexor pollicis brevis (superficial head)	Median	C8, T1	Flexion of MCP joint of thumb
Flexor pollicis brevis (deep head)	Ulnar	C8, T1	Flexion of MCP joint of thumb
Opponens pollicis	Median	C8, T1	Opposition of thumb
Lumbricals I and II	Median	C8, T1	Flexion of MCP joints and extension of IP joints of digits
Lumbricals III and IV	Ulnar	C8, T1	Flexion of MCP joints and extension of IP joints of digits
Adductor pollicis	Ulnar	C8, T1	Adduction of MC and flexion of MCP joints of thumb
Abductor digiti minimi	Ulnar	C8, T1	Abduction of little finger
Flexor digiti minimi brevis	Ulnar	C8, T1	Flexion of MCP joint of little finger
Opponens digiti minimi	Ulnar	C8, T1	Opposition of little finger
Palmar interossei	Ulnar	C8, T1	Adduction of digits II, IV, and V; flexion of MCP and extension of IP joints of digits
Doral interossei	Ulnar	C8, T1	Abduction of digits II, IV, and V; flexion of MCP and extension of IP joints of digits

MCP, Metacarpophalangeal; **IP,** interphalangeal; **MC,** metacarpal.

(From Booher JM, Thibodeau GA: *Athletic injury assessment,* ed 3, St Louis, 1994, Mosby.)

thumb, index finger, long finger, and radial half of the ring finger (Figure 5-22). The radial nerve supplies sensation to the dorsum of the hand.

History and Physical Examination of the Hand

In taking the history of a patient who is having a problem with the hand, the clinician should focus on the following questions:

- Which hand is the dominant hand?
- How long has the patient had the problem?
- Which activities of daily living does it affect?
- Is there any swelling?
- Is there any tingling or numbness?
- Has there been a recent or past injury to the hand?
- Is the patient's problem worse at night?
- Is there any pain in the neck, shoulder, or elbow?

All this information is critical in the diagnosis and clinical decision making related to conditions of the hand.

Any physical examination of the hand should begin with an inspection of both hands placed together. It is important to look for any differences in color (e.g., redness or pallor) or size (e.g., swelling or atrophy). Determining whether there is increased sweating or dryness is also important.

After inspecting the hand, the clinician puts the hand through a range-of-motion examination. First, the patient flexes and extends all of the digital joints, including the thumb, to test the active range of motion. Then the clinician tests the passive range of motion by manipulating each joint of the finger and determining whether there are any limitations of motion.

Any acute injury mandates range-of-motion testing of the collateral ligaments of the joints as well. In evaluating the condition of the metacarpophalangeal joints, it is best to assess the integrity of the collateral ligaments when the metacarpophalangeal joint is flexed. In this position the normal ligament has little laxity. Under normal conditions, the integrity of the ligaments of the proximal and distal interphalangeal joints can be tested with the fingers in slight flexion and extension. Palpation of the hand for areas of tenderness is important in localizing the exact area of pathologic variations.

The clinician should also test all the active motions of the thumb, including extension, flexion, abduction, adduction, and opposition of the thumb to the little finger. The interossei and lumbrical muscles of the fingers and the abductor muscles of the thumb and little finger are tested against resistance to the clinician's hand. Asking the patient to spread the fingers apart against resistance and then asking the patient to hold a piece of paper between two fingers while the clinician tries to pull the piece of paper out are ways to test the interossei muscles of the hand. (The patient's inability to hold the paper when the clinician tries to take it away is called Froment's

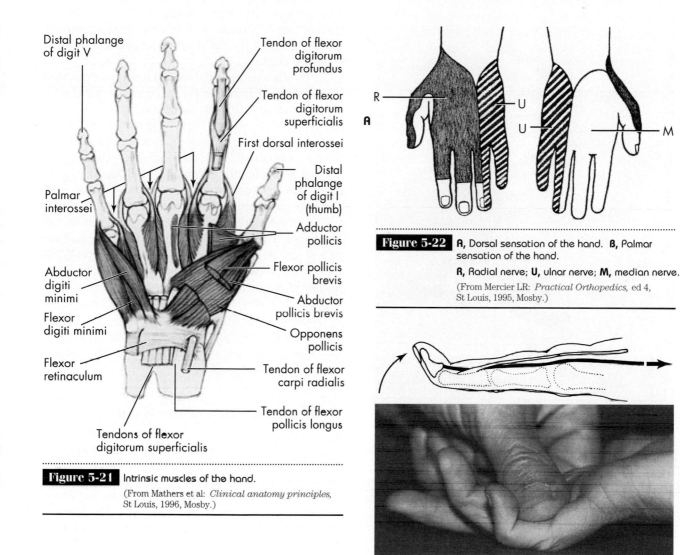

Figure 5-21 Intrinsic muscles of the hand.

(From Mathers et al: *Clinical anatomy principles*, St Louis, 1996, Mosby.)

Figure 5-22 **A,** Dorsal sensation of the hand. **B,** Palmar sensation of the hand.

R, Radial nerve; **U,** ulnar nerve; **M,** median nerve.

(From Mercier LR: *Practical Orthopedics*, ed 4, St Louis, 1995, Mosby.)

Figure 5-23 Profundus test.

(From Hunter JM, Mackin EJ, Callahan AD: *Rehabilitation of the hand: surgery and therapy*, ed 4, St Louis, 1995, Mosby.)

paper sign.) In addition, the clinician closely examines the patient's pinch strength between the thumb and index finger and visually inspects the muscle contour at the first dorsal interossei.

To test the flexor profundus tendon, the clinician simply asks the patient to make a fist or to bend each finger while the clinician assesses the flexion of the distal interphalangeal joint. The flexor digitorum profundus tendons, which insert into the bases of the distal phalanges, and the flexor pollicis longus, which inserts into the base of the distal phalanx of the thumb, flex the distal phalanges of the fingers and thumb.[78] The examiner secures the fingers in extension at the proximal interphalangeal joints as the patient attempts to bend the tip of the injured finger or thumb (Figure 5-23). The tendon of the flexor digitorum superficialis splits into two por-

tions and attaches to the middle phalanx of each finger; this tendon controls flexion of the proximal interphalangeal joint. Holding adjacent tendons in extension permits the clinician to isolate and test the function of the superficialis tendon in flexion. The flexion motion of the tendon is a function of the median nerve.

Testing of the motor function of the ulnar, median, and radial nerves can be done first without resistance, then with marginal resistance (Figure 5-24 *A-C*). Testing of the ulnar nerve includes tests of finger abduction and adduction strength. Testing the median nerve includes

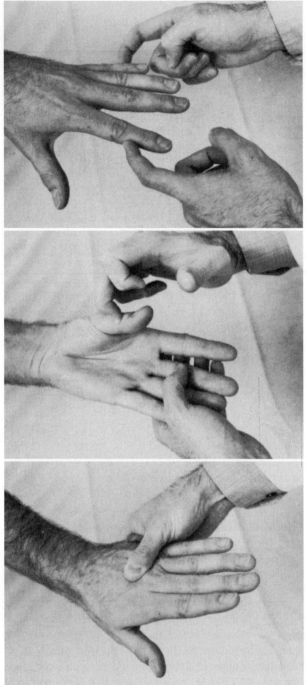

A

B

C

Figure 5-24   **A,** Testing for ulnar motor function. **B,** Testing for median nerve function by determining thenar muscle strength. **C,** Testing for radial nerve function by examining wrist extension against resistance.

(From Mercier LR: *Practical Orthopedics*, ed 4, St Louis, 1995, Mosby.)

tests of thumb opposition and thenar muscle strength. Finally, testing of the radial nerve includes tests of wrist extension ability.

The clinician tests the sensory function of the hand with a light touch from the other hand, examining all sides of each finger. Two-point discrimination can elicit fine loss of sensory function. The normal two-point discrimination of the hand is approximately 4 to 6 mm, and anything greater than 6 mm is considered abnormal.

In examining the alignment of the fingers (e.g., to investigate the possibility of fracture), the clinician compares the two hands and searches for any gross abnormalities in the injured hand. A finger that lies underneath or separate from the others is grossly malaligned. If the patient can flex the fingers (without undue pain), all the fingers should point toward the navicular bone. Asking the patient to place all the fingers together and inspecting the alignment of the tips of the fingernails allows the clinician to check rotational alignment. The tips of the fingernails should form basically a straight line. A severe angle in one fingernail suggests a rotational malalignment of that finger.

Traumatic Injuries of the Hand

Sprains

Injuries to the ligaments, joint capsules, and adjacent structures of the hand are quite common, since hands are almost always in use. Many injuries are minor and do not require extensive treatment. Some injuries, however, lead to chronic disability and even to deformity.[14] Trauma frequently leads to sprains. Because joint injuries such as sprains can cause articular instability, it is important to identify them as early as possible. Early detection of complicated joint problems allows referral to the appropriate specialist.

Interphalangeal Collateral Ligament Sprain
The most common injury to the hand is a sprain of the collateral ligaments and structures that support the joints of the hand. Injuries to the hand can occur in a number of ways: fall, participation in a sport, or motor vehicle accident, among others. An object that hits the tip of the finger transmits a force down to the joints of the finger and often causes swelling over the metacarpophalangeal, proximal interphalangeal, and distal interphalangeal joints (Table 5-9). Isolated collateral ligament sprains are the result of a pure angulatory stress.[48]

Table 5-9	Sprains of the Hand	
	Interphalangeal Collateral Ligament Sprain	**Ulnar Collateral Ligament Sprain**
Physical examination findings	Swelling around MCP, DIP, or PIP joints Pain and laxity of ligament Limited range of motion because of pain and swelling	Laxity of ulnar collateral ligament in thumb abduction Palpable or point tenderness at MCP joint of thumb Swelling at MCP joint, especially at ulnar aspect
X-ray findings	Standard three-view series to rule out chip fracture	Standard three-view series to rule out avulsion fracture from base of proximal phalanx
Treatment plan	Splint immobilization Application of ice Buddy taping	For grades I and II, thumb spica immobilization for 4-6 weeks For grade III ruptures, referral to orthopedic surgeon

MCP, Metacarpophalangeal; **DIP,** distal interphalangeal; **PIP,** proximal interphalangeal.

In testing the movement and flexibility of the interphalangeal joints, the clinician should remember that one or more of the joints may have been dislocated and reduced either spontaneously or by the patient. Therefore it is necessary to test the volar and dorsal stability of the joint. X-ray films in these cases are usually normal; however, a small chip fracture is sometimes evident on either the side of the joint or its volar aspect.

Treatment is symptomatic and may include immobilization with a finger splint in severe cases. Most first-degree interphalangeal sprains do not need to be immobilized for more than 5 to 7 days; immobilization is primarily for patient comfort, since stress testing of the joint shows no instability. Second-degree sprains have more swelling, greater loss of motion, and some angulation. Treatment generally includes splint protection for 2 to 3 weeks. After that time, it may be helpful to use a "buddy system" in which the injured finger is taped to the adjacent finger in a way that allows movement in the joints. Taping may continue for 3 more weeks. Third-degree injuries involve capsule rupture, joint dislocation, gross deformity, and possible fracture.[48] These types of injuries are usually referred to an orthopedic or hand surgeon.

Ulnar Collateral Ligament Sprain

Sometimes called "gamekeeper's thumb" or "skier's thumb," an ulnar collateral ligament sprain is common in athletes. It is the most common injury among skiers, hence the name, and occurs when the individual attempts to break a fall with an outstretched hand while holding a ski pole.[42] Such a fall on an outstretched hand forcefully abducts the thumb and may rupture the ulnar collateral ligament.[53] An avulsion fracture may also occur at the base of the proximal phalanx. The injury affects the stability of the metacarpophalangeal part of the thumb, which is needed for pinch and grip strength.

The ulnar collateral ligament consists of a proper ligament and an accessory ligament. The proper ligament extends from the first metacarpal to the first proximal phalanx; the accessory ligament inserts into the sesamoid of the thumb. In metacarpophalangeal joint flexion, the proper ulnar collateral ligament tightens. During extension, the proper ligament is lax, and the accessory ligament is taut. The volar plate lends stability in extension as well.[55]

Physical examination reveals effusion at the metacarpophalangeal joint, especially at the ulnar aspect, as well as palpable tenderness over the ligament and painful abduction of the thumb.[14] The ulnar collateral ligament is lax in thumb abduction. An abduction stress test should be performed with the ligament at 20 degrees of flexion because this position relaxes the volar plate (Figure 5-25), which normally acts as a secondary restraint and tightens in full extension.[41] Motion is painful, especially thumb abduction. The patient has decreased pinch strength, and dissociation of the joint may cause a deformity. Routine or stress views visualize any fracture and concomitant articular instability.

Most sprains (i.e., grade I or II) can be treated conservatively with 4 to 6 weeks of immobilization in a thumb spica brace. Even stable chip fractures that are not associated with displacement can be treated in a closed fashion.

The appropriate treatment of complete ruptures of the ulnar collateral ligament (i.e., grade III sprain) is a source of controversy. Some tears may respond well to conservative care. Others, however, may require open repair, because the ulnar collateral ligament normally lies deep to the adductor pollicis muscle. The pull of the muscle can cause the torn ulnar collateral ligament to lie on top of the adductor, which leads to dysfunction of the thumb. Known as the Stenner lesion, this condition requires surgery to restore hand function.[68]

Arthrography or MRI and clinical examination permit the identification of this lesion.[68] Patients with grade III tears need a referral to an orthopedic or hand surgeon for an evaluation of the condition; open repair with Kirschner-wire fixation of the joint is common in patients with 35 degrees or more of laxity.[50] Arthrography and MRI can be useful in documenting and diagnosing ligament and joint disruption (Figure 5-26 *A, B*).

Fractures

Intraarticular fractures of the hand are important in that loss of the congruence of the joint may result in severe loss of motion. Very small intraarticular fractures of the hand can frequently be left to heal spontaneously without jeopardy to full hand function. Any large intraarticular fracture should be reduced, however. An open reduction is usually necessary to restore proper joint alignment.

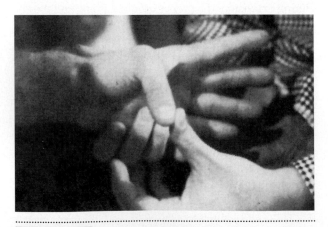

Figure 5-25 Torn ulnar collateral ligament of the metacarpophalangeal joint of the thumb.

(From Booher JM, Thibodeau GA: *Athletic injury assessment,* ed 3, St Louis, 1994, Mosby.)

Displacement and angulation, when viewed both radiographically and clinically, always steer the clinician toward a surgical referral and outcome. Despite the mechanical advantages of the rigid fixation that can be obtained through surgery, nonoperative methods of treatment frequently provide superior results for simple and nondisplaced fractures.[59]

Metacarpal Fracture

In primary care, metacarpal fractures are fairly common. The clinician should have a high index of suspicion when a patient exhibits dorsal swelling and has a history of trauma. Palpable tenderness, limitation of functional movement, and swelling are all signs of osseous injury. It is important to obtain an accurate radiologic assessment of the injury as soon as possible. Nonoperative treatment yields satisfactory results in most cases,[7] but confirmed fractures and displaced articulations require a referral to an orthopedic surgeon.

The most common metacarpal fracture is that of the fifth metacarpal (Figure 5-27). Because this type of fracture usually occurs when the individual gets into a fight or punches a wall, it is sometimes referred to as a boxer's fracture or barroom fracture. The site of the fracture is generally the neck of the metacarpal, just proximal to the metacarpal head, and the fracture usually results in the angulation of the head into the palm of the hand (Table 5-10). Swelling and ecchymosis become obvious. In contrast, fractures to the base of the fifth metacarpal are often missed and usually require an oblique x-ray projection for documentation. The pull of the extensor carpi ulnaris usually displaces the distal fragment and results in a carpometacarpal dislocation as well.[21]

A posteroanterior or anteroposterior x-ray film usually shows fracture lines. A good lateral x-ray film of the hand determines the amount of angulation at the fracture site. If the angulation exceeds 15 degrees, a closed reduction is necessary.[4] A lidocaine (Xylocaine) fracture block can be helpful in the reduction procedure. After completing the reduction, the clinician immobilizes the hand by applying an ulnar splint or short-arm cast, with extension to the little and ring digits and the metacarpophalangeal joint in approximately 90 degrees of flexion. As noted earlier, the collateral ligaments of the metacarpophalangeal joints are loose in extension; therefore immobilizing the joints in extension can allow the ligaments to shorten and make subsequent flexion of the joint difficult. The flexed position, however, minimizes such extension contractures of the collateral liga-

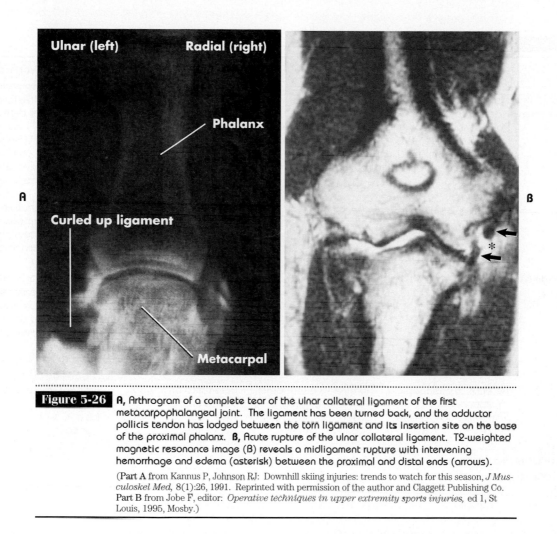

Figure 5-26 A, Arthrogram of a complete tear of the ulnar collateral ligament of the first metacarpophalangeal joint. The ligament has been turned back, and the adductor pollicis tendon has lodged between the torn ligament and its insertion site on the base of the proximal phalanx. B, Acute rupture of the ulnar collateral ligament. T2-weighted magnetic resonance image (B) reveals a midligament rupture with intervening hemorrhage and edema (asterisk) between the proximal and distal ends (arrows).

(Part A from Kannus P, Johnson RJ: Downhill skiing injuries: trends to watch for this season, *J Musculoskel Med*, 8(1):26, 1991. Reprinted with permission of the author and Claggett Publishing Co. Part B from Jobe F, editor: *Operative techniques in upper extremity sports injuries*, ed 1, St Louis, 1995, Mosby.)

ments at the metacarpophalangeal joints. The fracture should be immobilized for 4 weeks. After that, the patient should begin active range-of-motion exercises.

Fractures of the other metacarpals also tend to be angulated with the head directed toward the palm. The treatment should be the same as that for the fifth metacarpal. Again, 4 weeks of immobilization should allow the fracture to heal.

Bennett's Fracture

The most common injury to the thumb metacarpal is a Bennett's fracture, which occurs at the base of the thumb. This severe injury is actually a fracture dislocation from the dorsoradial displacement of the osseous fragment at the proximal first metacarpal.[67] The cause is usually a severe abduction of the thumb that dislocates the carpo-

metacarpal joint and frequently leaves a piece of bone attached to the volar ligaments of the joint. The pull of the abductor pollicis longus tendon displaces the remaining shaft of the metacarpal radially and dorsally.[14] X-ray films are the primary means of diagnosis. The insult to the physis of skeletally immature individuals must be further evaluated (Figure 5-28).

It is important to refer the patient with such a fracture to either an orthopedic or hand surgeon, because choices of care are complex. The dislocation component of the injury is of paramount importance. The anatomic reduction—via closed, percutaneous, or open methods— must be accurate and precise. A closed reduction should be the first procedure attempted, but many Bennett's fractures require the placement of a pin or a Kirschner wire to reduce the fracture.

Table 5-10 Fractures of the Hand

	Metacarpal Fracture	Bennett's Fracture	Rolando Fracture	Phalangeal Fracture
Physical examination findings	Pain and swelling over dorsum of hand Point tenderness over metacarpals Possible deformity, angulation	Palpable pain at base of thumb Swelling over dorsal aspect of metacarpal-carpal joint Loss of thumb abduction	Severe injury at thumb basal joint Carpal-metacarpal deformity Dorsal swelling at first metacarpal Loss of thumb movement	Swelling and visible deformity of digit Restriction of movement at PIP or DIP joints because of pain Pain during pressure testing along long axis of phalanx Sometimes anatomic subluxation because of volar plate injury (seen in fracture and dislocation)
X-ray findings	Three-view series Need to rule out angular deformity and displacement	Evidence of fracture at proximal first metacarpal Possible dorsoradial displacement	Evidence of intraarticular fracture at base of first metacarpal Often, mild-to-moderate displacement Need to assess size and alignment of fragment	Three-view standard series (anteroposterior, lateral, and oblique) Nondisplaced chip fracture above joint common* Need to rule out rotational deformity
Treatment plan	Referral to orthopedic surgeon Immobilization, closed reduction, if necessary	Referral to orthopedic or hand surgeon Closed, percutaneous, or open treatment	Referral to orthopedic surgeon Treatment by closed or open reduction	Referral to orthopedic surgeon Ice and buddy tape or splint

*Simple nondisplaced chip fractures are treated in a splint (finger cot or frog splint) for 7 to 14 days.
PIP, Proximal interphalangeal; **DIP,** distal interphalangeal.

Intraarticular fractures are especially unstable and, as such, require either pin fixation after reduction or open reduction with internal fixation. Extraarticular fractures, however, are generally stable after reduction and can tolerate up to 30 degrees of angulation.[4] Inaccurate reduction and improper maintenance of reduction may lead to malunion or even nonunion.

Outcome assessment is based on proper anatomic reduction. Healing in the proper position helps prevent osteoarthritic changes. The pin is usually left in place for 3 to 4 weeks, and the thumb is immobilized for another 3 or 4 weeks. Thus immobilization casting totals approximately 6 to 8 weeks.

Rolando Fractures

Like the Bennett's fracture, Rolando fractures occur at the base of the thumb. This injury is a severe intraarticular fracture in which the base of the metacarpal is shattered. These injuries are less common than a Ben-

nett's fracture and carry a worse prognosis (Figure 5-29). They also have varying degrees of comminution.[73] Because a Rolando fracture frequently leads to osteoarthritis of the joint, it is essential to obtain the best possible reduction and thus minimize the patient's risk of arthritis in the future.

If the fragments are large enough to hold screws, open reduction and internal fixation are appropriate. External fixation that provides traction across the joint may allow the pieces of the metacarpal to fall into a reasonable alignment. In certain cases, however, when the bone stock if too poor for rigid fixation, treatment by simple casting and early immobilization is the only option.

Phalangeal Fractures

Frequently, fractures of the proximal phalanges of the fingers are oblique in nature and cause a malrotation of the fingers. This deformity requires fixation with Kirschner wires to reestablish proper alignment and function of the

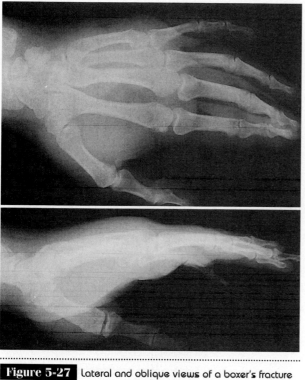

Figure 5-27 Lateral and oblique views of a boxer's fracture with 30 to 35 degrees of angulation. If there is no rotation, this fracture may be treated symptomatically with no reduction necessary.

(From Ruiz E, Cicero JJ: *Emergency management of skeletal injuries*, ed 1, St Louis, 1995, Mosby.)

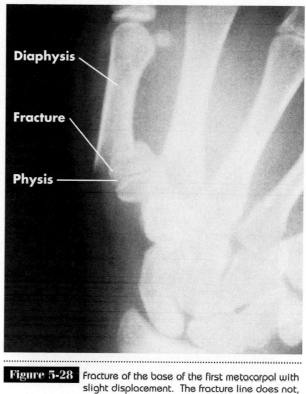

Diaphysis

Fracture

Physis

Figure 5-28 Fracture of the base of the first metacarpal with slight displacement. The fracture line does not, however, extend through the physis.

finger. A fracture of the proximal phalanx is more serious than a distal injury.

Fractures of the middle and distal phalanges are common injuries. Phalangeal fractures may cause associated ligament and/or tendon injuries.[61] Any rotational deformities of the fingers that result from such fractures need correction. Finger fractures generally require 3 weeks of immobilization. Again, the metacarpophalangeal joint should be immobilized in approximately 90 degrees of flexion to prevent extension contractures of the joint. The proximal and distal interphalangeal joints can be held in approximately 15 and 10 degrees of flexion, respectively, during immobilization.

Dislocations

Metacarpophalangeal Joints

The stability of the metacarpophalangeal joint is derived from the volar plate and the collateral ligaments. Although they are not very common, dislocations of the metacarpophalangeal joints do occur. These injuries are named according to the direction taken by the most distal bone in the dislocation. For example, a dislocation of the metacarpophalangeal joint that displaces the proximal phalanx dorsally over the metacarpal is called a dorsal dislocation of the joint; if the proximal phalanx is displaced volarly, the injury is a volar dislocation, which is quite rare.

A dorsal dislocation of the metacarpophalangeal joint results in severe pain and deformity of the hand. Careful examination of the x-ray films, especially the lateral view of the hand, reveals the dislocation. The practitioner should attempt a closed reduction with a lidocaine block, but this technique is frequently unsuccessful because the metacarpal head can become trapped between the flexor tendons, lumbricals, and neurovascular bundles in the palmar aspect of the hand. This event mandates an open reduction. Immobilization for 2 to 3 weeks may be necessary to maintain the joint reduction.

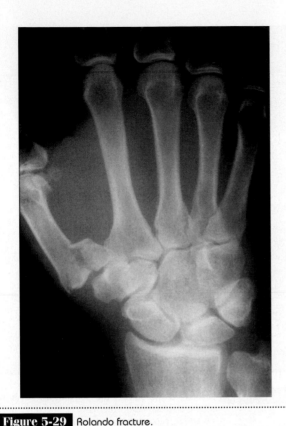

Figure 5-29 Rolando fracture.

(From Canale ST, editor: *Campbell's operative orthopaedics*, ed 9, St Louis, 1998, Mosby.)

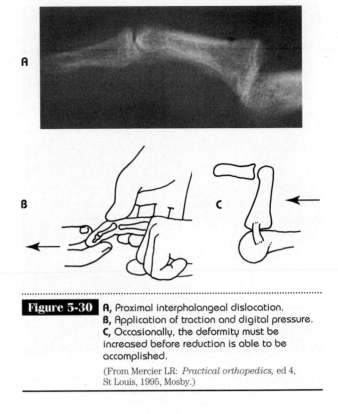

Figure 5-30 **A,** Proximal interphalangeal dislocation. **B,** Application of traction and digital pressure. **C,** Occasionally, the deformity must be increased before reduction is able to be accomplished.

(From Mercier LR: *Practical orthopedics*, ed 4, St Louis, 1995, Mosby.)

Phalangeal Joints

A strong force exerted on the tip of the finger can result in a dislocation of the phalangeal joints. Such dislocations are fairly common, especially in sports where a ball or another player can hit the fingertip. Dorsal displacement of the first or second joint causes capsular tearing and sometimes bone and tendon injury.[49]

In the proximal interphalangeal joints of the hand, dislocations are notorious for producing late severe deformities. Thus the clinician must be cautious in examining this joint, especially if there is any suggestion of a dislocation. In many cases, simple longitudinal traction on the finger after the administration of a lidocaine block permits reduction of the injury (Figure 5-30 *A-C*). Occasionally, however, there is a soft-tissue block that necessitates an open reduction.

Because dorsal dislocations of the proximal interphalangeal joint are usually associated with a rupture of the volar plate of the finger, it is important to test the volar plate's integrity. If the finger goes into severe hyperextension, the proximal interphalangeal joint should be immobilized after reduction in approximately 20 to 45 degrees of flexion. Immobilization in this position helps heal the volar structures and prevents permanent hyperextension of the joint.

Injuries to the Tendons

Flexor Digitorum Profundus Rupture

Closed ruptures of the flexor tendons frequently occur in football. Grabbing an opposing player's jersey, for example, can force a tackler's distal interphalangeal joint into extension and rupture the profundus tendon. This rupture usually occurs near the tendon's insertion into the distal phalanx. The patient has a swollen finger and is unable to flex the distal interphalangeal joint. A standard three-view x-ray series can rule out a concomitant avulsion fracture; the lateral projection usually reveals such a rupture.[67]

The tendons of an injured finger should be examined individually: first the sublimus (superficialis) tendon and then the profundus tendon. The function of the profundus tendon is evaluated by active flexion of the distal interphalangeal joint; the function of the super-

ficialis tendon is evaluated by active flexion of the proximal interphalangeal joint while the examiner maintains
the other digits in extension. Rupture or laceration of the
sublimus tendon is a very unusual injury.[80] It is not always repaired when it does occur, because the profundus
tendon can flex both interphalangeal joints. There may
be some residual weakness if the injury receives no treatment, however.

Repair of a ruptured flexor profundus tendon to
the digits, especially the thumb and the index, long, and
little fingers, is essential to ensure good hand function
(Table 5-11). If the repair does not take place within the
first 2 to 3 weeks, a two-stage operation and reconstruction of the tendon is necessary to restore the function of the distal interphalangeal joint.[88] Occasionally,
when the damage is severe and involves multiple sites,
the distal interphalangeal joint is fused in a flexed position in lieu of this secondary reconstruction procedure.

Mallet Finger

Rupture of the extensor tendon at the distal interphalangeal joint is very common; this injury prevents the
full extension of the joint and results in a condition called
a mallet finger. The mechanism of injury is the forcible
flexion of the extended distal interphalangeal joint.
Those who participate in sports, particularly baseball or
softball, are most likely to experience this injury. In fact,
the condition is sometimes called baseball finger.

In some cases a slough of bone that has separated
from the dorsal base of the distal phalanx is visible on an
x-ray film (Figure 5-31). Frequently, simply immobilizing the finger in extension for approximately 4 weeks
allows the tendon to heal. The patient must not remove
the splint, however; the distal interphalangeal joint must
be held in the extended position if the treatment is to be
successful.

Tendon Deformities

Swan Neck Deformity. If injured volar structures
heal in a lengthened position at the proximal interphalangeal joint, a swan neck deformity can develop. The hyperextension at the proximal interphalangeal joint has a
tethering effect on the profundus tendon, causing flexion
of the distal interphalangeal joint. The results are a finger
in which the proximal interphalangeal joint is in hyperextension and a distal interphalangeal joint is in flexion.

Chronic proximal interphalangeal sprains, untreated dislocations, and repeated sports trauma can all
damage the volar plate. Rheumatoid disease leading to
synovitis of the hand can also be a contributing factor in

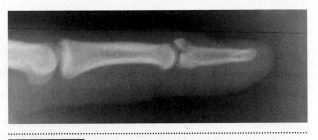

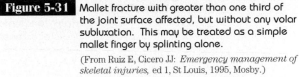

Figure 5-31 Mallet fracture with greater than one third of
the joint surface affected, but without any volar
subluxation. This may be treated as a simple
mallet finger by splinting alone.

(From Ruiz E, Cicero JJ: *Emergency management of
skeletal injuries*, ed 1, St Louis, 1995, Mosby.)

cases of swan neck deformity.[24] The degree of pain and
disability determines the appropriate treatment. Referral to a hand specialist may be necessary.

Boutonniere Deformity. A rupture of the central
extensor tendon slip frequently occurs in a volar dislocation of the proximal interphalangeal joint (Figure 5-32).
The mechanism of injury is a sudden and forceful flexion
movement of the extended proximal interphalangeal
joint. In this case the lateral bands of the tendon, which
extend the proximal interphalangeal joint, fall volar
(palmar) to the joint's center of rotation; the result is a
flexion deformity. The distal interphalangeal joint stays
in a hyperextended position because of the relative laxity
of the profundus tendon. The patient feels pain dorsally
over the proximal interphalangeal joint. Hyperflexion
of the proximal interphalangeal joint and hyperextension of the distal interphalangeal joint is called a boutonniere deformity (Figure 5-33).

If the patient can fully extend the finger at the time
of injury, the risk of boutonniere deformity is small. The
finger should be reduced and splinted in the extended
position for approximately 2 to 4 weeks, at which time
the clinician can prescribe active range-of-motion exercises. Untreated injuries often lead to a stiff proximal
interphalangeal joint, degenerative arthritis, and chronic
deformity.[48] At that time, referral to a hand specialist is
necessary.

An inability to extend the metacarpophalangeal
joint fully suggests an injury to the common tendon on
the dorsum of the hand; a lidocaine injection into the extensor tendon allows the clinician to determine whether
the loss of extension is the result of pain or an actual disruption of the extensor tendon. Any such injury should
be repaired.

Table 5-11 Injuries to the Tendons of the Hand

| | Flexor Digitorum Profundus Rupture | Mallet Finger | Tendon Deformities | |
			Swan Neck	Boutonniere
Physical examination findings	History of athletic trauma (e.g., jersey tackling in football) Swelling of finger Inability to flex DIP joint	History of trauma involving sudden flexion of extended fingertip Inability to extend finger at DIP joint Point tenderness at distal extensor tendon	Hyperextension deformity at PIP joint Flexion deformity at DIP joint (tethering of profundus tendon) Possible history of repetitive trauma	History of volar dislocation of PIP joint Dorsal tenderness over PIP joint Hyperflexion deformity at PIP joint with hyperextension deformity at DIP joint Difficulty in extending finger completely at PIP joint
X-ray findings	Soft-tissue swelling Need to rule out secondary avulsion fracture	Need to rule out concomitant avulsion fracture at distal phalanx	Need to rule out degenerative arthritis, old fractures, or rheumatoid disease	Need to rule out concomitant fracture, arthritis Need to confirm reduction after PIP dislocation
Treatment plan	Referral to orthopedic or hand surgeon for operative care	Splint immobilization of DIP joint in full extension for 4 weeks	Dependent on stage of deformity Referral to hand specialist according to degree of pain and disability	Reduction and splint immobilization of finger in extension for 2 to 4 weeks Referral to hand specialist according to degree of deformity and disability

DIP, Distal interphalangeal; *PIP,* proximal interphalangeal.

Lacerations and Crush Injuries

A lacerated finger should be examined closely for tendon injuries and neurovascular damage. The clinician can test the arterial supply to the finger by compressing the tip of the finger until it blanches, releasing it, and observing the briskness of the capillary refill. A delay in refill may indicate an arterial compromise. Sensory testing should include both sides of the finger, as well as the volar and dorsal aspects.

The patient's occupation affects the treatment of a lacerated nerve. If the patient is a musician who requires the fine feeling of the digit, for example, repair of the digital nerve is necessary. Nerves that definitely need repair are the digital nerves to the thumb, the radial digital nerve to the index finger, and the ulnar digital nerve of the fifth finger. The remaining digital nerves are not critical for hand function and are often left unrepaired. The patient and the surgeon must make such decisions together, however.

Injuries to the nailbed and matrix can lead to permanent disfiguring of the nail. A crush injury to the nail and nailbed frequently results in a hematoma underneath the nail (i.e., a subungual hematoma). If this is painful, the clinician can evacuate the hematoma by putting a hole in the nail with a large bore needle or even a heated paper clip, as long as there is no fracture.[60] Lacerations into the nail and nail matrix require suturing; otherwise, the patient will have permanent ridging of the fingernail. A forceful enough direct blow to the fingertip may cause a fracture of the distal phalanx.

If the fingernail has been avulsed from the nailbed, it is wise to pack a small piece of petroleum jelly gauze underneath the cuticle to prevent adhesions from the cuticle to the nail matrix. This packing can be changed every day, but the packing should continue for approximately 2 to 3 weeks. Soaking the fingernail in warm water (or a solution of one-half peroxide, one-half water) helps debride the tissue and allow a new nail to form.

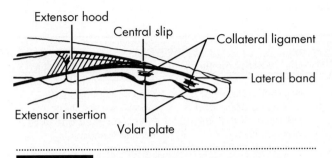

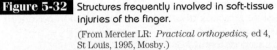

Figure 5-32 Structures frequently involved in soft-tissue injuries of the finger.

(From Mercier LR: *Practical orthopedics,* ed 4, St Louis, 1995, Mosby.)

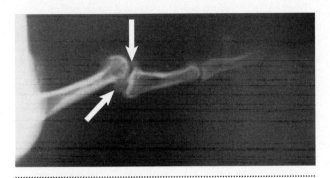

Figure 5-33 Boutonniere deformity in a 23-year-old man with a history of traumatic injuries. Lateral radiographic view shows a subluxed proximal interphalangeal joint with degenerative arthritis.

Nontraumatic Conditions of the Hand

Trigger Finger

In the 50-year-old age group and over, the condition called trigger finger is a very common hand problem (Table 5-12).[13,91] The patient complains that a finger gets locked into a flexed position and then snaps into an extended position. This can also occur in the thumb. The physical examination reveals a palpable nodule and tenderness on the volar aspect of the metacarpophalangeal joint of the involved digit. The finger locks when brought into extreme flexion, but unlocks when it is extended.

The cause of trigger finger is a swelling of the flexor tendon pulley (A-1 pulley) at the metacarpophalangeal joint, frequently as a result of arthritis in the joint. Occasionally, a benign swelling in the tendon causes the locking. X-ray findings are often normal, except for the evidence of mild arthritis.

Initially, treatment involves physiotherapeutic modalities, antiinflammatory medication, and gentle range-of-motion exercises. A cortisone injection into the volar aspect of the tendon sheath at the metacarpophalangeal joint may relieve the patient's symptoms,[44] but the symptoms can recur. If the patient's symptoms do not abate, the clinician may refer the patient to an orthopedic specialist for another injection or for a surgical consultation. The surgical release of the tendon sheath at the metacarpophalangeal level can resolve the problem.

Dupuytren's Contracture

Described as a contracture of the palmar fascia of the hand, Dupuytren's contracture typically begins when the patient is in the fifth decade of life and becomes a progressive problem. The condition is much more common in men.[84] The cause is unknown, but repeated trauma to the palm can increase a patient's susceptibility to this contracture. In addition, it may be associated with alcoholism and diabetes mellitus. Finally, it is generally recognized that Dupuytren's disease is inherited as a dominant gene with a variable degree of penetrance.[98]

Nodules, usually fusiform in shape, appear on the ulnar side of the hand, where they involve the ring finger, the little finger, or both. These nodules can contract, sometimes extending the contracture to the metacarpophalangeal or proximal interphalangeal joints. Conservative therapy is best in the early phases of the disease. Ultrasound treatment may help reduce the fibrosis in mild-to-moderate cases. Manipulation of the metacarpophalangeal and proximal interphalangeal articulations, along with mobilization of the digits, may aid in maintaining the mobility of the hand. When the contractures are so advanced that they interfere with the function of the hand, referral to an orthopedic or hand surgeon is indicated. When the flexion contracture of a joint is significant and disabling, surgical removal of the contracted palmar fascia is appropriate.

Arthritis

Various types of arthritic conditions can make it necessary for an individual to seek primary orthopedic care for the hand. Although psoriatic arthritis and erosive arthritis can cause severe destruction in the distal interphalangeal joints, degenerative arthritis and rheumatoid arthritis occur more commonly.

Table 5-12 Nontraumatic Injuries of the Hand

| | Trigger Finger | Dupuytren's Contracture | Arthritis | |
			Osteoarthritis	Rheumatoid Arthritis
Physical examination findings	Palpable nodule on volar aspect of hand Palpable tenderness over MCP joint of involved finger Locking of finger in flexion Fibrosis and swelling of flexor tendon sheath Age 50 years or older	Palmar contractures Stiffness and fibrosis of volar fascia Palpable nodules that can cause contractures at MCP and PIP joints Need to investigate functional capacity of hand	Bony deformity, most commonly at PIP and DIP joints and thumb basal joint Intermittent stiffness and swelling after use Possible previous trauma as causative factor Advanced deformity or instability in severe cases	Chronic pain and stiffness, especially at first MCP joint and wrist Nodule formation possible Ulnar deviation of digits; subluxation in advanced cases
X-ray findings	Often normal Mild osteoarthritis of MCP joint possible	Usually unremarkable	Three-view standard hand series Evidence of sclerosis, narrowing of joint space, or heterotopic bone formation Usually spur formation in digits Osseous malalignment or joint incongruity in severe cases	Three-view standard series of wrist or hand Evidence of bony erosion, especially at ulnar styloid Bony ankylosis of carpus in advanced disease Juxtaarticular osteoporosis
Treatment plan	Underwater ultrasound Range-of-motion and stretching exercises Medical referral for injection of cortisone, if needed Surgical release in severe cases	Underwater ultrasound Mobilization, passive stretching of MCP and PIP joints, manipulation Surgical referral only if hand is dysfunctional	Therapeutic modalities for pain and swelling Functional strengthening exercises with putty Cryotherapy Mobilization and manipulation to maintain joint mobility Bracing for unstable joints only NSAIDs for advanced pain and swelling	Cryotherapy, electrotherapy Rehabilitative exercises with putty Bracing and medication for flare-ups or exacerbating trauma

PIP, Proximal interphalangeal; **DIP,** distal interphalangeal; **MCP,** metacarpophalangeal; **NSAIDs,** nonsteroidal antiinflammatory drugs.

Osteoarthritis

The most common arthritic problem of the hand is osteoarthritis.[35] Often beginning when the patient is in the fourth or fifth decade of life, osteoarthritis is a degenerative joint disease in which there is a progressive loss of articular cartilage. It can occur at the wrist or hand as a result of years of wear and tear or because of an earlier traumatic event. Athletes or laborers commonly complain of arthritic pain in association with strenuous activity or weather change.

The interphalangeal articulations of the hand and the basal joint of the thumb are common sites of osteoarthritis.[51] Swelling of these joints may limit motion, particularly at the base of the thumb. Small nodules called Heberden's nodes may be noticeable on the dorsum of the distal interphalangeal joints. It is also common for nodules to form at the proximal interphalangeal joints; these are called Bouchard's nodes, which are a cystic degeneration of the joint capsule.

When a significant previous trauma in the wrist or digits has rendered a joint arthritic, the clinical evaluation should include both a physical examination and radiographic examination. A plain x-ray film can reveal joint subluxation, bony incongruency, osteophytosis, bony eburnation, and arthritic degeneration of the bone.[35] Treatment focuses on the symptomatology and functional ability of the patient.

Cryotherapy, gentle exercises, and therapeutic modalities such as ultrasound and electrotherapy may help many patients with arthritic pain.[16] In cases of severe pain, an over-the-counter antiarthritic medication may help. Patients should be aware of the gastric and other side effects of over-the-counter drugs, however. Furthermore, if they use a variety of medications, they must consult their medical physician or pharmacist about drug interactions.

Motion with manipulation, mobilization, and exercise are perhaps the best ways to (1) maintain joint and periarticular integrity and (2) prevent further degeneration by promoting diffusion and nutrient flow. Cases of severe instability, osseous destruction, and inability to complete common tasks should be referred to an orthopedic or hand surgeon for care. The lack of a satisfying life style and the inability to earn a living are important considerations in treating the patient with hand disability.

Rheumatoid Arthritis

Usually more destructive than osteoarthritis, rheumatoid arthritis affects both children and adults. The disease is inflammatory in nature, affecting the synovium and leading to joint destruction. It can affect all the joints of the hand, with the exception of the distal interphalangeal joints. Rheumatoid arthritis can involve one joint or many joints, as well as the surrounding soft-tissue structures.

Rheumatoid arthritis frequently appears first in the metacarpophalangeal joints of the fingers and hand. Destruction may be severe in the metacarpophalangeal joints, causing the joints to drift in an ulnar direction.[28] Ulnar drift makes grasping difficult and causes severe weakness of the hands. Swan neck deformities of the proximal interphalangeal joints can develop from degeneration of the volar plates. Although the history and physical examination are the clinician's primary tools in diagnosing rheumatoid arthritis, laboratory tests can be helpful. Patients with inflammation, swelling, and effusion in the joints should have a white blood cell count, erythrocyte sedimentation rate determination, urinalysis, and rheumatoid factor assay performed.[8]

The primary purpose of treatment for rheumatoid arthritis is to maintain the strength and mobility of the affected joints. The extent of the patient's disability and the degree of bony deformity and inflammation largely determine the appropriate adjunctive therapies.

The preferred treatments for acute flare-ups (i.e., swelling, stiffness, and pain) of rheumatoid arthritis in the hand are rest, cryotherapy, and electrotherapy in cool water, regardless of the patient's age. Patients may also benefit from antiinflammatory (antiarthritic) medication during acute flare-ups. Strengthening exercises are the key to a functional hand that is ready to handle everyday tasks.[11] Theraputty, Silly Putty, or Play-Doh are all easily manageable, pliable, and affordable. The frequency and duration of rehabilitation exercises should be predicated on the age, severity of symptoms, and osseous deformity of the individual's hand.[76]

Most cases of mild-to-moderate rheumatoid arthritis do well with the regimen of therapy described. Splinting a hand or finger that is developing a deformity may minimize the ulnar drift of the fingers; the patient can wear the splint at night. If the ulnar drift becomes severe, silicone (Silastic) replacements for the metacarpophalangeal joints may help restore the hand's function for the activities of daily living. Referral to a rheumatologic specialist for a medical evaluation is important for these patients.

In advanced rheumatoid arthritis, radiographic films of the wrist and hand show great bony deformity, severe anatomic subluxation of the carpal and metacarpophalangeal joints, and bony erosion (Figure 5-34). The pain and disfigurement may be great. Most of these patients have been or will be treated medically with a variety of medications and surgical procedures.

The goal of rehabilitation for patients with rheumatoid arthritis is similar to the goal of treatment for patients with other chronic debilitating diseases—helping these patients live with their illness. Many have been advised to take powerful drugs that adversely affect their immune system in an effort to control their illness. A patient with rheumatoid arthritis cannot depend on any treatment to correct the problem, but nonpharmacologic therapy regimens, especially gentle exercise, can help these people continue to lead productive lives.

Infections of the Hand

In general, infections of the hand occur as the result of a laceration or a puncture wound. Punching another person in the mouth notoriously causes transverse lacerations on the dorsum of the metacarpophalangeal joints. Such an injury is considered a human bite and should be treated very aggressively by irrigation, debridement of the joint, and the administration of a broad-spectrum antibiotic.[72] These wounds must be watched closely.

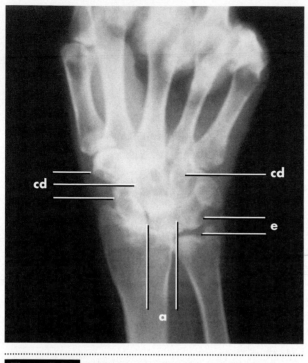

cd

cd

e

a

Figure 5-34 Radiographic view of the wrist of a 46-year-old woman with a 10-year history of rheumatoid arthritis. Bony erosion (e) and arthrosis (a) of the radiocarpal and intercarpal joints are clear. Cystic degeneration (cd) dominates the distal row of carpal bones.

A puncture wound or a laceration on the dorsum of the hand may lead to a collection of pus around the injured site. Because of the loose attachment of the dorsal skin to the underlying structures, the pocket of fluid can become quite large. The dorsum of the hand becomes very swollen, warm, and red. Frequently, pus may ooze from the wound. Such an injury should be evacuated surgically at once, and antibiotics should be administered to prevent osteomyelitis and extension of the infection into the flexor sheath or adjacent joint.[60]

Infections on the palm of the hand are more serious and more acute in their presentation. Although an infection can develop in this area without a laceration or puncture, such an injury most commonly precedes the infection. On the volar aspect of the hand, an infection in a digit can spread through the finger's tendon sheath and cause an acute bacterial tenosynovitis, resulting in severe pain, swelling, and redness of the finger.[37] Any movement of the finger, especially passive extension, is very painful. If the infection occurs in the thumb or little finger, it can spread from one to the other through a common tendon sheath in the wrist; this condition is called a horseshoe infection.

Osteomyelitis in the hand bones is unusual, although it can result from a compound wound of the hand. Symptoms include chronic pain, swelling, and redness. X-ray films may show a lucency in the bone. If osteomyelitis is confirmed, the dead and infected bone should be removed and antibiotics should be administered intravenously for 4 to 6 weeks.

Tumors of the Hand

Benign tumors of the hand are common. Similarly, ganglion cysts are prevalent; such a cyst is a secreting pocket in a joint that may be the result of a traumatic event or osteoarthritis. In the finger joints they are usually small, but they can occur in other joints where they cause pain and make it difficult for the individual to grasp objects in the hand. Treatment generally consists of hot or cold soaks, adjunctive therapies such as underwater ultrasound, the administration of antiinflammatory medication, and aspiration or surgical removal, if needed.

A giant cell tumor is a common tumor of the tendon sheath of the hand. It can occur on either the volar or the dorsal aspects of the hand. Usually, they are excised if they become unsightly or painful.

The most common bone tumor of the hand is an enchondroma, which usually occurs on a finger. It is a slowly expansive bone tumor that thins the cortex and makes the bone easily susceptible to fracture. As a result, a fracture through the enchondroma may be the initial presentation. The x-ray film shows the expanded and thinned cortex with speckled calcification within the lucent tumor. If the finger has fractured across the enchondroma, the fracture should be treated with a reduction and immobilization. Occasionally, when a finger has fractured through the tumor, the enchondroma can partially or completely fill in with bone during the fracture healing, which is helpful in stabilizing the area. If there is no fracture, treatment of an enchondroma involves curetting (i.e., removing) the tumor and filling the void with a bone graft.

Tumors in the hand are sometimes malignant. For example, a chondrosarcoma is a common malignant bone tumor of the hand; occasionally, the chondrosarcoma is a malignant degeneration of an enchondroma. Metastatic tumors of bone may appear in the hand. The most common metastatic tumor to the hand is from a carcinoma of the lung, however. Malignant bone tumors in the hand are usually treated by amputation.

Review Questions

1. (a) Standard radiography of the wrist includes which projections? (b) What should the clinician scrutinize in each view? (c) Name two supplemental projections and the pathologic abnormalities they confirm?

2. (a) What is De Quervain disease? (b) What are some pathomechanical factors in this condition? (c) What orthopedic test is positive during examination of the patient?

3. A 30 year-old woman complains of swelling on the dorsum of the hand and wrist after a fall. She has painful and limited dorsiflexion of the wrist with tenderness in the anatomic snuffbox. (a) What is your diagnosis? (b) What radiographic films should be taken? (c) What follow-up precautions should be followed?

4. (a) Name the common signs and symptoms of carpal tunnel syndrome. (b) What orthopedic tests would you perform to confirm this diagnosis? (c) What conservative treatment options are available to treat this condition? (d) What other conditions must be ruled out when diagnosing the patient?

5. (a) An individual with weakness or atrophy of the intrinsic muscles of the hand along with dysthesia at the fourth and fifth digits has what structure compromised? (b) What are some possible diagnoses for this clinical presentation?

6. (a) The term "gamekeeper's thumb" or "skier's thumb" denotes a traumatic injury to what structure of the hand? (b) Which joint is compromised, thus leading to a reduction of grip and pinch strength? (c) X-ray films are required for this clinical work-up to rule out what type of concomitant injury?

References

1. Abbaszadegar H, Johnson V, Sivers KV: Prediction of instability of Colles' fracture, *Acta Orthop Scand* 60(6):646, 1989.
2. Alfred R: *Wrist injuries in sports* (paper presented at the Sports Medicine Symposium), Cleveland, 1987, Cleveland Clinic Foundation.
3. Aro H, Koirunen J, Katevvo K et al.: Late compression neuropathies after Colles' fracture, *Clin Orthop* 233:217, 1988.
4. Ashkenaze DM, Ruby LK: Metacarpal fractures and dislocations, *Orthop Clin North Am* 23(1):19, 1992.
5. Ashton EB, Coffey D, Hyde T, Swenson R: Grand rounds: bilateral hand numbness, *JNMS* 3(2):99, 1995.
6. Atkinson LS, Baxley EG: Scapholunate dissociation, *Am Fam Physician* 499(8):1845, 1994.
7. Barton N: Conservative treatment of articular fractures in the hand, *J Hand Surg* 14A:386, 1989.
8. Baum J: Laboratory tests in rheumatoid arthritis, *J Musculoskel Med* 10(5):55, 1993.
9. Belsole RJ, Hess AV: Concomitant skeletal and soft-tissue injuries, *Orthop Clin North Am* 24(2):327, 1993.
10. Bishop AT, Beckerbough RD: Fracture of the hamate hook, *J Hand Surg* 13A:135, 1989.
11. Biundo JJ, Hughes GM: Rheumatoid arthritis rehabilitation: practical guidelines, *J Musculoskel Med* 8(7):37, 1991.
12. Blair WF: Regional anesthesia preferable for Colles' fracture, *Adv Orthop Surg* 15(1):20, 1991.
13. Bonnici AV, Spencer JD: A survey of trigger finger in adults, *J Hand Surg* 13B:202, 1988.
14. Booher JM, Thibodeau GA: *Athletic injury assessment*, ed 3, St Louis, 1994, Mosby.
15. Burkhart SS, Wood MB, Linscherd RL: Post-traumatic recurrent subluxation of the extensor carpi ulnaris tendon, *J Hand Surg* 7:1, 1982.
16. Calin A: What causes osteoarthritis? *J Musculoskel Med* 10(10):39, 1993.
17. Cervoni TD, Martire JR, Curl LA, McFarland EG: Recognizing upper extremity stress lesions, *Phys Sports Med* 25:8, 1997.
18. Chiv DTW, Ishii C: Management of peripheral nerve injuries, *Orthop Clin North Am* 17(3):365, 1986.
19. Conyers DJ: Scapholunate interosseous reconstruction and imbrication of palmar ligaments, *J Hand Surg* 15A:690, 1990.
20. Cookson JC: Musculoskeletal analysis: the elbow and hand. In Scully RM, Barnes MR, editors: *Physical therapy*, Philadelphia, 1989, JB Lippincott.
21. Corley FG: Commonly missed fractures in the hand and wrist, *J Musculoskel Med* 10(10):55, 1993.
22. Culver JE: Sports-related fractures of the hand and wrist, *Clin Sports Med* 9(1):104, 1990.
23. Culver JE, Anderson TE: Fractures of the hand and wrist in the athlete, *Clin Sports Med* 11(1):126, 1992.
24. D'Cruz D, Hughes G: Rheumatoid arthritis: the clinical features, *J Musculoskel Med* 10(1):85, 1993.
25. Dell PC: Traumatic disorders of the distal radioulnar joint, *Clin Sports Med* 11(1):148, 1992.
26. Donatelli R, Wooden MJ: *Orthopedic physical therapy*, New York, 1989, Churchill Livingstone.
27. Evans RC: *Illustrated essentials in orthopedic physical assessment*, St Louis, 1994, Mosby.
28. Ferlic DC, Clayton ML, Ries MD, Dennis DA: Surgery in rheumatoid arthritis: the upper extremity, *J Musculoskel Med* 7(10):12, 1990.
29. Friedman WA: The electrophysiology of peripheral nerve injuries, *Neurosurg Clin North Am* 2(1):43, 1991.
30. Gainor BJ: The pronator compression test revisited: a forgotten physical sign, *Orthop Rev* 19:888, 1990.
31. Garcia-Moral CA: Disorders of the hand and wrist. In Grana WA, Kalerak A, editors: *Clin Sports Med*, Philadelphia, 1991, WB Saunders.
32. Garrick JG, Webb DR: *Sports injuries: diagnosis and management*, Philadelphia, 1990, WB Saunders.
33. Giachino AA: Injury to the scapholunate ligaments, *Physician Sports Med* 21(5):57, 1983.
34. Gilula LA, Weeks PM: Radiological assessment of carpal instability, *Radiology* 129:641, 1978.
35. Greene MK, Hochberg MC: The epidemiology of osteoarthritis: what are the major risk factors? *J Musculoskel Med* 10(5):30, 1993.
36. Gutierrez G: Office management of scaphoid fractures, *Phys Sports Med* 24:8, 1996.

37. Hausman MR, Lisser SP: Hand infections, *Orthop Clin North Am* 23(1):171, 1992.
38. Hertling D, Kessler RM: *Management of common musculoskeletal disorders: physical therapy principles and methods,* ed 2, Philadelphia, 1990, JB Lippincott.
39. Johnson RK: Soft-tissue injuries of the forearm and hand, *Clin Sports Med* 5(4):701, 1986.
40. Jones JA, Burton RJ: Carpal tunnel syndrome: treatment, pitfalls, and failures. *Surg Rounds Orthop,* pg 37, 1988.
41. Kahlet DM, McCue FC III: Metacarpophalangeal and proximal interphalangeal joint injuries of the hand, including the thumb, *Clin Sports Med* 2(1):57, 1992.
42. Kannus P, Johnson RJ: Downhill skiing injuries: trends to watch for this season, *J Musculoskel Med* 8(1):26, 1991.
43. Kaplan SJ, Glickel SC, Eaton RG: Predictive factors in the nonsurgical treatment of carpal tunnel syndrome, *J Hand Surg* 15:106, 1990.
44. Kiefhaber TR, Stern PJ: Upper extremity tendonitis and overuse syndromes in the athlete, *Clin Sports Med* 11(1):39, 1992.
45. Kimura J: *Electrodiagnosis in diseases of nerve and muscle: principles and practice,* ed 2, Philadelphia, 1991, FA Davis.
46. Kozin SH, Urban MA, Bishop AT, Dobyns JH: Wrist ganglia: diagnosis and treatment of a bothersome problem, *J Musculoskel Med* 10(1):21, 1993.
47. Kulund DN: *The injured athlete,* ed 2, Philadelphia, 1988, JB Lippincott.
48. Kunkel SS: Basketball injuries and rehabilitation. In Buschbacher RM, Braddon RL, editors: *Sports medicine and rehabilitation: a sport-specific approach,* Philadelphia, 1994, Hanley & Belfus.
49. Lairmore JR, Engber WD: Serious often subtle finger injuries; avoiding diagnosis and treatment pitfalls, *Phys Sports Med* 26:6, 1998.
50. Lane LB: Acute grade III ulnar collateral ligament ruptures, *Adv Orthop Surg* 16(2):79, 1992.
51. Lewis CB, Knortz KA: *Orthopedic assessment and treatment of the geriatric patient,* St Louis, 1993, Mosby.
52. Linn MR, Mann FA, Gilula LA: Imaging the symptomatic wrist: Radiographic imaging in orthopedics, *Orthop Clin North Am* 21(3):515, 1990.
53. Loeb PE, Mirabello SC, Andrews JR: The hand: field evaluation and treatment, *Clin Sports Med* 2(1):27, 1992.
54. Louis DS, Hankin FM: Symptomatic relief following carpal tunnel decompression with normal electroneuromyographic studies, *Orthopedics* 10:434, 1987.
55. McCue FC, Nelson WE: Ulnar collateral ligament injuries of the thumb, *Physician Sports Med* 21(9):67, 1993.
56. Magee DT: *Orthopedic physical assessment,* 3 ed Philadelphia, 1997, WB Saunders.
57. Manga TN, Shanks GL, Poole BJ: Sensory palmar stimulation in the diagnosis of CTS, *Arch Phys Med Rehabil* 66:598, 1985.
58. Mariano KA, McDougle MA, Tanksley FW: Double crush syndrome: chiropractic care of an entrapment neuropathy, *J Manipulative Physiol Ther* 14:262, 1991.
59. Melone CP: Rigid fixation of phalangeal and metacarpal fractures, *Orthop Clin North Am* 17(3):421, 1986.
60. Mercier LR: *Practical orthopedics,* ed 4, St Louis, 1995, Mosby.
61. Meredith RM, Butcher JD: Field splinting of suspected fractures: preparation, assessment, and application, *Phys Sports Med* 25:10, 1997.
62. Miller SJ, Smith PA: Volar dislocation of the lunate in a weight lifter, *Orthop* 19(1):61, 1996.
63. Mirabello SC, Loeb PE, Andrews JR: The wrist: field evaluation and treatment, *Clin Sports Med* 11(1):1, 1992.
64. Mooney JF III, Siegel DB, Koman LA: Ligamentous injuries of the wrist in athletes, *Clin Sports Med* 11(1):129, 1992.
65. Moore KL: *Clinically oriented anatomy,* ed 2, Baltimore, 1985, Williams & Wilkins.
66. Nakamura R, Mori M, Imamura T et al: Method for measurement and evaluation of carpal bone angles, *J Hand Surg* 14A:412, 1989.
67. Neviaser RJ, Eisenfeld LS, Wiesel SM, Lewis RJ: *Emergency orthopaedic radiology,* New York, 1985, Churchill Livingstone.
68. Newland CC: Gamekeeper's thumb, *Orthop Clin North Am* 23(1):41, 1992.
69. Nielsen PT, Hedeboe J, Thommesen P: Bone scintiphotography in the evaluation of fracture of the carpus, *Acta Orthop Scand* 54:303, 1983.
70. Olehnik WK, Manske PR, Szerawk J: Median nerve compression in the proximal forearm, *J Hand Surg* 19:121, 1994.
71. Osterman AL, Moskow L, Low DW: Soft tissue injuries of the hand and wrist in racquet sports, *Clin Sports Med* 7(2):330, 1988.
72. Patzakis MJ, Wilkins J, Bassett RL: Surgical findings in clenched-fist injuries, *Clin Orthop* 220:237, 1987.
73. Pellegrini V: Fractures at the base of the thumb, *Hand Clin* 4(1)87, 1988.
74. Pennes DR, Jonsson K, Buckwalter KA: Direct coronal CT of the scaphoid bone, *Radiology* 171:870, 1989.
75. Peterson GW, Will AD: Newer electrodiagnostic techniques in peripheral nerve injuries, *Orthop Clin North Am* 19(1):13, 1988.
76. Phillips CA: Rehabilitation of the patient with rheumatoid hand involvement, *Phys Ther* 69:1091, 1989.
77. Pin PG, Semenkovich JW, Young VL et al: Role of radionuclide imaging in the evaluation of wrist pain, *J Hand Surg* 13A:810, 1988.
78. Post M: *Physical examination of the musculoskeletal system,* Chicago, 1987, Year Book Publishers.
79. Reeves RK, Laskowski ER, Smith J: Lunate dislocation, *Phys Sports Med* 26:2, 1998.
80. Rettig AC: Closed tendon injuries at the hand and wrist in the athlete, *Clin Sports Med* 11(1):89, 1992.
81. Rowland SA: Acute traumatic subluxation of the extensor carpi ulnaris tendon at the wrist, *J Hand Surg* 11A(6):809, 1986.
82. Schred ES: De Quervain's neuropathy in pregnant and postpartum women, *Obstet Gynecol* 68(3):411, 1986.
83. Schumacher HR: Occurrence of De Quervain's tendonitis during pregnancy, *Arch Intern Med* 145:2083, 1985.
84. Seyer AE, Hueston JT, editors: *Hand clinics: Dupuytren's contracture (monograph),* Philadelphia, 1991, WB Saunders.
85. Spooner GR, Desa HB, Angel JF, Reede BA, Donat JR: Using pyridoxine to treat carpal tunnel syndrome: randomized control trial, *Can Fam Physician* 39:2122, 1993.
86. Stanish W: Wrist-fracture repair in young athletes, *Physician Sports Med* 15(5):63, 1987.

87. Stark HH: Treatment of ununited fractures of the scaphoid by iliac bone grafts and Kirschner-wire fixation, *J Bone Joint Surg* 70A:982, 1988.

88. Steinberg DR: Acute flexor tendon injuries, *Orthop Clin North Am* 23(1):125, 1992.

89. Swenson RS: Double crush syndrome: what is the evidence? *JNMS* 1:23, 1993.

90. Taleisnik J: The ligaments of the wrist. In Taleisnik J, editor: *The wrist*, New York, 1985, Churchill Livingstone.

91. Thorson E, Szabo RM: Common tendinitis patterns in the hand and forearm, *Orthop Clin North Am* 23(1):65, 1992.

92. Trumble TE: Avascular necrosis after scaphoid fracture, *Adv Orthop Surg* 15(2):86, 1991.

93. Watson HK, Brenner LH: Degenerative disorders of the carpus. In Lichtman DM, editor: *The wrist and its disorders*, Philadelphia, 1988, WB Saunders.

94. Weinstein SM, Herring SA: Nerve problems and compartment syndromes in the hand, wrist, and forearm, *Clin Sports Med* 11(1):168, 1992.

95. Weissman B, Sledge C: *Orthopedic radiology*, Philadelphia, 1986, WB Saunders.

96. Whiteside JA: Field evaluation of common athletic injuries. In Grana WA, Kalenak A, editors: *Clinical sports medicine*, Philadelphia, 1991, WB Saunders.

97. Wilkes JS: Reconstructive surgery of the wrist and hand. In Donatell R, Wosden MJ, editors: *Orthopedic physical therapy*, New York, 1989, Churchill Livingstone.

98. Zemel NP: What you can do about Dupuytren's disease, *J Musculoskel Med* 9(5):89, 1992.

99. Zlatkin MB, Chao PC, Osterman AL et al: Chronic wrist pain: evaluation with high-resolution MR imaging, *Radiology* 173:723, 1989.

Chapter 6

Cervical Spine

Chapter Highlights

Not only is the cervical spine one of the most vulnerable sites for injury, but it is also a common area for everyday complaints and articular dysfunction. The vulnerability of the cervical spine is a result of the high level of mobility produced by its triplanar motion. This mobility also provides those engaged in manual therapy with a tremendous opportunity to correct postural and articular faults in the neck. Except in cases of advanced osseous or ligamentous trauma, corrective care that centers around early movement and aggressive restoration of joint mobility is the hallmark of treatment for mechanical disorders of the cervical spine.

Of the seven cervical vertebral segments (Figure 6-1), the third, fourth, fifth, and sixth vertebrae are typical. They possess a bifid (spinous) process and a foramen transversarium. These vertebrae have a broad body, superior and inferior articulating processes, and a foramen for the vertebral artery.[55] The first, second, and seventh cervical vertebrae are atypical. The atlas (C1) has no vertebral body and no spinous process. The axis (C2) has a dens or odontoid process. The atlantoaxial joint complex allows for rotation of the neck. The seventh cervical segment (C7) has a very prominent spinous process that is not bifid, and the vertebral artery does not enter the foramen transversarium at this point (Figure 6-2).

Biomechanical Perspectives of the Cervical Spine

Described as a complex region, the cervical spine has numerous articulations; intricate anatomic configurations of nerves, vessels, and joint structures; and a ligamentous network that provides vital support to mobile osseous structures. The cervical lordosis is a convex curve anteriorly and is known as a compensatory or secondary curvature.[29]

Cervical spine motions include flexion, extension, lateral (side) bending, and rotation. The latter seems to play a pivotal role in the degenerative process of the disk, and it is at the disk where cervical dysfunction and pain are prevalent.[41] In the cervical spine, the axis of rotation is superior to the disk, with the articular processes also aiding in the control of the motion.[57]

The nerve roots in the neck are particularly vulnerable to injury because of their relatively horizontal position in comparison with those of the lumbar spine. This is partly attributable to the angle of the upper extremities in relation to the neck, as opposed to the orientation of the lower extremity in relation to the lumbar spine (Figure 6-3). Furthermore, stretching of the spinal cord itself is greatest at the cervical spine, which also predisposes the cord and nerve roots to trauma. Excessive lateral flexion of the neck with sufficient loading forces can even avulse a nerve root, in addition to causing a brachial plexus traction injury from overstretching the neural elements at the thoracic outlet.

The height of the cervical disks and their relatively small diameter in both the sagittal and coronal planes contribute to the mobility of the neck. Motion segment degeneration begins at the disk, since the disk determines cervical motion.[65] Secondary changes then take place at the articular processes (joints of Luschka) and the facet joints.

Different regions of the cervical spine provide for different motion characteristics, a fact that supplies valuable information about the nature of an injury. The occipitoatlantal joint (C0-C1) ensures extensive movement in flexion and extension. On the other hand, the atlantoaxial complex (C1-C2) functions largely as a pivot point for posteroanterior rotation (Table 6-1). Stiffness of the ligaments, especially the ligamentum flavum, is also great.[109] The middle region of the cervical vertebrae contributes to the neck's considerable movement in flexion and extension, with the greatest range at the level of C5-C6.[109]

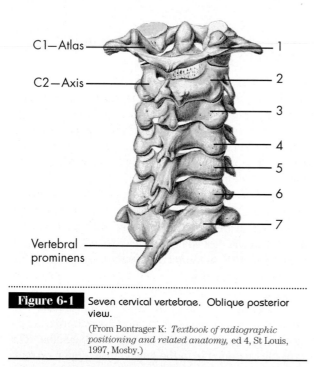

Figure 6-1 Seven cervical vertebrae. Oblique posterior view.

(From Bontrager K: *Textbook of radiographic positioning and related anatomy,* ed 4, St Louis, 1997, Mosby.)

The facet joints lie 45 degrees to the ventral, and motion involves a coupled movement along both the X and Y axes.[108] Lateral bending, for example, produces concomitant posteroanterior rotation, with spinous movement to the contralateral side of lateral flexion. The kinematics of the upper and lower cervical spine are different, however, because of the unique nature of disk, facet, and ligament arrangements in each area. Coupling movements actually decrease gradually from C2 to C7 as the incline of the facet joints change (Figure 6-4).[61]

The upper cervical complex is critically important in manual therapy because of the risks of vascular insult.[21] Several investigators have reported kinking of the vertebral arteries during moderate amounts of axial rotation,[98,127,141] even in individuals with no prior vascular disease. Most in the chiropractic profession are well aware of the cases of documented vertebrobasilar infarct following manipulation by various practitioners of manual therapy. Although Panjabi and White center their discussion on the "risk" of chiropractic manipulation of the cervical spine,[109] a review of the literature for the past several decades reveals few documented cases against chiropractors—despite the large number of manipulations they perform[27,132] and the almost constant scrutiny of the profession under the allopathic magnifying glass.[42,160] Nevertheless, a thorough practitioner of manual therapy should *always* screen patients for neurovascular disturbances, especially vertebrobasilar insufficiency, to ensure the safety and efficacy of cervical manipulation.

Mechanisms of Trauma to the Neck

Various types of exaggerated movements can cause cervical injury if accompanied by an external force (Table 6-2). Any exaggeration of normal coupling movement or excessive range of motion can potentially injure the

Table 6-1 Limits and Representative Values of Ranges of Rotation of the Occipital-Atlantoaxial Complexes

Unit of Complex	Type of Motion	Representative Angle (in degrees)
Occipital-atlantal joint (C0-C1)	Combined flexion and extension ($\pm\theta x$)	25
	One side lateral bending (θz)	5
	One side axial rotation (θy)	5
Atlantoaxial joint (C1-C2)	Combined flexion and extension ($\pm\theta x$)	20
	One side lateral bending (θz)	5
	One side axial rotation (θy)	40

(From Panjabi MM, White AA: *Clinical biomechanics of the spine,* Philadelphia, 1990, JB Lippincott.)

apophyseal (facet) joints, synovial capsule, and various soft-tissue structures that anchor the cervical region. Thus lateral bending, anteflexion (hyperflexion), extension loading, and extreme rotation are all capable of causing distress to the neck and its supporting elements.

Axial Compression and Flexion Loading

Normally, the elastic properties of the intervertebral disk allow it to withstand any movement or deforming force applied to it.[26] Tragic injuries to the neck and spinal cord, however, can occur when the head and neck are in flexion, thus segmentalizing the vertebral column and leaving the vertebral end-plates vulnerable to compression. The cortices of vertebral bone become fatigued be-

fore the intervertebral disk, thereby allowing for such types of compression fractures.

Flexing the neck to 30 degrees neutralizes the normal anatomic cervical lordosis and makes the segmented spinal column vulnerable to the brunt of axial loading by external forces.[170] If, for example, a defensive back in a football game makes a tackle head first in such a way that the initial contact occurs on the top of the helmet, the skull rapidly decelerates on impact with the other player; the torso and neck continue to accelerate, however. The result is axial loading of the cervical spine, which can lead to a fracture and cord damage. Diving into a pool or lake, bouncing on a trampoline, performing gymnastics, and playing hockey or rugby can produce a similar injury by a similar mechanism.[101] According to

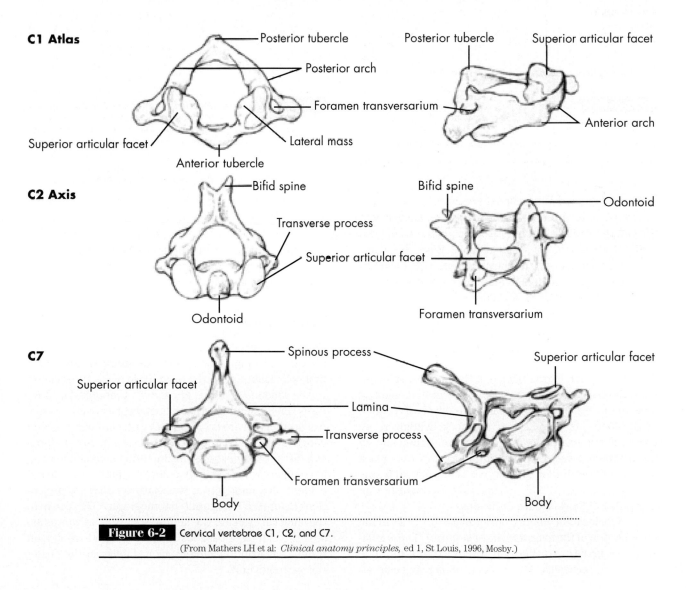

Figure 6-2 Cervical vertebrae C1, C2, and C7.
(From Mathers LH et al: *Clinical anatomy principles,* ed 1, St Louis, 1996, Mosby.)

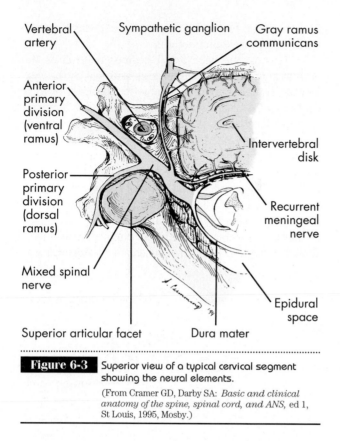

Figure 6-4 Coupled motions of the cervical spine. Lateral flexion is coupled to rotation in the same direction. When head and neck are bent to the left, the spinous processes go to the right, and vice versa.

Burstein, Otis, and Tory, when the cervical spine reaches total vertical compression as the segmented spine fails in flexion, the result is often vertebral body fracture, facet dislocation, or anatomic subluxation.[19] Even the strong secondary restraints of the spinal column (e.g., the intervertebral disk, paraspinal muscles, and ligamentous structures) cannot prevent injury during high-velocity axial loading and compression of the cervical spine.

Exaggerated Coupled Movements

As noted earlier, lateral flexion of the cervical spine incorporates axial rotation as well. Exaggerated coupling movement with traumatic loading can cause a dislocation of the facets on one side of the neck, leading to an anatomic subluxation or full dislocation, depending on the movement vectors. Such an injury can take place with or without fracture. The neck is often fixed to one side in a "cocked robin" position that distinguishes an overriding of facets from a dislocation.

A dislocation differs from an acute torticollis in the presentation of the ipsilateral musculature.[6] These muscles are relaxed in a dislocation, whereas they are spastic in an acute torticollis. Facet dislocations may occur ei-

ther unilaterally or bilaterally. Severe rotation with flexion can be pathomechanical, with the occasional occurrence of concomitant fractures.[161]

Flexion Injuries

Cervical compression fractures occur as a direct result of flexion loading. These fractures are related to vertebral body failure, with the magnitude of fracture related to the amount of force applied.[109] Compression fractures can be simple, with minimal displacement, or they can occur as severe bony defects with comminution and cord damage (burst or teardrop fractures). Severe force can disrupt the posterior ligamentous complex leading to complete vertebral body failure.[80] Injuries are clearly evident on a radiograph, especially on a lateral projection (Figure 6-5). Computed tomography (CT) can help the clinician evaluate the neurologic insult, as well as assess the extent of osseous injury.[111] Repetitive flexion trauma will lead to ligamentous instability at the posterior vertebral unit.

Table 6-2	Biomechanics of Cervical Injury
Mechanism	**Structures Affected**
Flexion or axial compressive loading	Posterior column elements Capsular ligaments Supraspinous ligament Interspinous ligament Erector spinae group Trapezius muscles
Lateral flexion	Nerve root Dorsal sleeve Brachial plexus Scalene muscles
Extension or axial rotation	Anterior column elements Anterior longitudinal ligament Outer annulus of disk Apophyseal joints Sternocleidomastoid muscle

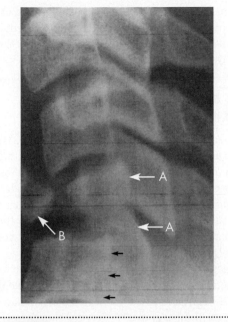

Figure 6-5 Lateral view of a cervical "teardrop" fracture with posterior displacement (arrow A) of the remaining body into the spinal canal. Displaced anterior vertebral body fracture fragment (arrow B); subjacent vertebral body cortex (small black arrows).
(From Watkins RG, editor: *Spine in Sports*, St Louis, 1996, Mosby.)

Lateral flexion injuries range from the volatile (e.g., an avulsed nerve root) to the benign (e.g., traumatic momentary paresthesia). Severe injuries are usually seen in the emergency department. In a motorcycle accident, for example, the rider may fall on the head while the shoulder is depressed and the neck laterally tilted. Total loss of specific motor function in a patient who has experienced such an injury generally indicates a disruption of the nerve root.

Mild-to-moderate lateral bending injuries cause a variety of nerve root or brachial plexus symptoms. These injuries usually result from automobile or sports trauma; both center around a relatively high-speed impact. Nerve roots C6 through C8 are most often affected. After this type of injury, patients commonly complain of a burning or numbness down the arm into the hand. Brachial plexopathy (sometimes called a "stinger," "burner," or "dead" arm) is also a possible result of a lateral flexion traction injury. The neurologic deficit may last for only a few seconds, or it may occur intermittently for several days. Swelling at the nerve root or distal to the spine can combine with traction to the nerve sleeves, making the deficit more severe.

Extension Injuries

In the laboratory, severe extension loading causes most cervical spine specimens to fail at the anterior longitudinal ligament or disk.[24,90,109] Thus a high-speed whiplash injury clearly has the potential to cause advanced ligamentous instability or a herniated or protruded disk. Overstretching or tearing the fibers at the sternocleidomastoid or scalene muscles can be quite painful and debilitating to the patient as well. Soft-tissue swelling and static contraction against gravity are also common sources of discomfort.

Fracture of the spinous process at the lower cervical spine (i.e., Clay Shoveler's fracture) is also the result of extension loading, although by a completely different mechanism. A ballistic and forceful contraction of the trapezius or rhomboid muscles, usually because of a fatigued spine, is typically responsible for this stable injury. Traumatic hyperextension may be responsible for compression of the posterior arch of C1 or the occiput, however. Odontoid fractures and *hangman's fractures* of C2 result from hyperextension.

Extension overloading of the cervical spine can also produce apophyseal sprain, mechanical facet imbrication, and synovitis—all common causes of mechanical neck pain. Individuals who participate in sports such as wrestling, football, and boxing often experience these types of injuries. Hyperextension is especially dangerous in those individuals with developmental or spondolytic narrowing of the spinal cord. Ligamentous infolding may further compromise the diameter of the canal during hyperextension.

Aging and Degeneration in the Cervical Spine

Certain aspects of the three-joint complex (i.e., the disk and two facet joints of the vertebra) that characterize the spinal motor unit have a strong impact on the degenerative processes associated with aging. First, high-tensile loads during macrotraumatic events can influence the rate of the degenerative process, especially at the level of the disk and the joints of Luschka. Second, constant low-level compressive loads alter the normal visco-elastic properties of the intervertebral disk.[109] Third, both stiffness coefficients and maximum loads are markedly limited for the elements of the cervical region compared with those of the lumbar spine.[100] Cervical spondylosis or degeneration of the three-joint complex centers around disk degeneration, loss of disk height, osteophyte formation, degenerative facet disease (arthrosis), ligamentum flavum hypertrophy, and finally cervical stenosis.[26]

The loss or alteration of the normal cervical lordosis, because of either repetitive cervical insult or articular hypomobility, may play a role in altered mechanics of the cervical spine and in the early degenerative process. Repetitive injury to the cervical spine, particularly from axial compression and flexion loading, is a definite risk factor in cervical degeneration. Individuals with a history of neck trauma often develop degenerative disk disease, including osteophytosis. In fact, fairly young adults who have been in multiple motor vehicle accidents (resulting in cervical whiplash syndrome) or who have participated in contact sports may show signs of early degenerative arthritis and intermittent clinical instability and stiffness in their cervical spines. Chronic synovitis of the facet joints, with or without joint capsule attenuation, combines with the affected disk to form a functional spinal unit that is less apt to withstand compressive loads or end-range tensile forces. Pathologic changes in the soft tissue, such as contractures, shortening, and fibrosis of the muscles, also alter mechanical function of the spinal unit.

Muscular Faults of the Cervical Spine

Over time, muscular pathologic variations can cause subtle and almost silent changes in joint motion and resting tension. At some point in this cycle, the individual feels twinges of discomfort, which, in time, may alter function in other nearby systems.

Postural faults at the neck, upper back, and shoulder girdle can affect the cervical spine directly because of the anatomic configuration of the musculature in the region. Most large muscles that impose leverage on the cervical spine span the upper dorsal spine and the back of the skull; the levator scapulae, trapezius, and erector spinae group all cover the suprascapular and suboccipital region (Figure 6-6). Therefore postural faults and muscular fatigue can easily cause suboccipital (cervical) muscle tension headaches.

Myofascial pain syndromes secondary to trauma can alter head, neck, and spine function as well.[51] Muscular fixation can result from both constant everyday positions at work and faulty sleeping positions at night. Muscular spasm, or hypertonicity, is thought to be the causative factor in the loss of the normal cervical lordosis.[56] Chronic hypertonicity of the cervicodorsal region and shoulder girdle can alter both neurologic and organic function via the sympathetic nervous system.[51,131,148]

Examination of the Cervical Spine

The physical findings largely determine the parameters of care for injury or disease of the cervical spine. The examining clinician has two priorities: (1) rule out advanced pathologic conditions and (2) identify any neurologic or osseous instability. Advanced pathologic abnormalities may result from soft-tissue trauma that has evoked a mechanical insult at the level of the brachial plexus, nerve roots, or spinal cord itself (e.g., traction avulsion) or has stimulated the body's exaggerated inflammatory response, causing extensive swelling just distal to the cord at the nerve root or ganglion level.

Although paresthesia and a dysthetic response are fairly common in patients with an injury to their cervical spine, motor changes indicate advanced tissue compromise. Compression impairment has an almost routine effect on follow-up recovery times at the afferent sensory level,[109,123] but it usually takes a larger compressive force to decrease conduction amplitude at the efferent motor level for any appreciable length of time.[106,112] Thus the trauma that causes motor effects is likely to be more severe than the trauma that causes sensory effects, and recovery is likely to be less predictable in the presence of motor effects.

Once the presence of motor weakness or atrophic change has been established, the condition must be doc-

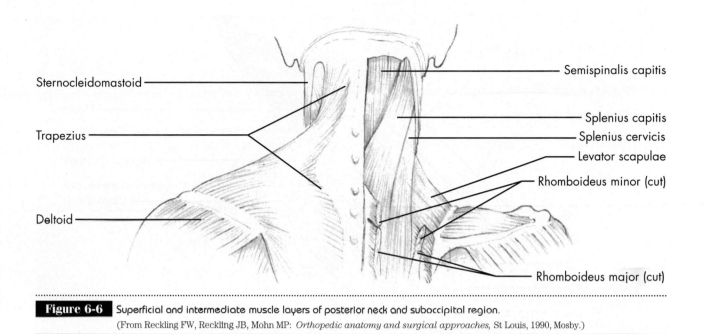

Sternocleidomastoid

Trapezius

Deltoid

Semispinalis capitis

Splenius capitis

Splenius cervicis

Levator scapulae

Rhomboideus minor (cut)

Rhomboideus major (cut)

Figure 6-6 Superficial and intermediate muscle layers of posterior neck and suboccipital region.
(From Reckling FW, Reckling JB, Mohn MP: *Orthopedic anatomy and surgical approaches*, St Louis, 1990, Mosby.)

umented, monitored, and treated with a multipronged approach. The case history should include detailed questions about sympathetic-mediated pathologic responses such as diplopia, nystagmus, vertigo, nausea, and sweating. Feelings of lightheadedness, tiredness, or altered body status are also common in patients with whiplash. The clinician should evaluate the brachial plexus (C5 to T1) through a neurologic examination for any motor, sensory, or reflex changes. Tests are also necessary to monitor the peripheral function of the radial, median, and ulnar nerves.

The clinician should palpate bony landmarks, such as the external occipital protuberance, mastoid and styloid process, axis, and the vertebral prominence at C7 or T1, for orientation (Figure 6-7). Because the posture of the head and shoulder can adversely affect cervical mechanics, it is important to rule out postural faults such as a forward head or shoulder (e.g., round-shoulders). From the lateral aspect, the external auditory meatus should not deviate much from the glenohumeral joint and acetabulum. From the rear of the patient (with the patient's hair out of the way and clothing clear of the cervical and thoracic region), the clinician should line up the mastoid and earlobe bilaterally, examine the shoulder levels bilaterally, and rule out a posterior or undescended scapula. These anatomic disturbances occur with scoliosis and Sprengel's deformity, respectively. The fol-

lowing childhood disorders may also cause distortion in the region:

- Congenital muscular torticollis (congenital wry neck)
- Klippel-Feil syndrome
- Atlantoaxial instability (Down syndrome, Still's disease)
- Brachial plexopathy in the newborn
- Erb's palsy
- Klumpke syndrome
- Erb-Duchenne paralysis
- Sprengel's deformity (cervicodorsal region)

The way the patient holds the head and moves around can also provide the clinician with significant information. Someone with ligamentous instability has difficulty maintaining the cervical spine in an erect position against the forces of motion and gravity (Rust's sign). For example, the patient may find it necessary to support the weight of the neck and head with the hands during the automobile ride to and from the office and may even need assistance in getting off the examination table. Rust's sign is pathognomonic for severe cervical injury, usually atlantoaxial instability or fracture.[38] The patient with this sign should undergo no further active or passive testing. Rather, the neck should be immobilized in a collar at once, and advanced diagnostic imaging should be ordered immediately.

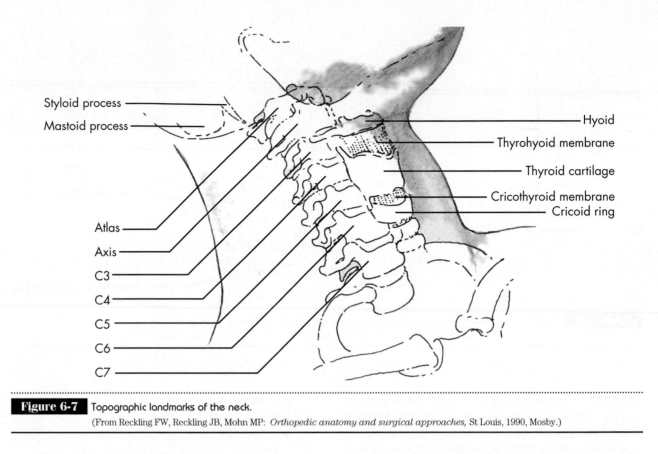

Styloid process
Mastoid process
Atlas
Axis
C3
C4
C5
C6
C7

Hyoid
Thyrohyoid membrane
Thyroid cartilage
Cricothyroid membrane
Cricoid ring

Figure 6-7 Topographic landmarks of the neck.
(From Reckling FW, Reckling JB, Mohn MP: *Orthopedic anatomy and surgical approaches,* St Louis, 1990, Mosby.)

A patient who appears to have an acute torticollis following trauma and maintains the head in a fused-coupled position (i.e., cocked robin position) should have an immediate radiographic examination to rule out dislocation or anatomic subluxation of the facet joints. An examination after high-speed trauma requires the clinician to test cognitive function and rule out medullary changes. The clinician should also assess fine movement, perform cerebral concussion tests, and examine the patient for the Romberg's sign (i.e., body sway, loss of balance when patient closes the eyes and stands still).

The paraspinal region must be examined and palpated for swelling or fullness of the musculature. Ecchymosis and swelling should be documented at both the anterior and posterior regions of the spine. Tape measurements are helpful in comparing the muscle contour immediately after injury with the muscle contour at various points during the recovery process. Patients typically have an anterior tenderness as a result of a violent hyperextension in an acceleration-deceleration accident; the sternocleidomastoid and scalene muscles are tender, swollen, and unable to pull the head forcefully or assist

the torso when the patient sits up from the recumbent posture (Rust's sign). These patients often complain of spasms or instability. The use of a soft collar can help alleviate these problems in the short-term.

The osseous integrity of the cervical spine is also of paramount importance. Plain-film radiographic studies are crucial. Anteroposterior and lateral views are standard (Figure 6-8 *A, B*), with an open mouth view of the upper cervical spine mandatory for patients who have experienced trauma. Oblique films may also be necessary in cases of peripheral pain (Figure 6-9). The foraminal canal is visualized on the oblique projection; the intervertebral joints are seen on the anteroposterior views.[118]

The lateral film screens for both osseous integrity and ligamentous stability.[125] The anterior longitudinal ligament may have buckled from progressive degenerative disease or from acute injury following trauma (Figure 6-10 *A, B*). Translation above or below a spondylitic motor segment is common; its hypermobility may be compensating for the hypomobility of the adjacent arthritic spinal unit.

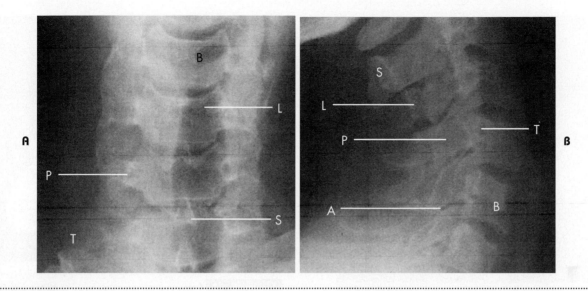

Figure 6-8 Radiographic films of the cervical spine. **A,** Anteroposterior view. **B,** Lateral view.

S, Spinous process; **T,** transverse process; **B,** body; **A,** articular (zygapophyseal) facet joint; **P,** pedicle; **L,** lamina. Note the slight lordosis and even spacing of the vertebrae and disks.

(From Mercier LR: *Practical orthopedics*, ed 4, St Louis, 1995, Mosby.)

Orthopedic Testing

To determine the parameters of disability and pain that are necessary to document an injury clearly, the examiner performs a variety of orthopedic tests. Range-of-motion testing allows the clinician to note the painful arcs of completed motion, for example (Table 6-3). Other tests make it possible to identify nerve root lesions secondary to compression or disk syndromes and to reproduce radiculopathy or radiculitis. Compression tests should be performed while the patient is in the neutral position (Figure 6-11), in the lateral bending position, and in the posture of the painful arc (e.g., flexion and rotation). If the patient has radicular symptoms or a history of arm pain following neck trauma, it is helpful to place the cervical spine in lateral flexion toward the side of pain with extension and provide axial compression; this procedure should reproduce the pain of a nerve root lesion in a patient with significant radiculopathy.

It is almost mandatory to place the neck under compressive loads during the examination procedure. Localized pain should be differentiated from more general arm and hand pain, and applying stress to the cervical spine structures is always helpful in determining the origin of referred pain patterns. The clinician should always refer back to cervical spine motion testing if there is a doubt about the cause of pain at the

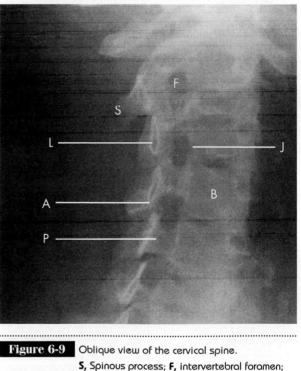

Figure 6-9 Oblique view of the cervical spine.

S, Spinous process; **F,** intervertebral foramen; **J,** joint of Luschka; **L,** lamina; **P,** pedicle; **A,** articular facet joint; **B,** body.

(From Mercier LR: *Practical orthopedics*, ed 4, St Louis, 1995, Mosby.)

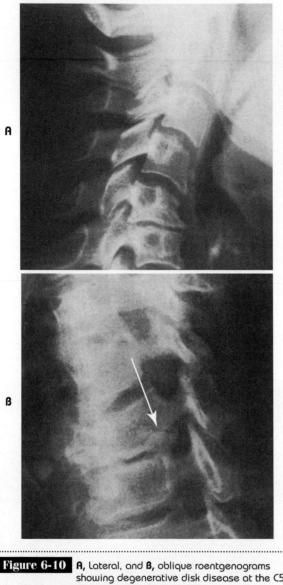

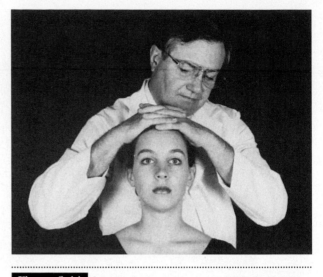

shoulder, elbow, wrist, or hand. The median nerve, for example, is sometimes compressed at the carpal tunnel distally or proximally between the two heads of the pronator teres muscle, but concomitant nerve root compression at the C5 to T1 levels of the spine occasionally clouds the diagnosis.

Investigation of the possibility of a central spinal lesion is also important for individuals who appear to have primarily peripheral nerve problems. In the upper extremity the clinician must differentiate between canal or nerve root lesions by physical examination and, if necessary, electrodiagnostic studies. Radial nerve lesions can produce posterior interosseous neuropathy at the elbow, but the clinician should rule out a cervical lesion at the levels contributing to the radial nerve (i.e., C6, C7).[155] Similarly, compression in the cubital tunnel at the elbow or near the hook of the hamate at the wrist can cause ulnar neuropathies. The clinician should rule out irritation of the lower trunk of the brachial plexus, if it is not possible to elicit a painful local response during the physical examination.[29] Although some peripheral neuropathies, such as the pronator teres syndrome, are difficult to document electrophysiologically, the physical findings and a careful case history can help fill in any diagnostic gaps.

Intersegmental Examination

After evaluating the osseous and neurologic components of injury, the meticulous clinician examines each level of the spine as a separate and distinct cause of disability and dysfunction. This approach to the assessment of the cer-

Table 6-3 Muscles Controlling Neck Motion

Muscle	Nerve(s)	Normal Function(s)	Paralysis	Test(s)
Rectus capitis anterior	Suboccipital C1-C3	Flexes head	Head flexion weakened	Resist head flexion
Rectus capitis lateralis	Suboccipital C1-C4	Bends head to same side	—	—
Rectus capitis posterior major and minor	Suboccipital C1	Both muscles acting bilaterally extend head; one acting alone turns face to same side	Weakens bend of head to side muscle	Resist bend of head to side of muscle
Obliquus capitis inferior	Suboccipital C1	Turns face to same side	—	—
Obliquus capitis superior	Suboccipital C1	Extends head and turns face to same side	Weakens head extension	Resist head extension and bend to same side
Splenius capitis	C2-C4	Extends head	Head extension weakened	Resist head extension
Splenius cervicis	C2-C4	Extends head	Head extension weakened	Resist head extension
Semispinalis capitis	C1-C4	Extends head	Head extension weakened	Resist head extension
Semispinalis cervicis	C3-C6	Extends head	Head extension weakened	Resist head extension
Longissimus capitis	C1-C8	Both muscles acting bilaterally extend head; acting alone head flexes toward same side	Head extension weakened	Resist head extension
Longissimus cervicis	C1-C8	Both muscles acting bilaterally extend head; acting alone head flexes toward same side	Head extension weakened	Resist head extension
Scalenus anterior	Anterior primary division lower cervical nerves C4-C7	Bends neck to same side	Weakens bending of head to side of muscle	Sitting or supine flexion of neck with chin on chest against resistance applied to forehead
Scalenus medius	C4-C8	Bends neck to same side	—	—
Scalenus posterior	C6-C8	Bends neck to same side	—	—

(From Post M: *Physical examination of the musculoskeletal system*, Chicago, 1987, Year Book Medical Publishers.)

vical spine—examining not only the region as a whole, but also the separate articulations and structural components at different spinal levels—distinguishes the chiropractic model of evaluation from the traditional allopathic model. The chiropractic physician checks total motion, as well as individual joint play, at different spinal levels. Combined with more traditional methods of ruling out osseous or neurologic instability, the intersegmental examination leads to the most thorough type of spinal assessment possible.

In the intersegmental examination, the clinician determines whether coupling characteristics have changed toward either hypermobility or hypomobility. Tenderness and joint blockage are common findings and are certainly major prerequisites for the initiation of manipulative therapy. A variation in muscle tone from one side of the spine to the other often indicates local muscular pathologic abnormalities (e.g., shortening, hypertonicity, contracture) or underlying articular dysfunction

(e.g., posterior joint syndrome). It is wise to examine the motion of the apophyseal joints in both the weight-bearing (i.e., sitting) and the non–weight-bearing (i.e., recumbent) positions. It is not uncommon for a joint to respond to stress differently in each position, and the difference may suggest the causative factor of fixation (i.e., myofascial versus articular).

Priorities of Neurologic Evaluation

Fortunately, most cases of cervical injury and dysfunction do not affect cognitive function or vital signs. Such a condition produces a variety of other signs and symptoms (Table 6-4), and the neurologic examination of the upper extremity and brachial plexus is the key to impairment screening in patients with cervical injury or disease (Figure 6-12). The presence of any risk factors, such as documented degenerative disk disease and traumatic ligamentous instability; the case history; and pertinent radiographic findings should support any neurologic findings.

Neurologically mediated pathologic responses to cervical injury range from benign to severe (Figure 6-13). The conditions of patients with evidence of such pathologic responses can be grouped into the following categories:

I.   Transient neurologic deficit (i.e., lasting less than 8 weeks) involving the nerve roots, trunk of the brachial plexus, or motor unit
II. Long-standing, consistent neurologic deficit (i.e., lasting more than 8 weeks)
III. Cervical myelopathy (i.e., clonus, lower or upper limb findings)
IV. Gross spinal cord impairment (i.e., quadriplegia)

Cervical plain films and stress studies in flexion and extension are a helpful first step in ruling out occult vertebral and ligamentous instability, as well as in diagnosing osseous injury[116] (Figure 6-14). Magnetic resonance imaging (MRI) following the plain films is valuable in determining the grade or severity of cervical spine lesions;[89] it facilitates the assessment of the spinal cord, vertebral disks, and nerve roots, because it reveals stenosis, anatomic defects, or lesions in the spinal canal (Figure 6-15).

Table 6-4	Signs and Symptoms of Neurologic Insult of the Cervical Region (Incomplete Spinal Cord Lesions)

Diagnosis	Signs and Symptoms
Central cervical cord syndrome	Upper extremity motor weakness greater than lower extremity weakness Lower extremity sensory changes fewer with motor weakness than those in upper extremity Sacral sparing
Cervical disk syndrome	Scapula, shoulder, arm, and hand pain Dermatome and motor changes Hyporeflexia
Cervical stenosis, myelopathy	Possible sensory changes in lower extremity Upper limb pain, weakness Clonus, Babinski's sign
Cervical nerve root avulsion	Dermatomal anesthesia Spinal level motor loss Areflexia
Anterior cervical cord syndrome	Bilateral motor loss below level of injury Loss of spinothalamic tract function Preservation of dorsal column function

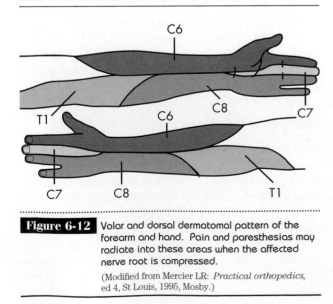

Figure 6-12 Volar and dorsal dermatomal pattern of the forearm and hand. Pain and paresthesias may radiate into these areas when the affected nerve root is compressed.

(Modified from Mercier LR: *Practical orthopedics,* ed 4, St Louis, 1995, Mosby.)

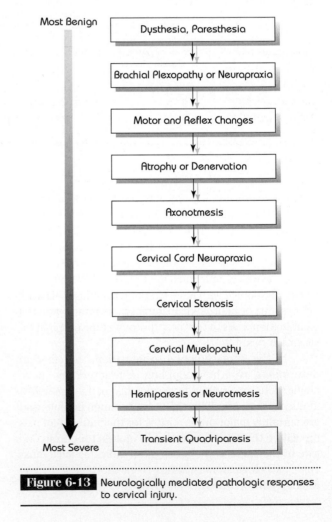

Most Benign

Dysthesia, Paresthesia

Brachial Plexopathy or Neurapraxia

Motor and Reflex Changes

Atrophy or Denervation

Axonotmesis

Cervical Cord Neurapraxia

Cervical Stenosis

Cervical Myelopathy

Hemiparesis or Neurotmesis

Transient Quadriparesis

Most Severe

Figure 6-13 Neurologically mediated pathologic responses to cervical injury.

Somatosensory-evoked potentials (SSEP) evaluate physiologic dysfunction of the sensory pathway (peripheral nerve or dermatome); computed tomography (CT) is useful in identifying bony defects, subtle osseous injury, or disk injury.

Patients with a history of neurologic impairment may be at greater risk for permanent injury, especially if there is underlying stenosis.[170] Cervical extension usually provokes pain in these patients. Evidence of cord compromise with MRI or CT, or altered function of the spinal cord documented by SSEP or motor-evoked potentials, combined with significant neurologic findings on physical examination, may preclude the patient from any future participation in contact sports or activities that have an increased risk of head or neck trauma.[92,143]

Manual Therapy

The healthy cervical spine is so mobile that even a slight alteration in its normal biomechanical function can have far-reaching consequences. Hands-on manual treatment for cervical ailments crosses the spectrum of several types of therapies, including exercise, acupressure, stretching or muscle-energy technique (i.e., a combination of contraction and relaxed stretching), mobilization, traction, and manipulation. Although manipulation is the centerpiece of spinal treatment in the chiropractic profession, other types of ancillary procedures are also helpful in correcting altered physiology of the spine.

There is no *single* scientifically proven effective treatment for neck pain, but there is no question that the

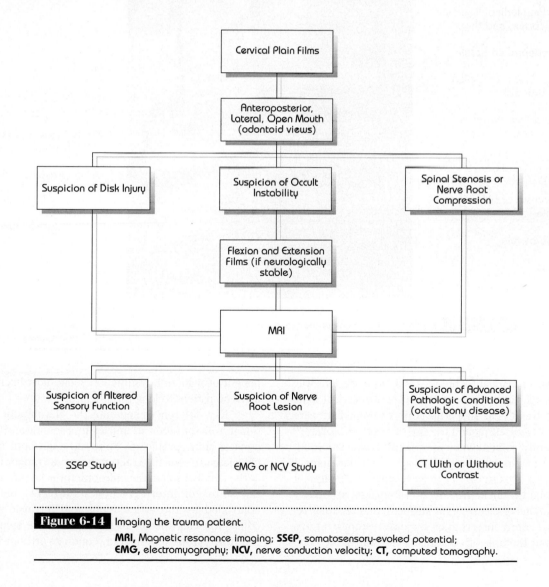

Figure 6-14 Imaging the trauma patient.

MRI, Magnetic resonance imaging; **SSEP,** somatosensory-evoked potential; **EMG,** electromyography; **NCV,** nerve conduction velocity; **CT,** computed tomography.

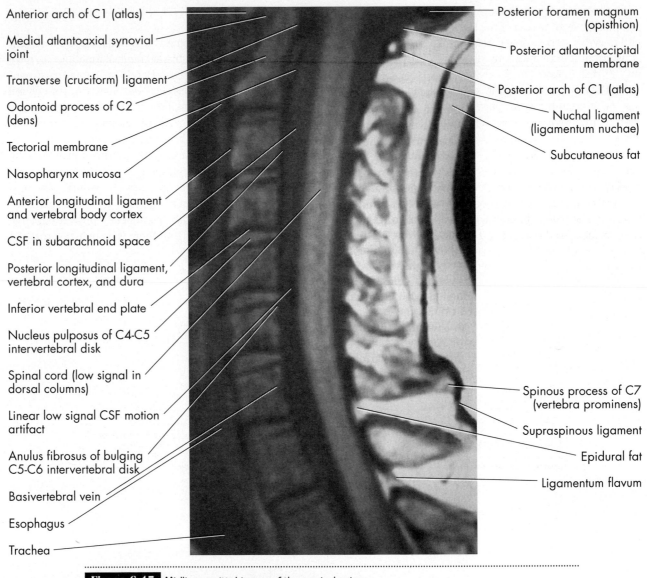

Anterior arch of C1 (atlas)

Medial atlantoaxial synovial joint

Transverse (cruciform) ligament

Odontoid process of C2 (dens)

Tectorial membrane

Nasopharynx mucosa

Anterior longitudinal ligament and vertebral body cortex

CSF in subarachnoid space

Posterior longitudinal ligament, vertebral cortex, and dura

Inferior vertebral end plate

Nucleus pulposus of C4-C5 intervertebral disk

Spinal cord (low signal in dorsal columns)

Linear low signal CSF motion artifact

Anulus fibrosus of bulging C5-C6 intervertebral disk

Basivertebral vein

Esophagus

Trachea

Posterior foramen magnum (opisthion)

Posterior atlantooccipital membrane

Posterior arch of C1 (atlas)

Nuchal ligament (ligamentum nuchae)

Subcutaneous fat

Spinous process of C7 (vertebra prominens)

Supraspinous ligament

Epidural fat

Ligamentum flavum

Figure 6-15 Midline sagittal image of the cervical spine.

(From Enzmann DR, DeLaPaz RL, Rubin JB: *Magnetic resonance of the spine,* St Louis, 1990, Mosby.)

active use of manual techniques is a more efficient way to address the intersegmental needs of the cervical spine than the traditional allopathic form of immediate care (i.e., rest, medication, and the use of a cervical collar).[94] Restoration of joint movement by gentle mobilization, adjustive or manipulative techniques, and encouragement of therapeutic exercise in the early stages of treatment can reduce the incidence of the often-seen secondary complications of disuse, joint stiffness, and articular reflex loss.[76] Early intervention by joint restoration techniques and therapies that address the soft-tissue component of pain and dysfunction seem most likely to return the patient to long-term health.[22,45,82,85]

Key differences separate the chiropractic practitioner from the medical clinician in assessing and treating cervical spine problems. First, although both types of clinicians are concerned about the overall range of motion at the cervical spine, the chiropractor is keenly aware of the status of intersegmental movement, since it is controlled by the articulations and intrinsic and extrinsic muscles specific to that level of the spine. As a rule, the chiropractor not only conducts orthopedic tests on the spine as a whole unit, but he or she also performs a series of stress tests on each individual articular facet.

Second, many medical physicians tend to diagnose cervical injury on an all-or-nothing basis. In the emergency department where many patients initially receive treatment following automobile-induced trauma, the physician may simply give a prescription for pain medication and a soft collar to the patient who has a cervical injury, but whose neurologic and radiographic findings are normal. Failure to provide follow-up instructions and to address the consequences of the injury leaves the patient helpless and uncertain, however.[168] Some patients live with subtle yet increasing after-effects of cervical injury for weeks or months before they seek additional care, thus increasing morbidity.

Chiropractic manipulative therapy (CMT) has been shown not only to have clinical merit,[4,31,132] but also to have several advantages over traditional, passive allopathic care:

- Early restoration of spinal function
- Early active rehabilitation therapy
- Less reliance on drug therapy
- Biomechanical principles of the spine as the basis for treatment
- Treatment of secondary myofascial component of neck, shoulder, and head pain
- Reduction of muscle spasm and joint stiffness, especially secondary to immobilization

Spinal manipulation has a high clinical yield with a most favorable margin of safety.[7,130] Research has shown that CMT may be more effective for acute neck and low back pain than for chronic pain.[64,73,81,115,150] Therefore to provide the best CMT possible, the chiropractic physician should possess the capacity for specific, differential diagnosis with early and aggressive active treatment within the constraints of patient tolerance. The proper use of chiropractic care, of course, hinges on the practitioner's ability to separate those who have suffered severe macrotrauma that requires a surgeon's care from those who are suffering the ill effects of more subtle soft-tissue disability.

Indications for Manipulation

Proper patient selection enhances the efficiency of CMT and minimizes the risks. The first step is to complete a thorough history and examination. Radiographic studies are important for patients who have a history of trauma. A patient with signs of vertebrobasilar insufficiency or carotid artery disease should have a vascular examina-

tion and Doppler studies. The findings obtained in the neurologic examination, together with those obtained in the radiologic, orthopedic, and chiropractic examinations, generally indicate the appropriateness of CMT for the individual patient.

Although some subjective complaints such as "tightness" or "pain" differ drastically among individuals, there are some objective findings that are indications for CMT:

- Alteration in gross range of motion of the cervical spine (This may include a pathologic change in movement either within the elastic zone of motion or in the neutral physiologic range. Causes of global hypomobility such as fracture and dislocation must be ruled out, but this is the function of the orthopedic, neurologic, and radiologic evaluations [Figure 6-16].)
- Physical evidence of muscular spasm, contracture, or myofascial hypertonicity in bilateral comparison
- Loss of proprioceptive reflexes or kinesthetic awareness of axial articulations combined with an alteration of normal joint biomechanics in the cervical spine
- Apophyseal fixation, hypomobile segments, or blocked vertebral motion
- Symptoms of tightness, stiffness, or pain in the absence of gross pathologic abnormalities

Cervical manipulation overcomes these problems essentially by restoring motion to the synovial joints of the spine, altering the existing tension of the myofascia,[64] lengthening connective tissue, disrupting adhesions, and relieving muscular hypertonicity.[151]

Contraindications for Manipulation

Gross contraindications for manipulation of the cervical spine are consistent for all techniques and practitioners. These contraindications include fractures, dislocations, carotid artery disease, vertebrobasilar insufficiency, signs and symptoms of Wallenberg's syndrome, malignant tumors, and infection. Relative contraindications vary from patient to patient and from practitioner to practitioner because of stark differences in individual pathologic conditions (e.g., frank herniations, severe muscle guarding and spasm, hematoma formation, psychologic status), and adjusting technique. Radiographic analysis, including flexion and extension stress views, enable the clinician to avoid manipulation of a hypermobile vertebral segment. Intersegmental instability is always a contraindication to local manipulation.[113]

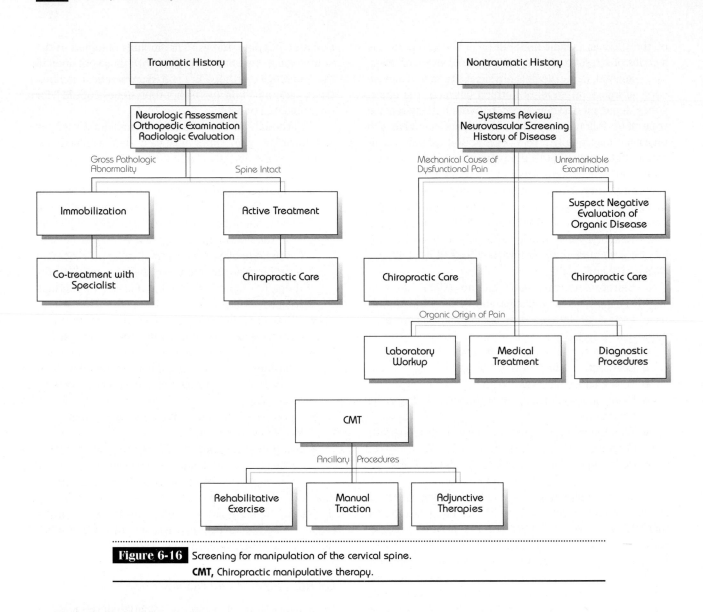

Figure 6-16 Screening for manipulation of the cervical spine.
CMT, Chiropractic manipulative therapy.

Mechanisms of Action in Manipulative Therapy

In addition to the mechanical action of CMT, there is a neurohormonal action (Figure 6-17). High-velocity, low-amplitude adjusting causes changes in joint capsule tension that, in turn, excites the mechanoreceptors of the synovial joints, primarily the type I and type II receptors (Table 6-5). The type I mechanoreceptors contribute to the perception of position and kinesthetic awareness, whereas the type II mechanoreceptors inhibit pain and exert a phasic (i.e., relaxing) effect on motor neurons. The endogenous opiate release that follows CMT, combined with nociceptor suppression at the cord level, also inhibits pain.[110,135]

Disorders of the Cervical Spine

Cervical Spine Trauma

Because the consequences of cervical trauma can be disastrous, a patient who has experienced an episode of cervical trauma requires special and immediate attention to make certain there is no clinical danger. Neurologic evaluation and orthopedic testing must be performed (within the patient's tolerance for pain). Immediately following trauma, a three-view series of plain x-ray films (i.e., anteroposterior, open mouth, and lateral) is a minimal standard procedure (Figure 6-18). Those who have more severe injuries may require additional film projec-

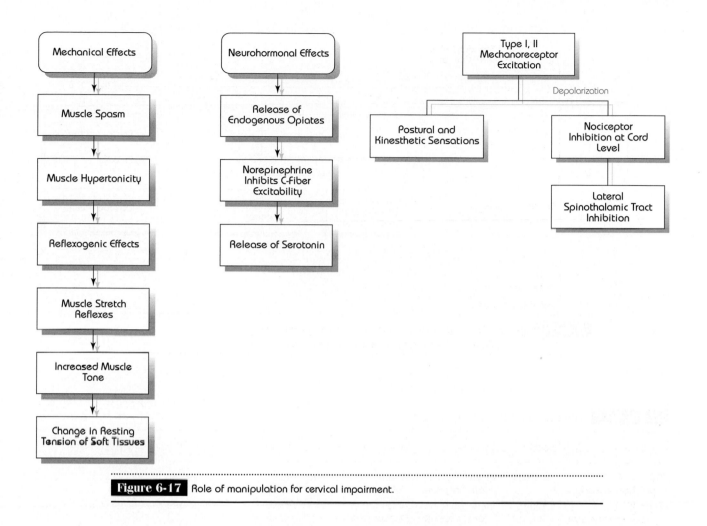

Figure 6-17 Role of manipulation for cervical impairment.

tions, such as oblique views or an anteroposterior Waters' projection with 10 degrees cephalad angulation under the mandible.[40] If there is any doubt about the neurologic, ligamentous, or osseous integrity of the cervical spine, the practitioner should order a thorough radiographic analysis.

After studying 775 motor vehicle accident victims, MacDonald and colleagues concluded that a single lateral x-ray film does not permit an accurate diagnosis of all cervical spine injuries.[88] It is necessary to take additional films and obtain a thorough neurologic assessment of the patient's condition. In most cases of trauma, however, the three standard projections are sufficient.

The open mouth view is essential for *every* patient who has experienced high-speed or high-impact trauma. The anteroposterior open mouth film, also called an odontoid projection, is helpful in identifying atlantoaxial instability, Jefferson fractures of the atlas, lateral mass dissociation, and odontoid fractures. Although most nondisplaced dens fractures are stable, atlas fractures may not be.

The chiropractic physician should monitor the patient's progress carefully following cervical trauma. If the findings of the initial radiographic examination are normal (Figure 6-19 *A-C*), but the patient continues to have significant symptoms referable to the cervical spine, further diagnostic investigation is necessary. A suspected osseous injury calls for CT. A patient who has sustained significant head trauma should be immobilized until a full radiographic examination has shown that immobilization is not necessary. A loss of consciousness following head or neck trauma mandates immobilization until the clinician can rule out cervical fractures. In such cases, tomograms of the cervical spine are helpful.[1] Tomography can define and delineate fine or questionable fracture lines, but soft-tissue (e.g., disk, ligament, or nerve root) injury

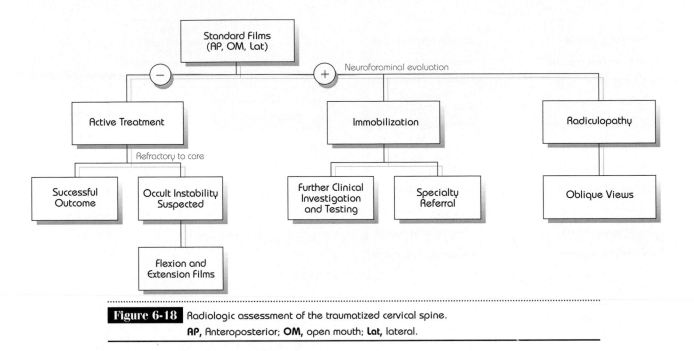

Figure 6-18 Radiologic assessment of the traumatized cervical spine.
AP, Anteroposterior; **OM,** open mouth; **Lat,** lateral.

Table 6-5 Characteristics of Mechanoreceptors

	Shape	Location	Neurologic Function	Adaptation	Motor Neuron Effect	Threshold
Type I mechanoreceptor	Globular	Outer layer of joint capsule	Monitoring of tension of joint capsule	Slow	Tonic effect	Low
Type II mechanoreceptor	Oblong, conical	Inner layer of joint capsule	Inhibition of nociception	Rapid	Phasic effect	Low
Type III mechanoreceptor	Fusiform	Ligaments and tendons	Inhibition of lower motor neurons by Golgi-like corpuscles	Slow	Inhibition of lower motor neurons	High
Type IV nociceptor		Joint capsule and ligaments	Pain production	Not active under normal conditions	Tonic reflexes, autonomic reflexes	Activated by pressure, adaptable to constant pressure

generally requires MRI for documentation.[36] Motion radiographic views (e.g., flexion and extension) and MRI are also helpful in diagnosing occult ligamentous instability.[83]

The translation of a single vertebra over the inferior vertebral segment greater than 3 or 3.5 mm is usually a radiographic signal of instability.[139,169] Acute anterior ligamentous tears, together with areas of hypermobility adjacent to degenerative, arthritic hypomobile spinal segments, are common findings. A standard lateral film or flexion and extension radiographic views reveal evidence of cervical spine instability:

- Anterolisthesis (i.e., flexion deformity or sagittal displacement of vertebral body more than 3.5 mm)
- Increased spinous spacing
- Subluxation of facet joints
- Acute angular deformity at level of injury (i.e., 11-degree angulation of adjacent vertebral bodies)
- Sagittal diameter of canal less than 13 mm

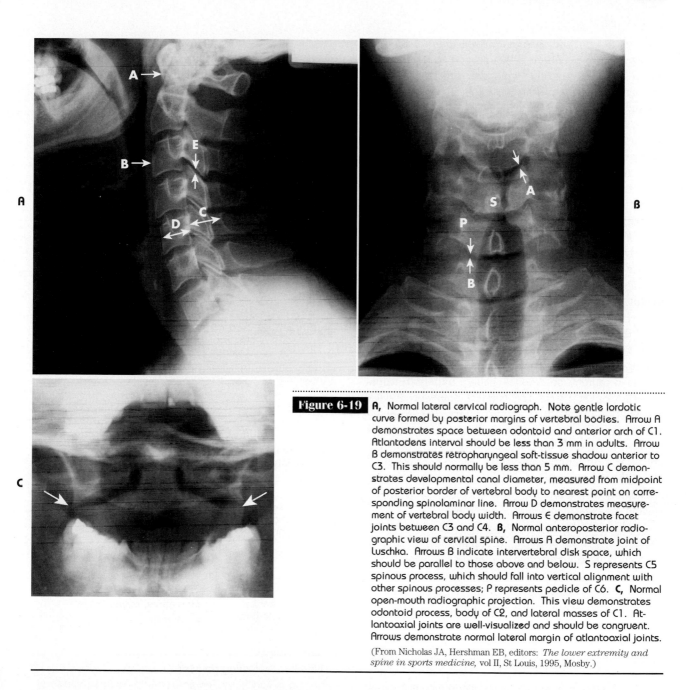

Figure 6-19 **A,** Normal lateral cervical radiograph. Note gentle lordotic curve formed by posterior margins of vertebral bodies. Arrow A demonstrates space between odontoid and anterior arch of C1. Atlantodens interval should be less than 3 mm in adults. Arrow B demonstrates retropharyngeal soft-tissue shadow anterior to C3. This should normally be less than 5 mm. Arrow C demonstrates developmental canal diameter, measured from midpoint of posterior border of vertebral body to nearest point on corresponding spinolaminar line. Arrow D demonstrates measurement of vertebral body width. Arrows E demonstrate facet joints between C3 and C4. **B,** Normal anteroposterior radiographic view of cervical spine. Arrows A demonstrate joint of Luschka. Arrows B indicate intervertebral disk space, which should be parallel to those above and below. S represents C5 spinous process, which should fall into vertical alignment with other spinous processes; P represents pedicle of C6. **C,** Normal open-mouth radiographic projection. This view demonstrates odontoid process, body of C2, and lateral masses of C1. Atlantoaxial joints are well-visualized and should be congruent. Arrows demonstrate normal lateral margin of atlantoaxial joints.

(From Nicholas JA, Hershman EB, editors: *The lower extremity and spine in sports medicine,* vol II, St Louis, 1995, Mosby.)

- Documentation of fracture or dislocation
- Atlantodens interval (ADI) greater than 3 mm in adults and 4 mm in children

Oblique projections make it possible to visualize the neuroforamina in cases of radiculopathy and are helpful in ruling out fracture or dislocation. Oblique views at 45 degrees also facilitate the visualization of the pedicles and lateral masses. Thus some authors advo-cate the routine use of oblique projections in trauma. It is preferable, however, to allow the status of the individual patient to determine this decision.[142] Routinely obtaining a full cervical series of plain films is expensive and has a poor clinical yield.[54] Oblique films usually offer the clinician little in cases of mild-to-moderate trauma, especially when the quality of the anteroposterior and lateral films is good.

In hospital and emergency department settings, it is easy to keep a patient with a suspected fracture immobile on the x-ray table while the clinician reads the standard films. If necessary, the clinician can then order oblique views. When the patient is in the chiropractic office, there should be physical evidence of neuroforaminal or osseous pathologic variations before the practitioner orders multiple films of the patient. The oblique projection can be extremely useful in cases of cervical spine trauma, but as noted earlier, the value of any ancillary radiographic procedure depends on the needs of the patient.

Four of the cervical spine conditions that result from trauma are germane to primary care and chiropractic practices: cervical whiplash syndrome, temporomandibular joint disease, cervical disk injuries, cervical strains, and cervical stenosis.

Whiplash Syndrome: Hyperextension-Hyperflexion Sprain or Strain

The age of the automobile has brought with it cervical whiplash injury, sometimes called hyperextension-hyperflexion injury to the cervical spine or cervical acceleration-deceleration (CAD) injury. Motor vehicle accidents are responsible for a significant number of neck injury cases in the offices of chiropractors, physical therapists, and orthopedic specialists. Since approximately 20 million U.S. citizens are suffering from some complaint associated with whiplash,[46] the condition is finally receiving the clinical attention it deserves.

Hirsch and associates noted that "whiplash has become an emotional term common in popular vocabulary, frequently used by attorneys, a term of derision by comedians, and sometimes the object of scorn by physicians.[71] They continued to say that, although patients with such complaints were once thought to "have partially imaginary or a magnified array of symptoms,...the evidence suggests that this syndrome is real and is manifested by symptoms consistent with the anatomic injury sustained."[71]

The vulnerability of the cervical region is so great that low-to-moderate trauma can compromise a multitude of systems.[23,44,162] As a result, a variety of signs and symptoms may develop; for example, electroencephalographic changes may appear following whiplash if brain injury has occurred.[20,72] The secondary, hidden effects of whiplash are sometimes as disabling, if not more so, than the soreness and muscular stiffness of the initial symptoms (Table 6-6). Cervical sympathetic insult, recurrent headaches, vestibular dysfunction, and chronic

myofascial pathologic changes are not present initially in many patients with whiplash (Figure 6-20).[17,43,60,70,78] The inappropriate and prolonged use of immobilization may cause or enhance secondary myofascial dysfunction as well. Active manual intervention, instituted as early as clinically possible during the course of care, is not a luxury, but a necessity to avoid long-term morbidity and impairment.

The fact that conventional diagnostic and radiologic imagery does not effectively document the magnitude of injury can complicate the management of whiplash trauma and may contribute to the poor track record of orthodox medical treatment in dealing with this clinical entity.[20,70] Although subtle changes appear in x-ray patterns, the array of equivocal or "normal" findings

Table 6-6 Secondary Complaints Associated with Cervical Whiplash and Its Causative Lesions

Complaint	Location of Lesion
Headache	Suboccipital muscles, greater occipital nerve, myofascial trigger points, facet point irritation
Disorientation, irritability	Brain
Visual disturbances	Vertebrobasilar artery network, brainstem, cervical spinal cord
Memory and concentration disturbances	Brain
Vertigo	Cervical sympathetic nerves, vertebral artery, inner ear
Arm and hand numbness	Brachial plexus, scalenes
Thumb, index finger, middle finger numbness; weakness; temperature changes	Median nerve, carpal tunnel
Difficulty swallowing	Pharynx
Ringing in ears	Temporomandibular joint, vertebral and basilar arteries, cervical sympathetic chain, inner ear
Dizziness, lightheadedness	Cervical sympathetic nerves, brain, inner ear
Neck and shoulder pain	Paravertebral muscles, apophyseal joints, cervical nerve roots, cervical disk
Poor balance, proprioception, and posture	Inner ear

seems endless and has perpetrated the myth of the "nonexistent" whiplash injury. Of course, the great void in diagnostic imaging capability lies in soft-tissue spinal injury. Most importantly, however, the entire health care community—including third-party payers—must understand that significant spinal soft-tissue injury can be present even in the absence of positive diagnostic signs.[34,115] A delay in the appearance of symptoms is common,[39] and chronicity of pain and dysfunction occurs in many cases.[8]

Pathomechanics of Whiplash. The supple and mobile cervical spine is open to insult and injury because of its position at the end of the long spinal lever and its inherent attachment to a head that weighs an average of 14 to 17 pounds. As the head whips into hyperflexion and hyperextension, the acceleration forces increase. In fact, small speeds can produce large acceleration impact forces during a rear-end collision.[91] Furthermore, the extent of automobile damage may not correlate with the seriousness of the patient's injuries.[34] In an 8-mph rear-end collision, for example, a 2-G vehicle force can result in a 5-G acceleration force at the occiput and head.[93] Although seat belts have proved to be extremely valuable in preventing injury to the head, skull, and chest wall, their use can potentially increase acceleration forces to the cervical spine because they fix movement at the lower body. The key automobile safety features that aid in preventing cervical whiplash injuries include a firm seat back, a high and stiff headrest, the use of a shoulder belt, and an air bag.[20]

Typically, whiplash occurs when the victim is hit from behind.[11] The cervical spine and head first whip into hyperextension as the torso and lower limbs are virtually fixed. A compensating force opposite to the initial movement of the head brings the cervical spine into retaliatory hyperflexion. The combination of an acceleration force followed by a deceleration movement (i.e., CAD injury) is exceptionally traumatic to the soft tissues of the paraspinal region, setting up a cycle of cervical structural damage, cord insult, and neurologically mediated pain cycles (Figure 6-21).

Hyperextension of the neck traumatizes the anterior soft-tissue structures of the cervical spine. For example, the anterior longitudinal ligament can be damaged.[140] The sternocleidomastoid muscles bear a large brunt of the load. Although the cervical sympathetic nerves are fairly immobile, their trunks lie in the prevertebral myofascia anterior to the transverse processes and are subject to stretch and irritation as well. Traumatic lesions to the sympathetic chain may occur without overt neurovascular compromise; thus careful physical examination is essential.

Physical Examination. The initial examination of a patient following neck and head trauma must address the potential for sympathetic-mediated dysfunction, focusing particularly on the brain, brain stem, and cranial nerves.[68,140] Among the procedures that should be routine in such an examination are the following:

- Assessment of pupillary function
- Evaluation of the fundus
- Bilateral measurement of blood pressure
- Examination for cardinal fields of gaze, ptosis, and nystagmus on fixed lateral gaze
- Evaluation of the function of the trigeminal nerve and the temporomandibular joint
- Questioning of the patient about lightheadedness, vomiting, confusion, excessive fatigue, sleep disturbances, and inability to concentrate to rule out concomitant concussion
- Full upper extremity neurologic examination, including an evaluation of motor, sensory, and reflex status
- Examination for concomitant injuries that may be silent or perceived as secondary to the spinal complaint, such as carpal tunnel syndrome, acromioclavicular and sternoclavicular sprains, costochondritis of the sternum, temporomandibular joint sprains, and cerebral concussion

The force of muscles is the primary protection of the cervical spine. Therefore the practitioner's initial inspection and observation of a patient who has a suspected injury should focus on the detection of muscle

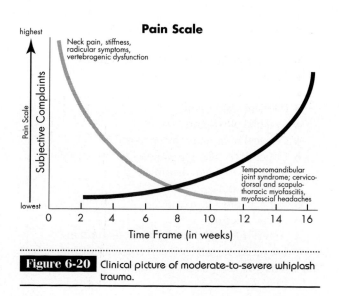

Figure 6-20 Clinical picture of moderate-to-severe whiplash trauma.

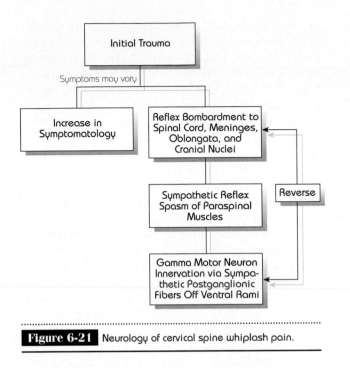

Figure 6-21 Neurology of cervical spine whiplash pain.

spasm, head tilt, neck swelling, and head position. It is important to palpate for tenderness at the sternocleidomastoids, trapezius, suboccipital, and spinal erector muscles. The inspection includes the temporomandibular articulation because the hyperextension of the head drops the mandible and exerts stress on the jawline. Palpation for supraspinous tenderness at the cervicodorsal region with the neck in flexion should also be part of the examination.

The practitioner should document bilateral comparisons of motion in all three planes. Measuring the circumference of the neck is helpful if moderate-to-severe swelling is present, because it establishes a baseline measurement for comparison at a later date.

While testing the facets for motion and "end-feel," the examiner checks the joint capsules for tenderness and notes the degree of fixation and coupled movement. It is wise to check for joint dysfunction in both the sitting (weight-bearing) and supine positions. Hyperextension pain over the facet indicates a localized sprain or synovitis. The disk and nerve roots are evaluated through the application of traction to determine whether it reproduces arm and hand pain, as well as the use of compression tests to determine whether there is a pattern of pain along a nerve root or dermatome. A complete neu-

rologic examination of the brachial plexus from the C5 through the T1 motor segments is essential. It is important to document any dysthetic response, along with any dermatome or motor and reflex changes.

Although soft-tissue findings associated with whiplash are not yet well-understood, recognition of subtle soft-tissue trauma is increasing. Khurana and Nirankari, a neurologist and ophthalmologist, respectively, documented such findings in two patients with bilateral postganglionic Horner's syndrome, complete with anterior neck tenderness, throbbing headache, and ptosis following a whiplash injury.[78] Although Horner's syndrome represents an especially severe cervical whiplash symptom, most primary care physicians (DC, DO, MD) have seen a wide variety of complications in patients who have a suspected whiplash injury:

- Posttraumatic vascular headaches
  - ❏ Basilar artery migraine
  - ❏ Common migraine
  - ❏ Suboccipital
- Cerebral contusion
- Chronic intermittent neck stiffness
- Tinnitus
- Paroxysmal extraocular muscle dysfunction
- Visual disturbances
- Vertigo
- Confusion or syncope
- Diplopia
- Intersegmental fixation, physiologic spinal subluxation
- Cervical myofascitis
- Nausea
- Vomiting
- Paresis
- Lightheadedness
- Facet dislocation (unilateral or bilateral)
- Early degenerative changes
- Laryngeal compromise
- Cervical disk lesion
- Brachial plexopathy
- Cervical radiculopathy or radiculitis
- Upper extremity paresthesia or dysesthesia
- Insomnia or sleep disturbance
- Photophobia
- Cervical muscle spasm
- Spinal fracture
- Anterior longitudinal ligament disruption

For medicolegal reasons, it is essential to document any inability of the patient to complete everyday tasks.

Head Injury

Although the mechanism of cerebral concussion and the countercoup mechanism (i.e., contact of the brain with the skull during rapid acceleration of head and neck) are well-known and accepted, the way in which a whiplash injury to the cervical spine may evoke a response similar to a central cerebral lesion is not clearly understood. Obviously, the brain may sustain a contusion when the neck is rapidly accelerated and decelerated. Although studies of patients who have experienced whiplash without direct head trauma are not plentiful, Ommaya and colleagues noted that this type of cervical insult produces hemorrhage and contusion at the brain surface and upper spinal cord.[107]

In patients with severe cervical whiplash trauma, it may be advisable that the clinician order *both* an x-ray film of the cervical spine and an MRI or a CT scan of the head and central nervous system to rule out such conditions as cerebral edema and hemorrhage. It is wise to check cerebellar function, evaluate the fundus for papilledema, and examine cranial nerve and pupillary response. It may be difficult to differentiate sympathetic from cervical dysfunction in certain areas, and the clinician should not hesitate to order either a diagnostic imaging study or a complete neurologic work-up if the results of the initial examination are ominous. After reviewing the possible sequelae from a hyperextension-hyperflexion injury, it is clear that the "simple" and "uncomplicated" cervical whiplash injury without a fracture or dislocation is neither simple nor uncomplicated.

Types of Cervical Whiplash Injury. It is possible to separate various grades of cervical whiplash injury according to the degree of external trauma, orthopedic and neurologic findings, and patient disability (Table 6-7).

Type I cervical whiplash injury always involves a small external force, although some patients have severe injuries as a result of seemingly small degrees of acceleration trauma. The patient experiences mild discomfort and stiffness of the cervical spine, accompanied by the loss of small increments in range of motion. The hypomobile segment usually appears to be a fixation in posterior-to-anterior rotation, with coupled lateral-

flexion loss. The findings of the neurologic examination are normal, and the results of a radiologic examination are unremarkable. There are no signs of instability and no peripheralization of pain. Orthopedic tests are normal, and the patient is able to participate successfully in all the activities of daily living.

The trauma that causes a type II cervical whiplash injury is generally more severe than the trauma that causes a type I injury. Type II injury culminates in palpable muscle splinting, restriction of motion, and mild-to-moderate spasm. The patient has no neurologic deficits, and there is no evidence of radiculopathy. Although the only radiographic sign is the loss of the normal cervical lordosis, the patient does exhibit mild physical findings of instability. Sympathetic-mediated findings (e.g., headache, dizziness, lightheadedness) may be present during the first week after the injury. Orthopedic tests such as Soto-Hall and cervical compression maneuvers all reproduce localized spinal pain in patients with a type II injury.

Type III cervical whiplash injury is a more serious trauma to the cervical spine. Its symptoms include moderate ligamentous sprain, advanced muscle swelling and spasm, and loss of range of motion in all planes. The patient may have a cervical disk lesion with subsequent nerve root signs. Radiculopathy without clear motor or reflex changes is the rule. Nerve root signs are present. All orthopedic tests contribute to nonspecific paravertebral pain secondary to myospasm. Complaints of vertigo, nausea, diplopia, and lightheadedness indicate sympathetic nerve injury and may continue for 7 to 10 days after injury. It may be necessary to obtain follow-up images of the cervical spine to confirm the diagnosis.

A type IV cervical whiplash injury is the most severe case that is usually treated in a clinician's office. Immediately after the injury, however, the patient is frequently transported via ambulance to the hospital emergency room, examined radiologically, and stabilized with a cervical orthosis (Figure 6-22 *A-C*). Radicular symptoms may be bilateral or unilateral, and motor and reflex changes are common. A more substantial herniated nucleus pulposus requires evaluation by MRI or CT. Electrodiagnostic studies can be performed at least 4 weeks after the nerve injury if needed. A patient with this type of injury is likely to need both chiropractic care and traditional medical treatment. Symptoms associated with this type of injury may continue for up to 2 or 3 years, with as many as 40% to 50% patients having some ongoing spinal dysfunction. Subsequent spinal

Table 6-16 Chronic Soft-Tissue Disorders

	Myofascial Pain Syndrome	Vertebrogenic Cephalgia	Cervical Facet Syndrome
Physical examination findings	Palpable trigger points paracervically Referral zone cephalad or down arm Muscular fixation paravertebrally Generally no motor or sensory deficit Often, history of cervical spine trauma Concomitant joint dysfunction and hypomobility	Dizziness, nausea, aura, and tinnitus common Cephalad referral of cervical pain Cervical posterior joint dysfunction Restricted movement of occipital or atlantoaxial region (C0-C2 axis) Suboccipital and para-vertebral tenderness Global immobility	Palpable tenderness and hypertonicity Restriction of joint play with hard end-feel at end range of motion Decrease in lateral bending with posteroanterior rotation Absence of nerve root signs Sclerotogenous referred pain to shoulder or upper arm Pain reproduced with early cervical extension
X-ray findings	Usually normal	Not usually helpful in diagnosis Need to rule out degenerative spondylosis as contributing factor	Standard two or three views, with or without stress films Need to rule out adjacent ligamentous instability
Treatment plan	CMT and PNF mobilization Stretching program, trigger point work Manual ischemic compression or combination of ultrasound and electrotherapy Postural exercise program Massage	CMT and postural alterations Acupressure or soft-tissue work Assessment of nutritional factors, if appropriate Massage	CMT and ancillary procedures for pain or spasm reduction Isotonic-accommodative resistance exercises

CMT, Chiropractic manipulative therapy; **PNF,** proprioceptive neuromuscular facilitation.

Vertebrogenic Cephalgia (Cervicocranial Syndrome)

According to Bogduk, the "neuroanatomical basis of cervical spine headache is overwhelming."[12] The paracervical sympathetic neural connections are responsible for a great many headaches. In addition, the upper cervical spine at the level of the C1, C2, and C3 vertebrae houses the trigeminal nerve, which can mediate head pain.[59] Both afferents and the trigeminal nucleus feed into the gray matter of the cord.[114] Because the C2-C3 facet causes upper cervical pain with referral toward the head,[15] headache may originate not only in the cervical musculature, but also in the functional spinal unit.

Frykholm stated that cervical migraine is common and often "erroneously diagnosed."[52] Vernon described a vertebrogenic model of migraine.[159] The periodicity of vascular headaches (e.g., migraines) may be helpful in differentiating them from vertebrogenic headaches. Chiropractic manipulation of the cervical spine may be helpful to those who suffer from migraine headaches, as well as for those who have experienced trauma, possibly because of sympathetic-mediated reflex changes that culminate in the upper neck.[137,157] Common aggravating factors include stress, poor positioning, biomechanical faults, and traumatic exacerbations.[156] A clinician should always beware of spontaneous headaches, which need to be thoroughly investigated at once.

Vertebrogenic headaches have a diverse array of clinical features. Some patients have posterior joint dysfunction; some have global immobility. In some cases the patient has a history of nerve root pain. Patients with muscle contraction (i.e., tension) headaches exhibit upper cervical articular restrictions.[86,128,152] Most patients with suboccipital tenderness and greater occipital neuralgia have a fixed spinal segment at the atloido-occipital or atlantoaxial junction. Pain may extend from the cervical spine toward the vertex of the head, or it may follow the course of the greater occipital nerve and temporalis muscle (Figure 6-27). In most cases the head pain is unilateral with neck involvement. It is important to confirm the level of dysfunction and pain pattern with palpation. Vertigo, nausea, aura, and tinnitus may be present; pupillary changes are not uncommon.[49]

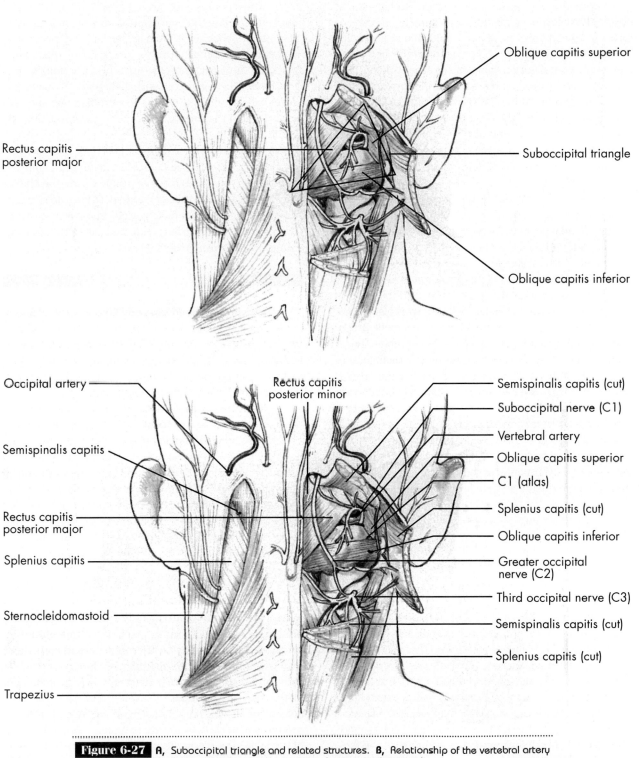

Oblique capitis superior

Rectus capitis posterior major

Suboccipital triangle

A

Oblique capitis inferior

Occipital artery

Rectus capitis posterior minor

Semispinalis capitis (cut)

Suboccipital nerve (C1)

Vertebral artery

Semispinalis capitis

Oblique capitis superior

C1 (atlas)

Rectus capitis posterior major

Splenius capitis (cut)

Oblique capitis inferior

B

Splenius capitis

Greater occipital nerve (C2)

Sternocleidomastoid

Third occipital nerve (C3)

Semispinalis capitis (cut)

Splenius capitis (cut)

Trapezius

Figure 6-27 **A,** Suboccipital triangle and related structures. **B,** Relationship of the vertebral artery and suboccipital and greater occipital nerves to the triangle.

(From Reckling FW, Reckling JB, Mohn MP: *Orthopedic anatomy and surgical approaches,* St Louis, 1990, Mosby.)

Radiographic findings are often ambiguous at best.[50] Hypolordosis occurs consistently in various forms of "mechanical neck pain," and this radiographic aberration frequently accompanies chronic headache, many times secondary to whiplash or other trauma. Expensive testing procedures such as electroencephalograms, electromyograms (EMGs), CT scans, or MRI scans are not helpful unless the clinician suspects a neurologic disease process or a neoplasm. Spontaneous headaches or drastic changes in headache pattern warrant clinical evaluation with such imaging procedures, however, (Figure 6-28).

A significant portion of the adult population experiences cervicogenic headaches.[2,119] Many patients with chronic headache have been medicated needlessly or treated allopathically without success. The primary treatment method should be manual therapy. Recent studies have showed spinal manipulation to be an effective form of treatment.[103] Postural and behavioral changes are desirable, especially in the workplace. Biofeedback techniques, chronic pain management procedures, and counseling can help patients overcome the attitudes and stress factors that present a roadblock to effective treatment. The application of ice to the cervical spine is helpful during acute exacerbations. CMT to the cervical spine is paramount. The practitioner should look carefully for primary restrictions in the upper cervical spine and for compensatory joint fixation in the lower cervical spine. Correction of the biomechanical faults or intersegmental dysfunction of the cervical spine can interrupt the neurochemical cycle of autonomic dysfunction.

Charting the Course of Headaches

It is helpful if patients with cervical headaches who are about to undergo chiropractic care keep daily charts on the frequency, duration, and intensity of their pain. These charts may make it easier to rule out biomechanical and nutritional factors that may be triggers for their headaches. Hard cheeses, red wine, chocolate, and shellfish are common culprits, as are all food substances high in tyramine and monosodium glutamate. Dairy products may increase the production of mucus and clog sinus passages. Smoking and excessive alcohol consumption often increase the frequency of headaches. Estrogen, certain cardiac medications, and prolonged periods of fasting can all be contributing factors to headache.

The spontaneous development of headaches may be a red flag that warns the individual of a disease process. Headaches that have periods of remission and exacerbation are rarely a cause for medical concern, but those that increase linearly in unremitting intensity may be consistent with neoplasm. Blood pressure measurements, pulse determinations, and an evaluation of the fundus are imperative to rule out organic disease.

The clinician should examine every patient with headache thoroughly and should take a clear, concise history. As the centerpiece of primary care, the chiropractor should work in close association with family medical practitioners, neurologists, and psychologists, if necessary, to improve the life and ease the suffering of the patient with headaches.

Cervical Facet Syndrome and Chronic Cervical Sprain

Some cervical patients continue to exhibit mechanical joint problems of the neck such as recurrent hypomobility, synovitis, and pain. Secondary muscular findings may not be found, or they may be localized only to the segmental level of involvement.

Richly innervated structures such as the articular capsule provide a convenient pathway for nociception, since the number of mechanoreceptors is greater in the cervical spine than in the lumbar spine, for example.[14,58] Synovitis of the facet leads to stiffness, loss of cervical function, and pain.[74] Secondary cephalgia and recurrent spasm of the paravertebral musculature may be part of the symptom complex. Patients with recurrent, disabling pain may be candidates for repeat plain-film analysis or stress projections in flexion and extension to rule out instability.

On manual examination, the facet involved possesses a hard end-feel with discomfort or pain at the end-range (mechanical joint block). Muscular hypertonicity or alteration in local tone is palpable. Although not always referred, pain may be sclerotogenous in nature and may extend toward the shoulder or upper arm. Facet pain from the C2-C3 level may refer toward the occiput or the back of the head.[28,35] Nerve root signs are conspicuously absent, but extension of the cervical spine reproduces pain early in the arc of motion. A combination of the facet's coupled motion with extension of the spine exacerbates the pain response as well. The manipulatable lesion can usually be isolated unilaterally. Posteroanterior rotation with lateral bending is usually restricted.

Disorders of the Cervicobrachial Region

The junction between the shoulder joint and the cervical spine is commonly known as the cervicobrachial region or the thoracic outlet. Transversed by delicate neurovascular structures, this zone is often the site of complaints that affect both the neck and upper extremity (Figure 6-29).

Faulty posture, awkward sleeping positions, and trauma to the shoulder and neck can all lead to cervicobrachial syndrome. Because muscular structures such as the scalenes abut the neurovascular bed of the brachial plexus, muscular strains and myospasm in this area can cause neurovascular compromise. Vascular deficiencies can also mimic mechanical brachial pain, as can cardiac disease. Traction injuries to the nerve roots and to the trunks of the brachial plexus can be quite disabling, causing neurologic pain similar to that associated with herniated disks. Mechanical disorders can lead to symptoms of thoracic outlet syndrome, such as with cervical ribs or lateral flexion disorders of the spine seen with arm hyperabduction during some faulty sleeping postures.

Diagnosis of problems at the cervicobrachial junction is often difficult. The history plays a key role, and the clinician should ask questions about previous trauma (e.g., lateral bending injuries), as well as about the time, place, and site of neurologic signs (e.g., numbness, tingling, and swelling of the hand). A careful and systematic history is particularly important in the older patient.

In addition, a thorough diagnostic work-up is essential to rule out systemic disorders, such as metabolic and peripheral vascular disease (Table 6-17). The use of neurodiagnostic tests, such as EMGs or determinations of nerve conduction velocities, is often quite helpful. Palpatory findings, orthopedic tests, and radiologic studies all contribute to a working diagnosis.

Although most problems at the thoracic outlet are mechanical in nature and involve soft tissue, manipulation may not always totally alleviate the patient's symptomatology. Methodical strengthening and stretching of

Table 6-17	Diagnostic Work-Up for Disorders of the Cervicobrachial Region
To Rule Out	**Procedure**
Venus insufficiency	Venogram
Subclavian artery compression	Auscultation, arteriogram
Collagen vascular disease	Laboratory work (ANA test)
Degenerative spondylosis	X-ray films
Apical lung disease	Examination, history, x-ray films
Cardiac disease	Auscultation, electrocardiogram, laboratory work, stress testing

ANA, Antinuclear antibody.

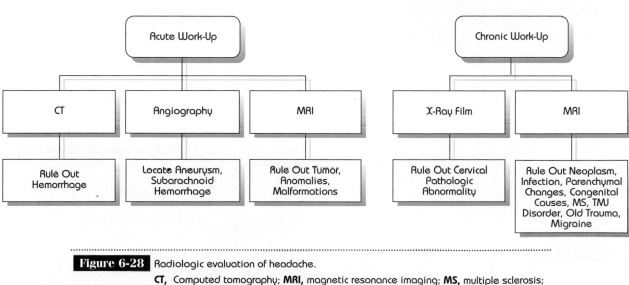

Figure 6-28 Radiologic evaluation of headache.

CT, Computed tomography; **MRI,** magnetic resonance imaging; **MS,** multiple sclerosis; **TMJ,** temporomandibular joint disorder.

the paracervical muscles, along with biomechanical correction of joint play and posture, may also be necessary in the total treatment of cervicobrachial disease.

Thoracic Outlet Syndrome

Although considered a neurovascular condition, the symptoms of thoracic outlet syndrome are primarily neurogenic. Physical examination is the central basis for diagnosis.

Certain types of referred brachial pain are tell-tale signs of thoracic outlet syndrome. First, the patient's symptomatology is positionally related. For example, hyperabduction of the arm may exacerbate the pain, and the radial pulse may disappear during external rotation and abduction.[18] Second, because of the involvement of the C8 and T1 nerve roots, the distribution of pain is almost always over the medial arm and forearm. The thenar and hypothenar regions are commonly affected. Third, pure cervical testing procedures or movements do not reproduce the pain. *It takes a combination of shoulder girdle and arm motions to replicate the pain and localize the problem.*

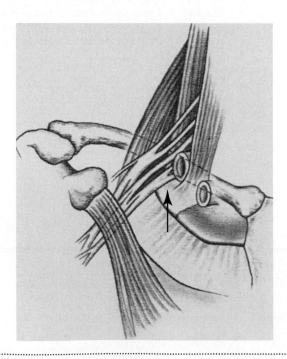

(From Mercier LR: *Practical orthopedics*, ed 4, St Louis, 1995, Mosby.)

Figure 6-29 Cervicobrachial anatomy. Note that the lower trunk of the brachial plexus lies on the first rib (arrow).

In addition to pain and paresthesia at the medial aspect of the brachium, the patient may have pain referred to the fourth and fifth digits, weakness of the intrinsic hand muscles, numbness with hand swelling, and a feeling of heaviness of the arm. The subclavian vessels may be compressed as they leave the thoracic outlet, producing signs and symptoms that vary according to the site of the compression (Table 6-18). Edema, cyanosis, and discoloration may appear in cases of venous obstruction; coolness, numbness, and fatigue may occur in cases of arterial occlusion. In rare instances a Raynaud's phenomenon may occur.[77] Although thoracic outlet syndrome was originally thought to affect all three components of the costoclavicular compartment (i.e., vein, artery, and nerve), this is not always the case.

The neurovascular problems associated with thoracic outlet syndrome may appear most often at night, particularly if the patient sleeps with the arm in hyperabduction. Numbness, tingling, and swelling of the digits may occur. The pain, like that arising from carpal tunnel syndrome, may wake the patient in the middle of the night. Thus it is important to advise the patient to avoid sleeping in positions that may impinge on the neurovascular bundle of the thoracic outlet.

Routine electrodiagnostic tests are normal for many patients with thoracic outlet syndrome. Nerve conduction velocities are almost always normal. Patients with repeated episodes of thoracic outlet syndrome may show some C8 innervated muscle changes, but active denervation on an EMG is rare. Classic neurogenic findings in thoracic outlet syndrome include normal median nerve sensory action potentials with normal amplitude,

Table 6-18 Sites of Compression at the Thoracic Outlet

Anatomic Site	Structures Affected
Interscalene space (anterior or middle scalenes, first rib)	Brachial plexus, subclavian artery
Costoclavicular space (clavicle, first rib)	Neurovascular bundle
Proximal axilla (smaller pectoral muscle, coracoid process)	Neurovascular bundle
Paracervical region (C7 transverse processes, C7 ribs)	Neurovascular bundle

and normal median nerve motor (large C8 component) potentials with reduced amplitude. It is not uncommon for the ulnar nerve to be spared.[173] Plain films are not helpful except for documenting neurovascular compression caused by the presence of a cervical rib. MRI and magnetic resonance angiography (MRA) have shown some promise in helping to diagnose this condition.[37] The cost versus the clinical benefits of the study must always be weighed.

The clinician palpates the supraclavicular fossa carefully for pulsations, muscle spasm, and tenderness. If there was previous trauma, the clinician feels along the clavicle for any osseous deformity or acromioclavicular aberrations. Scalene spasm can trigger myotomal referral down the arm, or it can cause neurovascular compression as in thoracic outlet syndrome. Lower cervical joint fixation, especially in lateral bending, is a common manual finding. Cervical compression tests are not helpful in the absence of disk or nerve root disease. Shoulder depression, hyperabduction, and costoclavicular tests may prove useful.

The proper management of thoracic outlet syndrome depends on an accurate diagnosis and the exclusion of various other pathologic forms that can mimic this syndrome:

- Raynaud's phenomenon
- Cervical radiculopathy from a herniated disk
- Stroke
- Angina pectoris
- Carpal tunnel syndrome
- Peripheral vascular disease
- Paracervical myofascial pain syndrome

Collagen vascular disease may mimic the findings of thoracic outlet syndrome, but may have, in addition, peripheral dermatitis or other findings. It is necessary to rule out subclavian artery compromise or venous insult; the presence of bruits on a stethoscopic examination may be indicative of atherosclerosis or congestive heart disease. Plain radiographic films make it possible to exclude cervical spondylosis and organic disease.

It is important to investigate thoroughly the differential diagnosis of thoracic outlet syndrome, since misdirected therapy may prolong the course of disability and treatment program. CMT aimed at increasing the mobility of the lower cervical region and shoulder girdle is the primary treatment. If radiologic studies indicate the presence of a cervical rib, adjustment of the first rib with the patient in the prone, sitting, or supine position (whichever is most comfortable) is helpful, along with scrutiny of the joint mechanics at C7 and T1.

Muscular rehabilitation is also crucial in the treatment of thoracic outlet syndrome, however, (Tables 6-19 and 6-20). Stretching should be geared toward the lateral flexors of the cervical spinal column and the pectoral muscles. Proprioceptive neuromuscular facilitation, static stretching performed at home, and moist heat are helpful. Postural changes initiated at home and in the workplace are key components of total patient care. Structural characteristics, such as a low carriage of the shoulder girdle, may predispose an individual to thoracic outlet syndrome via a depressed shoulder. In this case the muscles that provide suspension of the scapula should be strengthened as well.[87]

Brachial Plexopathy and Neurapraxia

From its position at the thoracic outlet, the brachial plexus is the neurologic switchboard responsible for transferring the sensory and motor impulses from the cervical nerve roots to the peripheral nerves of the upper limbs. In most individuals, cervical roots 5 through 8 and thoracic root 1 contribute to the plexus. Occasionally, C4 also contributes to the brachial plexus; less commonly, T2 does.

Sensory ganglia usually lie near or within the neuroforamen outside the canal, whereas motor ganglia lie at the anterior horn cells within the spinal cord. Lesions proximal to the dorsal root ganglia are considered preganglionic lesions; lesions distal to the dorsal root ganglia are postganglionic. Clinically, injuries that involve avulsed nerve roots (i.e., preganglionic lesions) undergo Wallerian degeneration (i.e., disruption and breakdown of nerve material) and do not recover.[5] Postganglionic lesions may recover spontaneously, depending on the severity of the injury.

The examination of a person with a brachial plexopathy should begin with observation for round shoulders, forward neck, or obvious swelling. The practitioner should palpate the paraspinal region for spasm or hypertonicity in the musculature. Similarly, it is necessary to palpate the supraclavicular area for swelling, spasm, or masses that can adversely affect the brachial plexus.

A thorough evaluation of the brachial plexus includes upper extremity testing for motor, sensory, and reflex changes. Compression and range-of-motion maneuvers are necessary to rule out nerve root radiculopathy from a spinal source. Lateral bending of the spine stretches the scalenes and usually reproduces discomfort or peripheral pain from a brachial plexus lesion. The practitioner places the patient into cervical compression, rotation, and extended position toward the side of

Table 6-19 Disorders of the Cervicobrachial Region

	Thoracic Outlet Syndrome	Brachial Plexopathy	Brachial Neuralgia
Physical examination findings	Pain and paresthesia along medial arm, forearm Lower trunk involvement most common Night pain with postural symptomatology Pain reproduced by shoulder depression or arm hyperabduction Pectoralis, scalene hypertonicity Lower cervical spinal restriction Need to rule out vascular insufficiency	Pain, burning, and numbness into arm (neurapraxia) History of cervical stretch or neck injury Temporary or transient paresis Neck, shoulder, and arm pain Need to rule out motor, sensory loss after 24 hours	Somatic pain referred from paracervical region to shoulder and arm Pain reproduced by lateral flexion of neck Segmental articular fixation of lower cervical region Soto-Hall maneuver an indication of localized spinal pain No true motor or sensory deficit
X-ray findings	Standard cervical series Need to rule out cervical spondylosis, cervical ribs, and organic pathologic abnormalities	Standard cervical series Need to evaluate vertebrae for fractures, assess disk spaces Need to rule out ligamentous instability, spinal stenosis, and degenerative disk disease	Standard cervical series Need to rule out chronic ligamentous instability, degenerative disk disease, and organic illness
Treatment plan	CMT Exercise and strengthening of shoulder girdle Counseling on postural and sleep faults	Modalities (e.g., ice) for reducing pain and swelling CMT or manual traction MRI, if HNP or spinal stenosis suspected Electrodiagnostic testing, if signs of nerve injury are present for 4-6 weeks with abnormal MRI	CMT Myofascial trigger point therapy Spinal exercise, postural correction Electrotherapy, ice, and moist heat for acute care

CMT, Chiropractic manipulative therapy; **MRI,** magnetic resonance imaging; **HNP,** herniated nucleus pulposus.

involvement (e.g., Spurling's maneuver) to determine whether pain occurs. Any pain, numbness, or paresis that lasts longer than 24 hours warrants a careful physical and radiologic reexamination.

The individual with brachial plexopathy usually has transient paresis of the upper limb because of an excessive lateral flexion injury of the cervical spine, with or without shoulder depression.[154] Paresthesia generally emanates from the middle or lower cord of the plexus, reproducing the usual distribution of the dysthetic response seen in football injuries called "burners" or "stingers."[105] Sometimes, the entire hand goes numb and weak, and the individual tries to shake the limb to reduce the pain. A blow to the shoulder girdle that drives it in a caudad direction can also stretch the plexus. Follow-up EMG studies show some axonal injury in many athletes with traumatic injuries to the brachial plexus.

Individuals with simple, uncomplicated neurapraxia have normal EMG and nerve conduction velocity studies.[32]

Brachial neurapraxia involves demyelination of the axon sheath without disruption. In some neuronal injuries, there is an interruption of the axon, but the surrounding tissues remain intact. Called axonotmesis, degeneration of the affected muscles appears on electrodiagnostic studies 2 to 3 weeks after neural injury. Patterns of reinnervation frequently develop after a period of time, however. In contrast, recovery from neurotmesis, a severe injury that destroys the axon and supporting structures, is unlikely.

After cervical disk herniation or spinal stenosis has been excluded from the working diagnosis, the patient with brachial plexopathy should undergo a combination of chiropractic manipulation, gentle manual traction, and therapeutic modalities to reduce pain and swelling. Ice

Table 6-20	Muscular Rehabilitation in the Treatment of Thoracic Outlet Syndrome

Muscle	Goal of Rehabilitation
Levator scapula	Strengthen on low shoulder side
Greater and lesser rhomboids	Strengthen on symptomatic side
Posterior deltoid	Strengthen bilaterally
Rotator cuff	Strengthen bilaterally
Greater and smaller pectorals	Stretch and strengthen bilaterally
Scalenes	Stretch and strengthen on symptomatic side
Sternocleidomastoid	Stretch and strengthen bilaterally
Anterior serratus	Strengthen bilaterally

followed by the application of moist heat is appropriate for 24 to 72 hours after injury. If the patient does not respond to conservative care in the first 2 to 4 weeks, MRI is useful to rule out a cervical disk lesion. Electrodiagnostic tests are helpful in identifying denervation or axon regeneration 4 to 6 weeks after an abnormal MRI scan. No athlete who participates in a contact sport should return to play with arm pain, neck immobility, or significant neurologic findings.

Football players should consider using a neck roll to prevent extreme ranges of motion.[165] Once injury has occurred, the prevention of further injury centers around the restoration of neck flexibility through manipulation and other techniques. The patient can perform strengthening exercises isometrically at first and then progress to accommodative resistance and isotonic movements. In organized athletics it is wise to encourage the entire team to participate in stretching and neck-strengthening exercises. Performing cervical spine exercises after practice teaches the athletes to work when they are tired and helps offset the "fatigue factor" that often plays a key role in spinal injury during competitive sports.

Brachial Neuralgia (Cervicobrachial Syndrome)

In general, brachial neuralgia connotes a physical impairment involving the paracervical region and extending to the shoulder, upper arm, and possibly forearm. Unlike patients with brachial plexopathies, patients with brachial neuralgia rarely have pain in the hand. Somatically referred pain can arise from ligamentous and capsular sprains to the cervical spine. Patients usually describe the pain as dull, achy, or diffuse. Impairment of

the shoulder and arm is usually vague and not well-localized. The thoracic outlet region is often tender to palpation, as are the lateral stabilizers of the cervical spine.

Patients with brachial neuralgia usually have no signs of nerve root traction. The Soto-Hall maneuver (i.e., hyperflexion of the neck) reproduces local spinal pain, but lateral flexion of the cervical spine stretches the brachial region and is generally more accurate in reproducing paracervical, shoulder, and arm pain. Motor and sensory function is normal in most cases.

The differential diagnosis includes rotator cuff disease with reflex muscle spasm to the neck, degenerative disk disease of the cervical spine, and chronic ligamentous instability of the cervical spine. The clinician should rule out organic disease if orthopedic and range-of-motion testing of the cervical spine and shoulder does not significantly reproduce pain.

Repetitive lateral flexion or rotation of the neck, as required in the clerical and computerized workplace, can be responsible for brachial neuralgia. This syndrome is often chronic in nature, with periods of exacerbation determined by the degree of stress placed on the upper extremity or cervical spine. Radiographic findings are not usually consistent with physical findings. Changes in home and work habits and strengthening of the upper limb are helpful in prevention and treatment.

Chiropractic care should focus on articular fixation of the lower cervical spine and cervicodorsal junction. Ancillary procedures, including electrotherapy and the application of ice or moist heat, may play a role in acute care. It is important to advise the patient to avoid extreme lateral flexion of the neck and hyperabduction of the shoulder. Postural habits and the presence of myofascial pain are usually closely related.

Arthritides

Axial arthropathies commonly stem from the arthritides, with cervical spine involvement no exception. It has been estimated that rheumatoid arthritis produces symptomatology related to the cervical spine in 60% to 70% of patients,[120] and the seronegative spondyloarthropathies can also contribute to spinal pain and dysfunction. Atlantoaxial subluxation and instability have been associated with both rheumatoid disease and ankylosing spondylitis.[167] Flowing ossification or calcification along the anterior and lateral aspects of the spine, tagged diffuse idiopathic skeletal hyperostosis (DISH) is common in elderly men.[122] Degenerative cervical spondylosis may occur as a result of past traumatic episodes or as an incidental finding consistent with the aging process.

Most patients with arthritic involvement of the cervical region complain of a generalized stiffness of the neck, loss of functional mobility, and pain. Specific motions may affect different patients in various ways, according to their specific arthritis; however, most patients use the term *stiffness* to describe their condition to the treating physician. The clinician should take a careful history, noting (1) which daily activities (e.g., driving, shaving, reading) are most affected, (2) whether the patient has any polyarthropathies or recurrent peripheral joint swelling, (3) if there is any evidence of dermatitis, and (4) whether any other members of the family have the condition. It is also helpful to ask if the patient has been using over-the-counter medication or has seen a health care provider for treatment.

The physical examination of the arthritic patient should include a complete neurologic and orthopedic work-up. Radiographic evaluation should include the standard anteroposterior and lateral views, as well as any other films needed to ensure an accurate diagnosis. If the advisability of manipulative therapy is not clear and the clinician suspects ligamentous instability, a stress or motion series with extension and flexion films may be helpful. The consequences of cervical spine involvement in some arthritides can be quite severe; for example, erosion, inflammation, and instability are possible sequelae. Proper sequencing of imaging modalities and a thorough physical examination can be helpful in identifying patients at greatest risk for such events.

Rheumatoid Arthritis

Although rheumatoid arthritis seems to affect the hands first in most cases, Conlin reported an incidence of 60% to 70% for cervical spine involvement in patients with this condition.[25] Patients with rheumatoid arthritis complain of cervical stiffness, neck pain, and immobility that can range from mild to severe joint restriction. The patient with cervical involvement usually has concomitant hand or wrist pain.

Mild rheumatoid disease of the spine may involve articular dysfunction and stiffness of the muscles and joints; advanced disease may include inflammatory and erosive changes, as well as ligamentous instability. Physical findings may not be consistent with the history or radiographic assessment of the patient's condition. There may be radiographic evidence of osteoporosis, spinal joint erosion, and minimal osteophyte (i.e., new bone) formation. Entrapment neuropathies and spinal

cord involvement are common.[30] All patients with rheumatoid arthritis must be screened radiographically for atlantoaxial joint instability before they enter into a treatment trial of manipulation. Subtle radiographic signs of cervical spine instability include a widened odontoid and hyperplasia of the vertebrae.[66]

The possible complications of rheumatoid disease of the cervical spine include cervical myelopathy, craniocervical and atlantoaxial anatomic subluxations, and facet erosion or collapse.[30,163] Patients who have overt signs of myelopathy should not be routinely subjected to extreme motion studies for obvious reasons. Individuals with suspected vertebral or ligamentous instability and no neurologic abnormalities may benefit from lateral cervical stress films, since such films may uncover occult cases of anatomic subluxations. Anterior anatomic subluxation of C1 or C2 is documented in adults by separations of 2.5 mm or more at the anterior arch of the atlas inferiorly and the adjacent odontoid process.[167] MRI is helpful in patients who show progressive neurologic deficits, sensory changes, or signs of cervical compression.

Once the patient's condition is neurologically stable, a reasonable treatment program can be outlined. The program not only should address peripheral arthropathies, but it should also include palliative and stabilizing therapy for the cervical spine. Chiropractic manipulation with supportive adjunctive therapies and soft-tissue techniques are safe for the neurologically stable patient. Neurologic instability is an indication for more passive methods of treatment, such as physiotherapeutic modalities for pain, application of moist heat, and gentle soft-tissue mobilization. It is helpful to instruct patients on neck positioning for sleep and for household tasks and to review their medical and pharmaceutical history with them. Frequent blood work is necessary for patients on gold therapy, penicillamine, or any autoimmune medications to monitor liver function (Table 6-21).

Degenerative Arthritis (Cervical Spondylosis)

A myriad of pathoanatomic factors are associated with the development of degenerative joint disease. Age-related changes at the level of the C5-C6 intervertebral disk are common. Synovial joint changes, conversely, occur over a larger area, ranging from the C2 to C6 levels.[13] (One major reason for the lack of degenerative changes at the cervicocranial junction is the absence of an intervertebral disk.)

Joint immobility, morning stiffness, lack of rotation and lateral bending capability, and neck pain are all common complaints of patients with arthritis. Pain does

Table 6-21 Arthritides

	Rheumatoid Arthritis	Degenerative Arthritis	DISH
Physical examination findings	History of neck pain and discomfort Morning stiffness Concurrent hand or wrist complaints Intermittent loss of cervical mobility Need to rule out neurologic signs in extremities	History of chronic or intermittent neck stiffness Pain or discomfort at end-range of movement History of trauma or disk lesions (e.g., from sports, motor vehicle accidents) Need to screen for radicular symptoms Morning stiffness, muscle hypertonicity Loss of posteroanterior rotation and lateral bending	Prolonged history of cervical stiffness Immobility in multiple planes Men over age of 60 years of age commonly affected
X-ray findings	Minimum of three standard views Need to evaluate ADI for atlantoaxial subluxation Stress films are sometimes needed to diagnose occult instability	Minimum of anteroposterior and lateral views Additional oblique views, if radiating symptoms are present Need to rule out osseous encroachment at intervertebral foramen	Dense calcification at multiple vertebral levels Disk spaces and facet joints well-preserved Concomitant extraspinal findings at tendon attachments and entheses
Treatment plan	CMT Laboratory work is sometimes needed to monitor drug therapy Physiotherapy modalities	CMT Manual traction Application of moist heat, electrotherapy Range-of-motion exercises	CMT Soft-tissue mobilization Therapeutic exercise Physiotherapy modalities

DISH, Diffuse idiopathic skeletal hyperostosis; *CMT,* chiropractic manipulative therapy; *ADI,* atlantodens interval.

not normally radiate peripherally unless the patient has signs of radiculopathy or myelopathy from nerve root or spinal canal compromise. Individuals with severe arthritis may experience spinal canal compression because of heterotopic bone formation, disk protrusion, or advanced facet disease. Other individuals at increased risk for cord compression include those with anterior longitudinal ligament buckling and vertebral (anatomic) subluxation attributable to severe degeneration.[118]

Patients with a history of multiple, repetitious, or gross trauma generally show radiographic signs of spondylosis. Degenerative spondylosis appears radiographically as a decrease in disk height and calcification of the annulus and vertebral body margins, with the appearance of heterotopic bone adjacent to the vertebrae and in the anterior longitudinal ligament (Figure 6-30 *A, B*). The disk spaces are usually well-preserved, however.

The symptoms of arthritis do not necessarily coincide with its radiographic appearance. Patients with advanced radiographic evidence of degenerative spondy-losis may benefit from additional plain-film projections. Oblique films make it possible to visualize the neuroforamina for osseous impingement and pathologic abnormalities (see Figure 6-30 *B*). Right and left films should always be taken together. However, CT or MRI may be necessary to assess the neurologic status of the spine thoroughly.

In patients with severe degenerative arthritis, manipulative therapy should not be directed at the level of anatomic instability. Age and physical findings must play a particularly strong role in the treatment of these patients. Manual traction in the office or a prescription for an over-the-door home traction unit is helpful in the treatment of cervical spondylosis. Intervertebral traction for 5 to 10 seconds with a gradual release time of 3 seconds is usually safe, but manipulation through axial traction is not advisable for patients with osteoporosis, neurologic deficits, or instability. Gentle chiropractic manipulation can begin to include higher velocity adjustments as treatment progresses. Ancillary therapy,

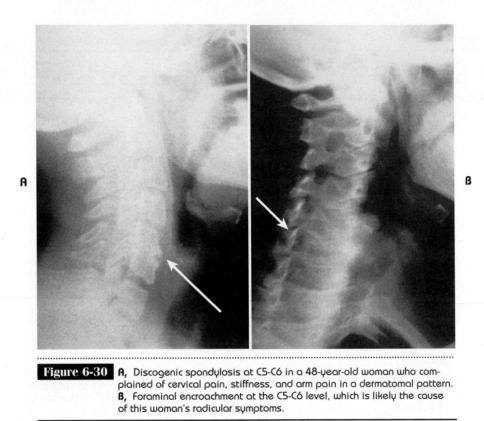

Figure 6-30 **A,** Discogenic spondylosis at C5-C6 in a 48-year-old woman who complained of cervical pain, stiffness, and arm pain in a dermatomal pattern. **B,** Foraminal encroachment at the C5-C6 level, which is likely the cause of this woman's radicular symptoms.

such as electrotherapy and the application of moist heat, are soothing to the patient with arthritis.

The key to effective patient care is to restore, maintain, and improve the quality of spinal motion. Range-of-motion exercises are helpful in this effort. It is typical for the patient with neck arthritis to attain a moderate increase in spinal mobility and cervical rotation from only a few manipulations. Those who drive often remark on their noticeably improved ability to back a car out of their driveway.

Diffuse Idiopathic Skeletal Hyperostosis

Sometimes called Forestier's disease or ankylosing hyperostosis, DISH is generally an incidental finding on radiographic films taken of men over 60 years of age. The cervical and thoracic regions are most commonly affected.[10] These patients complain of spinal pain, stiffness, and immobility. Individuals with cervical involvement may also complain of dysphagia because of osteophytic compression of the hypopharynx.[164]

Hyperostosis and large areas of flowing calcification at the anterior aspect of the vertebral motor unit are visible radiographically (Figure 6-31). Disk spaces and apophyseal joints are usually well-preserved. Certain groups of patients who exhibit cervical spine involvement have calcification of the posterior longitudinal ligament as well.[164] Extraspinal findings concomitant with DISH include calcification of tendon sheaths and heterotopic bone formation at entheses.

Physical findings are similar to those in a patient with advanced osteoarthritis, except that by the time patients with DISH become symptomatic and seek help, they usually have severely restricted mobility that may span all planes of motion. The diagnosis is made radiologically, and the patient is then placed on a treatment program to aid or maintain the range of motion. The patient who has a mild case of DISH is likely to have a more marked improvement from chiropractic manipulation than the patient who is older and has advanced disease.

Mobilization, manual traction of the spine, stair stepping, and range-of-motion exercises are all helpful in treating the severe hypomobility associated with DISH. Adjunctive therapy consisting of heat, ultrasound therapy, or electrotherapy is soothing to the musculature

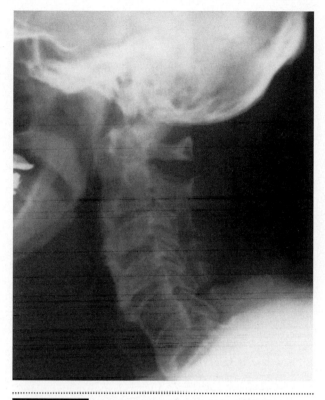

Figure 6-31 Diffuse idiopathic skeletal hyperostosis visualized on a lateral cervical film of a 68-year-old man with a history of global neck stiffness. Note the flowing anterior calcification at C2 through C5 and C7. A congenitally blocked vertebrae at C5-C6 contributes to the impaired cervical motion of this patient.

and palliative for discomfort, but it does not produce a pathologic change. The practitioner should instruct the patient in proper sleep and task posture. The patient may need supportive care over an extended period to ensure freedom of movement and function.

Review Questions

1. (a) Discuss the biomechanical differences at various points along the cervical spine. (b) What is biomechanically responsible for the mobility of the cervical spine? (c) Describe the coupled movement of the facet joints.

2. (a) Describe flexion loading of the neck in contact sports. (b) What are some possible injuries that arise from this type of trauma?

3. Match the cervical pathologic conditions with its appropriate diagnostic procedure:

1. Occult vertebral or liga-   a. Oblique plain films
   mentous instability   b. Flexion-extension
2. Assessment of spinal cord,   stress films
   nerve roots, and vertebral   c. SSEP
   disk   d. MRI
3. Evaluation of physiologic
   dysfunction of sensory
   pathways
4. Neuroforaminal encroachment

4. (a) What mechanical corrections are made through CMT administered to the injured cervical spine? (b) What are some contraindications for cervical manipulation?

5. A CAD trauma is often disabling and difficult to predict. (a) Name some secondary causes of disability. (b) What factors in case management can successfully decrease the chances of long-term morbidity? (c) What studies are poor predictors of whiplash injury?

6. (a) Patient's that exhibit peripheral pain on cervical compression tests, relief on distraction, and arm, hand, or scapula pain in a radicular pattern are usually suffering from what type of condition? (b) What are some conservative acute treatment options for this injury?

7. (a) What are some orthopedic conditions that may lead to cervical spinal stenosis? (b) With what abnormalities has developmental stenosis of the cervical spine been associated? (c) What procedures produce a definitive diagnosis?

8. (a) A patient with neurogenic pain of the medial arm and forearm that is positionally related and with no signs of pain during cervical testing procedures may have what condition? (b) What structures are most commonly involved? (c) What findings are usually seen with electrodiagnostic studies? (d) What orthopedic tests are useful in patients with this diagnosis?

References

1. Abitbol JJ: Commentary on diagnosis of cervical spine injury, *Adv Orthop Surg* 14(3):162, 1990.
2. Alders EE, Hertzen A, Tan CT: A community-based prevalence study on headache in Malaysia, *Headache* 36(6):379, 1996.
3. American Academy of Pediatrics Committee on Accident and Poison Prevention: *Trampolines*, Evanston, Ill, 1976, The Academy.
4. Anderson R et al: A meta-analysis of clinical trials of spine manipulation, *J Manipulative Physiol Ther* 15:181, 1992.

5. Archambault JL: Brachial plexus stretch injury, *J Am Coll Health* 31:256, 1983.

6. Arnheim DD, Prentice WE: *Principles of athletic training*, ed 8, St Louis, 1993, Mosby.

7. Assendelft WJJ, Bouter LM, Knipschild PG: Complications of spinal manipulation: a comprehensive review of the literature, *J Fam Pract* 42:475,1996.

8. Balla JI: The late whiplash syndrome, *Aust NZJ Surg* 50:610, 1980.

9. Bannister G, Gargan M: Prognosis of whiplash injuries: a review of the literature, *Spine: State of the Art Reviews* 7(5):557, 1993.

10. Boden SD, Wiesel SW, Laws ER, Rothman RH: *The aging spine: essentials of pathophysiology, diagnosis and treatment*, Philadelphia, 1991, WB Saunders.

11. Bogduk N: The anatomy and pathophysiology of whiplash, *Clin Biomech* 1:92, 1986.

12. Bogduk N: *Cervical cause of headaches*, Toronto, Canada, 1991, The American Back Society.

13. Bogduk N: *Free communication on the clinical anatomy of the spine*, Toronto, Canada, 1991, The American Back Society.

14. Bogduk N, Marsland A: The cervical zygapophyseal joints as a source of neck pain, *Spine* 13:610, 1988.

15. Bogduk N, Windsor M, Inglis A: The innervation of the cervical intervertebral discs, *Spine* 13:2, 1988.

16. Bovim G: Cervicogenic headache, migrane and tension-type headache: pressure-pain threshold measurements, *Pain* 51:169, 1992.

17. Braaf MN, Rosner S: Meniere-like syndrome following whiplash injury of the neck, *J Trauma* 2:494, 1962.

18. Bradley JP, Tibone JE, Watkins RC: History, physical examination, and diagnostic tests for neck and upper extremity problems. In Watkins RG, editor: *The spine in sports*, St Louis, 1996, Mosby.

19. Burstein AH, Otis JC, Tory JS: Mechanisms and pathomechanics of athletic injuries to the cervical spine. In Tory JS, editor: *Athletic injuries to the head, neck and face*, Philadelphia, 1982, Lea & Febiger.

20. Carroll C, McAfee PC, Riley LH: Whiplash injuries and how to treat them, *J Musculoskel Med* 9(6):97, 1992.

21. Carver G, Willits J: Comparative study and risk factors of a CVA, *J Amer Chiropractic Assoc* 32(10):65, 1996.

22. Cassidy JD, Lopes AA, Yong-Hing K: The immediate effect of manipulation versus mobilization on pain and range of motion in the cervical spine: a randomized controlled trial, *J Manipulative Physiol Ther* 15:570, 1992.

23. Chester JB: Whiplash, postural control, and the inner ear, *Spine* 16:716, 1991.

24. Coffee MS et al: *Hyperextension injury patterns in the human cadaveric cervical spine*, 1989, Cervical Spine Research Society.

25. Conlin PW: Rheumatoid arthritis of the cervical spine. In Resnick D, Niwayama G, editors: *Diagnosis of bone and joint disorders*, ed 2, Philadelphia, 1988, WB Saunders.

26. Connell MD, Wiesel SW: Natural history and pathogenesis of cervical disk disease, *Orthop Clin North Am* 23(3):369, 1992.

27. Coulter I, Hurwitz E, Adams A, Meeker W, Hansen D, Mootz R, Aker P, Genovese B, Shekelle P: *The appropriateness of manipulation and mobilization of the cervical spine*, Santa Monica, Calif, 1996, RAND Corporation.

28. Cramer GD, Darby SA: Anatomy related to spinal subluxation. In Gatterman MI, editor: *Foundations of chiropractic: subluxation*, St Louis, 1995, Mosby.

29. Cramer GD, Darby SA: *Basic and clinical anatomy of the spine, spinal canal, and ANS*, St Louis, 1995, Mosby.

30. D'Cruz D, Hughes C: Neurologic manifestations of rheumatoid arthritis, *J Musculoskel Med* 9(2):35, 1992.

31. Difabio RP: Efficacy of manual therapy, *Phys Ther* 72:853, 1992.

32. Dossett AB, Watkins RG: Stinger injuries in football. In Watkins RG, editor: *The spine in sports*, St Louis, 1996, Mosby.

33. Ducker TB: Post-traumatic progressive cervical myelopathy in patient with congenital spinal stenosis, *J Spinal Disord* 9:76, 1996.

34. Dvorak J, Valach L, Schmid S: Cervical spine injuries in Switzerland, *J Manual Med* 4:7, 1989.

35. Dwyer A, Aprill C, Bogduk N: Cervical zygapophyseal joint pain patterns: I. A study in normal volunteers, *Spine* 15:453, 1990.

36. Enzmann DR, DeLaPaz RL: Trauma. In Enzmann DR, DeLaPaz RL, Rubin JB, editors: *Magnetic resonance of the spine*, St Louis, 1990, Mosby.

37. Esposito MD, Arrington JA, Blackshear MN, Murtagh FR, Silbiger ML: Thoracic outlet syndrome in a throwing athlete diagnosed with MRI and MRA, *J Magn Reson Imaging* 7:598, 1997.

38. Evans RC: *Illustrated essentials in orthopedic physical assessment*, St Louis, 1994, Mosby.

39. Evans RW: Some observations on whiplash injuries, *Neurol Clin* 10(4):975, 1992.

40. Farah M, Matasar K, Cacciarelli A, Wong P: Radiographic evaluation of the acutely traumatized cervical spine, *Spine* 3(2):281, 1989.

41. Farfan H, Crossette J, Robertson G et al.: The role of torsion in disk degeneration, *J Bone Joint Surg* 52A:4, 1970.

42. Ferezy J: Neural ischemia and cervical manipulation: an acceptable risk, *J Amer Chiropractic Assoc* 25(8):61, 1988.

43. Fitz-Ritson D: Assessment of cervicogenic vertigo, *J Manip Physiol Ther* 14(3):193, 1991.

44. Fitz-Ritson D: Cervicogenic sympathetic syndromes: etiology, treatment, and rehabilitation. In Gatterman MI, editor: *Foundations of chiropractic subluxation*, St Louis, 1995, Mosby.

45. Fitz-Ritson D: Chiropractic management and rehabilitation of cervical trauma, *J Manipulative Physiol Ther* 13:17, 1990.

46. Foreman SM, Croft A: *Whiplash injuries: the cervical acceleration/deceleration syndrome*, Baltimore, 1988, Williams & Wilkins.

47. Fourre M: On-site management of cervical spine injuries, *Phys Sports Med* 19(4):53, 1991.

48. Fredriksen TA, Hovdal H, Sjaastad O: Cervicogenic headache: clinical manifestation, *Cephalgia* 27:147, 1987.

49. Fredriksen TA et al: Cervicogenic headache: pupillometric findings, *Cephalgia* 8:94, 1988.

50. Fredriksen TA, Fougner R et al: Cervicogenic headache: radiological investigations concerning head/neck, *Cephalgia* 9:139, 1988.

51. Friction JR: Myofascial pain and whiplash, *Spine: State of the Art Reviews*, 7(3):403, 1993.

52. Frykholm R: Cervical migraine: the clinical picture. In Hirsch C, Zotteman Y, editors: *Cervical pain*, Oxford, England, 1972, Pergammon Press.

53. Funk FJ, Wells RE: Injuries of the cervical spine in football, *Clin Orthop* 109:50, 1975.

54. Garfin SR: Which x-ray views are needed for neck injuries in the ER? *J Musculoskel Med* 10(10):11, 1993.

55. Gargan MF, Fairbank JCT: Anatomy of the spine. In Watkins RG, editor: *The spine in sports,* St Louis, 1996, Mosby.

56. Gay RE: The curve of the cervical spine: variations and significance, *J Manipulative Physiol Ther* 16(8):591, 1993.

57. Gertzbein S, Seligman J, Holtby R et al.: Centrode patterns and segmental instability in degenerative disc disease, *Spine* 10:257, 1985.

58. Giles LC: The surface lamina of the articular cartilage of human zygapophyseal joints, *Anat Rec* 233:350, 1992.

59. Goadsby PJ, Zagani AS, Lambert GA: Neural processing of craniovascular pain: a synthesis of the central structures involved in migraine, *Headache* 31:365, 1991.

60. Gold B, Brickner D, Sukerik S: Reflex sympathetic dystrophy syndrome following minor trauma, *Isr J Med Sci* 25:107, 1989.

61. Gracovetsky S: Biomechanics of the spine. In White A, Schofferman JA, editors: *Spine care: diagnosis and treatment,* St Louis, 1994, Mosby.

62. Granges G, Littlejohn G: Prevalence of myofascial pain syndrome in fibromyalgia syndrome and regional pain syndrome: a comparative study, *J Musculoskel Pain* 1(2):19, 1993.

63. Greenan TJ: Diagnostic imaging of sports-related spinal disorders, *Clin Sports Med* 12(3):487, 1993.

64. Haldeman S: Spinal manipulative therapy in sports medicine, *Clin Sports Med* 5(2):283, 1986.

65. Hardarl JA, Knapp J, Poletti S: The cervical spine. In White AH, Schofferman JA, editors: *Spine care: diagnosis and treatment,* St Louis, 1994, Mosby.

66. Henderson DJ: Radiographic evaluation of the upper cervical spine. In Vernon H, editor: *Upper cervical syndrome: chiropractic diagnosis and treatment,* Baltimore, 1988, Williams & Wilkins.

67. Herzog RJ, Wiens JJ, Dillingham MF, Sontag MJ: Normal cervical spine morphometry and cervical spinal stenosis in asymptomatic professional football players, *Spine* 16(6):178, 1991.

68. Hildingsson C, Wenngren BI, Bring G, Toolanen G: Oculomotor problems after cervical spine injury, *Acta Orthop Scand* 60(5):513, 1989.

69. Hinck VC, Hopkins CE, Savara BS: Sagittal diameter of the cervical canal in children, *Radiology* 79:97, 1962.

70. Hinoki M, Niki H: Neurological studies on the role of the sympathetic nervous system in the formation of traumatic vertigo of cervical origin, *Acta Otolaryngol Suppl* 330:185, 1975.

71. Hirsch SA et al: Whiplash syndromes: fact or fiction? *Orthop Clin North Am* 19(4):791, 1988.

72. Hohl M: Soft tissue injury of the neck in automobile accidents: factors influencing prognosis, *J Bone Joint Surg* 56A:1675, 1974.

73. Howe DH, Newcombe RG, Loade MT: Manipulation of the cervical spine—a pilot study, *J R Coll Gen Pract* 33:574, 1983.

74. Jackson R: *The cervical syndrome,* ed 4, Springfield, Ill., 1978, Charles C Thomas.

75. Jaeger B: Are cervicogenic headaches due to myofascial pain and cervical spine dysfunction? *Cephalgia* 9(3):159, 1989.

76. Janda V: Muscle spasm: a proposed procedure for differential diagnosis, *Manual Medicine* 6:136, 1991.

77. Karas SE: Thoracic outlet syndrome: neurovascular injuries, *Clin Sports Med* 9(2):297, 1990.

78. Khurana RK, Nirankari US: Bilateral sympathetic dysfunction in post-traumatic headaches, *Headache* 26:183, 1986.

79. Kidd RF, Nelson R: Musculoskeletal dysfunction of the neck in migrane and tension headache, *Headache* 33:566, 1993.

80. Kingston RS: Radiology of the spine. In Watkins RG, editor: *The spine in sports,* St Louis, 1996, Mosby.

81. Kirkaldy-Willis WH, Cassidy JD: Spinal manipulation in the treatment of low back pain, *Canadian Family Physician* 31:535, 1985.

82. Koes BW et al: Spinal manipulation and mobilization for back and neck pain—a blinded review, *Br Med J* 303:1281, 1991.

83. Kulkarni MV, McArdle CB, Koparicky D et al: Acute spinal cord injury: MR imaging at $1^{1}/_{2}$T, *Radiology* 164:837, 1987.

84. LaBan MM, Macy JA, Merschaert JR: Intermittent cervical traction: a progenitor of lumbar radicular pain, *Arch Phys Med Rehabil* 73(3):295, 1992.

85. Lewit K: Management of muscular pain associated with articular dysfunction. In Frictor JR, Awad EA, editors: *Advances in pain research and therapy,* vol 17, New York, 1990, Raven Press.

86. Lewit K: Pain arising from the posterior arch of the atlas, *Eur Neurol* 16:263, 1977.

87. Lutz FR, Gieck JH: Thoracic outlet compression syndrome, *Athletic Training* 21(4):302, 1986.

88. MacDonald RL et al: Diagnosis of cervical spine injury in motor vehicle crash victims: how many x-rays are enough? *J Trauma* 30(4):392, 1990.

89. Mackeag DB, Cartu RD: Neck pain in a football player, *Phys Sports Med* 18(3):115, 1990.

90. MacNab I: Acceleration injuries of the cervical spine, *J Bone Joint Surg* 46A:1797, 1964.

91. MacNab I: The whiplash syndrome, *Orthop Clin North Am* 2:389, 1971.

92. Marion DW: *Definitive care of the cervical spine: diagnostic techniques and management,* proceedings from the 49th annual meeting, 49th Annual Meeting and Clinical Symposium, Baltimore, 1998, National Athletic Trainers' Assoc.

93. McKenzie JA, Williams IF: The dynamic behaviour of the head and cervical spine during whiplash, *J Biomech* 4:477, 1971.

94. Mealy K, Brennan H, Ferelan G: Early mobilization of acute whiplash injuries, *Br J Med* 292:656, 1986.

95. Mennell J: Myofascial trigger point as a cause of headaches: commentary, *J Manipul Physiol Ther* 12(4):308, 1989.

96. Meschan I: *Roentgen signs in diagnostic imaging,* ed 2, Philadelphia, 1985, WB Saunders.

97. Miller B: Manual therapy treatment of myofascial pain and dysfunction. In Rachlin ES, editor: *Myofascial pain and fibromyalgia,* St Louis, 1994, Mosby.

98. Miller RG, Burton R: Stroke following chiropractic manipulation of the spine, *JAMA* 229:189, 1974.

99. Moldofsky H et al: Musculoskeletal symptoms and non-REM sleep disturbances in patients with fibrosis syndrome and healthy subjects, *Psychosom Med* 37:341, 1975.

100. Moroney SP, Schutte AB, Miller JA, Andersson CBJ: Load displacement properties of lower cervical spine motion segments, *J Biomech* 21(9):767, 1988.

101. Mueller FO, Cantu R: Catastrophic injuries and fatalities in high school and college sports: Fall 1982–Spring 1988, *Med Sci Sports Exerc* 22(6):737, 1990.

102. Nagata K: Clinical value of MRI for myelopathy, *Spine* 15(11):1088, 1990.

103. Nilsson N, Christensen HW, Hartvigsen J: The effect of spinal manipulation in the treatment of cervicogenic headache, *J Manipulative Physiol Ther* 20(5):326, 1997.

104. Norris SH, Watt I: The prognosis of injuries resulting from rear-end vehicle collisions, *J Bone J Surg* 65B(5):608, 1983.

105. O'Connor CE, Pekow PS, Klingersmith MT: Brachial plexus injury (burners) incidence and risk factors in collegiate football players: a prospective study, *J Athletic Training* 33(2):(suppl)5, 1998.

106. Olmarker K, Rydevik B, Holm S: Edema formation in spinal nerve roots induced by experimental graded compression: an experimental study on the pig cauda equina, *Spine* 14(6):569, 1989.

107. Ommaya AK, Faas F, Yarnell P: Whiplash injury and brain damage: an experimental study, *JAMA* 204:75, 1968.

108. Panjabi MM, Oxland T, Parks E: Quantitative anatomy of the cervical spine ligaments, Part II. Middle and lower cervical spine. *J Spine Disord* 4:277, 1991.

109. Panjabi MM, White AA: *Clinical biomechanics of the spine,* ed 2, Philadelphia, 1990, JB Lippincott.

110. Parker GB, Tupling H, Pryor DS: A controlled trial of cervical manipulation for migraine, *Aust N Z J Med* 8:589, 1978.

111. Pedowitz RA, Garfin SR, Roberts WA, White AA: Evaluating the causes of neck, shoulder and arm pain, *J Musculoskel Med* 5(6):61, 1988.

112. Pedowitz RA et al: *The effects of magnitude and duration of acute compression upon impulse conduction in the pig cauda equina,* Miami, 1988, International Society for the Study of the Lumbar Spine.

113. Peterson CK: The nonmanipulable subluxation. In Gatterman MI, editor: *Foundations of chiropractic: subluxation,* St Louis, 1995, Mosby.

114. Pfeffenrath V, Dardekar R, Pollman W: Cervicogenic headache: the clinical picture, radiological findings, and hypotheses on its pathophysiology, *Headache* 27:495, 1987.

115. Potter GE: A study of 744 cases of neck and back pain treated with spinal manipulation, *J Can Chiropractic Assoc* 21(4):154, 1977.

116. Przybylski G, Marion DW: Injury to the vertebrae and spinal cord. In Moore EE, Mattox KL, Feliziano DV, editors: *Trauma,* ed 3, Stanford, Conn, 1996, Appleton & Lange.

117. Radanov BP, Sturzenegger M, Stefano GD: Long-term outcome after whiplash injury: a two-year follow-up considering features of injury mechanism and somatic, radiologic, and psychosocial factors, *Medicine* 74(5):281, 1995.

118. Rahim KA, Stambough JL: Radiographic evaluation of the degenerative cervical spine, *Orthop Clin North Am* 23(3):395, 1992.

119. Rasmussen BK, Jensen R, Schroll M, Olsen J: Epidemiology of headache in a general population: a prevalence study, *J Clin Epidemiol* 44(11):1147, 1991.

120. Resnick D, Niwayama G: Rheumatoid arthritis. In Resnick D, Niwayama G, editors: *Diagnosis of bone and joint disorders,* ed 2, Philadelphia, 1988, WB Saunders.

121. Rothman RH, Simeone FA: *The spine,* ed 3, Philadelphia, 1992, WB Saunders.

122. Resnick D, Niwayama G: Radiographic and pathologic features of spinal involvement in diffuse idiopathic skeletal hyperostosis, *Radiology* 1:559, 1976.

123. Rydevik B, Brown MD, Lundborg G: Pathoanatomy and pathophysiology of nerve root compression, *Spine* 9(1):7, 1984.

124. Saal JA, Dillingham MF: Nonoperative treatment and rehabilitation of disk, facet, and soft tissue injuries. In Nicholas JA, Hershman EB, editors: *The lower extremity and spine in sports medicine,* vol II, St Louis, 1995, Mosby.

125. Sartoris DJ, Resnick D: What radiology reveals about the painful neck, *J Musculoskel Med* 5(10):52, 1988.

126. Schaefer DM, Flanders A, Northrop BE et al: Magnetic resonance imaging of acute cervical spine trauma: correlation with severity of neurologic injury, *Adv Orthop Surg* 13(4):156, 1990.

127. Schellas KP et al.: Vertebrobasilar injuries following cervical manipulation, *JAMA* 244:1450, 1980.

128. Schimek JJ, Mohr Y: The importance of manual therapy in the treatment of chronic headache, *Manual Med* 22:41, 1984.

129. Seghof D, Curl DD: Chiropractic manipulation of anteriorly displaced temporomandibular disc with adhesion, *J Manipulative Physiol Ther* 18(2):98, 1995.

130. Shekelle PG, Adams AH, Chassin MR, Hurwitz EL, Brook RM: Spinal manipulation for low back pain, *Ann Intern Med* 117(7):590,1992.

131. Skootsky SA, Jaeger B, Dye RK: Prevalence of myofascial pain in internal medicine practice, *West J Med* 151:157, 1989.

132. Shekelle PG et al: Spinal manipulation for low back pain, *Ann Intern Med* 117:590, 1992.

133. Simons DG: Clinical and etiological update of myofascial pain from trigger points, *J Musculoskel Pain* 4(1/2):93, 1996.

134. Simons DG: Myofascial pain syndrome: one term but two concepts; a new understanding (editorial), *J Musculoskel Pain* 3(1):7, 1993.

135. Sloop PR et al: Manipulation for chronic neck pain: a double blind controlled study, *Spine* 7:532, 1982.

136. Sokoloff R, Sartoris DJ, Resnick D: Uncovering the sources of temporomandibular joint malfunction, *J Musculoskel Med* 5(3):69, 1988.

137. Stodolny J, Chmielewski H: Manual therapy in the treatment of patients with cervical migraine, *Manual Med* 4:49, 1989.

138. Tall RL, DeVault W: Spinal injury in sport: epidemiologic considerations, *Clin Sports Med* 12(3):441, 1993.

139. Taylor JAM: The role of radiology in evaluating subluxation. In Gatterman MI, editor: *Foundations of chiropractic: subluxation,* St Louis, 1994, Mosby.

140. Teasell RW: The clinical picture of whiplash injuries: an overview, *Spine: State of the Art Reviews* 7(3):373, 1993.

141. Terret AG: Vascular accidents from cervical spine manipulation: report on 107 cases. *J Amer Chiropractic Assoc* 17:15, 1987.

142. Thomas M, Bell GR: Radiologic evaluation and imaging of the spine. In Nicholas JA, Hershman EB, editors: *The lower extremity and spine in sports medicine,* ed 2, vol II, St Louis, 1995, Mosby.

143. Torg JS, Glasgow SG: Criteria for return to contact activity following cervical spine injury, *Clin J Sport Med* 1:12, 1991.

144. Torg JS, Naranja RJ, Pavlov H, Galinat BJ, Warren R, Stine RA: The relationship of developmental narrowing of the cervical spinal canal to reversible and irreversible injury of the cervical spinal cord in football players, *J Bone Joint Surg Am* 78:1308, 1996.

145. Torg JS, Pavlov H: Cervical spinal stenosis, *Clin Sports Med* 6(1):115, 1987.
146. Torg JS, Pavlov H, Genvarro SE et al: Neurapraxia of the cervical spinal cord with transient quadriplegia, *J Bone Joint Surg* 68A(9):1354, 1986.
147. Torg JS, Vegso JJ, Sennett B et al: The natural football head and neck registry: 14-year report on cervical quadriplegia, 1971-1984, *JAMA* 254:3439, 1985.
148. Travell J: Myofascial trigger points: a clinical review. In Bonice J, Albe-Fessard D, editors: *Advances in pain research and therapy,* vol 1, New York, 1976, Raven Press.
149. Travell J, Simons DG: *Myofascial pain and dysfunction: the trigger point manual,* Baltimore, 1983, Williams & Wilkins.
150. Triano JJ et al: *A randomized controlled clinical trial of manipulation for chronic low back pain patients,* London, 1993, World Federation of Chiropractic Congress.
151. Triano JJ, Skogsbergh D, McGregor M: Validity and basis of manipulation. In White AH, Schofferman JA, editors: *Spine care,* vol I, St Louis, 1995, Mosby.
152. Turk Z, Ratkolb O: Mobilization of the cervical spine in chronic headache, *Manual Med* 3:15, 1987.
153. Verditti PP, Rosner AL, Kettner N, Sanders G: Cervical traction device study: a basic evaluation of home-use supine cervical traction devices, *J Neuromusculoskeletal Syst* 3(2):82, 1995.
154. Vereschagin K: Burners, *Physician Sports Med* 19(9):96, 1991.
155. Verhaar J, Spaars F: Radial tunnel syndrome: an investigation of compressive neuropathy as a possible cause, *J Bone Joint Surg* 73A:539, 1991.
156. Vernon H: Cervicogenic headache. In Gatterman MI, editor: *Foundations of chiropractic: subluxation,* St Louis, 1995, Mosby.
157. Vernon H: Spinal manipulation and headaches of cervical origin, *J Manipulative Physiol Ther* 12(6):455, 1989.
158. Vernon H: Spinal manipulation and headaches of cervical origin, *Manual Med* 6:73, 1991.
159. Vernon H: *Upper cervical syndrome: chiropractic diagnosed treatment,* Baltimore, 1988, Williams & Wilkins.
160. Wardwell W: Why has chiropractic survived? In Wardwell W, editor: *Chiropractic history and evolution of a new profession,* St Louis, 1992, Mosby.
161. Watkins RG: Neck injuries in football. In Watkins RG, editor: *The spine in sports,* St Louis, 1996, Mosby.
162. Weinberg S, La Pointe H: Cervical extension-flexion injury (whiplash) and internal derangement of the TMJ, *J Oral Maxillofac Surg* 45:653, 1987.
163. Weissman BN, Aliabad P, Weissman M et al: Prognostic features of atlantoaxial subluxation in rheumatoid arthritis, *Radiology* 144:745, 1982.
164. Weissman B, Sledge C: *Orthopedic radiology,* Philadelphia, 1985, WB Saunders.
165. Wells RP, Bishop PJ: The inappropriateness of helmet drop tests in assessing neck protection in head-first impacts, *Am J Sports Med* 18(2):201, 1990.
166. Wesolowski DP, Wang AM: CT and myelographic evaluation of spinal trauma, *Spine: State of the Art Reviews* 3(2):313, 1989.
167. Westmark KD, Weissman BN: Complications of axial arthropathies, *Orthop Clin North Am* 21(3):427, 1990.
168. White AH: Conservative care: pulling it all together. In White AH, Schofferman JA, editors: *Spine care,* vol I, St Louis, 1995, Mosby.
169. White AA, Johnson RM, Panjabi MM, Southwick WO: Biomechanical analysis of clinical stability in the cervical spine, *Clin Orthop* 109:85, 1975.
170. Wilberger JE, Maroon JC: Cervical spine injuries in athletes, *Phys Sports Med* 18(3):56, 1990.
171. Yu YL, Stevens JM, Kendall B et al: Cord shape and measurements in cervical spondylitic myelopathy and radiculopathy, *Am J Neuroradiol* 4:839, 1983.
172. Yunus MB: Research in fibromyalgia and myofascial pain syndrome: current status, problems, and future directions, *J Musculoskel Pain* 1(1):23, 1993.
173. Zahn C: *Electrodiagnosis of the cervicobrachial region,* Toronto, Canada, 1991, American Back Society.

Chapter 7

Thoracic Spine

Chapter Highlights

Anatomy of the Thoracic Spine
Biomechanics of the Thorax
Examination of the Thoracic Spine
Conditions that Affect the Thoracic Spine
Conditions that Affect the Thorax and Rib Cage

Often overlooked and underassessed, the thoracic or dorsal spine is an area that requires evaluation both in isolation and in conjunction with the cervical and lumbar spine. The thoracic region and rib cage not only protect the heart and lungs, but they also provide osseous support. Unfortunately, however, the region is frequently a site for postural deformity.

Anatomy of the Thoracic Spine

The thorax consists of the sternum, twelve pairs of ribs, spine and associated cartilage, muscles, and ligaments required for internal stability. Sternal articulations include (1) the sternocostal joints between the costal cartilage of the ribs and sternum, and (2) the costochondral articulations between the ribs and cartilage. The upper seven pairs of ribs are called *true* ribs, because they articulate directly with the sternum. The remaining five pairs of ribs do not articulate with the sternum and are called *false* ribs. The eighth, ninth, and tenth pairs are attached to cartilage that is linked to the costal cartilage of the superior (seventh) pair of ribs and thus to the sternum. Because they have no anterior attachment, the eleventh and twelfth pairs are termed *floating* ribs (Figure 7-1).

The vertebrae of the dorsal spine are closely related to the ribs, as exemplified by the diarthrodial articula-

tions that are present. The sixteen articular facets are almost totally vertical in their orientation, allowing for sagittal translation and rotation. The thorax itself is a limiting factor for lateral flexion of the thoracic spine, since the ribs articulate with the demifacet of the vertebrae and the articulating groove at the broad transverse process (Figure 7-2 *A-C*).

The first thoracic vertebra articulates with both the first and second ribs. The two most inferior dorsal vertebrae tend to exhibit lumbarlike features, and they lack the structure necessary to provide any support for the final two ribs. Ribs nine through twelve tend to be anchored along the vertebral body as opposed to the transverse process and vertebrae.[40]

As a primary curve, the dorsal kyphosis forms early and should ultimately take a moderately posterior position. The kyphotic curve can become severe, however, because of infection, biomechanical problems (e.g., scoliosis), metabolic disorders, or disease (e.g., Scheuermann's disease). A delicate balance of anterior compression at the functional spinal unit and the static forces of the postural elements and dorsal tissues contribute to the formation and maintenance of the thoracic kyphosis.

The muscular system of the dorsocostal interface is responsible for a myriad of functions, including, but not limited to, respiration, chest and thorax expansion, postural integrity, and spinal stabilization (Figure 7-3). The serratus and intercostal muscles support the rib cage of the thorax. The serratus posterior muscles are responsible for inspiration as well. The intercostal muscles are supplied by the intercostal nerves, and they are arranged in three layers: external, internal, and innermost.[32] At the superior aspect of the thoracic spine are muscles that aid in respiration and stabilization of the

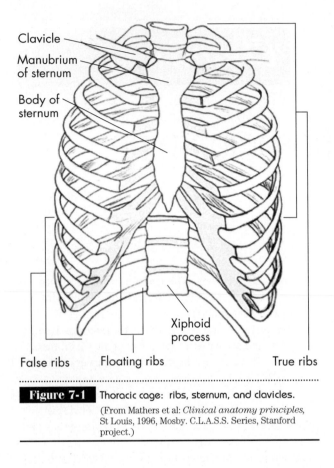

Clavicle

Manubrium of sternum

Body of sternum

Xiphoid process

False ribs   Floating ribs   True ribs

Figure 7-1 Thoracic cage: ribs, sternum, and clavicles.

(From Mathers et al: *Clinical anatomy principles,* St Louis, 1996, Mosby. C.L.A.S.S. Series, Stanford project.)

scapula to the thoracic wall. The subscapular muscle, along with the serratus, rhomboid, and intercostal muscles, all aid in static posture. The iliocostal muscle of the thorax and the erector muscle of the spine not only stabilize the spine, but with the ribs and synovial joints, they check rotation. The iliocostal muscle of the thorax also aids in the lateral flexion and extension of the thoracic spine.[14]

Biomechanics of the Thorax

The mobility of the thoracic spine varies according to the region involved. The upper dorsal spine (i.e., T1-T2) mimics the cervical region, although the presence of the ribs limits movement of this region somewhat; the upper thoracic spine exhibits greater freedom in rotation than in flexion and extension. In the lower thoracic spine (i.e., T7-T12), there is a definite increase in sagittal motion, with a subsequent increase in vertebral body size. The articular facets tend to become more sagittally oriented in the dorsolumbar transition, and as expected, rotation is decreased.

The costovertebral region includes a dynamic set of joints that involve intervertebral and rib movement. Inspiration requires muscular activity at the thorax, although expiration may not. Forced respiration requires contraction of the accessory muscles.

The attachment of the ribs to the spine posteriorly and sternum anteriorly limits (with the exception of the floating ribs) rib motion significantly. The motion of the ribs is primarily rotation with a slight gliding movement.[14] The transverse diameter of the thorax is greater than the anteroposterior diameter in adults, but not in infants; in all groups, however, elevation of the ribs to increase the transverse diameter of the thorax improves vital capacity and everts the ribs. The sternum moves upward and forward as the anterior ribs are elevated. The lower ribs move laterally to increase the stretch on the diaphragm and increase its power capacity.[41]

When the ribs move horizontally, the anteroposterior diameter of the thorax increases. The contraction of the diaphragm and elevation of the first two ribs produce vertical movement. Extending the thoracic spine during forced inhalation improves this movement. The erect position of the spine allows for spinal and pelvic stabilization against the pull of the abdominal musculature. The rib cage increases the axial stability of the spinal column.[39] Other stabilizers of the thorax include the greater and smaller pectoral muscles, which aid in sternal elevation and first rib dynamics; the quadrate muscle of the lumbar spine, which stabilizes the twelfth rib and improves the motion of the diaphragm; and the trapezius muscle, which aids in the balance of scapula rotatory forces, thus allowing smooth scapulothoracic rhythm.[7]

Any fixation or aberrant movement of the costovertebral articulations or ribs can have an impact on the synovial joints of the dorsal spine. It is not uncommon to find concomitant loss of joint play at the rib angle and corresponding vertebral motor unit. Even so, some authors believe that the dorsal spine is in a way protected from some of the detrimental forces and resultant pathologic conditions of the cervical and lumbar spine. Boden and colleagues, for example, suggested that the rib cage may act as a splint to the thoracic spine.[9] This splinting effect may perhaps prevent stresses placed directly on the midspine. In addition, it may be one of the reasons that thoracic disk herniations are less common.[24] Because costovertebral and intervertebral changes directly affect the dorsal region as a whole, however, this area can play a major part in either the cause or the effect of mechanical dysfunction.

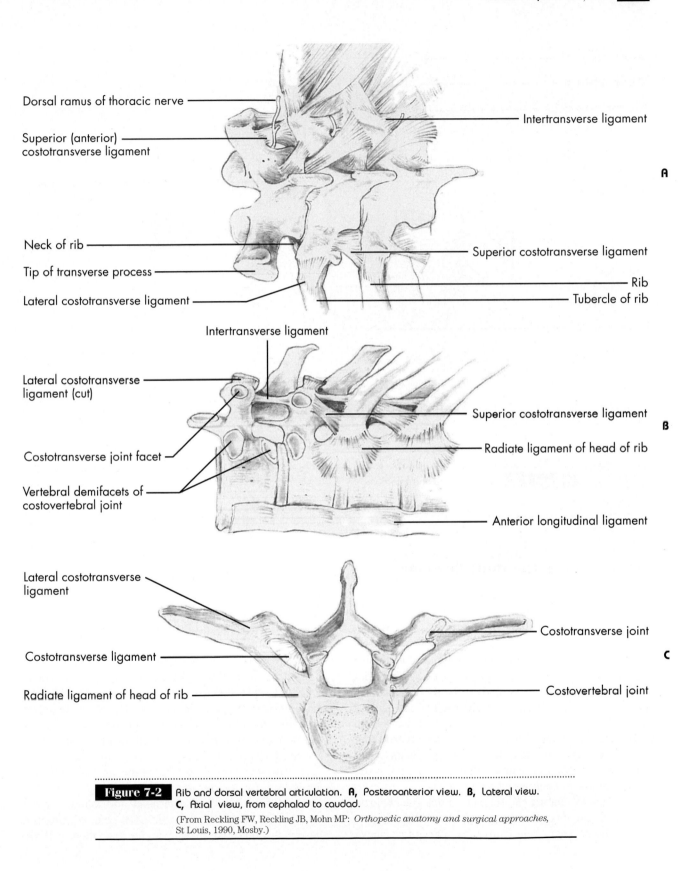

Dorsal ramus of thoracic nerve

Superior (anterior) costotransverse ligament

Neck of rib

Tip of transverse process

Lateral costotransverse ligament

Intertransverse ligament

Superior costotransverse ligament

Rib

Tubercle of rib

A

Intertransverse ligament

Lateral costotransverse ligament (cut)

Costotransverse joint facet

Vertebral demifacets of costovertebral joint

Superior costotransverse ligament

Radiate ligament of head of rib

Anterior longitudinal ligament

B

Lateral costotransverse ligament

Costotransverse ligament

Radiate ligament of head of rib

Costotransverse joint

Costovertebral joint

C

Figure 7-2 Rib and dorsal vertebral articulation. **A,** Posteroanterior view. **B,** Lateral view. **C,** Axial view, from cephalad to caudad.

(From Reckling FW, Reckling JB, Mohn MP: *Orthopedic anatomy and surgical approaches,* St Louis, 1990, Mosby.)

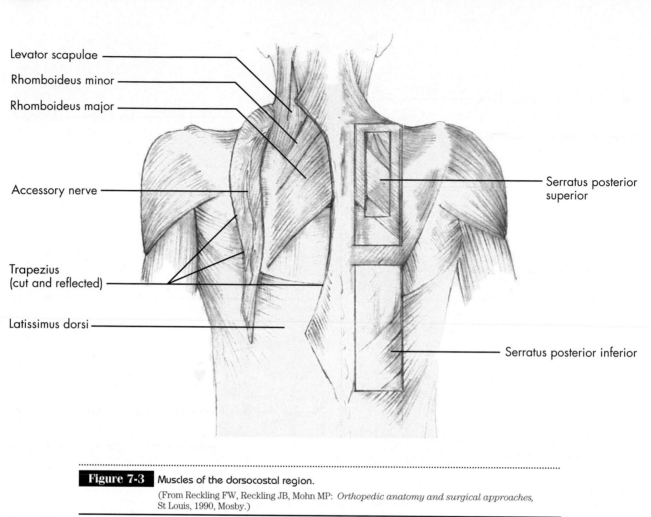

Levator scapulae

Rhomboideus minor

Rhomboideus major

Accessory nerve

Trapezius
(cut and reflected)

Latissimus dorsi

Serratus posterior
superior

Serratus posterior inferior

Figure 7-3 Muscles of the dorsocostal region.

(From Reckling FW, Reckling JB, Mohn MP: *Orthopedic anatomy and surgical approaches*, St Louis, 1990, Mosby.)

Examination of the Thoracic Spine

Physical Examination

In a visual inspection of the thoracic spine, the clinician screens the patient for scoliosis, rib humping, vertebral asymmetry, shoulder girdle deformity, and excessive kyphosis (Figure 7-4). After looking at the midline from the front and rear, the clinician then places the dorsal and dorsolumbar spine through the three planes of motion: (1) rotation, (2) lateral flexion, and (3) extension-flexion in the sagittal plane. The cervical spine controls the upper dorsal spine motion, and the rib cage limits lateral bending. Rotation is full, enacted by the muscles of the spinal column and controlled by the facets.

When evaluating the thoracic spine, the clinician must make an effort to inspect, palpate, and check motion at the rib cage. The intercostal spaces that house the neurovascular and muscular components of the costovertebral system are sensitive to positional and dynamic changes in movement and tension. Thus the chance of injury and referred pain from the ribs to the spine is very real. In addition, the cervicodorsal and thoracolumbar transitional areas should always be monitored for proper movement and muscle tone.

It is essential to palpate carefully over the vertebrae and supraspinous ligament, the paravertebral region, and over the ribs themselves. The chest should be evaluated for deformity, such as pectus excavatum or pectus carinatum, and the costal cartilage should be screened for any tender points. Bony landmarks on the dorsal surface of the vertebral column are also assessed for deformity or tenderness (Figure 7-5).

Raising both arms overhead and taking a deep breath exacerbates rib or intercostal pain. Placing the head in flexion causes more pain for the patient with rib

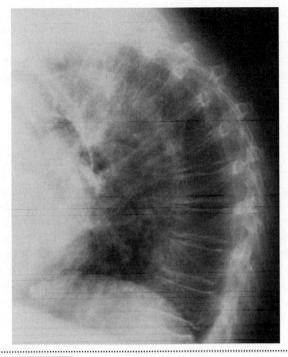

Figure 7-4 Roentgenogram of an elderly patient with senile kyphosis.

(From Mercier LR: *Practical orthopedics*, ed 4, St Louis, 1995, Mosby.)

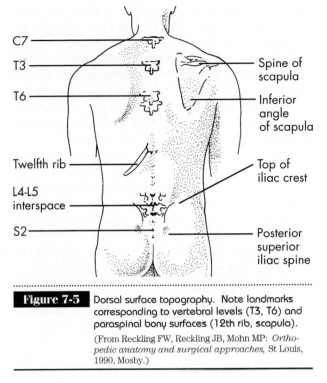

C7

T3

T6

Twelfth rib

L4-L5 interspace

S2

Spine of scapula

Inferior angle of scapula

Top of iliac crest

Posterior superior iliac spine

Figure 7-5 Dorsal surface topography. Note landmarks corresponding to vertebral levels (T3, T6) and paraspinal bony surfaces (12th rib, scapula).

(From Reckling FW, Reckling JB, Mohn MP: *Orthopedic anatomy and surgical approaches*, St Louis, 1990, Mosby.)

dysfunction. The examiner may place a tape measure around the thorax and spine to determine rib expansion. It is also possible to check rib expansion visually by placing the thumbs in the midline at the superior border at T8-T9 and watching as the patient expands the chest to see whether the excursion of the thumbs from the posterior thorax is symmetric. It is also necessary to examine the thorax for conditions that may limit movement, such as arthritides or systemic (infectious) illness.

Using motion palpation techniques to check the dorsal vertebral segments in flexion and extension, the examiner searches for areas of fixation or tenderness. Dorsal vertebrae that are palpable inferiorly are associated with tenderness over the supraspinous ligament. These vertebral subluxations may correspond with adjacent rib hypomobility and, as such, can be manually corrected while the patient is in a sitting, standing, or prone position. Spinal unit fixation can be checked by assessing the motion of the segment for a springy "end-feel."

The strength of the dorsal erectors can be tested with the patient lying in the prone position. As the patient raises one arm in front of him or her and holds it for 5 seconds, the examiner palpates for muscle tone. The examiner repeats the procedure on the contralateral side and compares the spinal erectors on the two sides for symmetry of strength and tone. Most individuals can maintain a static contraction of the erector muscles of the spine for at least 5 seconds.

Radiologic Evaluation

To confirm a suspected diagnosis and ensure proper case management, a radiologic assessment of the thorax may be necessary (Figure 7-6). X-ray films should be routine for patients who experience spinal pain after significant trauma; patients who have a moderate-to-severe deformity; patients whose range of motion is unusually impeded; and patients who may have underlying disease processes, such as previously diagnosed cancer or certain arthritides, that affect the thoracic region. Ankylosing spondylitis, for example, affects the sacroiliac joints, dorsal spine, and thoracolumbar transition area. Radiographic studies of the thoracic spine also show osteoarthritis secondary to cumulative trauma, obesity, or surgery.

Patients who are known to have breast, lung, or colon cancer and have new spinal complaints should undergo a radiologic examination that includes plain films and, if warranted, bone scans or computed tomography (CT) to rule out metastatic disease. Individuals with suspected neurologic involvement of the thoracic dermatome band or with a confirmed disease process who have new peripheral pain that can be traced back to the thoracic spine may be candidates for magnetic resonance imaging (MRI). If necessary, MRI or CT can be used to differentiate benign from pathologic entities.

A radiographic assessment can reveal underlying conditions (e.g., curvatures, arthritis, osteoporosis) that will delay the patient's recovery from soft-tissue complaints (Table 7-1). This knowledge aids the clinician in providing the patient with a more appropriate treatment plan and a more accurate prognosis. Such an assessment may also lead to incidental findings, such as end-plate irregularities as a result of previous trauma or indications of degenerative changes.

Conditions that Affect the Thoracic Spine

Musculoskeletal injuries to the thoracic spine can vary not only in their etiology, but also in their presentation (Table 7-2). Trauma, for example, can affect the thoracic spine and adjacent structures, as well as the viscera. Sprains and strains to this area of the spine are common sequelae to sporting and motor vehicle accidents and to the lifting injuries that sometimes occur in the workplace. Repetitious microtrauma can affect the spine, as evidenced by isolated regions of fixation and discomfort. In these areas of pinpoint dysfunction and tenderness, altered articular and soft-tissue physiology often set up aberrant neural cycles that can develop into chronic pain patterns.

Faulty posture and poor soft-tissue dynamics play a key role in dorsal spine pain and disability. Round shoulders, forward head, and exaggerated kyphosis all place great loads on the posterior stabilizing elements of the midspine. Proper postural alignment, along with the early identification of muscle insufficiency and imbalance, is the cornerstone of a proper treatment program. Care should center around soft-tissue rehabilitation. The importance of postural changes and rehabilitation exercises cannot be overemphasized.

Thoracic Sprain and Strain

Several mechanisms of injury to the thoracic spine can lead to a sprain or strain disability (see Table 7-2). Flexion and extension loading in a ballistic fashion, as may occur in a motor vehicle accident, can damage the joints and paravertebral soft tissues of the thoracic spine. Usually a sprain or strain results from the head being whipped (i.e., cervical acceleration-deceleration [CAD]), so there is often a cervical impairment as well. Lifting can also injure the midspine if the weight is too heavy or the mechanics are incorrect. Excessive contraction and rotation can place undue strain on the facet joints and erector muscles of the spine.

An evaluation of the individual's posteroanterior rotation reveals an altered end-play of the spinal joints and muscle splinting. Other physical findings include tenderness over the supraspinous ligament, bogginess or overt spasm of the dorsal erector muscles, and loss of gross movement in at least one plane of motion. Flexion of the head and thoracic spine usually produces pain over the posterior elements of the spine. Motor and sensory deficits are rare.

Radiographic studies are not usually helpful. They may reveal incidental findings or asymmetries such as scoliosis, arthritic changes, or spinous deviations, however. Acute fractures of the thoracic spine proper are uncommon, except at the thoracolumbar junction where flexion loading trauma may cause axial "compression" loads through the transitional region.

Treatment involves ruling out adjacent osseous and soft-tissue disability and allowing proper healing time for

---

Table 7-1   Common Radiographic Findings of the Thoracic Spine

Idiopathic or Congenital	Traumatic	Pathologic Condition
Spinal curvatures (scoliosis)	Osteoarthritis	Metastatic disease
Vertebral apophysitis	Spastic scoliosis	Osteoporosis
Transitional vertebrae	Compression fracture	Vertebral compression deformities
Rib anomalies (hypoplasia, asymmetry)	End-plate irregularity	Hemangioma
Ankylosing spondylitis		

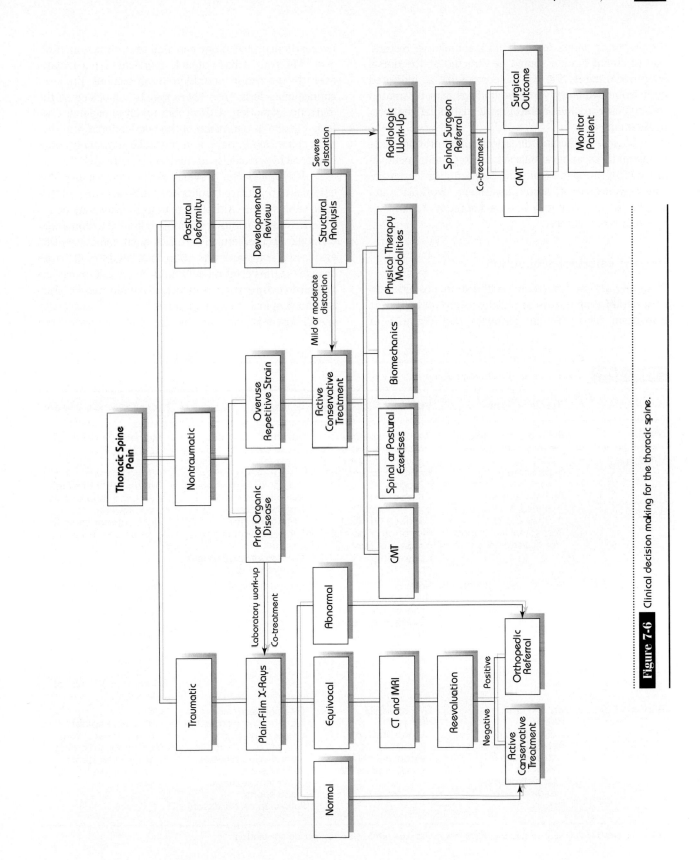

Figure 7-6 Clinical decision making for the thoracic spine.

the posterior joints. Manual and manipulative restoration of spinal motion should be directed at the dorsal apophyseal joints. Flexion malpositioning, as indicated by inferior palpatory vertebral findings, can be treated through osteopathic or chiropractic manipulative therapy techniques.[52]

Muscle retraining and postural alteration, centering on the scapula stabilizers, are key components in preventing thoracic sprain and strain injuries from becoming a chronic soft-tissue impairment. Workplace and activity modification may be essential parts of follow-up care and rehabilitation.

Thoracic Vertebral Subluxation

Generally, thoracic vertebral subluxation produces no peripheralization of pain or radicular signs and no overt myospasm. The potential chronicity and alteration of neuroarticular physiology can lead to dysfunction, however. The patient has palpable tenderness, particularly over the posterior neural arch or spinous process–supraspinous ligament. There may be a blockage of the end range of motion, with an abnormally nonspongy end-feel. Flexion or extension of the cervicodorsal and thoracic spine causes pain, and muscular asymmetry with unilateral hypertonicity is common (see Table 7-2).

Postural faults, previous rib or spinal injury, and episodes of repetitive trauma are common causes of thoracic subluxation. Although pain in the ribs may be referred from spinal injury, it is more common to find a concomitant rib problem. There has been some scientific evidence of somatic dysfunction translated to soft-tissue changes at the vertebral column from disorders that are organic in nature, such as myocardial infarction.[5,35] Furthermore, spinal manipulation has been associated with specific viscerosomatic and biochemical responses.[10,20,51]

Table 7-2	Conditions of the Thoracic Spine			
	Sprain or Strain	**Vertebral Subluxation**	**Scoliosis**	**Scheuermann's Disease**
Physical examination findings	Palpable tenderness over intervertebral joint Supraspinous ligament tenderness Pain on twisting, cervical flexion, or extreme extension Paraspinal myospasm or hypertonicity	Pain over spinous process or supraspinous ligament Flexion or extension fixation; malposition Loss of normal springy end-feel Alteration of normal muscle or joint physiology	Structural deformity, such as hip or pelvis unleveling, leg length discrepancy, posterior scapula, high shoulder Muscular asymmetry and unilateral hypertonicity Lateral curvature of spine Chronologic age versus skeletal maturity	Kyphotic deformity of dorsal spine Rigid musculature of thoracic spine Discomfort of back in growing children and adolescents Tight anterior shoulder girdle and thorax
X-ray findings	Usually unremarkable	Normal Need to rule out concomitant mechanical factors that can delay recovery	Lateral deviation of spine (D1 to S1 view)	End-plate irregularity, abnormal vertebral ossification patterns, anterior plate or body deformity, involvement of three or more vertebral bodies More than 40°-45° of kyphosis
Treatment plan	Ice and CMT HMP and electrotherapy Rehabilitation with static-postural exercise for dorsal spine and rib cage	CMT and EMS HMP and rehabilitation exercises for extensors and scapula stabilizers	CMT and exercise Traction and derotation Spinal orthosis for curves of 20°-40° in skeletally immature youngsters Symmetric activities and sports Follow-up as necessary	CMT Orthosis or spinal brace, if necessary Myofascial stretching of shoulder girdle, pectoral, and spinal muscles

CMT, Chiropractic manipulative therapy; **HMP,** hot moist pack; **EMS,** electrical muscle stimulation.

A knowledge of the zones of referral for both mechanical and internal pathologic conditions is important in differential diagnosis. For example, costovertebral dysfunction often correlates to a problem with an inferior dorsal vertebra, which is almost always tender over the supraspinous ligament.

The treating physician determines the need for x-ray films of the dorsal spine. In nontraumatic cases they may not yield much pertinent information. A history of multiple injuries or sufficient antecedent trauma is an indication for a radiographic study of the thoracic spine, however. Thoracic x-ray films most often reveal osteoarthritic changes or a lateral curvature of the spine. Arthritic spurring may be the cause of intermittent stiffness and hypomobility; scoliosis may be an incidental finding, or it may be the cause of an asymmetric biomechanical function that is responsible for soft-tissue injury.

The patient may need advice about posture and sleeping position. The shoulders should not be rounded, and the thorax should not be in a static flexed posture for prolonged periods. Sleeping on the stomach almost invariably makes a dorsal problem worse, and the patient often awakens with midback muscle stiffness.

Chiropractic manipulative therapy is the basic treatment and should begin as soon as possible to prevent chronic articular dysfunction and spinal immobility. Moist heat and electrotherapy can alleviate the patient's pain response after the first adjustment or two. Static postural exercises, such as scapular isometrics, are helpful in supportive care.

Scoliosis

The spinal column centers the mass of the torso and head in line along the vertical axis that drives through the pelvis. Theoretically, this structure allows for a more efficient use of energy in maintaining the upright posture. Disturbances of the spine, such as the curvatures associated with scoliosis, may significantly alter the normal balance and coordination of the spine, however, predisposing the individual to possible neurologic impairment and premature degeneration of the spinal column[37] (see Table 7-2).

The normal thoracic kyphosis averages approximately 35 degrees. Patients with scoliosis lose their physiologic kyphotic curve, along with convex vertebral body rotation and lateral bending. The physiologic alteration tends to decrease the spine's inherent resistance to deforming loads, especially in rotation.[32] In addition,

secondary curves or half-curves often develop because of the body's attempt to center the head and accommodate the primary curve.

Asymmetry of gross joint motion is probably more apparent in the skeletally mature adult population than in youngsters, where the incidence of pain may be more significantly related to scoliosis. In fact, until they develop some sort of back pain that requires care, most adults who have mild-to-moderate curves are not aware that they have scoliosis, largely because they were asymptomatic as children and teenagers and because screening procedures may have been inadequate. Mechanical back pain may be the result of a spinal curvature in the mature patient. Trapezius tightness, medial scapula pain, midthoracic complaints, especially at the thoracic curve convexity region, and lumbar pain are all common in adults.[54] Furthermore, it appears that the more inflexible the spine (especially in association with poor muscle tone), the more discomfort the patient experiences as a result of spinal curvature.

Although the cause of most spinal curvatures remains elusive, medical treatment to correct the aberrant biomechanical forces has improved over the second half of the twentieth century. Curvatures of great magnitude may require orthopedic surgery, but various forms of nonsurgical treatment for mild-to-moderate scoliosis are in the trial stages. Furthermore, there are well-documented clinical trials involving the use of chiropractic manipulation that are beginning to clarify the proper application and effective use of manual therapies for mechanical back pain that may be associated with spinal curvature.[15,46,47]

Types of Scoliosis

Curvatures of the spine incorporate a peculiar combination of mechanical and biologic factors that disturb the human frame. Scoliosis may be idiopathic, congenital, or neuromuscular in origin.

Idiopathic Scoliosis. According to Panjabi and White, idiopathic scoliosis is responsible for 85% to 95% of all cases of scoliosis.[39] Various theories have ascribed idiopathic scoliosis to the following:

- Handedness
- Malalignment of spinal elements
- Hormonal or stress changes associated with rapid periods of growth
- Equilibrium disturbances
- Decompensation via lumbopelvic disturbances

Infantile idiopathic scoliosis spans the ages of 0 to 3 years. It is referred to as juvenile idiopathic scoliosis in patients aged 4 to 10 years and to adolescent idiopathic scoliosis in those older than 10 years. An evaluation of rib cage posture is important in formulating short- and long-term prognoses for these youngsters (Figure 7-7).

Congenital Scoliosis. Pathologic anomalies at birth are responsible for scoliosis in some individuals. Usually, the problem results from either a "failure of formation" (e.g., a wedge vertebra or a hemivertebra; Figure 7-8) or a "failure of osseous segmentation," as may occur in Klippel-Feil syndrome.

Patients with congenital scoliosis usually have unique medical anomalies that require a great deal of attention. Concomitant conditions may include kidney disorders (20% to 30% of patients) and cardiac abnormalities (15% of patients); genitourinary tract anomalies are also common.[12]

Neuromuscular Scoliosis. Although it appears in several disease processes, the neuromuscular type of scoliosis is not as common as the idiopathic type. Neuromuscular scoliosis can be further classified as neuropathic or myopathic.

Neuropathic scoliosis is attributable to neurologic disease. The patient may have an upper motor neuron lesion, such as multiple sclerosis, for example. Imaging, laboratory testing, and evaluating the cerebral spinal fluid may be necessary to formalize the diagnosis.

Myopathic scoliosis results from disease processes of the muscular system. Entities such as muscular dystrophy, hypotonia, or dystonia may be the causative factor in these spinal curvatures.

Evaluation of Scoliosis

A complete and thorough case history is essential in the evaluation of scoliosis. The history should include the chronologic age of the patient, incidence of pain (if present), any neurologic or visceral complaints (e.g., pulmonary problems), and physiologic maturity. Any previous treatment, such as bracing, manipulation, or observation, should be noted; the location of the curve, age of onset, and pain pattern or radiation should also be investigated.

The physical examination should include an assessment of the spinal column and rib deformity (Figure 7-9 *A,B*), measurements of leg length, and comparison of skeletal versus chronologic age. It is possible to assess

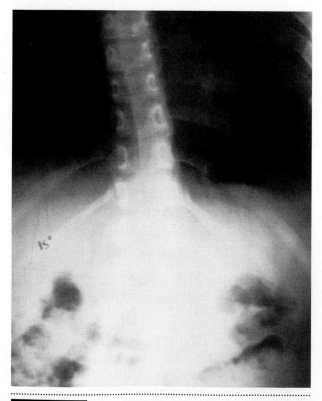

Figure 7-7 Scoliosis in a 9-year-old boy. Compensation is fairly good, since the ribs remain in a horizontal position.

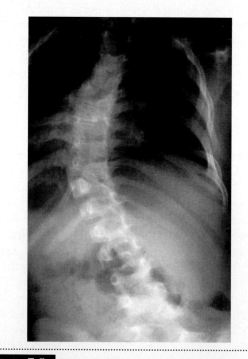

Figure 7-8 Thoracolumbar curve with hemivertebra.

(From Canale ST, editor: *Campbell's operative orthopedics,* ed 9, vol 3, St Louis, 1998, Mosby.)

skeletal age by rating the iliac apophyseal ring according to the Risser sign (on x-ray analysis) and comparing the anteroposterior roentgenogram of the left hand and wrist with the standards of the Greulich and Pyle radiographic atlas.[19] Excursion of the iliac apophysis starts at the anterosuperior iliac spine and correlates with cessation of spinal growth (Figure 7-10). Grading ranges from 0 (complete skeletal immaturity) to 4 (complete excursion) and 5 (ossification to the ilium).

The clinician visually inspects the patient from the front, watching for equal excursion of the clavicle, shape of the chest and thorax, and height of the shoulder. From the posterior, the clinician then evaluates the alignment of the patient's ear and mastoid, shoulder, scapula, rib hump, lumbar prominence, and cosmetic curve deformity, if present. Plumb line analysis can also be helpful.

The patient stands in the forward flexed position in the Adam's test position for functional scoliosis (Figure 7-11 *A, B*). Then, again from behind the patient, the clinician bends the patient laterally to the convex side of any visible curve to see whether this will reduce the curve. Both testing postures give the clinician a clue as to the flexibility of the scoliosis.

The clinician rates spinal curvatures per progression of growth and curve, taking into consideration the skeletal maturity of the patient. The onset of menarche usually signals a slowing of a girl's growth process, and skeletal growth generally ceases altogether 1 year after menarche. At the time of puberty, a boy's skeletal growth is 84% completed; this increases to approximately 90% 2 years later.[2]

Curves are usually described by the area of spine, direction of vertebral body rotation, and apex of the curve. For example, a right curvature with the apex at T7 with vertebral body rotation to the right is termed a

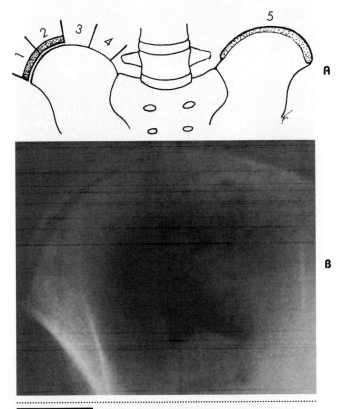

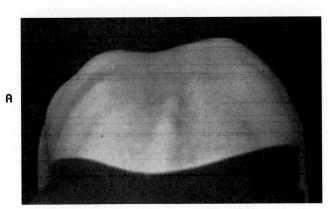

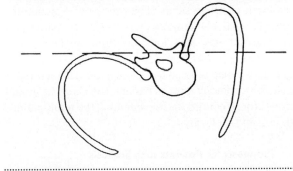

Figure 7-9 **A,** Scoliosis with rib prominence attributable to vertebral rotation best exhibited on forward bending. **B,** Cross-section of chest showing rib distortion attributable to vertebral rotation.

(From Mercier LR: *Practical orthopedics*, ed 4, St Louis, 1995, Mosby.)

Figure 7-10 Iliac apophysis. **A,** Initial ossification of the apophysis at the anterosuperior iliac spine. The excursion or stage of maturity on the left is 50% complete; thus the Risser sign is 2. On the right, the excursion is complete, and the apophysis has fused with the iliac crest—a Risser 5. **B,** A Risser 2 excursion.

(From Bradford DS, Lonstein JE, Ogilvie JW, Winter RB: *Moe's textbook of scoliosis and other spinal deformities*, ed 2, Philadelphia, 1987, WB Saunders.)

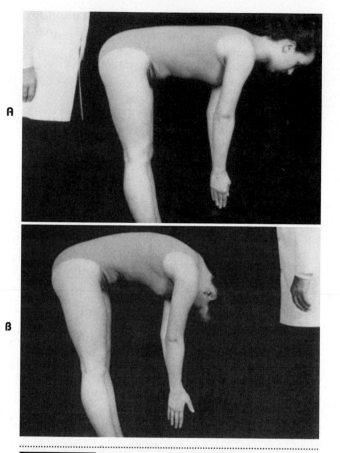

Figure 7-11 Examining a patient for scoliosis. **A,** for Adam's position posterior, the patient flexes forward at the waist. The arms are allowed to hang toward the floor, and the hands are placed together in a prayer position. The examiner, who is posterior to the patient, observes the thoracolumbar spine for deformity, which includes persistent scoliotic curvature, rib humping, and muscular atrophy. **B,** In Adam's position anterior, the patient assumes the Adam's position by flexing the spine at the waist and additionally flexing the cervical spine. The examiner, who is anterior to the patient, observes for upper thoracic scoliosis defects.

(From Evans RC: *Illustrated essentials in orthopedic physical assessment,* St Louis, 1994, Mosby.)

(either direction) double major (lumbar and thoracic) and double thoracic major.[31]

Double major curves usually involve a left lumbar and right thoracic scoliosis. It may be difficult to distinguish this condition from a right thoracic scoliosis with a compensatory left lumbar curve without side-bending films, however. Such films may facilitate an assessment of flexibility of the curvature as well.

Children with back pain need an examination for other pathologic conditions as well, because scoliosis in children does not usually produce the same symptoms that occur in adults. Scheuermann's disease and tumor may appear in children as scoliosis, for example. If the patient is a youngster or adolescent who is undergoing a growth spurt, he or she may have not only a spinal distortion, but also an extreme (although transient) muscle-tendon tightness at the hip flexors, hamstrings, and erectors of the spine. The clinician should ask if anyone in the family has or has had a spinal distortion. It is often helpful to compare a child's spine with that of one or both parents (Figure 7-13 *A,B*).

Very mild curves in juveniles who are prepubescent may not require radiologic examination. Moderate cases of scoliosis or marked structural distortion probably warrant such an examination, however. A 14- x 17-inch film from the superior aspect of the thoracic spine to the pelvis (D-1 to S-1 projection) is generally sufficient. The clinician or technician should try to include the pelvis to investigate the possibility of obliquity.

If the patient is an adult, the clinician assesses the status of spinal deformity, including any progression since the previous examination; concomitant health problems; and intersegmental compromise. Radiographic examination and comparison with any prior films facilitates the assessment of progression. The presence of symptoms warrants a manual examination of the facets, paravertebral musculature, and joint motion. Because poor muscle tone, gross weakness, posterior joint fixation, and degenerative disk disease can all be causative factors for pain in the skeletally mature patient, the clinician should consider these conditions in examining the adult patient with possible scoliosis.

Prognosis for Patients with Scoliosis

According to Lonstein and Carlson, it is possible to determine the likely progression of a spinal curvature on the basis of the following equation involving curve magnitude, skeletal maturity, and age[27]:

$$\text{Progression factor} = \frac{\text{Cobb angle} \times \text{Risser's sign}}{\text{Chronologic age}}$$

right thoracic dextrorotatory scoliosis with convexity to the right. Primary curves are large, generally rigid in lateral bending, and pronounced in their cosmetic deformities (Figure 7-12). Compensatory curves are generally smaller, allow more flexibility, and pose less of a cosmetic deformity. The most common curve patterns for idiopathic scoliosis are right thoracic, thoracolumbar, lumbar

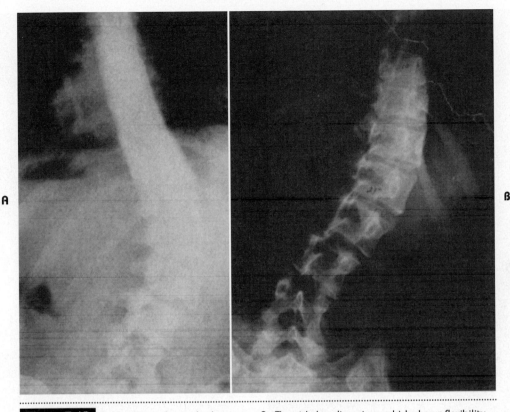

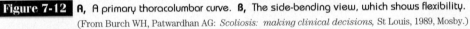

Figure 7-12 **A,** A primary thoracolumbar curve. **B,** The side-bending view, which shows flexibility.
(From Burch WH, Patwardhan AG: *Scoliosis: making clinical decisions,* St Louis, 1989, Mosby.)

An increase of 5 to 10 degrees on radiographic films 6 to 12 months apart indicates a significant progression of scoliosis.

The prognosis is different between male and female patients, as well as between adults and children. Progression is more common in women than in men; furthermore, in a woman's young adult years, pregnancy may exacerbate her scoliosis. Blount and Mellencamp, and Berman and associates all demonstrated the adverse effects of pregnancy on scoliotic progression.[6,8] Although there are no data to suggest that scoliosis is an obstetric complication, the hormonal changes and spinal stress associated with pregnancy can aggravate the scoliosis.[34]

Most children are asymptomatic, particularly those with minor curvatures, and scoliosis may not progress before the onset of puberty. This may not be true of young, competitive female athletes such as gymnasts.[50] It is not recommended that all these children undergo regular radiologic examination every 6 to 12 months, but skeletally immature children who have moderate-to-severe curva-tures or who have a history of curve or distortion progression may need such close monitoring. The condition is likely to progress in those who are skeletally immature. Lonstein and Carlson showed that scoliosis progressed in 36% of the patients who have a Risser grading of 0.[25]

There is also some evidence that progression is more likely in curves with greater magnitudes. Weinstein noted that, although thoracic curves less than 30 degrees at skeletal maturity do not progress, curves greater than 30 degrees at maturation progress an average of 19.6 degrees (average follow-up of 40 years).[53] Double curves (e.g., thoracolumbar curves) have an even greater incidence of progression. Single thoracic curves progress more than single lumbar curves.[26]

Prognostication has also centered around clinical entities such as spinal morphology, muscular physiology, and aberrant facet movement. Schultz and associates described progression in slender spines,[45] whereas Redford and colleagues claimed to find a difference in the electromyographic activity of paravertebral muscles in

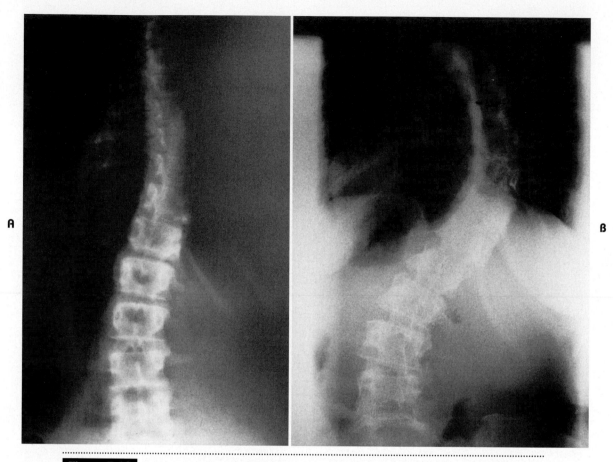

Figure 7-13 A, Moderate primary curvature of the dorsolumbar spine in a 15-year-old girl, measured at 23 degrees. B, Double major curve (left lumbar, right thoracic) in the girl's 40-year-old mother, measured at 62 degrees.

progressive and nonprogressive curves.[43] Armstrong and associates reported that spinous rotation to the convexity of the curve correlates with a lower risk of progression.[3]

Treatment of Scoliosis

Flexibility, strength, and muscular endurance are important concerns in the rehabilitation and overall treatment of the patient with scoliosis. The age of the individual patient is one of the primary considerations in determining the appropriate treatment. A child with an aggressive scoliosis requires a treatment different from that appropriate for an adolescent or adult with a mild curvature, for example. Among the other important clinical features that must be considered in planning treatment are the following:

- Sex
- Skeletal maturity
- Chronologic versus physiologic age
- History of progression
- Prognostication status of the curvature

Exercise. Although the orthopedic literature clearly states that exercise alone does not convert curves, properly prescribed spinal exercise can help stabilize the spine and allow the patient with scoliosis to attain a higher level of function.[28,48] Strengthening the spinal erector muscles is useful in the maintenance of correct posture and static positioning of the trunk. It is unlikely to correct the curve, however, because the spinal erector muscles cannot effectively exert the continuous, prolonged force necessary for the correction of a spinal deformity.

The patient can begin to work the spinal erector muscles while in the prone position, then progress to the "all fours" position. Working the opposite arm and leg in extension will strengthen the dorsal and scapular muscles and the hip and lumbar extensors (Figure 7-14 *A,B*). Pelvic tilts and abdominal curls can improve lumbar stability. Static stretching is helpful for the hamstrings, quadriceps, and erectors of the spine. Williams' flexion exercises—knee-to-chest stretches with the person in the supine position—are benign and easy to perform. Hip and lumbopelvic flexibility must be increased, especially for thoracolumbar and lumbosacral curves.

To help maintain curve flexibility, lateral bending exercises are appropriate. For a right thoracic curve, the patient first places the left arm over the head, presses the right hand tightly against the rib cage or lumbar region, and bends to the right. Children and young adults can also be instructed to stand on a stool or chair, bend the knees so that the legs can help support the body weight, and hang from a chinning or pull-up bar several times a day for 30 seconds to 2 minutes. Holding the arm on the same side of the curve over the head flexes the spine laterally toward the side of the convexity and stretches the muscles.

Exercise may play a positive role in curve flexibility and spinal strength—two factors that may reduce the risk of progressive distortion or back pain. In young girls who have yet to reach skeletal maturity, exercise may play a multifunctional role. First, increased flexibility may reduce the likelihood of a structural curve. Second, the flexibility and strength gained through the spinal stabilization program may combat the adverse effects of the hormones associated with pregnancy and childbearing in the young adult years.

Electrical Muscle Stimulation. The clinical use of electrotherapy for the patient with scoliosis has received both favorable and unfavorable reviews in the literature.[1,11,40] It was postulated that stimulation of the muscles by means of electrodes implanted on the convex side of the curve musculature would reduce the hypertonicity or holding elements responsible for the distortion, but the evidence gathered in studies of nocturnal stimulation and other procedures has been inconclusive.

The use of electrotherapy in the office-based practice one to three times per week is not likely to affect a spinal curve. Electrical stimulation may be beneficial for an adult as a treatment for pain, but its effect on the natural history of idiopathic adolescent scoliosis is not clear. Under some circumstances, youngsters with a mild-to-moderate curve may derive some benefit if electrical stim-

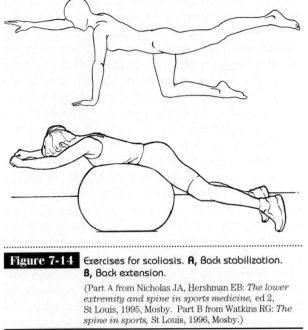

Figure 7-14 Exercises for scoliosis. **A,** Back stabilization. **B,** Back extension.

(Part A from Nicholas JA, Hershman EB: *The lower extremity and spine in sports medicine*, ed 2, St Louis, 1995, Mosby. Part B from Watkins RG: *The spine in sports*, St Louis, 1996, Mosby.)

ulation is used in conjunction with a spinal orthosis. The most important goals of conservative care are to improve or maintain curve flexibility and spinal strength, however. Therefore electrotherapy is best limited to an ancillary treatment modality in clinical practice.

Spinal Orthoses. The use of spinal orthoses dates back centuries. Their effectiveness rests on the biomechanical principles of joint creep and relaxation. Bracing can stabilize moderate curves in children and adolescents with scoliosis; however, because curves greater than 40 degrees are likely to progress, bracing may not be an efficient treatment for those with this degree of curvature.[39] For patients who need a brace, an orthotist must take meticulous measurements and impressions to ensure the proper fit. The two most commonly used appliances in the United States today are the Milwaukee brace and the Boston brace.

The Milwaukee brace is a cervicothoracolumbosacral orthosis (CTLSO) that has been used since the late 1940s when it was introduced as an alternative to postoperative casting. It supports the spine from occiput to pelvis, and it must include axillary and thoracic pads to be most effective. The thoracic pads are placed at the apex of the curve. The brace should be worn while the patient is recumbent, as well as upright, although it need not be worn during certain athletic events (e.g., baseball).[56] The Milwaukee brace may be quite helpful for those with moderate degrees of scoliosis, particularly when used with an exercise program.[13]

Described as a thoracolumbosacral orthosis (TLSO), the Boston brace requires only measurements or an impression from the xiphoid to the greater trochanter. It is usually applied to thoracolumbar and lumbar curvatures. Because it is smaller and easier to conceal, patient compliance with recommendations to wear the Boston brace may be higher than that associated with the Milwaukee brace.[4]

Spinal orthoses are used primarily to halt or slow the progression of scoliosis.[17] Factors that are directly related to successful outcomes include degree of curve, skeletal maturity, timing of initiation of therapy, and patient compliance. Recent studies have also shown that children with large curves need their curves reduced by half to have a good outcome.[29,36]

Traction. By itself, traction has never been considered a viable alternative to more conventional methods of nonoperative care for scoliosis. Edgar and associates studied 175 patients with adolescent idiopathic scoliosis and concluded that, although traction may be beneficial for those with smaller curvatures, scoliosis greater than 70 degrees rendered traction unnecessary.[16] There is statistical evidence, however, that traction may have a beneficial effect on severe scoliotic deformities preoperatively, which further suggests that it may be helpful for moderate curves.[33] Pelvic traction may improve the distortion of pelvic obliquity.

Spinal manipulation through a traction or distractive force may be an excellent alternative for those adult patients with inflexible, structural curves with severe hypomobility. Gaining audible releases (i.e., joint click or pop) from the posterior joints can be difficult. It is often effective to place the spine under an axial traction force by distracting the pelvis, laterally flexing the spine to the side of convexity to reduce the deformity and applying even force through manual traction. The patient may experience significant relief as a result of this axial traction force, especially in rigid curvatures of greater magnitude.

Manipulation and Clinical Biomechanics. The chiropractic physician can apply certain biomechanical principles through the use of the manipulative model of spinal care. Creep and relaxation of the joints and soft tissues of the vertebral column can be induced through distractive loads. The patient can be placed into rotation, flexion, and axial traction to relieve pressures placed at the spine.

Chiropractic manipulation can take advantage of the fact that transverse loads have been proved helpful in converting bending movements to coupled movements.[42,55] Most chiropractic adjustive procedures induce the normal biomechanical coupling movements at the functional spinal unit; therefore the combination of joint distraction, transverse loads, and axial loads help not only restore the normal mechanism of the intervertebral segment, but also increase the overall flexibility of the spine.

Panjabi and White summed up the biomechanical principles that the clinician should include in a treatment protocol for scoliosis as follows[39]:

- Maintain lumbar lordosis
- Maintain thoracic kyphosis
- Use distraction and axial loading forces
- Use creep-and-relaxation techniques in mechanical treatment
- Introduce coupling movements through manipulation
- Apply traction in the form of distraction and transverse loading
- Use manipulation to maintain or improve spinal flexibility
- Recommend exercise to maintain or improve static and postural strength and endurance of the inherently inefficient muscle system of the spine

Surgery. Consultation and co-treatment with a spinal surgeon is appropriate under the following conditions:

- Curvatures greater than 20 degrees in a boy under the age of 10 years or a girl under the age of 9 years
- Curves that show marked progression before the onset of pubescence (i.e., 6 to 10 degrees per year)
- Significant scoliosis (greater than 20 degrees) in a child who has back pain of an undetermined cause
- Spinal curvatures greater than 40 degrees, as well as organ compromise, in an early adolescent
- Progressive curves of more than 40 degrees in a child or adolescent who has been enrolled in a conservative care program

Surgical care of adult scoliosis is usually reserved for those patients who exhibit physiologic compromise from their spinal curvatures. Conservative treatment aimed at pain reduction, restoration of spinal mobility, and muscular flexibility is preferable for most patients.

Scheuermann's Disease (Juvenile Kyphosis)

In 1920, Holger Scheuermann postulated that kyphotic deformity in some adolescents and juveniles is the result of abnormal growth.[44] He based this theory on radiographic evidence of an anterior end-plate irregularity that was markedly different from that observed in tuberculous spondylitis (Figure 7-15). This unique abnormality of growing children also differed from other causes of kyphotic deformities, such as scoliosis or metabolic conditions.

There is as yet no certain cause for Scheuermann's disease. Probably a host of mechanical, nutritional (metabolic), and biologic (hormonal) factors result in postural round back. The osteochondrosis of Scheuermann's disease is similar to other forms of chondral defects of apophyseal anomalies, such as Blount disease. Biologic factors, such as end-plate changes during growth, may be a triggering factor. In fact, it is possible that the dynamics of the vertebral end plate, rather than the ring apophysis, may be primarily responsible for Scheuermann's disease.[38] Muscular and postural factors (e.g., tight or contracted pectoral muscles, shoulder girdle inflexibility) also seem to play at least a secondary role in Scheuermann's disease. Trauma can be a significant factor, as can intense, early stresses on skeletally immature spines.[18]

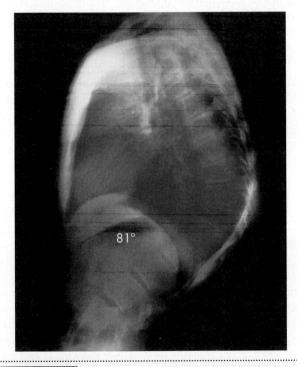

Figure 7-15 Scheuermann's kyphosis. Kyphotic deformity of 81 degrees and Schmorl nodes.

(From Canale ST, editor: *Campbell's operative orthopedics*, vol 3, ed 9, St Louis, 1998, Mosby.)

Physical Examination

Adolescent boys make up the majority of patients with Scheuermann's deformity. Parents may seek an examination because of their child's progressively worsening posture. Some patients seek help as a result of scoliosis screening at school or because of stiffness or discomfort in the middle to upper back, generally caused by compensatory muscular hypertonicity (see Table 7-2).

Excessive lordosis, with or without a concomitant scoliosis of the thoracic or thoracolumbar spine, warrants investigation. Progressive thoracic kyphosis may occur hand in hand with a curvature of the dorsal spine. The deformity of the middle and upper back is not flexible and therefore is not reducible through manual means. The anterior shoulder girdle is usually tight; in addition, as in spondylolysis or scoliosis, the hamstring and hip flexor muscles are tight. Neurologically, the children are usually normal.

The clinician places the patient in the forward bending position to see whether the deformity is flexible (i.e., not caused by structural pathologic variations). Ligamentous laxity or mechanically poor posture may be the cause. Scheuermann's deformity can be manually converted by positioning or postural changes. Any kyphosis greater than 50 degrees in a growing child is certainly abnormal.[30]

Radiographic Findings

In Scheuermann's disease, the vertebral end plates exhibit spotty and irregular patterns of ossification. Fragmentation may occur, and the front portion of the plates do not seem to ossify. There are signs of notching, which may cause the vertebrae to develop a typical "slant" appearance. As the condition worsens, the intervertebral disk begins to show signs of degeneration, and the anterior portions of the bodies collapse. Defective end plates are the pathomechanical basis of anterior disk collapse, anterior epiphyseal disease, and anterior growth defects with vertebral wedging.

Three or more adjacent vertebrae are involved, although one level begins the process. Wedging of 5 to 8 degrees with a kyphosis of 40 to 45 degrees is usually sufficient radiographic evidence of Scheuermann's disease. Other possible findings include excessive lumbar lordosis, scoliosis of the thoracic or thoracolumbar spine, and osteoporosis.

Treatment

Most cases of Scheuermann's disease are treated conservatively unless the youngster has a progressive distortion that is not responding to treatment. Severe scoliosis (i.e., greater than 40 to 60 degrees) is the causative factor in many cases of Scheuermann's disease. Thus postural exercises can play an important role in supporting the spine and controlling the deformity. Antilordotic exercises are the key; Williams' flexion exercises, pelvic tilts, and hamstring stretches are indicated. The shoulder girdle and pectoral muscles must be effectively stretched as well. Corner stretching on the wall (push-up posture) is also beneficial.

Manual care and chiropractic manipulation should focus on restoring intervertebral mobility and myofascial flexibility. Proprioceptive neuromuscular facilitation patterns of the hamstring, spinal erector, and hip flexor muscles are important in maintaining or improving hip and low back flexibility, as well as reducing contractions that can transfer loads inappropriately to the lumbar spine. Chiropractic manipulative therapy for the thoracic spine should incorporate extension adjustments (inferior and anterior moves) to reduce kyphosis. These patients should be taught to sit up straight, follow good posture habits, and avoid sleeping on their stomach. These steps may help prevent excessive deformity and discomfort for these patients in their adult years.

Children who have moderate, flexible deformations should wear a brace. If the curvature is a thoracolumbar scoliosis, a TLSO is helpful. Extension braces can reduce lumbar lordosis and thoracic kyphosis. Braces should be prescribed only if absolutely necessary, however, because they are associated with decreased patient compliance and other psychosocial problems. If the patient is not experiencing pain or if the prescribed exercises are improving the condition, the patient may participate in recreational, noncontact athletics.

Surgical treatment is warranted only for patients with progressive distortions and large, inflexible scoliotic curves of more than 60 degrees.[25] Rod implementation in the surgical treatment of Scheuermann's disease may have a complication rate of 40%.[21] There have been reports of pseudoarthrosis, correction failure, and disability.[22,23] Therefore posterior instrumentation should be used only in individuals with excessive spinal deformity or disability.

Conditions that Affect the Thorax and Rib Cage

Strain as a result of repetitive movements, joint stress, physiologic subluxations, or inflamed nerves in the surrounding structures can all cause pain in the thorax and rib cage. Postural distortions, especially at the shoulder girdle or thoracic spine, can also have adverse effects on the thorax. For example, excessive kyphosis or round-shoulderedness can alter rib cage function and impair the breathing apparatus. Poor muscle tone and poor conditioning predisposes individuals to scapulothoracic strain and intercostal injuries when they are under physical stress.

Individuals who have anterior chest pain may belong in the group of patients with thoracic conditions. The clinician must quickly distinguish mechanical pain at the sternum or osteochondral junction from substernal or apical pain of cardiac origin. The differential diagnosis of costochondritis, angina pectoris, and anxiety can be difficult if the clinician does not take the time to examine and question the patient carefully.

Arthritides such as ankylosing spondylitis or cardiopulmonary diseases such as emphysema can impose their treacherous effects on the biomechanics of the thoracic spine and rib cage. It is essential to evaluate and document the lack of proper ventilation, an inability to expand the chest fully, or any limitation of thoracic spine movement. In some cases, particularly if there is any evidence of pulmonary compromise, consultation and co-treatment with an internist is necessary.

Costochondritis

Also known as Tietze's syndrome, costochondritis is an inflammation of the rib cartilage at the costosternal junction. Both the unknowing patient and clinician may have difficulty identifying this "chest" pain. The differential diagnosis includes angina pectoris, intercostal strain and neuralgia, rib subluxation, and in cases of substantial trauma, rib fracture. Although many individuals report a prior exertion with their chest muscles or a sudden forced hyperabduction movement, a certain percentage of patients are unaware of any episode of exertion that could be the cause of their pain.

The patient with costochondritis complains of point tenderness over one or two rib heads or costal junctions lateral to the sternum (Table 7-3). Symptoms are most commonly localized to the second, third, or fourth costochondral junctions.[57] Abduction of the arm reproduces the patient's pain, which may radiate down the arm. Acute inflammation causes discomfort or pain on deep inspiration as the rib cage expands. Bogginess or swelling over the costal cartilage is possible, but does not always occur. Although patients do not usually experience referred pain around the intercostal space toward the posterior as in intercostal neuralgia, such an event is a possibility. Bilateral costochondritis is rare. If a blunt trauma precedes a moderate-to-severe injury, the clinician should order x-ray films to rule out an anterior rib fracture.

Treatment to reduce the inflammation should be prompt and aggressive, since the relative avascularity of cartilage may prolong the time required for the condition to resolve. The application of ice and electrotherapy over the costochondral junction is helpful, and the patient should avoid repetitive and resisted abduction of the affected arm. If the condition is recalcitrant to conserva-

tive therapy, it may be necessary to place the patient on an oral regimen of a nonsteroidal antiinflammatory drug. It is also wise to tell the patient that the condition may require a protracted period of time to heal.

Intercostal Strain

The intercostal muscles lie between the ribs and are responsible for aiding in respiration and maintaining the integrity of the rib cage. During times of exertion, this muscle group acts as strong accessory muscles of respiration along with the abdominal and scalene muscles.

Table 7-3 Conditions of the Thorax and Rib Cage

	Costochondritis (Tietze's Syndrome)	Intercostal Strain	Intercostal Neuralgia	Costovertebral Syndrome	Pectoralis Strain
Physical examination findings	Painful arm abduction Palpable tenderness at costosternal junction Commonly at 2nd to 4th rib cartilage Normal results on cardiac examination Exacerbation of pain on stretching of pectoralis muscle	Palpable tenderness at rib interspace Splinting or spasm of affected intercostal muscle Reproduction of pain at deep inspiration with arms overhead	Painful rib interspace Possible strain of intercostal muscle Referral of pain from anterior to posterior or vice versa Exacerbation of pain with deep inspiration or spinal rotation Need to rule out infection (e.g., herpes zoster) and organic disease	Tenderness over rib angle or head Fixation of costovertebral articulation Inferoanterior subluxation of corresponding dorsal vertebral level Muscle guarding, spasm over affected rib cage Palpable spinal rotation or cervicodorsal fixation Referral to anterior thorax possible	Pain on examination at pectoralis muscle, either proximally or distally Swelling or bogginess of muscle belly Discomfort on abduction of arm Ecchymosis at injury site possible Pain reproduced by adduction against resistance Need to rule out costochondral injury, avulsion of pectoralis tendon at proximal humerus
X-ray findings	Usually normal Need to rule out rib fracture in cases of blunt trauma	Not applicable	Only needed for suspected organic disease or rib trauma	Not applicable	Not applicable unless rupture or avulsion is suspected
Treatment plan	Ice and electrotherapy Manual care to dorsal spine and rib cage in presence of secondary joint dysfunction (e.g., hypomobility)	Ice or moist heat Electrotherapy Active and passive mobilization of rib cage, massage CMT of dorsal spine or ribs	CMT and HMP Electrotherapy Medical referral for suspected infectious or organic disease	CMT, HMP, and OMT Application of ice with acute pain Postural corrective exercise program	Ice and ultrasound Activity modification

CMT, Chiropractic manipulative therapy; **HMP**, hot moist pack; **OMT**, osteopathic manipulative therapy.

Excessive exertion or straining usually causes the intercostal muscle injury. Athletes often have intercostal injuries, since forcefully swinging a baseball bat, throwing the discus or javelin, twisting or cutting in football, or sprinting are common causes of such injuries.

On examination, the clinician may feel muscle guarding or listing of the rib cage to one side. Fine palpation reveals the tenderness to be at the rib interspace rather than directly over the ribs. It is important to check chest expansion and rule out any pleural, cardiac, or lung abnormalities via auscultation. If the muscle strain and spasm are severe, the patient may experience referred pain around the thoracic cage toward the spine. Pain may occur at both the anterior and posterior margins of the thorax. Flexing the trunk or extending the arms overhead while taking a deep breath will reproduce the pain.

Treatment initially should consist of ice (for acute pain) or moist heat (for subacute, chronic pain), gentle stretching, and electrotherapy. Case management can progress to passive and active mobilization of the rib cage, chiropractic manipulation of the dorsal spine and rib, if necessary, and moist heat with electrical stimulation. Soft-tissue mobilization and massage are also helpful in reducing myospasm and promoting circulation. Water therapy can be used as a conduit to sports rehabilitation before the athlete actually participates in racquet or batting activities.

Intercostal Neuralgia

The intercostal nerve runs with the intercostal artery, vein, and muscle from the posterior thorax to the anterior rib cage. Pain in this nerve, called intercostal neuralgia, may have an infectious, osseous, muscular, or metabolic cause. Rib fractures, intercostal strains with myospasm, rib subluxations, and herpetic lesions can all cause intercostal neuralgia.

At first, it may be difficult to determine whether the pain is originating in the thoracic dermatome band or in a musculoskeletal structure. Respiration, rib cage stretching, and rotation of the spinal column may provide helpful evidence. Shingles, a herpetic condition that is quite contagious when the vesicles are active, may erupt after being harbored in neural ganglia and may cause pain along a dermatome. Manual pressure on a tender spot or trigger point can elicit pain from front to back. The dorsal and cervical spines are commonly affected. The possibility of gastric, esophageal, or lung disorders warrants investigation as well.

Treatment should first address the cause of the neuralgia. It may be necessary to arrest a muscle spasm, adjust a rib subluxation or fixation, or refer the patient with herpes zoster to a dermatologist. Moist heat and electrotherapy may reduce muscle spasm and guarding, thus facilitating manual therapy. The patient should avoid sleeping in the prone position and should maintain an erect posture of the neck and shoulder girdle.

Costovertebral Syndrome (Rib Subluxation)

Injury and dysfunction of the costovertebral complex is one of the more painful mechanical syndromes of the thorax. Concomitant derangement to the rib head and dorsal vertebrae is common. The costovertebral articulation is usually tender, and protective muscle spasm exacerbates the pain. Deep breathing may radiate pain to the anterior or may cause an exquisite tenderness at the cupola of the diaphragm. Forward flexion and posteroanterior rotation of the trunk makes the pain worse. The rib angle is usually painful when the examiner checks for joint play. The corresponding thoracic vertebral segment is usually palpated as inferior (anterior) with exquisite tenderness over the supraspinous ligament.

Treatment usually consists of the application of moist heat or ice (depending on the severity of the pain), along with manipulation of the affected rib and thoracic vertebra. Although quite tender to the manipulative thrust, the joint fixation must be addressed to reduce the cycle of spasm, physiologic subluxation, and spasm. The more chronic the pattern, the more difficult it is to address. Several treatments may be necessary to break a chronic rib subluxation.

In cases of severe muscle splinting, it may be helpful to apply moist heat for 10 to 15 minutes before the manipulation, as well as 15 to 20 minutes after the treatment. Although most chiropractic manipulative techniques involve adjustment of the rib while the patient is in the prone position, many patients are more comfortable in the supine position for an osteopathic rib maneuver (Figure 7-16 A,B). It is imperative that the patient's head is in neutral or slight extension and that the patient exhales and relaxes on the clinician's thrust. Long axis mobilization of the thorax in extension is also palliative for costovertebral syndrome (Figure 7-17).

The patient should be advised to maintain the neutral or slightly extended position of the shoulder, scapula, and neck while driving or sitting to take pressure off the rib cage. In addition, the patient should sleep in the supine position with a small pillow placed directly

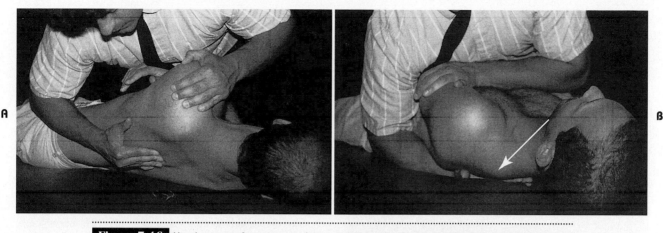

Figure 7-16 Hand position for posterior rib manipulation. **A,** The rib malposition and fixation is first palpated and then cupped with the thenar eminence. **B,** The patient's arms are crossed for traction and tissue pull. The thrust is a body drop, anterior to posterior on expiration.

under the cervical spine. Manipulation and postural-static exercises, such as scapula retraction and cervical extension work, are appropriate for problems such as forward head and rounded shoulders (Figure 7-18).

Pectoralis Muscle Strain

The presentation of pectoralis muscle strain resembles that of a costochondral injury. Both conditions can occur close to the sternum. Some pectoralis strains are in the middle of the muscle, however, and certain strains are closer to the pectoralis-deltoid triangle. Most pectoralis strains result from sudden overuse, such as performing an intense weight-training workout or moving heavy objects.

Palpation reveals a ropiness or swelling of the muscle. The sternum is not usually tender to palpation. Adduction of the arm against resistance is helpful in the diagnosis, since it reproduces the pain in the pectoralis muscle. Motor and sensory function are intact.

The initial treatment of a pectoralis strain includes the application of ice, pulsed ultrasound, and active rest. Symptoms usually resolve in 2 or 3 days. At first, the patient should avoid bench pressing movements or other motions that stretch or involve the pectoralis. Continuous ultrasound and electrotherapy are often beneficial as the patient makes a graded return to full activities.

Rarely, a complete rupture of the muscle occurs at the attachment of the pectoralis tendon at the lesser tubercle of the proximal humerus. This type of injury is most likely to occur in athletes (e.g., football players or

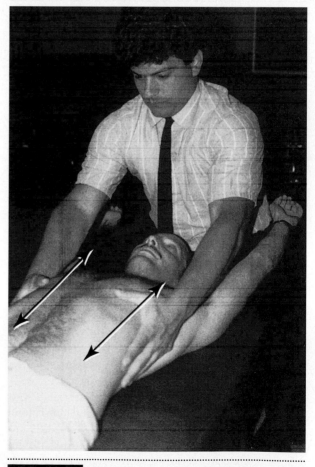

Figure 7-17 Mobilization of the thoracic spine and rib cage in long axis extension.

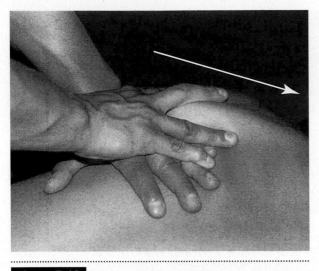

Figure 7-18 Hand contact for scapulothoracic manipulation. The patient is prone, and the adjustive thrust is in a superior direction.

competitive weight lifters and power lifters) taking androgens. The avulsion causes a severe ecchymosis at the chest and upper arm. The muscle belly usually "rolls up" like a window shade. Treatment is most often surgical in competitive athletes, and a cosmetic deformity remains even after the restoration of function.

Study Questions

1. (a) What curve classification is the dorsal kyphosis? (b) What conditions may accentuate the kyphotic curvature? (c) Name the anatomic structures that are responsible for checking rotation and stabilizing the spine.

2. (a) Which ribs are called true? (b) Which are called false? (c) Which rib pairs are called floating?

3. A 50-year-old man with a history of progressive loss of spinal mobility, decreased chest expansion, and significant radiographic changes at the thoracolumbar junction should be worked up for what diagnosis?

4. (a) Name the clinical findings associated with vertebral subluxation (posterior joint dysfunction) of the thoracic spine. (b) What are some causes of this impairment? (c) Where will a patient with costovertebral dysfunction and an inferior vertebral segment exhibit palpable tenderness?

5. (a) What is the most common type of scoliosis? (b) What are some biomechanical features of scoliotic curves? (c) What is the progression factor equation proposed by Lonstein and Carlson? (d) What are some goals for conservative case management of scoliotic patients?

References

1. Akbarnia BA, Kepple L, Price EA, Gote T: Lateral electrical stimulation for the treatment of adolescent idiopathic scoliosis: an analysis based on progression risk, *Orthop Trans* 10:3, 1986.
2. Andersen J, Hwant S, Greer WT: Growth of the normal trunk in boys and girls during the second decade of life, related to age, maturity, and ossification of the iliac apophysis, *J Bone Joint Surg* 47A:1554, 1965.
3. Armstrong GWD, Livermore NB III, Suzuki N, Armstrong JG: Nonstandard vertebral rotation in scoliosis screening patients: its prevalence and relation to the clinical deformity, *Spine* 7:50, 1982.
4. Asher MA: Non-operative treatment of scoliosis, *Spine: State of the Art Reviews* 1(2):213, 1987.
5. Beal MC: Palpatory testing for somatic dysfunction in patients with cardiovascular disease, *J Am Osteopath Assoc* 82(11):822, 1963.
6. Berman AT, Cohen DL, Schwertker EP: The effects of pregnancy on idiopathic scoliosis: a preliminary report on eight cases and review of the literature, *Spine* 7:76, 1982.
7. Bigliani LV, Compito CA, Duralde XA, Wolfe IN: Levator scapula and rhomboid transfer for trapezius paralysis, *J Bone Joint Surg* 78A(10):1534, 1995.
8. Blount WP, Mellencamp DD: The effect of pregnancy on idiopathic scoliosis, *J Bone Joint Surg* 62A:1083, 1980.
9. Boden SD, Wiesel SW, Laws ER, Rothman RH: *The aging spine: essentials of pathophysiology, diagnosis and treatment*, Philadelphia, 1991, WB Saunders.
10. Brennan PC, Kokjohn K, Kaltinger CJ, Lohn GE, Glendening C, Hordras MA, McGregor M, Triano JJ: Enhanced phagocytic cell respiratory burst induced by spinal manipulation: potential role of substance P, *J Manipulative Physiol Ther* 14:399, 1991.
11. Brown JC, Alexgaard J, Howson DB: Multicenter trial of a noninvasive stimulation method for idiopathic scoliosis: a summary of early treatment results, *Spine* 9:382, 1984.
12. Burch WH, Patwardhan AG: *Scoliosis: making clinical decisions*, St Louis, 1989, Mosby.
13. Carr WA, Moe JN, Winter RB, Lonstein JE: Treatment of idiopathic scoliosis in the Milwaukee brace, *J Bone Joint Surg* 62A:599, 1980.
14. Cramer GD, Darby SA: *Basic and clinical anatomy of the spine, spinal cord and ANS*, St Louis, 1995, Mosby.
15. Deyo RA, Cherkin D, Conrad D, Volinn E: Cost, controversy, crisis: low back pain and the health of the public, *Annu Rev Public Health* 12:141, 1991.
16. Edgar MA, Chapman RH, Glasgow MM: Pre-operative correction in adolescent idiopathic scoliosis, *J Bone Joint Surg* 64B:530, 1982.

17. Gavin TM, Shurr DG, Patwardhan AG: Orthotic treatment for spinal disorders. In Weinstein SL, editor: *The pediatric spine,* New York, 1993, Raven Press.

18. Green T, Hensinger RN, Hunter LY: Back pain and vertebral changes simulating Scheuermann's disease, *J Pediatr Orthop* 5:1, 1985.

19. Greulich WW, Pyle SI: *Radiographic atlas of skeletal development of the hand and wrist,* ed 2, Stanford, Calif, 1959, Stanford University Press.

20. Herzog W: Mechanical and physiological responses to spinal manipulative treatments, *J Neuromusculoskeletal Syst* 3(1):1, 1995.

21. Kostuik JP: Adult scoliosis. In Weinstein J, Wiesel SW: *The lumbar spine,* Philadelphia, 1990, WB Saunders.

22. Kostuik JP, Lorenz M: *Long-term results of posterior instrumentation for the treatment of Scheuermann's kyphosis in adults,* Montreal, 1981, The Scoliosis Research Society.

23. Kostuik JP, Lorenz M: Long-term follow-up of surgical management in adult Scheuermann's kyphosis, *Orthop Trans* 7:28, 1983.

24. Krag MH, Seroussi RE, Wilder DC: Internal displacement distribution from in vitro loading at human thoracic and lumbar spinal motion segments: experimental results and theoretical predictions, *Spine* 12:1001, 1987.

25. Lemire JJ, Mierau DR, Crawford CM, Dzus AK: Scheuermann's juvenile kyphosis, *J Manipulative Physiol Ther* 19:195, 1996.

26. Lonstein JE: Natural history and school screening for scoliosis, *Orthop Clin North Am* 19(2):227, 1988.

27. Lonstein JE, Carlson MJ: The prediction of curve progression in untreated idiopathic scoliosis during growth, *J Bone Joint Surg* 66A:1061, 1984.

28. Lonstein JE, Winter RB: Adolescent idiopathic scoliosis: nonoperative treatment, *Orthop Clin North Am* 19(2):239, 1988.

29. Lonstein JE, Winter RB: Milwaukee brace treatment of adolescent idiopathic scoliosis—review of 1020 patients, *J Bone Joint Surg* 76A:1207, 1994.

30. Marrero GH: Juvenile kyphosis, *Spine: State of the Art Reviews* 4(1):173, 1990.

31. Meade K, Burch W, Vanderby R, Patwardhan A, Knight G: Progression of unsupported curves in adolescent idiopathic scoliosis, *Spine* 12:520, 1987.

32. Moore KL: *Clinically oriented anatomy,* Baltimore, 1980, Williams & Wilkins.

33. Morrissy RT, Busch MT: Neuromuscular scoliosis, *Spine: State of the Art Reviews* 1(2):283, 1987.

34. Nachemson A, Cochraon TP, Irstam L et al: Pregnancy after scoliosis treatment, *Orthop Trans* 6:5, 1982.

35. Nicholas AS: Somatic component to myocardial infarction, *J Am Osteopath Assoc* 87(2):123, 1987.

36. Noonan KJ, Weinstein SL, Jacobson WC, Dolan LA: Use of the Milwaukee brace for progressive idiopathic scoliosis, J Bone Joint Surg 78A:557, 1996.

37. Ogilvie JW: Biomechanics of the spine. In Bradford DS, Lonstein JE, Ogilvie JW, Winter RB: *Moe's textbook of scoliosis and other spinal deformities,* ed 2, Philadelphia, 1987, WB Saunders.

38. Ogilvie JW, Millar EA: Comparison of segmental spinal instrumentations devices in the correction of scoliosis, *Spine,* 8:416, 1983..

39. Panjabi MM, White AA: *Clinical biomechanics of the spine,* ed 2, Philadelphia, 1990, JB Lippincott.

40. Parke WW: Applied anatomy of the spine. In Rothman RH, Simeone FA, editors: *The spine,* ed 2, Philadelphia, 1982, WB Saunders.

41. Piscopo J, Baley JA: *Kinesiology: the science of movement,* New York, 1981, John C. Wiley.

42. Ransfort AO, Edgar MA: A transverse system to supplement Harrington instrumentation in scoliosis, *J Bone Joint Surg* 64B:226, 1982.

43. Redford RB, Butterworth TR, Clements EL: Use of electromyography as a prognostic aid in the management of idiopathic scoliosis, *Arch Phys Med Rehabil* 50:443, 1969.

44. Scheuermann HW: Kyphosis dorsalis juvenilis, *Ugesk Langer* 82:385, 1920.

45. Schultz AB, Ciszewski DJ, DeWald RL et al: Spine morphology as a determinant of progression tending in idiopathic scoliosis, *Orthop Trans* 3:52, 1979.

46. Shekelle PG, Adams AH, Chassin MR, Hurwitz EL, Brook RH: Spinal manipulation for low back pain, *Ann Intern Med* 117(7):590, 1992.

47. Stano M, Ehrhart J, Allenburg TJ: The growing role of chiropractic in health care delivery, *J Am Health Policy* 3(6):39, 1992.

48. Stone B, Beekman C, Hall V et al: The effect of an exercise program on change in curve in adolescents with minimal idiopathic scoliosis: a preliminary study, *Phys Ther* 59:759, 1979.

49. Sullivan JA, Davidson R, Renshaw TS, Emans JB, Johnston C, Sussman M: Further evaluation of the Scolitron treatment of idiopathic adolescent scoliosis, *Spine* 11:903, 1986.

50. Tofler IR, Stryer BK, Micheli L et al: Physical and emotional problems of elite female gymnasts, N Engl J Med 335(4):281, 1996.

51. Vernon HT, Khami MSI, Howley TP, Annett R: Spinal manipulation and beta-endorphin: a controlled study, *J Manipulative Physiol Ther* 9:115, 1986.

52. Walton WJ: *Osteopathic diagnosis and technique,* ed 2, Colorado Springs, Colo, 1970, American Academy of Osteopathy.

53. Weinstein SL: Natural history of scoliosis in the skeletally mature patient, *Spine: State of the Art Reviews,* spinal deformities 1(2):195, 1987.

54. Winter RB, Lonstein JE, Denis F: Pain patterns in adult scoliosis, *Orthop Clin North Am* 19(2):339, 1988.

55. Wolf AW, Brown JC, Barrett CA, Nordwall A, Sanderson R: Transverse traction in the treatment of scoliosis: a preliminary report, *Spine* 6:134, 1981.

56. Wynarsky GT, Schultz AB: Trunk muscle activation in braced scoliosis patients, *Spine* 14(12):1283, 1989.

57. Zohn DA: *Musculoskeletal pain: diagnosis and physical treatment,* ed 2, Boston, 1988, Little Brown.

Lumbosacral Spine

Chapter 8

Chapter Highlights

Socioeconomic Aspects of Back Pain

Anatomic Model of the Lumbar Spine

Evaluation of the Lumbosacral Spine

Chiropractic Manipulation

Manual and Mechanical Traction

Spinal and Pelvic Mobilization

Physiotherapeutic Modalities and Ancillary Procedures

Exercise and Spinal Rehabilitation

Lumbar Disk Disease

Lumbar Spinal Stenosis

Posterior (Zygapophyseal) Joint Disorders

Sacroiliac Joint Disorders

Lumbopelvic Myofascial Pain Syndromes

Arthritic and Metabolic Disorders

PART ONE: INTRODUCTION TO LOW BACK DISORDERS

Allopathic methods and traditional medical care have been ineffective at worst and inconsistent at best in treating low back ailments. Substantial research into clinical biomechanics and causes of lumbar pain was not well-implemented until the 1970s. Perhaps these inadequacies were part of the reason so many people began to consider alternative therapies for the treatment of back pain. Although empirical data and statistical analyses based on multistudy environments are still not plentiful to show the effectiveness of long-term chiropractic care in comparison with various other treatment models, it is clear that improving the patient's quality of life and func-

tional capacity plays a major role in determining how the patient feels about chiropractic care.

In their study of patient perceptions of medical physicians and chiropractors, Cherkin and MacCornack found clear evidence of the satisfaction of chiropractic patients with personalized "hands-on" care.[41] This type of therapy may be the buffer needed to promote early ambulation and speedy return to the workplace of the patient with low back pain.

Socioeconomic Aspects of Back Pain

Low back pain is one of the most common disorders in human beings. Not only does it account for extensive morbidity among individuals, but it has a significant impact on society. Yet, it continues to puzzle patients, practitioners, and researchers. Does the problem of low back pain originate in the evolutionary process through which humans have become biped, or is the environment of an industrialized and high technologic society the crux of the problem?

Epidemiologic Perspectives

Low back pain and sciatica have been common since Biblical times, but the rate of occurrence has been increasing in recent decades. This increase in the incidence of low back pain is consistently larger than the rate of population growth, and the cost of spinal treatment has increased faster than the rate of inflation.[66,162,168] Frymoyer clearly described the "magnitude" of the problem: 50% to 70% of the adult population exhibit lifetime prevalence; 14.3% of new patient visits to physicians are for low back complaints; and these complaints are responsible for millions of visits to chiropractors, physical therapists, and orthopedic specialists.[65,69,150,168] Industrialized nations consistently have a higher rate of low back pain and disability.

Although both women and men commonly experience lumbar problems, the rate of disability differs between the two sexes beyond the age of 50 years. Men have a high incidence of low back pain between the ages of 25 and 55, after which there is a drop-off in the incidence. Rates among women tend to continue to increase past 50 years, however.[65]

The natural course of biologic factors in human beings, such as spinal aging, does not necessarily correlate with the incidence of back pain. Acute back pain differs from chronic back pain in its causative factors and in the appropriate modes of treatment. Usually biologic causes of acute pain can be isolated or understood, facilitating treatment for individuals with acute pain. These patients require immediate aggressive treatment to both eliminate early pain and restore function in a fairly short window of time to avoid the development of chronic conditions. Bed rest, long-term medication, and constant passive treatments are more likely to lead to chronic disability than to return patient function.[200] Chronic pain perpetuates itself, and many psychosocial elements contribute to despair, fear, and disability. Environmental and mental health factors, which can be difficult to identify, may play a particularly significant role in chronic low back conditions.[179] A program of weight reduction and aerobic fitness is a key component in treating and preventing chronic low back pain.

Properly executed clinical trials conducted by individuals who have no financially vested interest in the results are necessary to determine the best methods of prevention for acute and chronic lumbar spinal problems. The need for this research is urgent because of the potential threat of financial catastrophe that back pain poses for individuals and for the health care delivery system.

Economic Perspectives

Although most cases of acute low back pain subside within 4 weeks, the economic consequences of the condition are enormous. In 1991 the American Chiropractic Association estimated that low back pain costs the United States approximately $40 billion every year.[6] Health care costs from 1980 to 1985 *alone* rose 310%, with the per capita expenditure rising to $1364. The treatment costs for injured workers *alone* was estimated at $4.4 billion in 1991.[168]

A combination of economic and medicolegal factors has changed the medical care customarily provided to patients with low back disability. Surgical procedures such as laminectomies and lumbar fusions were once commonplace, but in the 1990s, even orthopedic surgeons and neurosurgeons tend to advocate conservative care and to adopt a wait-and-see approach. Some surgeons now declare that perhaps they were too quick to perform surgery on patients with motor signs of spinal injury. Failed back syndrome, a condition in which patients experience progressively disabling back pain postoperatively, is frustrating for all those involved. Back pain is so prevalent, however, that even with the shift to conservative therapies, back problems continue to be the third most common reason for surgery.[9]

It is difficult to extrapolate the mean costs per back problem. According to some authors, only one third of the total costs of low back problems are from treatment, whereas two thirds are from disability.[11,118,178] An upward trend in the pattern of utilization may contribute to spiraling medical costs as well.[33] Andersson and other researchers suggested that back injuries average 21% of all compensable work injuries, but average 33% of the cost.[11] Although total compensation approached $5 to $13 billion and the cost per case may be $6,000, only one fourth of the cases accounted for 90% of the total costs.[11]

Trends in health care expenditures continue to shift from high technology and a surgical and hospital-based treatment for spinal problems to low technology and manual approaches in an office-based outpatient setting.[137] Passive care continues to diminish in importance, whereas active treatment options such as exercise and manipulation play a vital role in cost-saving rehabilitation.[138]

Occupational Health

With continuing industrialization and advancing technologies has come a wave of work-related spinal injuries. The mechanisms for potential lumbar failure in occupational tasks include the following:

- Excess compression forces from erector spinae loading
- Resistance of shearing forces on the lumbar facets and posterior ligamentous structures in lifting objects in exaggerated flexion
- Large moment forces in flexion and exaggerated twisting of the lower lumbar disks
- Inability to maintain a small horizontal distance of the load to the L5-S1 disk

- Muscular fatigue, postural alterations, and accelerated disk degeneration because of repetitive vibration.

As a result of these and other mechanisms, back complaints are the leading cause of disability in workers under age 45.[105,183] The subsequent chain of events has been ominous: higher employee contributions to health insurance, higher cost of insurance premiums for everyone, and higher retail price index because of the increased cost of doing business (Figure 8-1).[147]

In spite of the tremendous opportunities for ergonomic and industrial consultation, those in the health care professions have failed to reduce the problems associated with spinal injuries in the workplace.[17,203] Pre-employment physical examinations and radiographic screening have proved to be poor predictors of spinal injury and disability.[17] There are, however, certain constant factors that are important in predicting the incidence of low back injury in the workplace, such as spinal weakness in jobs that require lifting, vehicle vibrations, cigarette smoking, and job satisfaction.[17,64,145]

Pressure exerted on the lumbar disks during work tasks performed in the sitting posture is the reverse of that exerted in the upright or recumbent posture.[141,148,155] Seats that distribute load more evenly between the pelvis and buttocks, and chairs that reduce the degree of backward pelvic rotation and forward torso-lumbar movement are helpful in reducing this pressure.[11] Arm supports are also beneficial in distributing load, as are chairs with a backrest.

When work requires the performance of manual lifting tasks from the upright posture, the employee should follow certain basic biomechanical principles (Figure 8-2). For example, the worker should keep the load close to the spine and should maintain the lifted material in a position that is not so high or low that it changes the trunk angle. The spinal erector muscles show negligible contractibility at 90 degrees of trunk flexion; this posture isolates statically the secondary ligamentous restraints of the lumbopelvic spine. The spinal erector muscles provide large contributory compressive forces to the lumbar spine. Shearing forces at the facet joints and

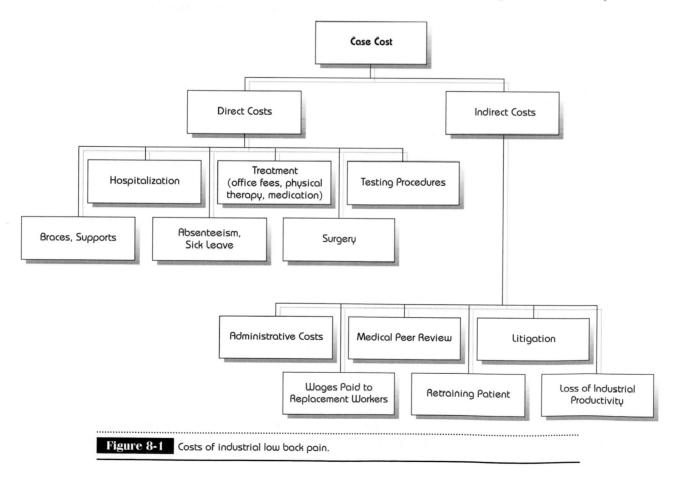

Figure 8-1 Costs of industrial low back pain.

clearly determining the source of the patient's pain. Unlike pathologic changes at the body surface, which are clear indications of medical conditions, the evidence of disk degeneration on an x-ray film may, in fact, have very little to do with the low back pain that the patient is experiencing. Although the focus has been on the normal versus abnormal degeneration processes of the spine, the chemistry of pain that has so elusively evaded spinal scientists for years may actually be the key factor. Only in the last few years have researchers discovered the biochemical mediators of back pain.

Another gray area is the differentiation between the normal aging process of the spine and abnormal pathologic processes. The disk goes through certain normal stages related to aging, including desiccation and loss of shock-absorbing capacity, but some advanced stages of pathologic changes or injury are beyond the body's inherent capability to make adjustments. Those disabilities may include disk herniation, protrusion, or extruded fragments (sequestered disk).

Intervertebral Disk and Intervertebral Joint

Healthy intervertebral disks act together as a hydraulic system that absorbs not only shocks between adjacent vertebrae, but also compressive loads. Each disk is composed of the vertebral end plate, annulus fibrosus, and nucleus pulposus. The annulus fibrosus contains collagen fibers in concentric lamellae arranged in parallel fashion at an angle of 60 degrees to the axis of the spine. Collagen is quite stiff and has a fairly high tensile strength. The nucleus pulposus consists of mostly proteoglycans, which bind large amounts of water and convert the matrix into a gel. Proteoglycans are largely glycosaminoglycan (95%), but have a small percentage of protein (5%).[193] Proteoglycan attaches to hyaluronic acid in a chainlike fashion, absorbing pressure in the disk by squeezing out fluid. The disk represents the center of the three-joint complex with injury occurring at the level of either facet joint (posterior) or the disk.

The combined effects of aging, degeneration, or injury may cause biochemical changes in the intervertebral disk that alter its ability to function in the hydraulic system. Degenerated disks may undergo internal resorption, loss of both water content and hydraulic power, carbohydrate binding, and finally failure under axial loading and compression (Figure 8-4). Loss of nuclear contents may place the weak link in this system—the vertebral end plate—at further risk when compression forces are particularly intense. Compression fractures

(as a result of disk dehydration) or fissures of the end plate (as a result of peripheral compressive forces) can lead to an improper transfer of loads at the intervertebral joint. This ultimately places greater demands in weight-bearing posture on the facet joints of the lumbar spine.

Mechanical Pathways for Failure

The lumbar spine is subject to compression, shear, and torsion stresses (Figure 8-5), and there is a delicate balance of restraining forces at the three-joint complex. Although soft-tissue structures such as the ligaments and muscles act as secondary restraints to the spine, the intervertebral disk and the corresponding two facet joints represent the main support structures. Farfan has described the stress at the intervertebral joint in the following fashion[55]:

$$\text{Intervertebral stress} = \sqrt{C^2 + S^2}$$

$$\text{where: } C \text{ is compression force, and}$$
$$S \text{ is shear force}$$

The facet joints (zygapophyseal joints), which are responsible for the planes of motion at the intervertebral joint, resist shearing forces. The iliolumbar ligament assists the facets in limiting rotation.[43] Shear, repetitive or excessive flexion-extension, and accentuated weight bearing can all cause mechanical injury to the posterior joints. Like an insult to other diarthrodal joints, insult to the facet joint can cause a synovial effusion and inflammatory response, distending the capsule and posterior joint ligaments. Thus tissues served by the primary dorsal ramus of a lumbar spinal nerve are sensitive to mechanical and chemical stimulation.[32] Thinning of the hyaline cartilage and subsequent fibrillation lead to dysfunction of the posterior joints that later appear in diagnostic studies as posterior arthrosis. Stiffness and immobility at the vertebral level usually precede the degenerative process, which may ultimately encroach on the viability of the lateral recess.

The sagittal plane orientation of the zygapophyseal joints aids in flexion and extension movements, while limiting torsional motion. The thoracolumbar junction possesses facet joints that lie midway between the coronal and sagittal planes.

Because the spine is essentially a closed kinetic chain consisting of motion segments, dysfunction or degeneration in either the disk or posterior joint usually produces a deleterious chain reaction in the other components of the three-joint complex (Figure 8-6). It has

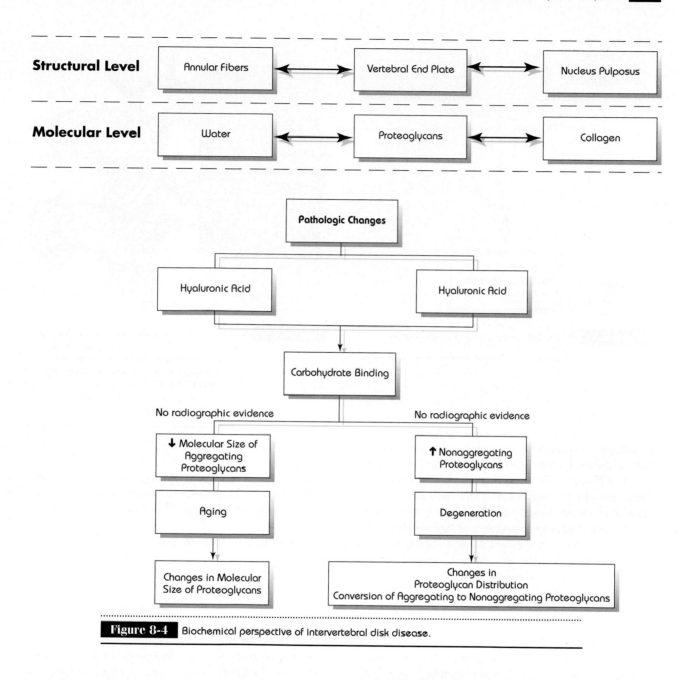

Figure 8-4 Biochemical perspective of intervertebral disk disease.

been shown in the laboratory that degenerative disks have altered patterns of creep and reduced viscoelastic behavior as well.[101] If this should occur, it seems likely that the facets would bear an unaccustomed level of shock absorption for the functional spinal unit. This has been shown by such researchers as Yong and King[221]; Liu, Rang, and Hirsch[125]; and Lorenz, Patuardham, and Vanderberg.[127]

The increased load is one reason that symptoms associated with degenerated, protruded, and even herni-

ated disks may suggest problems with the facet joints. Therefore chiropractic manipulative therapy that centers around high-velocity thrusts and provides greater freedom of movement for the posterior joints may be highly effective in cases of this nature.[38] After all, once a disk lesion heals and connective tissue infiltrate appears and muscle shortening occurs, the patient is left with a highly immobile and dysfunctional spinal unit. The restoration of motion to the facets tends to restore normal coupling, muscular elasticity, and joint receptor

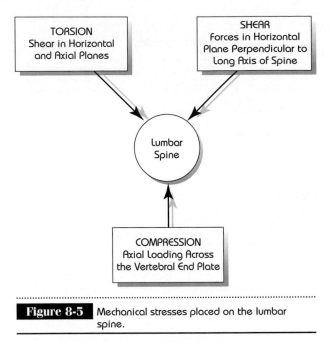

Figure 8-5 Mechanical stresses placed on the lumbar spine.

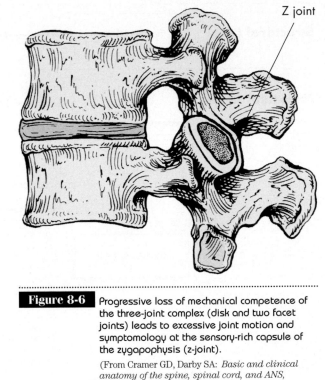

Figure 8-6 Progressive loss of mechanical competence of the three-joint complex (disk and two facet joints) leads to excessive joint motion and symptomology at the sensory-rich capsule of the zygapophysis (z-joint).

(From Cramer GD, Darby SA: *Basic and clinical anatomy of the spine, spinal cord, and ANS,* St Louis, 1995, Mosby.)

stimulation[217]—all effective for combating low back pain, even in the patient with disk disease.

Torsion places stress at the outermost portion of the annulus fibrosus first. Combined with axial rotation, torsion renders the disk vulnerable, especially at the posterolateral edges. The posterior longitudinal ligament cannot protect this structure at the caudal end of the spine at the lumbosacral junction. On the other hand, strong abdominal muscles and thoracolumbar fascia take pressure off the intervertebral joint structure. The abdominal muscles have the ability to increase intra-abdominal pressure, and the thoracolumbar fascia serves as an anchoring mechanism for the transmission of forces up the vertebral column via the pelvic chain.[24,163] Both increase the overall stability of the spine and reduce stress at the three-joint complex.[79]

A multitude of forces can break down the various structural components of the intervertebral joint. The culmination of compression, shear, and torsion adds to the momentum of the effects of aging. Loss of disk space may lead to compression at the intervertebral foramen.[163] Injuries may be macrotraumatic in nature, or they may be microtraumatic (i.e., stemming from years of wear and tear). Although the possible causes for injury and disease of the human spine are extensive, three pathways may be major conduits for biomechanical failure: (1) repetitive sagittal motion, (2) excessive torque on the functional spinal unit, and (3) axial over-

loading on the lumbar spine. Any injury that causes mechanical failure, alone or in combination with other conditions, can precipitate lumbar pathologic abnormalities.

Repetitive Sagittal Motion

Constant flexion and extension of the lumbar spine have been shown in biomechanical studies to increase the likelihood of failure at the posterior joints, especially at the pars interarticularis.[94,161,215] Young, skeletally immature athletes are especially prone to injury as a result of repetitive loading of the lumbar spine. Athletes in certain sports, such as football and gymnastics, seem to have a higher incidence of low back complaints and subsequent diagnoses of spondylolysis or spondylolisthesis.[82,206] Interestingly, the incidence of fatigue fractures of the spine is much higher through childhood and adolescence in female gymnasts than in male gymnasts.[161] Evidently, the adverse effects of repetitive hyperextension are more pronounced in female adolescents than in male adolescents. Youngsters of both sexes seem particularly vulnerable to a fatigue fracture at the ages of 5 to 11 years, and such an injury is usually superimposed upon a congenital defect or developmental anomaly.

Cyclic loading of the functional spinal unit has been shown to be the fatiguing load that causes a defect in the neural arch.[94,215] It is certainly a distinct possibility that sufficient lordotic loading in a young lumbar spine may be a predisposing factor in pars defects and subsequent spondylolisthesis and back pain in later teenage years.

Effects of Torque on the Functional Spinal Unit

Torsion is the combination of shearing forces that act on the spine in the horizontal and axial planes. Pure shearing stresses that are perpendicular to the direction of the annular fibers of the disk can cause the intervertebral disk to fail, and torsion can produce breakdown in the zygapophyses as well.

Flexion at the lumbopelvic junction during lifting (stooped posture) does not necessarily increase compressive forces on the lumbar spine. With the back flexed, however, shear forces greatly increase, which places significant pressure on the posterior structures of the functional spinal unit, including the articular facet capsules and posterior ligaments (Figure 8-7).[12] Further flexion of the trunk to 90 degrees over the femur heads almost completely eliminates the action of the spine in the lift and places the ligaments of the pelvis under tremendous loading potential.

Asymmetry in either posture or the actual act of lifting may cause uneven amounts of torsion on the back and associated joints. The lack of symmetry in weight distribution during lateral bending and twisting movements can injure the facet joints, causing sprain and synovitis of the articular capsules. In addition, unequal lifting movements in flexion and unilateral rotation can lead to greater torsion, further breakdown at the three-joint complex, and disk injury. The individual who lifts a heavy object too far away from the body and twists to one side commonly experiences such an injury.

There are several ways to prevent spinal failure during lifting tasks. First, because the spinal load during manual lifting is directly related to the amount lifted in each task motion, lifting lighter objects several times can be easier on the spine than lifting a heavy object once. Second, keeping the object to be lifted as close to the spine and pelvis as possible will drastically reduce the chance of excessive torsion on the functional spinal unit, especially the posterior elements. Third, if the object can be placed near or between the legs, then a semi-squatting posture that takes advantage of the hip extensors and leg muscles in the lifting task is best for reducing the chance of back injury. If the object cannot be placed close to the lower limbs, however, then the external force associated

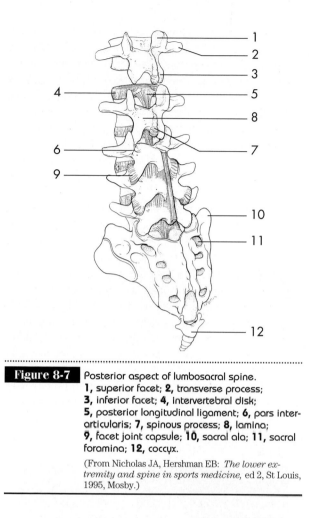

Figure 8-7 Posterior aspect of lumbosacral spine. **1,** superior facet; **2,** transverse process; **3,** inferior facet; **4,** intervertebral disk; **5,** posterior longitudinal ligament; **6,** pars interarticularis; **7,** spinous process; **8,** lamina; **9,** facet joint capsule; **10,** sacral ala; **11,** sacral foramina; **12,** coccyx.

(From Nicholas JA, Hershman EB: *The lower extremity and spine in sports medicine,* ed 2, St Louis, 1995, Mosby.)

with lifting may be too far away from the spine and pelvis, and this position may ultimately be detrimental.[10]

Axial Loading on the Lumbar Spine

Compressive loads of various magnitudes can inflict damage on the intervertebral disk and functional spinal unit. Both short duration–high amplitude and long duration–low magnitude loads can be harmful. An element of rotation with axial loading may be more likely than a pure compressive force to cause an acute disk lesion, however.[212]

Long-term repetitive loading on the intervertebral disk has a time-dependent degenerative effect. The disk exhibits creep, relaxation, and viscoelasticity over years. Because the biomechanical behavior of the disk ultimately affects the stage or status of its degeneration, the age and traumatic history of the patient are all pertinent in the management of low back pain.

Under extreme clinical loading conditions, the vertebral end plate will fail well before the disk.[1,164] The extrusion of nuclear contents in a case of Schmorl's nodule, as well as fissures and fractures of the end plate, can alter the instantaneous axis of rotation at the functional spinal unit and therefore make the motion segment unable to attenuate and transfer axial loads properly. At this stage of weakness at the three-joint complex, bending and torsional loading is particularly devastating to the functional spinal unit, especially the lumbar intervertebral disk (Figure 8-8).

The role, if any, that the lordotic curve plays on axial compression and the incidence of low back pain continues to be less than clear. Frymoyer and colleagues and Ferrand and Fox reported no association between low back pain and significant increases in lordosis.[57,67] Even if it is not related to low back symptomatology, the lordosis or restoration of lordosis is probably biomechanically significant in rehabilitating the lumbar spine, however. The coupled motion of a nonstraight spine (lordotic spine) is helpful in converting pelvic movement into axial torque for locomotion.[75,77,128]

Methods of lifting incompatible with proper load transfer not only increase the compressive load, but they also may add deleterious torsion. *Poor use of the pelvic girdle, once again, may allow inappropriate transfer of load to the vertebral column in the absence of an efficient spinal muscular system.*

Overview of Lumbopelvic Kinetics

Musculoligamentous structures act to mobilize and protect spinal motion segments. The three-joint complex consists of two synovial joints—the posterior facets. Anteriorly, the intervertebral disk represents the anterior intervertebral joint. The disk is structured to provide maximum stability with a small amount of motion.[120]

Ultimately, compression and shearing forces may adversely affect these structures through acute or repetitive trauma. Proper transfer of loads through efficient muscular action, including hip extensor recruitment and static supportive contractions of paravertebral muscles,[194] produces effective spinal movement and protects the intervertebral joint and lumbopelvic ligaments from failure.

Motion Segment Failure in Lumbar Flexion

Electromyographic (EMG) studies have consistently shown poor spinal erector activity at 90 degrees of lumbar flexion.[25,59] If the pelvis rotates around the femoral heads sufficiently to flex the spine, the posterior ligamentous structures become extremely taut; conversely, the erector muscles of the spine become inactive or relaxed. The inefficient spinal erector muscles can then exert only torsional loads and certainly cannot generate the movements necessary to complete a significant lifting task.

The proper transfer and sequencing of forces are commonly evident in elite athletes. The lumbodorsal fascia increases with load, compensating for the transmission of load, especially to the upper extremity as in athletic endeavors. This compensation occurs primarily in conjunction with extension of the legs and pelvis in the absence of independent spinal erector muscular recruitment. Soft-tissue injury at the spinal level can result from excessive forces, a biomechanically incorrect lifting posture, the lack of articular coordination in novice task performers, or repetitive loading on a degenerated functional spinal unit. *Because the coordination of spine and pelvis is a key component to safe task completion in patients with low back problems, elements of lumbar rehabilitation that require isolation of the spine with harnessing of the pelvis are questionable.*

Disk and Ligamentous Loading of the Lumbar Spine

In the lower portion of the lumbar spine, the function and hydration of the disks are crucial, because the ability

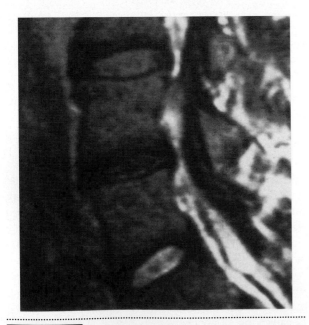

Figure 8-8 T2-weighted image showing a dehydrated disk at L4-L5. The disks at L3-L4 and L5-S1 are relatively normal.

(From Watkins RG: *The spine in sports,* St Louis, 1996, Mosby.)

of the posterior joints to absorb axial compression is inefficient (approximately 20% support). The facets may bear 16% of the axial load in the erect posture, but pressure between the disks increases in the sitting position. Axial load also increases the stiffness of the intervertebral joint; conversely, distraction of the spine decreases intervertebral joint stiffness. The healthy disk is able to transfer load from one adjacent vertebral segment to the next, as well as handle compressive forces and shock absorption.

Repetitive loading of the intervertebral disk through flexion and rotation fatigues collagen fibers.[23] Radial and circumferential tears weaken the annulus, making rupture a possibility.[175] Although normal disks do not succumb to these forces, degenerated disks may finally fail under axial loading and compression. End-plate fracture usually occurs before rupture of the disk during excessive movements in axial compression.[56,166] Loss of disk height may lead to spinal stenosis.

The release of inflammatory markers in the epidural space or the introduction of proteoglycans outside the internal boundaries of the nucleus may be the result of excessive loading of the disk. The capsular distention associated with swelling and fibrosis of the articular capsules may lead to pain in a referred or local pattern.

Torsional strains are great at the annulus, especially if the axis of rotation is distant to the peripheral fibers. Weaker fibers at the posterolateral region of the annulus are most vulnerable to injury, however. Lack of muscular protection places an increased strain on the entire disk-facet interface, making the likelihood of a disk or posterior ligamentous injury more common.

Excessive shear or flexion loading of the spine with rotation not only may tear the annular tissue of the intervertebral disk, but either may strain the ligaments. In the synovial joints, ligamentous laxity may develop as a result of either chronic breakdown of the three-joint complex or excessive twisting movements that are checked by the facet joints. Chronic synovitis of the articular capsule leads to chronic laxity and anatomic subluxation of the posterior joints. This may occur concomitantly with internal disk degeneration or from maximal loading and failure of the facet joints.

Protective Role of the Hip Extensors

Most rehabilitation clinics that treat low back injuries have isokinetic systems that require strapping the pelvis and immobilizing the lower quarter while the spinal column translates back and forth during repetitive flexion-extension exercises. Such a posture places the spine at a clear disadvantage. Without the muscular restraints that span the hip and pelvis, the spine must rely on the intervertebral joint and the poor working action of the inefficient erector spinal mass, which lies parallel to the vertebral column and has only a short lever arm (Figure 8-9).[78] The facet joints are left in a vulnerable state, and the pelvis' normal mechanical advantage in providing the forces that drive the spine through the lumbodorsal fascia is removed by its immobility.

Other than ambulation, the squatting posture is perhaps the most natural movement in the human lower extremity. A fast glance at a child between the ages of 8 and 18 months reveals the squatting motion to be a natural and ingenious way to commence the standing and walking process. The head makes up a large percentage of the child's body weight. To balance the head over the center of gravity, the child who is learning to stand and walk takes a relatively wide stance and drops the hips to compensate for the lack of development in the legs and spine (Figure 8-10). Therefore the more powerful hip extensors perform the bulk of the work.

In the adult the powerful hip extensor muscles are also primarily used in the squatting motion, with slight modification. *The adult's gluteal muscles place the spine in a more advantageous posture, sparing both the knee and lumbar joints detrimental loads during lifting and movement.* In the dead lift, for example, the extensor muscles of the hip are the key components of safe completion (Figure 8-11 *A-D*). The hip extensors begin to lift the object, and the muscles that extend the spine (e.g., multifidi, longissimus) are electrophysiologically silent. The fibers of the gluteus blend into the thoracolumbar fascia, which transfers the movement to the upper limb. When the shoulder bears the weight, the erector muscles relax. The movement of the trunk into the erect position originates primarily in the hip extensors. According to Gracovetsky, the "erectors are incapable of lifting anything above 20 kg...the tightening of the lumbodorsal fascia must increase with load, so that the forces generated by the powerful hip extensors may be transmitted all the way to the upper extremities."[76]

Evaluation of the Lumbosacral Spine

If performed in a concise and systematic fashion, screening an individual for the cause of low back pain is not the monstrous problem that it may first appear to be. The screening process begins when the patient enters the office to discuss the problem. Key points in the case history and definitive clinical impressions developed during the orthopedic and neurologic examination form the working diagnosis.

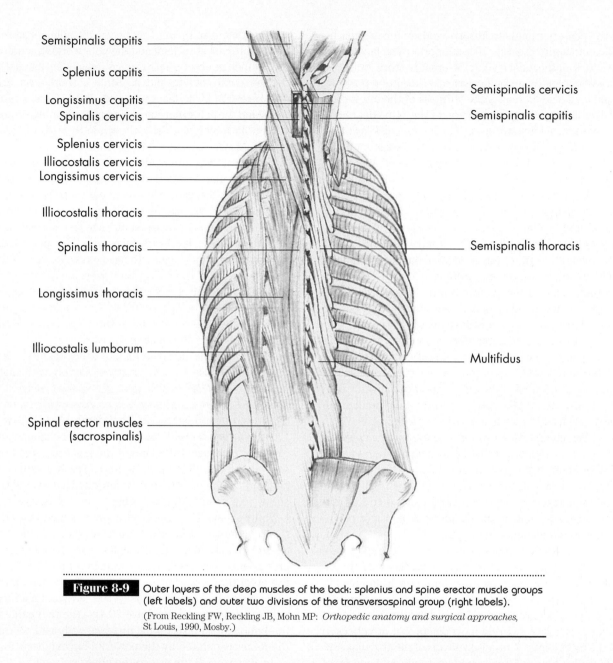

Semispinalis capitis

Splenius capitis

Longissimus capitis

Spinalis cervicis

Splenius cervicis

Illiocostalis cervicis

Longissimus cervicis

Illiocostalis thoracis

Spinalis thoracis

Longissimus thoracis

Illiocostalis lumborum

Spinal erector muscles (sacrospinalis)

Semispinalis cervicis

Semispinalis capitis

Semispinalis thoracis

Multifidus

Figure 8-9 Outer layers of the deep muscles of the back: splenius and spine erector muscle groups (left labels) and outer two divisions of the transversospinal group (right labels).

(From Reckling FW, Reckling JB, Mohn MP: *Orthopedic anatomy and surgical approaches,* St Louis, 1990, Mosby.)

Initial Assessment

One of the priorities of the initial examination is to obtain a history. The clinician needs to know the details of the events leading up to impairment; the nature of the pain, including its site and severity; and any other symptoms that the patient is experiencing. Most patients clarify key points about the origin of their pain. Repetitive occurrences of injury or dysfunction often signify a chronic soft-tissue impairment of the vertebral column. If the condition is clearly a soft-tissue injury, it is necessary to document the date, time, place, and mechanism of the accident or injury.

Not all patients have local signs that explain their low back pain, but the following are some common signs of organic disease:

- Prior neoplasm or infection
- Lack of reproducible orthopedic or neurologic findings
- Full range of motion in the presence of pain

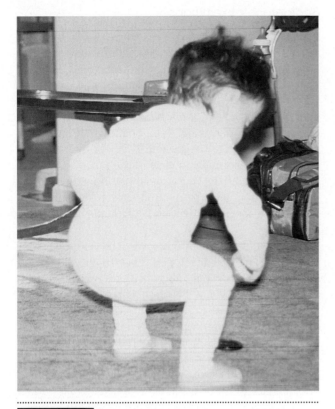

Figure 8-10 Baby squatting. Because of their supreme flexibility, toddlers can easily achieve a biomechanically correct squatting position.

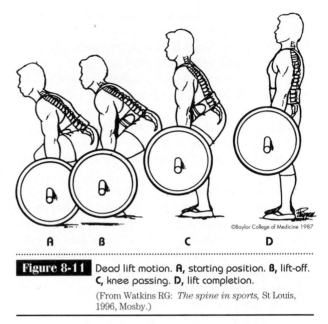

A   B   C   D

©Baylor College of Medicine 1987

Figure 8-11 Dead lift motion. **A,** starting position. **B,** lift-off. **C,** knee passing. **D,** lift completion.

(From Watkins RG: *The spine in sports*, St Louis, 1996, Mosby.)

- Unremitting pain or pain that consistently increases in frequency
- Pain that is constant or worse at night
- Weight loss accompanied by disturbance in bowel or bladder habits

In patients who lack the signs and symptoms of a mechanical low back injury, it is important to examine the peripheral joints and limbs for sensory or motor loss, upper tract signs (i.e., neurologic signs of brain injury), and joint effusions. Clinical signs of systemic illnesses such as diabetes, vascular insufficiency, or pelvic disease should be investigated to determine whether the source of the low back pain is organic (Table 8-1).

The gait and face of the patient may be revealing. Is the patient worried? Does the patient show signs of extreme anxiety? Neurotic movements and speech may cloud the diagnosis. For example, many individuals with mental health problems (e.g., clinical depression) have concomitant low back complaints that may be clinically related to or exacerbated by their mental outlook.

The life style and occupation of the individual is key. For instance, male smokers have a much higher incidence of low back pain.[67,89,126] If the patient works in a job that requires physical labor, it is helpful to ask if the patient must lift heavy or light objects repeatedly. Does the job require pushing, pulling, or twisting? An activity that the patient performs 8 hours a day, 5 days a week may correlate with the nature and severity of the problem. Truck drivers, for example, often suffer chronic lumbar disk disease attributable to long-term, repetitive vibration of their vehicles and a prolonged sitting posture.[20,88,201]

The following is a guide to questions to be asked during an interview with the patient who complains of low back pain:

- How long have you had the complaint or disturbance?
- What daily activities does it impair?
- Have you ever experienced this pain before at the same site?
- What is the mechanism of injury if antecedent trauma was the cause of disability?
- Where is your pain, and does it travel to any other region?
- Have you taken any medication or seen any other physician for the pain?
- Do you have any other complaints, concomitant fever, weight loss, rash, or joint swelling?

- Did anyone in your immediate family ever suffer from the same complaint?
- What is your occupation—more specifically, what are the tasks related to your job?
- Are you satisfied at work, and have you lost any appreciable amount of time recently or before being injured?
- Do you have any loss of bowel or bladder function or any sexual dysfunction?
- Have you had any prior back examination or spinal radiographic films?
- What are the dates of the visits?

Screening patients who may have motives other than a desire to return to full capacity may place the clinician in an unenviable position. Clinician-patient relationships are built largely on trust and honesty, and malingerers are rarely straightforward with the treating physicians. Clinicians should be wary if patients have seen several physicians or specialists in a short-time span following an injury. Many visit a physician simply to hear, "Stay out of work indefinitely." If there is a long list of practitioners who have already treated the patient, it is essential to practice defensively, insist on prior records (e.g., x-ray films), and ask the exact reason why the patient has switched clinicians so frequently.

Table 8-1   Clinical Picture of Organic Back Pain

Area or Problem	Symptoms
Gastrointestinal system	Nausea, vomiting, constipation and diarrhea, abdominal pain
Genitourinary system	Pain, hesitation during urination, frequency or urgency, costovertebral pain, flank pain, hematuria
Upper abdomen	Dorsolumbar pain, midback pain, intercostal neuralgia, anteroposterior referral, reflux
Neoplasm	Constant pain, night pain, unusual referral zones, laboratory or diagnostic evidence, weight loss
Infection	Fever, lymphadenopathy, painful movement, elevated erythrocyte sedimentation rate, possible elevation of white blood cell count

Radiographic Examination

In recent years the scrutiny of case reviews and risk:value ratios has finally eroded the traditional standard of ordering x-ray films for almost every patient.[51,52,189] Peer reviews have indicated that practitioners who own x-ray equipment tend to perform imaging procedures more frequently.[92] The use of x-ray films for so-called "patient education" or "marketing" (i.e., pointing out an abnormality to encourage the patient to accept treatment) is unforgivable, especially in view of the radiation dose of lumbopelvic films.[144] There are far better methods of patient education, and the method chosen should be tailored to the specific patient and magnitude of the injury sustained.

Patients who are over the age of 50 years or are experiencing newly developed back pain should be screened for pathologic abnormalities both physically and radiographically *if* their disability is not in any way related to trauma or overuse. Patients with a history of metabolic disease or neoplasm should also have a radiographic examination routinely if they develop back pain.[51,104] In addition, it is appropriate to order x-ray films for those individuals with back pain who have undergone prior spinal surgery or sustained significant gross trauma to the region if their earlier films are older than 3 years.

Any suspicion of ankylosing spondylitis that arises during the case history or physical examination may warrant ordering plain films. Patients whose blood findings are abnormal may also need to undergo an x-ray examination to rule out pathologic anomalies. Individuals with acute low back pain and abnormal neurologic findings should, in some cases, have a radiographic examination. Acute episodes of mechanical low back pain with normal neurologic findings do not mandate an immediate radiologic work-up, especially for younger individuals.

The overwhelming number of patients with low back pain who seek treatment makes the proper use of radiography a critical challenge to the chiropractic physician. According to Phillips, the implications to chiropractic are three-fold:

"The lack of scientific evidence supporting the use of x-rays in acute low back pain patients, the potential for abuse of x-rays when imaging equipment is owned by the treating physician, and the high frequency of back pain in the population offers a challenge to justify the use of plain film radiography for the evaluation of spinal pain."[160]

The following guidelines permit the clinician to order the necessary radiologic tests while providing cost-effective care that protects the patient's health:

1. Plain radiographic films of the lumbar spine are usually of little clinical value *early* in the course of low back pain.

2. When the results of a neurologic examination are normal, plain radiographic films are not clinically helpful in patients with mechanical low back pain.

3. Patients who are between 20 and 50 years of age, have no pathologic signs and symptoms, describe no remarkable history, and complain of low back pain need *not* routinely undergo an x-ray examination.

4. Patients with mechanical low back pain who exhibit neurologic deficits or whose condition is refractory to care are likely to benefit from a standard x-ray series in 2 to 4 weeks after undergoing a trial of conservative therapy.

5. Individuals with unexplained weight loss; significant trauma; suspicion of ankylosing spondylitis; drug or alcohol abuse at age 50 years or older, since it may have begun many years earlier; history of cancer, metabolic disease, or prolonged corticosteroid use; and a temperature higher than 100° F should have a radiographic examination before the initiation of manual treatment.

Standard lumbar x-ray films include anteroposterior and lateral views (Figure 8-12). Oblique projections should be used with gross trauma or if the diagnosis or symptomatology is unclear. Oblique films are often necessary in screening patients with suspected pars abnormalities. Advanced diagnostic imaging studies may be necessary for individuals with suspected nonmechanical or neurologically compromised pathologic conditions (Figure 8-13). For example, CT and MRI scans may be necessary to confirm soft-tissue masses, space-occupying lesions, and nerve root disorders (Figure 8-14). CT is particularly useful in revealing bony elements, such as fracture lines and fragments, and in determining the condition of multitraumatized patients. MRI is better at demonstrating intramedullary and extradural processes, and it is especially helpful in the diagnosis of discoligamentous injuries.

Orthopedic Examination

Although the orthopedic examination has several purposes (e.g., screening for joint instability, nerve root signs, and myospasm), one of the most important features is to ascertain whether the patient is a candidate for conservative care. Fortunately, most patients with mechanical low back pain are prime candidates for conservative care, including spinal manipulation.

The timing of the orthopedic examination is extremely important. Tenderness or pain in multiple planes, spasm, and cloudy nerve root test findings often accompany acute episodes of low back pain (Figure 8-15). It may be easier to make a definitive diagnosis or identify the specific pain-producing structure in the patient with subacute or chronic pain. For the patient with acute low back pain, a tentative, working diagnosis

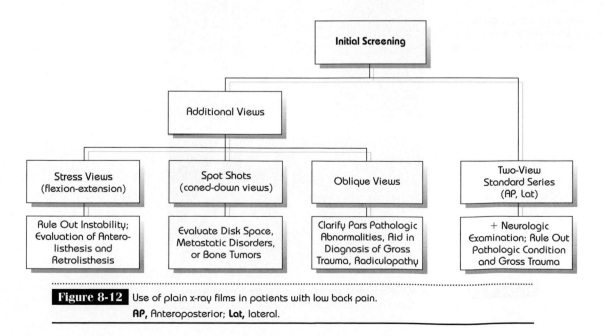

Figure 8-12 Use of plain x-ray films in patients with low back pain.
AP, Anteroposterior; **Lat,** lateral.

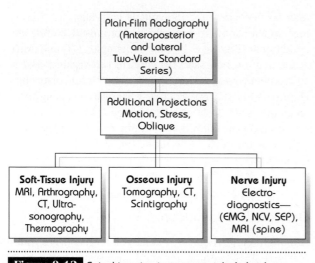

Figure 8-13 Spinal imaging in neuromusculoskeletal care.

EMG, Electromyography; **NCV,** nerve conduction velocity; **SEP,** somatosensory-evoked potential; **MRI,** magnetic resonance imaging, **CT,** computed tomography.

with a commitment to reevaluate the patient's condition as needed may be the best initial diagnosis.

Musculoligamentous Instability

It is often difficult to examine individuals with musculo-ligamentous instability because of the pain. Spasm may mask the true cause of dysfunction and disability. The intensity of a generalized pain or an alteration in freedom of movement of the spine and limbs can also complicate the collection of true hard data through the orthopedic procedures normally used.

Lumbar instability may result from muscle spasm or from ligamentous or capsular sprain of the synovial joints in the posterior vertebral unit. Although patients with muscle spasm in the low back often experience severe pain, the causative condition is often benign and self-limiting. Causes of acute lumbar spasm include the following:

- Acute sacroiliac sprain
- Acute facet sprain

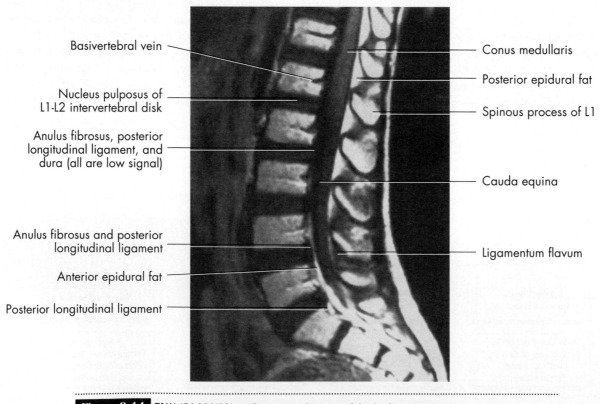

Figure 8-14 T1W (SE 800/20) midline sagittal image of the lumbar spine.

(From Enzmann DR, DeLaPaz RL, Rubin JB: *Magnetic resonance of the spine,* St Louis, 1990, Mosby.)

- Acute lumbar strain
- Lumbar disk protrusion
- Herniated nucleus pulposus (HNP)
- Fracture

Those who suffer from chronic low back pain often exhibit signs of ligamentous instability. There is a host of possible medical causes for this instability, including the following:

- Degenerative disk disease
- Facet syndrome (chronic)
- Chronic sacroiliac sprain
- Spondyloarthropathies

The signs and symptoms of lumbar instability resulting from muscle spasm can be similar in some respects to those of lumbar instability resulting from ligamentous problems. Disk degeneration, synovitis of the posterior joints, and biochemical irritants at the spinal level all contribute to the pain-spasm cycle, clouding the initial lumbar diagnosis even further (Figure 8-16). Difficulty getting out of a chair or seated position is a common complaint with either muscle or ligamentous pain, especially in chronic sufferers who sit for prolonged periods of time. In addition, forward flexion in the standing posture aggravates the pain of musculoligamentous instability, because this position stretches both the posterior joint capsules and lumbar erector muscles, causing reflex spasm. Breathing difficulty can also add to the pain. Although acute spasm and structural instability cause significant distress, treatment includes a support or brace for a short period of time, physiotherapy, and reassurance.

Range-of-Motion Testing

Probably the most valuable of all orthopedic testing procedures are the range-of-motion tests. Not only do these tests usually make it possible to distinguish mechanical back pain from organic back pain, but they facilitate the assessment of the condition of patients who are suspected of malingering. In fact, combined with a thorough knowledge of applied spinal anatomy, carefully administered range-of-motion testing can be the key component to the physical examination.

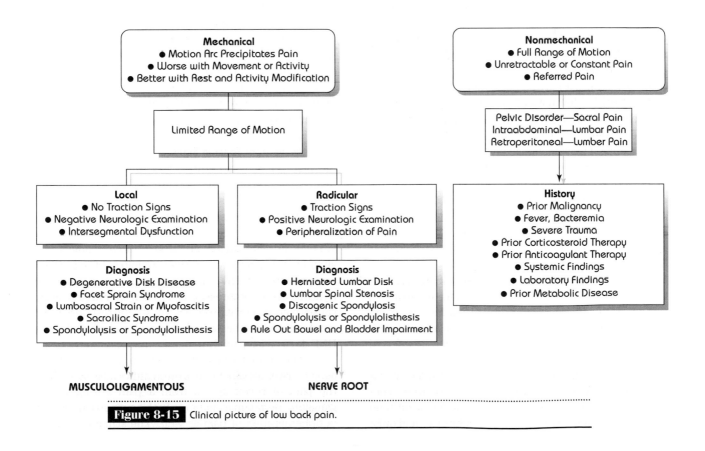

Figure 8-15 Clinical picture of low back pain.

in nature, and the clinician should seek the underlying mechanical problem carefully.

It is important to document any unilateral muscular changes; asymmetry in soft tissue, list, or gait; limitation in spinal motion; and changes in levels of perceived tenderness found during the examination. These findings aid in the diagnosis of a mechanical dysfunction or injury. Palpation can be performed while the patient is sitting, standing, or even lying on one side if the patient cannot be moved. The patient should be advised to relax as much as possible and encouraged to inform the clinician of any unusual sensations.

Neurologic Examination

The orthopedic examination may be the key to confirming the presence of mechanical back pain, but it is the neurologic examination that reveals the extent of the problem. During the neurologic examination, the examiner determines what other orthopedic tests and imaging procedures may be necessary (Figure 8-18). Furthermore, the results of the neurologic evaluation provide the information that the clinician needs to decide whether to treat the patient with conservative manual therapy or to refer the patient to another type of practitioner.

Signs of neurologic deficits warrant careful screening, documentation, and close follow-up. The practitioner should always thoroughly investigate any pain, as well as any visceral signs in conjunction with significant neurologic findings and correlate these signs with the patient's history. More proximal and anterior leg (thigh) and pelvic (hip) pain usually originates in the nerve root levels L1-L3. More distal leg and foot pain can usually be traced back to the lower nerve root levels L4-S1 (Figure 8-19).

The evaluation procedures that a chiropractor uses in a neurologic examination are the same as those used by the neurologist, orthopedic surgeon, and neurosurgeon, and the chiropractor's office is frequently the hub of care. Trials of conservative care and manipulation are often evaluated through follow-up neurologic examinations.

Motor Function

Perhaps no other component of the neurologic examination has received more attention than the detection or presence of motor signs. Muscle weakness, atrophy, or the inability to perform functional testing maneuvers all suggest the presence of nerve root compression that is more significant than the alteration of sensation. Although nerve root compression can lead to hypersensitivity and functional loss, sensory or motor changes can be evaluated by physical examination and objective electrophysiologic testing (Table 8-2). The excitability of the spinal nerves, particularly the dorsal root ganglion, cannot.

Table 8-2 Typical Pattern of Dysfunction Seen With Specific Radiculopathies

Nerve	HNP	Foramen	Muscle	Reflex	Sensation
T10					Umbilicus
T12					Pubis
L1	T12-L1	L1-2			Upper anterior thigh
L2	L1-2	L2-3			Midanterior thigh
L3	L2-3	L3-4	Quadriceps femoris		Lower anterior thigh
L4	L3-4	L4-5	Quadriceps femoris Anterior tibial	Patella	Anterior thigh Medial leg Foot (occasionally)
L5	L4-5	L5-S1	Anterior tibial EHL	Posterior tibial	Lateral leg Dorsum of foot Big toe
S1	L5-S1		Heel raise Peroneal	Achilles' tendon	Posterior leg Sole of foot Lateral foot Little toe

HNP, Herniated nucleus pulposus; **EHL,** extensor hallicus longus.
(Adapted from Watkins R: *The spine in sports,* St Louis, 1996, Mosby.)

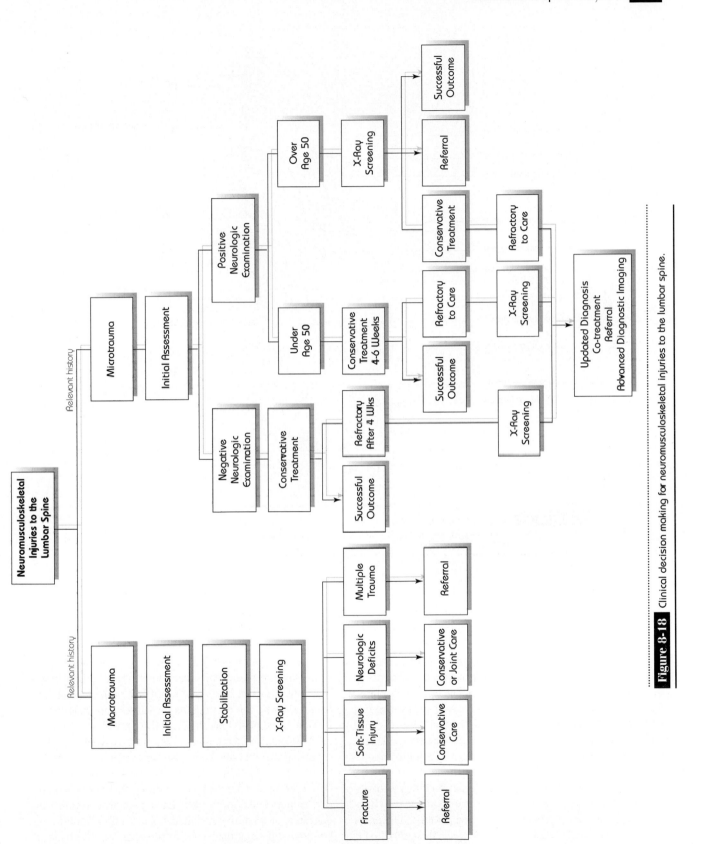

Figure 8-18 Clinical decision making for neuromusculoskeletal injuries to the lumbar spine.

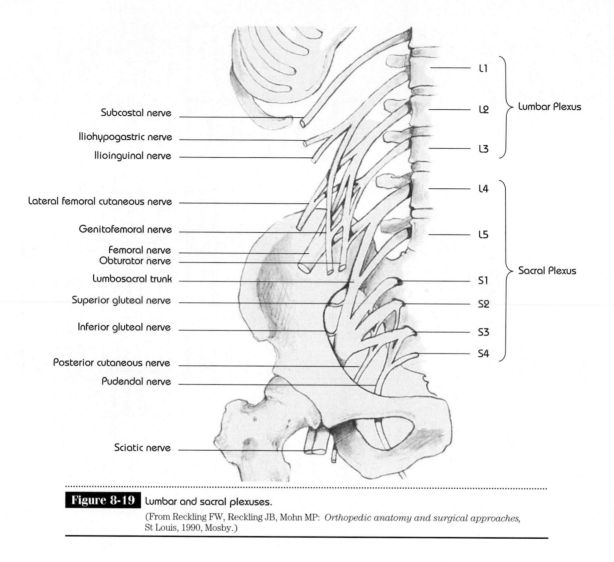

Subcostal nerve

Iliohypogastric nerve

Ilioinguinal nerve

Lateral femoral cutaneous nerve

Genitofemoral nerve

Femoral nerve
Obturator nerve

Lumbosacral trunk

Superior gluteal nerve

Inferior gluteal nerve

Posterior cutaneous nerve

Pudendal nerve

Sciatic nerve

L1

L2 Lumbar Plexus

L3

L4

L5

S1 Sacral Plexus

S2

S3

S4

Figure 8-19 Lumbar and sacral plexuses.

(From Reckling FW, Reckling JB, Mohn MP: *Orthopedic anatomy and surgical approaches,* St Louis, 1990, Mosby.)

To begin the examination for motor function, the clinician palpates the lower extremities for muscle tissue, bulk, and symmetry. If in doubt about muscle atrophy, the clinician may take circumferential measurements. The clinician then moves the muscles so that they perform in passive repetitive contractions with and without resistance, checking for the strength of the contraction and fatigue. Repetitive stressing brings out subtle motor weakness. Heel and toe walking tests, for example, may reveal asymmetry in gait or foot function.

An evaluation of spasm, rigidity, and clonus is also important to rule out neurologic disease. Gait should be analyzed, especially in the presence of disability. The patient should be asked to heel walk (for assessment of L5)

and toe walk (for assessment of S1); foot inversion strength (for assessment of L4) should be determined.

It has long been recognized that true nerve root signs, weakness, and pain over 6 months are serious in nature, but the guidelines for identifying patients with low back pain who are candidates for surgery are narrowing. Kahanovitz stated that, although the clinical presentation of neurologic impairment includes sciatica, weakness, loss of sensation, and bowel and bladder dysfunction, only 1% to 2% of low back pain patients may require surgery.[97] Other prominent surgeons have stated that not only is the percentage of patients with back pain who require an operative procedure very small, but also practitioners may be moving for aggressive care "too soon" on the basis of motor signs alone.[84,151] Saal and Saal found exercise treatment successful, even for a group of patients disabled with lumbar HNP with radiculopathy who experienced pain on a single leg raise of less than 60 degrees, neurologic loss, and an abnormal MRI or CT scan.[174] The Agency for Health Care Policy and Research (AHCPR) concluded that conservative measures such as manipulation should be pursued before surgical intervention or oral administration of steroidal drugs are considered.[3]

The patient who consistently shows *progressive* motor loss, atrophy, or loss of functional abilities (e.g., walking, sitting, working) requires a surgical consultation.[58] Patients with a diagnosed lumbar intervertebral disk lesion that does not respond in any favorable way to conservative care within 4 weeks should be sent for either a second opinion regarding their clinical status or further diagnostic testing procedures to confirm or exclude the diagnosis.[3]

Sensory Patterns and Pain Modalities

Compression and deformation of the spinal nerve roots lead to specific alterations in sensory patterns and pain modalities, such as paresthesia, dysthesia, and dermatomal pain. These sensory changes appear before motor signs, since they result from lesser degrees of nerve root compression than motor signs.

Soft-tissue swelling and intraneural edema lead to pressure in the dorsal root ganglion, which, in turn, may decrease the blood flow to the sensory nerve bundles.[157] When this occurs, the patient experiences radicular pain, most likely in a typical dermatomal pattern. Several authors have alluded to the vulnerability of the spinal nerves and the difference between these nerves and the popliteal nerve.[153,222] Although there are no exact pathophysiologic explanations for sciatica, it is likely that a combination of compression and vascular impairment produces the sensory disturbances associated with lumbar spine disease (Figure 8-20).

If there is any disturbance in the sensory system, the goal of testing is not only to confirm sensory deficit or loss, but also to determine the type of sensory dysfunction and spinal structure (if any) likely to have caused the disturbance. Testing procedures include manual pinwheel testing for sensory alteration along typical dermatomes, investigation of the history of pain patterns along with the exact site and quality of pain, and the reproduction of spinal and leg complaints.

When performing sensory testing, the clinician keeps a careful watch on the patient and lower extremity. If an individual must pause to consider whether there is

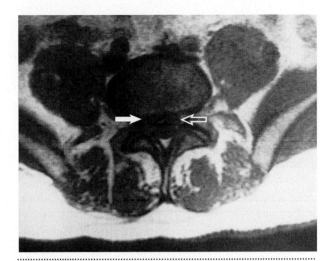

Figure 8-20 Axial lumbar magnetic resonance image depicting obliteration of the right nerve root. Seen at the L5 level, there is a loss of high signal intensity from fat, usually visualized around the nerve root (closed arrow). The left nerve root is unaffected (open arrow).

a difference from one side to the other during testing, then the results are equivocal. Only clear-cut disturbances should be recorded as positive results.

Radicular Pain. Patients generally describe radicular or dermatomal symptoms as sharp, stabbing, or shooting, with a pinpoint zone of pain patterns approximately 1 to 2 inches in width.[48] Radicular problems may be associated with sensory distribution (paresthesias, dysthesias), motor changes (weakness, atrophy), reflex changes (hyporeflexia), or pain radiating outward from the spine (radiculopathy).[154] Disk disease, trauma, space-occupying lesions, and infection can each cause radicular pain.

Somatic-Referred Pain. Structures of the vertebral column sometimes produce pain that is felt in areas distant to the pain-generating structure, and it is necessary to differentiate this type of referred pain from radicular (nerve root) pain. Structures that may be responsible for somatic-referred pain include the disk, neural elements, and posterior joint itself, as well as the synovial joint capsules, ligaments, cartilage, and vertebrae.

Somatic-referred pain causes constant discomfort, has no motor component, and is often mediated through the posterior primary division of the dorsal root. Most patients describe somatic-referred or scleratogenous pain as a dull, deep, achy pain that is hard to localize. The reason for the difficulty in localizing the pain is that a multitude of multilevel sensory afferent impulses converge on single tract neurons.[49] Although the pain may be difficult to pinpoint, spinal motion, lower extremity movement, or intersegmental stressing at the vertebral column can reproduce it. Pressure on the dorsal root ganglion from structures such as the posterior intervertebral disk and ligamentum flavum can actually cause somatic-induced referral without radiculopathy.[48] Further complicating an already cloudy diagnostic dilemma is the possibility of discogenic pain occurring via sympathetic afferents from the sinuvertebral nerves.[149]

Physiologic segmental subluxation of the lumbar spine, sacroiliac sprain, musculoligamentous sprain or strain injuries, synovitis of the apophyseal joints, chronic facet syndromes, and degenerative joint disease of the lumbosacral spine can each cause somatic referral to the lower extremity. A possible neurophysiologic effect of vertebral joint dysfunction is to mimic visceral disease.[180] Chiropractic adjustment of the spinal segment that exhibits pathomechanical features is usually palliative to the patient's complaint, and symptoms usually resolve in a shorter time span than with radicular syndromes. With only approximately 10% of all patients with mechanical low back pain exhibiting signs of true nerve root compression, it is clear that many patients are experiencing pain referred from the deep somatic structures of the spine, and the clinician should take this possibility into consideration.

Dermatomal Patterns versus Myotogenous Referral. Although muscles can actually produce somatic-referred pain, they have referral zones all by themselves and are usually termed myotogenous pain or myofascial trigger points. Myotogenous-referred pain from active trigger points differs distinctly from the traditional paresthesia and dysthetic response in the patient with nerve root compression. In contrast to the sharp, well-localized dermatomal pain, myofascial-referred pain is usually poorly localized; in this respect, it is similar to somatic-referred pain.

Patients with quadratus lumborum syndrome and chronic low back pain are the most likely candidates for myotogenous-referral zones (Figure 8-21 *A-D*). Often mimicking dermatomal pain, the myotogenous-referred pain may travel toward the hip, thigh, or even beyond. Palpation of the paravertebral structures, including deep palpation, is often necessary to uncover the subtle culprit. All other neurologic tests often prove fruitless.

The rotators of the hip, including the gluteus maximus, gluteus medius, and piriformis, are often the cause for gluteal, hip, and thigh pain (Figure 8-22 *A-E*). This

leg and hip pain is generally dull, achy, yet deep. Usually, only compressing the trigger points or stretching the muscle can reproduce the pain.

Deep Tendon Reflex Pathology

Checking reflexes of the lower extremity to pinpoint abnormal lumbar spine responses often brings past spinal injuries to the surface. It is not uncommon to encounter a patient who has simple mechanical low back pain and a completely normal neurologic examination except for a weak or absent reflex in the lower extremity. In the majority of cases this clinical finding will do little to alter the clinical course of treatment or the prospects of future testing procedures.

The L4, L5, and S1 spinal nerves can be evaluated through an examination of the corresponding motor reflexes of the lower extremity (Table 8-3). The common "knee jerk" reflex test reflects predominantly the condition of the L4 motor level. A patient with a remarkable neurologic examination that includes a decreased knee jerk (i.e., weak knee extension), hypoesthesia of the medial leg, and quadriceps weakness is likely to have an L3-L4 disk herniation.

Table 8-3	Neurologic Changes Associated With Common Lumbar Disk Herniations	
Lesion	**L4 Herniation Between L4-L5**	**L5 Herniation Between L5-S1**
Affected nerve root	Fifth lumbar	First sacral
Pain pattern	Lateral thigh, anterolateral leg, dorsal aspect of foot	Posterior thigh, posterolateral leg, lateral aspect of foot, including heel and fourth and fifth toes
Sensory changes	Hypesthesia or anesthesia in areas where pain is felt	Hypesthesia or anesthesia in areas where pain is felt
Common muscle weakness	Extensor hallucis longus, extensor digitorum brevis, and tibialis anterior	Plantar flexors of foot (triceps) and atrophy of posterior calf muscles
Reflex change	Tibialis posterior may be absent	Decreased or absent Achilles' reflex

(From Post M: *Physical examination of the musculoskeletal system,* St Louis, 1987, Mosby.)

The L5 reflex is not always routinely tested. When necessary (because of an elusive diagnosis or a suspected injury), the clinician can perform such a test at two sites: the medial hamstring (semitendinosus) or the posterior tibialis. In both cases, the examiner strikes the tendinous portion of the lower extremity muscle with the reflex hammer. Tests at both sites are superficial and should evoke a movement that is typical of the muscle action. Tapping the medial hamstring should evoke a slight knee flexion; tapping the posterior tibialis should cause a slight inversion. Patients with an L4-L5 herniated disk usually have no reflex changes accompanying their dermatomal pain or sensory changes.

The S1 nerve root can be tested through the Achilles' or ankle reflex. The clinician taps the tendon of the gastrocnemius muscle, which normally causes a plantar flexion response at the ankle. This response can be correlated with toe walking (S1 nerve level) during motor testing. Again, reflex findings need to be carefully correlated with the rest of the neurologic and orthopedic evaluations. A decreased ankle jerk reflex, decreased sensation on the lateral side of the foot, and decreased plantar flexion are the typical signs of a L5-S1 disk lesion.

Cauda Equina Syndrome

The continuation of the neurologic structures distal to the end of the spinal cord at the L1-L2 level is the cauda equina. Giving rise to the dorsal root ganglia and rootlets, the cauda equina is subject to compromise from thecal sac encroachment and deformation attributable to a central disk lesion. Tumors, infection, and trauma all may result in neurologic compromise of the cauda equina.

Cauda equina insult commonly leads to the loss of bowel or bladder function, and the clinician must routinely ask about these functions in individuals who complain of neuromusculoskeletal low back or leg pain. The examiner must differentially diagnose cauda equina syndrome from radiculopathy secondary to a herniated disk.

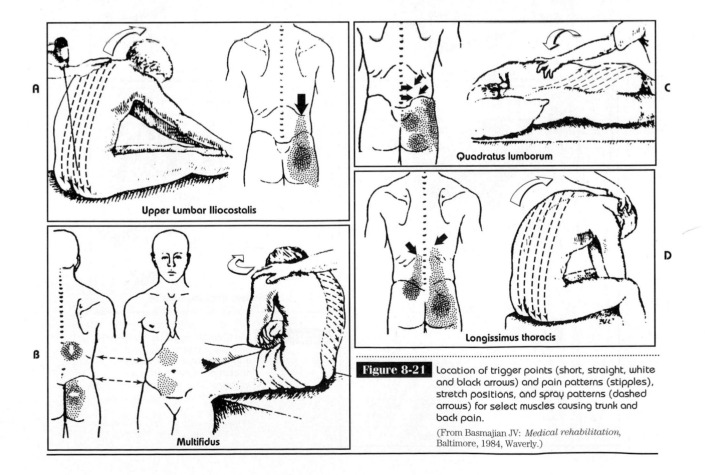

A   Upper Lumbar Iliocostalis

B   Multifidus

C   Quadratus lumborum

Longissimus thoracis

D

Figure 8-21 Location of trigger points (short, straight, white and black arrows) and pain patterns (stipples), stretch positions, and spray patterns (dashed arrows) for select muscles causing trunk and back pain.

(From Basmajian JV: *Medical rehabilitation*, Baltimore, 1984, Waverly.)

Both can raise intrathecal pressure, which can prove painful as the patient attempts to move the bowels. Dyspareunia in women and erectile difficulties in men are also possible consequences. S2-S4 sensory dysfunction or loss of the anal wink reflex are not as commonly noted in the literature, however.

Several authors have alluded to the relative hypovascularity of the cauda equina.[158,170] It is also possible that blockage of the cerebrospinal fluid from arachnoiditis and stenosis can lead to vascular and nutritional alterations that could cause further neurologic compromise in the patient with low back pain.

Signs of Myelopathy

Signs and symptoms of spinal cord compression resemble those of central stenosis. Compression symptomatology warrants evaluation for cauda equina syndrome. Myelopathy resulting from disk lesions in the cervical and lumbar spine may cause sensory disturbances in the lower extremities and abnormal cortical tract signs (e.g., a Babinski reflex or clonus). Significant lumbar disk herniation in patients who are anatomically compromised at the spinal canal may describe pain on walking relieved by rest, feelings of weakness or "giving way," and coldness and numbness in the legs (Figure 8-23 *A-D*).

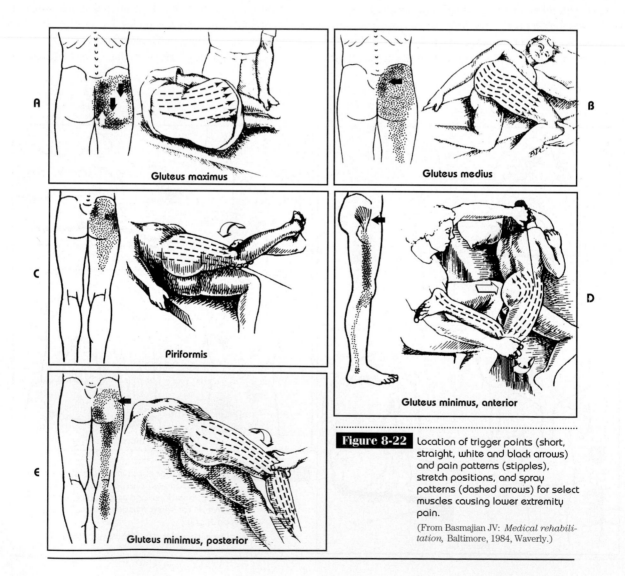

Figure 8-22 Location of trigger points (short, straight, white and black arrows) and pain patterns (stipples), stretch positions, and spray patterns (dashed arrows) for select muscles causing lower extremity pain.

(From Basmajian JV: *Medical rehabilitation*, Baltimore, 1984, Waverly.)

Extension narrows the intervertebral foramen, thus increasing the likelihood of neurogenic claudication and back or leg pain. Flexion may in fact be palliative to the patient.

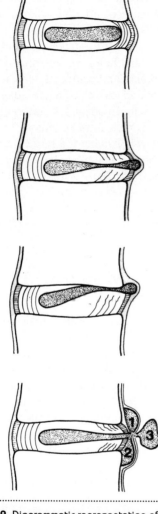

Figure 8-23 **A,** Diagrammatic representation of disk bulge; **B** and **C,** disk herniation; **D,** "free" disk fragment. Disk bulge refers to bulging, but intact, anulus (**A**). In herniated disks, nucleus pulposus material ruptures through a discontinuous anulus (**B, C**), but remains contiguous with native disk space. Tear in anulus may be radial (**B**) or transverse (**C**). The latter interrupts Sharpey's fibers. Free disk fragment or sequestered disk (**D**) refers to nucleus pulposus material that migrated under posterior longitudinal ligament (**2**), between ligament and dura (**1**), or through dura (**3**).

(From Enzmann DR, DeLaPaz RL, Rubin JB: *Magnetic resonance of the spine*, St Louis, 1990, Mosby.)

Chiropractic and Biomechanical Evaluation

Static and dynamic evaluations give the examiner a general idea of the cause-and-effect relationship between the condition of the spinal segments and the pain or chief complaint of the individual. Gross motor or sensory disturbance, along with nerve tension and nerve root signs, are red flags for neuromusculoskeletal compromise. A large percentage of patients have so-called simple mechanical low back pain that has never fit into an allopathic or chiropractic model, however. Therefore after examining the patient with low back pain from an orthopedic and neurologic perspective, the practitioner uses manual techniques such as palpation and motion analysis to determine the relationship between structural distortion and functional breakdown (Figure 8-24).

Few practitioners of allopathic medicine have studied intersegmental dysfunction of the vertebral column and pelvis. Thus the chiropractic (manual) and biomechanical evaluation may be the distinguishing factor in reaching an appropriate neuromusculoskeletal diagnosis and providing the hands-on conservative care that is appropriate for the patient's lumbar spine.

Evaluation for Pelvic Obliquity

Synonymous with the term *tortipelvis,* the term *pelvic obliquity* connotes a tilt of the pelvis or hip region (Figure 8-25). The development of a sufficient obliquity of the pelvis changes a person's functional leg length in the absence of a "true" anatomic discrepancy. This so-called functional short leg may, in time, subtly change lumbopelvic and lower extremity mechanics in a way that alters both gait and load distribution to the joints of the lower quarter. Running athletes, in particular, are usually able to discern these subtle differences in hip height and recognize differences in stride length as they hear a different cadence in their heel strike.

A biomechanical examination of the lumbopelvis should be performed with the patient in both the supine and prone positions. First, the examiner measures the legs with the patient in the supine (or standing) position. Tape measurement for anatomic leg length discrepancy covers bony point (anterosuperior iliac spine) to bony point (medial malleolus). Functional leg length discrepancy (pelvic obliquity) involves measurements from the umbilicus to the medial malleolus. It is essential to obtain all leg length measurements bilaterally. (Radiographic measurement is more accurate, but it is not feasible in practice.)

Then, with the patient in the prone position, the practitioner examines the lumbopelvis, analyzes the motion of the lumbar spine, and checks the sacroiliac joints for fixation. Next, the examiner places the patient in the supine position and palpates the anterior superior iliac spines bilaterally to check for anterior pelvic tilt. Manipulation to level the pelvis can be carried out via muscle energy techniques in a fashion similar to proprioceptive neuromuscular facilitation (PNF) mobilization. Finally, the patient stands in the weight-bearing position while the examiner checks the patient's hips for leveling.

An unlevel sacral base is *not* synonymous with pelvic tilt. Although sacral unleveling may accompany pelvic obliquity to varying degrees, they are different postural and structural imbalances. It is common for patients with sacral unleveling to have a concomitant or resultant lumbar scoliosis, although a certain percentage of individuals with spinal curvatures have compensated through their lumbopelvic articulation. The functional leg lengths may be different in either sacral unleveling or pelvic tilt. Low back pain may or may not be present, however.

Other screening procedures for pelvic distortion include checking gluteal folds, asymmetry in gait or static weight bearing, or unilateral asymmetry of muscle tone of the hip or spinal extensor mass.[132] It is also necessary to rule out hip flexor tightness or contracture on the side of the functional short leg. The clinician should keep in mind the need to evaluate both subjective symptomatology and objective orthopedic and neurologic testing with findings of pelvic distortion.

When Is a Short Leg a Short Leg?

Both functional and structural (anatomic) leg length discrepancies can lead to biomechanical imbalances at the pelvis. Short leg syndromes can alter gait, cause pelvic tilt or obliquity, place abnormal loads on the sacroiliac joint and psoas muscle, and predispose individuals to low back pain, sciatica, and muscle spasm. The lumbar spine may compensate by curving to the side of deficiency. This, in turn, can shift the individual's center of gravity.[63]

An anatomically short leg is less common than a functionally short leg. Functional leg length discrepancies occur as a structural or mechanical problem in lumbosacral disorders such as scoliosis and sacroiliac dysfunction. Measurements can be performed in the supine or prone positions via leg checks, tape measurements, or radiographic evaluations. Although the center of gravity can shift toward the short leg side, the patient may be prone to sacroiliac dysfunction and muscle imbalance, especially at the hip flexors and hamstring muscles.

Patients with an anatomically short leg as a result of a congenital variant, an orthopedic injury, or a previous orthopedic surgery of the lower quarter may require a small heel lift. Lifts should be introduced subtly (i.e., $1/16$-inch thickness) and left in place for 4 to 6 weeks to allow the individual to grow accustomed to each increment before proceeding to the next.

Functional leg length syndromes should be aggressively treated with chiropractic adjustments to the lumbopelvic spine, manual mobilization and stretching of the hip and pelvic muscles, and strict monitoring of gait, as well as balancing the sacrum and pelvis. Manipulative therapy can alter the articular dysfunction that occurs in short leg syndromes and restore proper alignment of the pelvis, sacral base, and lumbar spine.

Ambulation and Motion Analysis of the Lumbopelvis

Dynamic vertebral motion and function of the locomotor system are both interrelated and symbiotic. Subtle changes during ambulation may, in fact, be the direct result of lumbopelvic dysfunction. Determining whether the dysfunction originates in the myofascia or articular spinal elements is not an easy diagnostic task and requires specific screening procedures of the lumbopelvis in dynamic or movement functions. (The patient must be properly dressed so that the lower extremity is visible in form and function.)

Sacroiliac Dyskinesia. The sacroiliac joint can be checked for hypomobility in a variety of positions:

1. Place the patient in a prone position. With one hand, grasp the anterior iliac spine; with the other hand, press down over the sacrum on the same side. Spring the ipsilateral lumbopelvis to check for quality of motion. Use the same technique on the contralateral side and compare the findings.
2. Stand or sit behind the patient as he or she stands. Have the patient lock the legs fully and stand fully erect. Place your thumbs on the posterior superior iliac spine bilaterally. Instruct the patient to bend forward from the waist. Watch the excursion of your thumbs on the skin, checking to see if both

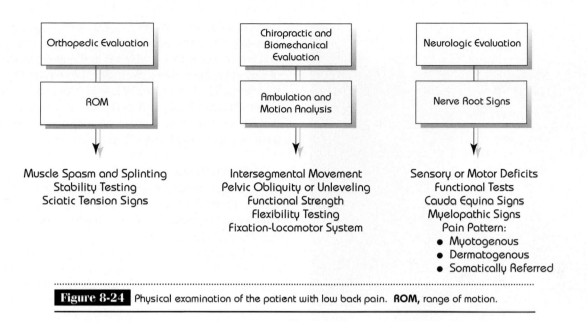

Figure 8-24 Physical examination of the patient with low back pain. **ROM,** range of motion.

sacroiliac joints drop.[73] If one thumb "rides high," the sacroiliac joint on that side is usually fixed or hypomobile.

3. Relative movement of the sacroiliac joint may also be tested by placing one thumb over the ipsilateral posterior superior iliac spine and the other thumb over the second sacral tubercle. Have the patient bend the knee and thigh of the ipsilateral side and raise the leg as in Figure 8-26 *A-D*. With normal mobility, the posterior superior iliac spine moves in a downward fashion 1 to 2 cm as the leg is raised. If the sacroiliac joint is fixed, the posterior superior iliac spine does not move downward. The lower sacroiliac joint and ischial excursion can be checked as well.

4. Have the patient sit to eliminate the hamstring muscles as a contributing factor to pelvic dysfunction. Once again, have the patient bend forward at the waist and repeat the test as described in #2.

Ambulation Screening. Wearing a gown or shorts so that the clinician can observe clearly, the patient performs the normal movements of walking. The patient should be observed both coming toward the clinician and walking away. The clinician looks for the following:

1. EQUALITY OF STRIDE LENGTH. A shortened excursion of the thigh may be attributable to pelvic dysfunction, psoas shortening, or hamstring contracture.

2. EXCESSIVE PELVIC TILT OR LEAN DURING AMBULATION. Severe muscle imbalance as a result of hip flexor con-

traction can be a major cause of asymmetric pelvic loading.[30]

3. ANTALGIC LEAN OF THE LUMBOPELVIC SPINE. Occult degenerative disk disease or bony sciatica may cause the patient to favor one side or develop an antalgic gait.

4. EXCESSIVE SWAYBACK OR HYPERLORDOSIS. Congenital distortion or functional muscle weakness, such as weak abdominal muscles, may cause excessive swayback. A lateral view is the best vantage point for evaluation, because it allows the clinician to see the trunk and spine behind the arms as they swing during ambulation. This condition is often associated with a forward head, since the spine attempts to correct the posture. Subsequently, the low back is usually stressed.

5. CHANGES IN PELVIC INCLINATION (TILT). From the back and side of the patient, the clinician can see how the femora rotate with an increase or decrease in pelvic inclination. Excessive anterior tilt usually involves medial rotation of the femur; decrease in pelvic tilt can lead to external rotation of the femur. Changes in pelvic inclination can alter knee and foot function. Pronation and faulty patella tracking should be checked as well.

Intersegmental Movement of the Lumbar Spine

The traditional medical practitioner evaluates spinal motion through gross ranges of motion for the spinal region;

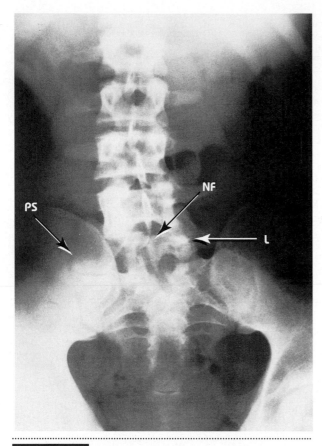

Figure 8-25 Levorotatory scoliosis with mild pelvic obliquity. There are multiple congenital variants at the lumbosacral junction, including a nonfusion defect (NF), lumbarization (L), and a pseudoarthrosis (PS).

the manual practitioner evaluates gross spinal mobility, but evaluates intersegmental movement as well.

Although motion palpation methods may vary, it is possible to check spinal segment movement while a patient is in the seated or prone position. First, the clinician can flex and extend the lumbar spine while the patient is seated with the spine exposed to see if there are any blocks or fixations to the movement. Opening and closing of the interspinous spaces suggest the status of sagittal dynamics.

Next, with the patient face down and the lumbar spine exposed, the clinician takes the thigh and abducts it to induce lateral bend at the lumbar spine. Placing the thumb of the superior hand on the ipsilateral side of the spinous process allows the clinician to check freedom and spring of movement. Actually, the clinician is checking the coupled motion of rotation and lateral bending. The spinous process should move to the ipsilateral side as lateral flexion takes place, which is in direct contradiction of cervical spine motion. Springing the spinous process, the clinician feels for block or loss of joint play. Fixation or vertebral block can be freed by means of manipulative techniques with the patient in the side-bending or side-posture position with the afflicted joint up.

Functional Muscle Strength

The clinician should palpate the paravertebral musculature to check for tone, spasm, and hypertonicity. The muscles of the trunk and pelvis should be evaluated for functional ability and strength.

The gluteal and erector muscles aid in stabilizing the spine and provide extension. To evaluate functional strength in spinal extension, the clinician asks the patient to take a prone position, raise one arm out straight in front of him or her, and simultaneously lift the leg on the opposite side out straight. The patient holds this position for 5 to 10 seconds, and the clinician notes any fatigue or inability to gain a healthy contraction, especially on the side of the leg lift. This side activates the hip and spinal extensor mass. The patient repeats the exercise on the opposite side, and the clinician compares the observations.

Next, the patient lies supine on the examining table with the legs bent at the knee at approximately a 90-degree angle. The feet should not be held down. The subject then crosses the arms over the chest while attempting to sit up. The trunk should be flexed to approximately a 30-degree angle or until the scapulae are off the table. The clinician then palpates the abdominal muscles for strength and tone, especially the rectus abdominis.

Finally, the patient lies in the lateral decubitus position and attempts to flex the trunk laterally in a side sit-up position. This maneuver will indicate the strength of the oblique muscles and the quadratus lumborum.

All the muscles that have been mentioned contribute to the stability and integrity of the lumbosacral spine. The findings of these tests reflect the capabilities of these muscles in the functional movements of the spine and are closely related to the findings of the palpatory and orthopedic examinations.

Flexibility Testing

Because many patients who suffer with chronic low back pain have a diverse array of neuromusculoskeletal faults,

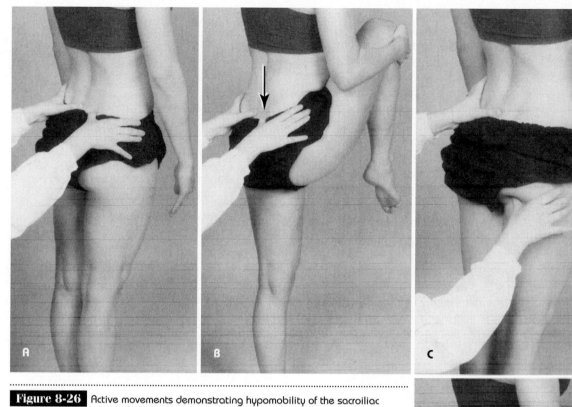

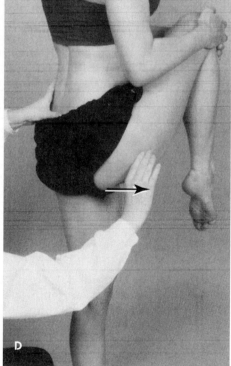

Figure 8-26 Active movements demonstrating hypomobility of the sacroiliac joints. **A,** Starting position for sacral spine and posterior superior iliac spine. **B,** Hip flexion; the illium drops as it normally should (arrow). **C,** Starting position for sacral spine and ischial tuberosity. **D,** Hip flexion; ischial tuberosity moves laterally (arrow) as expected.

(From MaGee DJ: *Orthopaedic physical assessment,* Baltimore, 1997, WB Saunders.)

their care requires a comprehensive approach. Flexibility testing will help the clinician identify any myofascial faults, muscle contracture or shortening, or general loss of mobility.

Patients with chronic lumbar pain usually have lumbopelvic myofascitis, which prevents normal excursion of the pelvis. In addition, their hip inflexibility leads to a vicious cycle. Their inability to use proper lumbopelvic and lower-quarter biomechanics makes it impossible for them to achieve the proper posture to lift an object[30]; as a result of their faulty spinal mechanics, these patients are constantly injuring and reinjuring themselves. Failure to recognize myofascial disorders that lead to chronic hip and lumbar spine inflexibility perpetuates the provision of futile, revolving-door health care that exasperates the sufferer of chronic low back pain.

Flexibility testing should address the culprits commonly responsible for chronic back pain. The examiner should check the following muscle groups for tightness or hypertonicity, as well as for contracture or shortening:

1. SPINAL ERECTOR MUSCLES. With the patient in the supine position, the clinician gently bends the patient's knee to the chest. This stretches the muscles required for extension of the lumbosacral spine, namely the erector muscles of the spine. The gluteals are also stretched. As always, a bilateral comparison is advisable.

2. HIP FLEXOR MUSCLES. The best way to stretch or test for tightness of the iliopsoas muscle is first to bend the knee to slacken out the quadriceps muscles. With the patient prone, the clinician places the affected hip into extension, then abducts the thigh. Stabilizing the patient facilitates stretch of the hip extensor muscles. Active stretching of the quadriceps muscles can precede iliopsoas stretching to reduce the effect of the rectus femoris during testing of the hip flexor muscles.

3. HAMSTRING MUSCLES. If tight, the hamstring muscles can pull eccentrically on the pelvis. Combined with tight erector muscles of the spine, this can place the low back under a good deal of stress. Placing the patient supine and keeping the patient's hips and buttocks down to the table, the clinician performs a straight leg raise with the knee held in extension. A bilateral comparison should indicate any hamstring contracture or tightness.

4. GLUTEAL MUSCLES. The patient should be supine and placed in hip flexion with a bent knee. The lower leg can be internally rotated with thigh adduction to facilitate a stretch of the rotator muscles of the hip, such as the gluteus medius and piriformis.

5. QUADRICEPS MUSCLES. With the patient prone and the clinician's inferior hand on the affected knee, the clinician uses his or her shoulder to move the lower leg gently toward the ipsilateral buttock to induce knee flexion. The patient's pelvis can be stabilized as needed. The clinician then compares the lack of excursion with the buttocks from one side to the other.

Fixation and the Locomotor System

There are two types of fixation to be considered during a musculoskeletal examination: muscular and articular (Table 8-4). Many patients with low back pain have both

Table 8-4	Muscular versus Articular Fixation	
Muscular Fixation	**Articular Fixation**
Spasm or splinting of large muscle groups such as hip and spinal extensors and knee flexors	Loss of joint play as opposed to affected arc of normal movement
Pain or tightness when muscle system in doubt is placed on stretch in absence of joint play	Restoration of normal articular mechanisms
Lesions with somatic dysfunction on passive movement that do not respond to joint gapping in neutral position	Motion restriction in articulations that do not possess intrinsic muscles
	Movement restriction in positions of relaxed musculature
Shortening or overt contracture of muscle or muscle group that limits excursion in body part with evidence of taut and tender fibers or trigger points	Lack of springy end feel in a vertebral segment that signifies joint blockage

muscular and articular restrictions, and it is not always easy to distinguish one from the other. In the case of the sacroiliac joint, however, there are no intrinsic muscles involved, and the presence of restricted joint play indicates fairly clearly the presence of an articular lesion.[123] Thus manipulation of the sacroiliac joint will most likely restore lumbosacral mechanics.

The physiologic impact of fixation, both muscular and articular, can begin at the lumbar spine and be felt as far distal as the foot and as proximal as the cervical spine. Altered gait and biomechanical transfer of loads help accentuate local pathologic responses at distant sites. During the observation and examination of the patient with a problem in the lumbar spine, the clinician should always keep in mind the probability of locomotor dysfunction at different sites of the lower extremity.[122]

PART TWO: TREATMENT MODALITIES FOR LOW BACK PAIN

Although there is a wide spectrum of treatment modalities available to combat low back pain, few have empirical evidence to support their efficacy.[117] Modern, clinically controlled trials are now demonstrating the effectiveness of spinal manipulation, however, and this type of therapy seems to be gaining widespread acceptance within the academic and research communities.[42,117] Most randomized clinical trials conducted to study acute episodes of low back pain of a mechanical origin have shown that spinal manipulation provides both pain relief and functional improvement faster than other methods of treatment or the natural history of illness.[14,31,86,199] Recent cost profile analysis of chiropractic treatment as compared with medical treatment (i.e., outpatient versus inpatient care) has been quite favorable to chiropractic treatment.[190] Exercise, life-style modification, weight control, and physical fitness are also important considerations in planning the care of the patient with low back pain.

There are five major classifications of treatment and rehabilitative modalities for low back pain: (1) chiropractic spinal manipulation, (2) manual and mechanical traction, (3) spinal and pelvic mobilization, (4) physiotherapeutic modalities and ancillary procedures, and (5) exercise and spinal rehabilitation. All or none of these treatment options may be appropriate for a particular patient, depending on the clinical picture.

Traditional medical treatments (e.g., bed rest and medication) are not included here, because recent changes in standards of care have rapidly moved treatment away from such passive forms of intervention. Furthermore, passive modalities such as electrical stimulation, hot and cold therapy, and ultrasound have no proven effectiveness as long-term treatments; therefore they should be used only in conjunction with other recommended treatment in the acute inflammatory phase of spinal dysfunction. This recommendation is extended to medication as well.

The treatment of low back pain has three stages of care, each addressing different issues:

1. Initial acute care addresses the individual's pain and may include treatment to combat swelling, spasm, and inflammation.
2. Secondary biomechanical corrections address myofascial and articular dysfunction, loss of functional abilities (both static and dynamic), and the mechanical system of the spine and pelvis as a unit.
3. The tertiary stage of rehabilitation addresses the strength of the supporting structures of the spine and pelvis, as well as spinal flexibility in relation to proper fundamental lifting and task patterns, the individual's overall level of physical fitness, and the dynamic coordination of the locomotor system as a whole.

Chiropractic Manipulation

In the treatment of mechanical disorders of the spine, chiropractic manipulative therapy can be quite effective.[40] Pain control, stretching of myofascial structures, increased spinal and articular mobility, and improvements in muscular stretch reflexes and tone are just some of the possible favorable results of spinal manipulative therapy.[38,113] Patients with myofascial disorders, osteoarthritis, or degenerative disk disease may experience an increase in spinal motion and a decrease in stiffness, discomfort, and pain with chiropractic manipulation.[38,85]

By changing tension in the joint capsule, manipulative techniques activate the type I and type II receptors found at the outer joint capsule.[218] Type I mechanoreceptors negate joint tension through static and dynamic modes; type II mechanoreceptors monitor movement of the articulation. Manipulative therapy not only can affect the spinal pain response through nociceptive influence, but it also seems to influence muscle tone and cord reflexes.[90,177] Spinal manipulative therapy may also positively affect plasma beta-endorphin levels,[44,202] as well as other immune and biologic markers.[29,136]

Joint manipulation differs from mobilization in physiology and function. Manipulative techniques bring a diarthrodal articulation beyond the physiologic range of motion without exceeding the anatomic limit. Long- or short-lever thrusts can force movement beyond an elastic barrier into the paraphysiologic space. This is usually associated with an audible pop or crack that is caused by cavitation of the joint.[195] It is believed that a sudden release of gases in the joint's synovial fluid is responsible for the "click" heard during manipulation. Mobilization, on the other hand, takes place within the physiologic joint space and does not go beyond the elastic barrier.

Distractive Techniques

Flexion distraction and other manual techniques allow distraction of the lumbopelvic spine while the patient is in the prone position (Figure 8-27). As with intermittent traction, the practitioner separates the intervertebral units and places the spine in a palliative position of derotation.

Distractive techniques make it possible for the clinician to treat the patient who cannot tolerate rotational thrusts because of acute pain, muscle spasm, or inflamed nerve roots. Other advantages include separation and restoration of motion into the facet joints and early, active intervention with mobilization and manipulation. These techniques have few adverse side effects.[181] Distraction procedures also allow the clinician to "buy time" while the patient's nerve roots or disks "calm down." For example, some cases of HNP in the lumbar spine may need to undergo distraction before high-velocity rotational manipulation can be initiated. As soon as adjunctive therapy, distraction, and rest reduce the inflammation, the patient may be a candidate for appropriate high-velocity thrust adjustments.[119]

High-Velocity Rotational Techniques

When directed at the posterior joint component of the three-joint complex, adjusting procedures in side posture place motion in the spine. Most chiropractic adjustments are delivered with a high-velocity, low-amplitude thrust. A short- or long-lever arm can be used to move the (fixed) hypomobile joint lesion into the paraphysiologic space. Spinal manipulation is directed at connective tissues because of their viscoelastic properties.[16] The patient may be placed in several different positions, but the most common is the lateral recumbent posture (Figure 8-28). Side-posture manipulation of the lumbar spine causes elongation and elastic deformation of contracted tissues,

such as capsular fibers, ligamentous fibers, discal material, tendons, and articular cartilage.[15]

Among the many lesions that seem to respond to this type of adjusting are disk lesions with sufficient spinal canal clearance, facet syndrome, muscle strains and myofascitis, and sacroiliac dysfunction.[19] The ability of high-velocity rotational manipulation to correct biomechanical spinal faults, such as joint blockage and facet immobility, cannot be overestimated.

Manual and Mechanical Traction

Spinal traction involves the administration of a series of longitudinal forces directed at the spine. Only 20 years ago, continuous hospital-based traction for 2 to 3 weeks was advocated for the treatment of lumbar spine disease. This is no longer an appropriate treatment. Manual techniques and mechanical traction are still used for intermittent periods of traction in chiropractic and physical therapy clinics around the world, however.

A clinician can easily initiate manual traction through hand or ancillary techniques. Dutchman's rolls and table inclination angles, combined with manual stretching or pressure, can effectively distract the elements of the vertebral column. Intersegmental manual traction may produce a pumping effect to increase

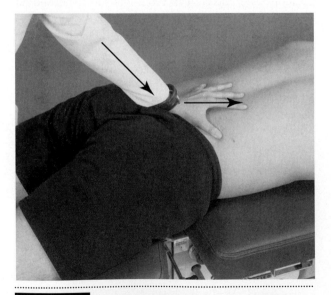

Figure 8-27 Graded loading of lumbar spine with flexion distraction technique.

(From Bergmann TF, Davis PT: *Mechanically assisted manual techniques: distraction procedures,* St Louis, 1998, Mosby.)

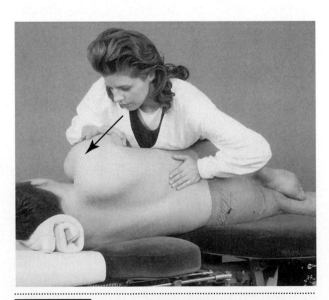

Figure 8-28 Clinician demonstrating a typical side-posture lumbar manipulative procedure.

(From Bergmann TF, Davis PT: *Mechanically assisted manual techniques: distraction procedures,* St Louis, 1998, Mosby.)

vascular and lymph flow at the spinal unit, as well as stretch and mobilize the articular joint capsules.

Many physiotherapy companies manufacture mechanical traction tables that make it possible to place a harness around the patient's pelvis and apply traction force to the spine while the patient is in either the prone or supine posture. Lumbar mechanical traction usually involves poundage no greater than one quarter to one half of the patient's body weight. Traction can be programmed to induce static, intermittent, or continuous pressure. Patients with subacute and chronic disk disease may benefit from this therapy.

Once the craze of fitness fanatics, inversion therapy has lost some of its former popularity. It requires very careful patient selection. Contraindications include advanced age, neurologic instability, peripheral vascular disease, hypertension, ocular problems, and certain peripheral orthopedic injuries. Younger, healthier patients can usually achieve an effective stretch and traction force at the lumbar spine with few adverse side effects. Because it helps ensure that the stretch or traction force is placed at the spine instead of at the lower limb, an inversion unit with a roller for the hips and pelvis (so that the patient is suspended from the unit at the pelvis) is preferable to a unit with ankle boots from which the patient is suspended.

Spinal and Pelvic Mobilization

For patients with chronic low back pain, mobilization or stretching patterns are crucial in restoring the myofascial tissues to a healthy state. The use of these patterns eventually leads to the return of lumbopelvic flexibility, which enables the subject to achieve the full active range of motion and proper mechanical postures conducive to lifting. Mobilization techniques for the lumbopelvic region include PNF patterns and muscle energy techniques. Contract-relax patterns may be developed through an isometric muscle contraction or an accommodative resistance arc. After muscle contraction, a period of reflex relaxation occurs, and the joint is then mobilized or stretched to a new resting position or length.

The practitioner may prescribe static stretching to be done at home to supplement the work performed in the office or during rehabilitation. Williams' flexion exercises, for example, are fairly benign movements that mobilize the lumbar apophyseal articulations and gently stretch the spinal erector and hip extensor muscles (Figure 8-29). Static stretches for the hamstring, quadriceps, and gluteal muscles can also supplement the

Williams' program. All stretches should be performed on both sides, with one leg or hip stretched at a time. Stretches should be held for a minimum of 10 to 20 seconds with slow, deliberate increases in range of motion consistent with joint creep and capsular relaxation.[114] Ballistic or fast stretches may not be appropriate, since they do not provide a controlled environment for patients with spinal injuries.

A muscle energy technique or PNF is helpful as an ancillary procedure to chiropractic manipulation of the lumbosacral spine. The technique is most efficient for rehabilitation patterns of muscular recruitment, and it helps overcome the secondary muscular component of joint dysfunction and pain. With a working knowledge of applied anatomy, the clinician can effectively carry out proper proprioceptive arcs in the office before manipulative therapy (Table 8-5). Gentle control of movement and muscle contraction is essential at all times.

Physiotherapeutic Modalities and Ancillary Procedures

Acute care of the lumbar spine often necessitates the use of adjunctive therapy (e.g., electrotherapy, ultrasound, cryotherapy, moist heat) for the control of pain, swelling, and inflammation (Table 8-6). These three sequelae of acute soft-tissue injury are barriers to manual therapy. Thus the limited use of physiotherapeutic techniques in acute care not only facilitates healing by controlling and limiting the inflammatory response of the tissue, but physiotherapeutic modalities may enable the clinician to institute manual or manipulative therapy earlier. As a result, the patient can improve his or her mobility and function in a shorter time period. Similar to rest and medication, physiotherapeutic modalities are treatment

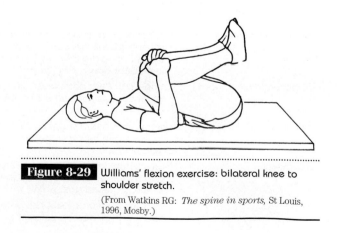

Figure 8-29 Williams' flexion exercise: bilateral knee to shoulder stretch.

(From Watkins RG: *The spine in sports,* St Louis, 1996, Mosby.)

methods with short-term objectives, because they do not prevent long-term morbidity in patients with low back pain.

Clinical considerations for the use of these modalities include the following:

- What is the age and medical status of the patient?
- What are the indications and contraindications for the modality?
- What is the patient's fitness level?
- Which positions are palliative, and which are provocative?
- Which modality is most efficient for the injury?

Table 8-5 Proprioceptive Mobilization Patterns of the Lumbopelvis

Muscle Involved	Position for Mobilization and Stretch
Psoas	Prone, knee flexed, hip extended, thigh abducted
Hamstring	Supine, knee extended, hip flexed
Quadriceps	Prone, knee flexed, hip neutral
Hip or spinal extensors	Supine, knee flexed, hip flexed
Gluteal or pelvic rotators	Supine, knee flexed, leg rotated, hip adducted
Quadratus lumborum	Sitting, trunk bent, hip stationary

- Does the patient have a metallic implant, wear contact lenses, or have a pacemaker?
- Is the patient pregnant?

Electrotherapy

With the experience of post–World War II care, the physical therapy profession entered the spotlight of medical treatment. The therapeutic use of electrical stimulation also became more common. In the 1940s and 1950s, most electrotherapy units were low-voltage, high-amperage. Galvanic current, as it was known, was used in direct current devices that emitted a flow of electricity in one direction for 1 second or longer. Thus they were not quite as comfortable as today's electrical stimulation units, which involve shorter bursts of electrical current, emit many pulses per second, and have varying wave forms for each type of unit[4]:

Monophasic: High-voltage stimulation (HVS)

Biphasic: Variable muscle stimulation (VMS)

Polyphasic: Sine wave, faradic or Russian stimulation, interferential currents (IFC)

Currents can be continuous, interrupted, or modulated for pain or muscle recruitment.[99]

The clinical uses of electrical stimulation include the following:

- Acute or chronic pain control through desensitization or endogenous opiate release
- Reduction of swelling and inflammation through mechanical means
- Breaking the spasm-pain-spasm reflex cycle

Table 8-6 Clinical Use of Modalities for Low Back Pain

Modality	Clinical Use	Contraindications
Electrical stimulation	Control of pain, muscle spasm, swelling; counterirritant, desensitization; muscle re-education in disuse atrophy and immobilization	Pacemaker, malignancy, dermatitis, metallic implant, gravid uterus
Ultrasound (continuous)	Chronic low back pain, muscle hypertonicity or contracture, adhesions or fibrosis	Open growth plates, treatment requiring application directly over spinal cord, acute care, swelling, metallic implants
Ultrasound (pulsed)	Chronic myofascial trigger points, acute spinal strain injuries, acute pain or inflammation	Treatment requiring application directly over spinal cord, metallic implant
Cryotherapy	Acute spinal injuries, acute or chronic peripheral joint injuries, muscle sprains, swelling, neuralgias, pain	Treatment for longer than 15-20 minutes or on areas of desensitized skin
Moist heat	Subacute or chronic low back pain, muscle strain or tightness, myofascitis	Acute care, swelling, treatment requiring direct application on fair skin or desensitized areas

- Muscle reeducation and recruitment patterns of unused atrophied muscles or postmanipulation soft tissues[98]

Electrical stimulation can be used in conjunction with either moist heat or ice therapy, because moisture can increase the depth of penetration of the electrotherapy.

Ultrasound

Musculoskeletal ultrasound can be useful in both chronic and acute soft-tissue injuries. Continuous ultrasound (100% duty cycle) should be used for chronic conditions only. It has a deep penetrating heating component. In addition, continuous ultrasound has chemical and physical tissue properties that increase cell permeability and thus promote the absorption of the products of inflammation.

The typical duty cycles of pulsed ultrasound are 25% or 50%. Because its duty cycle is less than 100%, pulsed ultrasound does not possess a thermal effect. Rather, it has an antiinflammatory effect, which is the result of its ability to absorb tissue exudates and precipitates, and it can also help reduce muscle spasm. Pulsed ultrasound is used in cases of acute injury or in conjunction with high-voltage stimulation for chronic myofascial trigger points (trigger point ultrasound or combination therapy).

Cryotherapy

The therapeutic use of cold is common in the care of acute trauma and the appendicular skeleton. Because of the likelihood of swelling in injured dependent joints, cryotherapy should always be used for their care. In the case of spinal injury, however, the particular circumstances determine whether heat or cold is appropriate.

For the lumbar spine, cryotherapy is used primarily in the first 72 hours of treatment for acute traumatic spinal injury or acute exacerbations of sprain and strain. The use of traction or electrical stimulation can accompany the application of cold packs placed over the injured area for 15 minutes. A cloth dampened with warm water can protect the skin and add comfort. The cold pack should remain off for a full hour between applications. A second treatment option is the application of ice by means of a massage performed in a circular fashion for 5 minutes until the area is numb; such a massage may be repeated every hour. The application of ice provides the following:

- Reduces muscle spasm
- Acts as a localized anaesthetic to control pain

- Localizes antiinflammatory and control of swelling (augmented with the use of concomitant compression)
- Prevents the widespread extravasation of extracellular fluid in the trauma injury region when used with rest, compression, and elevation (RICE)[115]

Vapor coolant sprays (e.g., fluoromethane and ethyl chloride) are helpful in the treatment of myofascial pain disorders and in efforts to mobilize the spine. Cold has been shown to be a potent counterirritant to trigger point pain in dysfunctional muscles, and the spray-stretch technique (i.e., first spraying the contracted muscles with a coolant and then stretching them) is a viable alternative in treatment.[198]

Ice should not remain in place longer than 15 to 20 minutes to prevent a reflex vasodilation response. Extra care is necessary when ice is applied to desensitized areas or to patients who are very young or very old.

Moist Heat

For centuries, heat has been used to alleviate pain and heal wounds. The local physiologic effects include not only vasodilation, but heat also increases the metabolic rate of tissues, the flow of blood, and the supply of nutrients to the tissues. Moist heat allows for greater tissue and skin penetration than dry heat, because convection is greater with moist heat. Without moisture, heat has a tendency to dry out tissues, which can lead to vasocongestion and edema.

Wet or moist heat can be applied to the lumbar spine by means of a hot shower, hot whirlpool, hydrocollator pack (150° F to 170° F), or hot towel. Treatment time is usually 15 to 30 minutes. In the office, hydrocollator packs are applied over a towel and can be used in conjunction with manual or electrotherapy.

Subacute and chronic low back disorders are well-suited for treatment with moist heat. Caution is essential to prevent burns when using heat with patients who are fair-skinned, desensitized (e.g., because of a prior injury or questionable mental status), very young, or very old.

Exercise and Spinal Rehabilitation

Rehabilitation of the lumbar spine encompasses various aspects of spinal health, including flexibility, functional capacity, paravertebral strength, muscular endurance, and dynamic power. In view of the potentially wide range of treatment needs, clinicians should establish realistic goals for patients with low back disability. Sometimes, teaching a patient to sit, stand, and walk properly is an enormous feat.

Exercise is being used more and more as a primary treatment mode for spinal dysfunction and as an alternative to surgery in cases of herniated lumbar intervertebral disks.[174] Three major components of a lumbar exercise program are (1) the spinal stabilization series of exercises, (2) a functional therapeutic squatting program, and (3) mobility training of the lumbopelvic spine.

Spinal Stabilization Program Series

As noted earlier, the hip extensor muscles function partly to protect the inefficient erector muscles of the spine in the lumbopelvic region. The spinal stabilization program series of exercises not only strengthens the hip and spinal extensor group, but it also coordinates the cooperative movements of the region (Table 8-7).

The patient begins by gently contracting the buttocks while in the supine position, then tilts the pelvis, and ends by performing abdominal work with the knees bent. In this supine position the patient can progress to unilateral leg lifts with gluteal contraction (Figure 8-30) and lumbosacral arches, which can be performed with or without a medicine ball.[167]

Prone leg lifts can begin, provided that extension is palliative. In the prone position the patient performs a series of stabilization exercises, including single leg lifts, opposite arm–opposite leg lifts, and tandem movements in the "all fours" position. The patient can be placed simultaneously in the McKenzie extension program to improve low back flexibility in extension and strengthen the spinal erector muscles in this arched-extended posture (Figure 8-31). All these exercises, which can be performed in the office or at home, aid greatly in finding the "neutral" or stable position of the spine and trunk in space.[53] The extensors of the hip and pelvis and spine all work together, and they relate to the multijoint-multiregional movements of everyday living. Dynamic pelvic stabilization and balance exercises aid in kinesthetic awareness and proper biomechanical transfer of muscular activity to the lower limb and pelvis.[54]

The key to a successful strengthening program of the lumbopelvic region is to strengthen and activate the hip extensors, not to isolate the spinal erector muscles. Back flexion-extension devices that immobilize the pelvis to inactivate the hip extensors do not permit functional movements during rehabilitation, however. Variability of measurements in isokinetic testing is also a common problem.[74]

Table 8-7	Spinal Stabilization Series of Exercises	
Position	**Exercise**	**Muscles Affected**
Supine, knees bent	Crunches, abdominal curls	Rectus abdominis, thoracolumbar fascia
	Pelvic tilt	
	Single leg lift	Gluteals, spinal erectors
	Back and hip extension (arch)	Thigh, gluteals, spinal erectors
		Gluteals, spinal erectors, quadriceps
Prone	Single straight leg raises	Hamstrings, gluteals, ipsilateral spinal erectors
	Tandem opposite arm or leg raises	
	McKenzie extension program	Spinal erectors, gluteals, hamstrings
		Spinal extensors

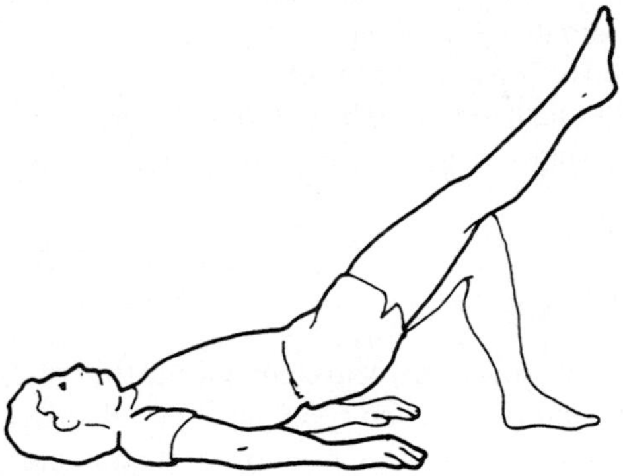

Figure 8-30 Single leg raise with pelvic extension from the supine posture.

(From Watkins RG: *The spine in sports,* St Louis, 1996, Mosby.)

Functional Therapeutic Squatting Program

Inherent in human beings, the squatting movement appears at a very early age. A toddler squats to balance his or her weight in attempting to stand erect and begin to walk. Because of a wonderfully flexible trunk-pelvis-hip movement, a toddler performs a perfect biomechanical squat that makes it possible for the toddler to achieve a low center of gravity and to balance his or her disproportionately large head. Adults, on the other hand, develop such inflexibility at the hips and trunk that they

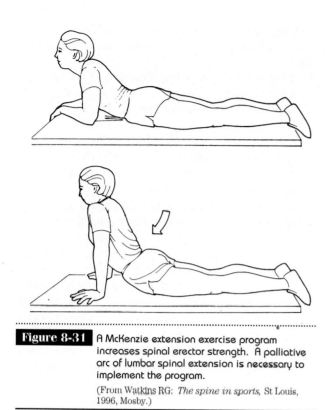

Figure 8-31 A McKenzie extension exercise program increases spinal erector strength. A palliative arc of lumbar spinal extension is necessary to implement the program.

(From Watkins RG: *The spine in sports*, St Louis, 1996, Mosby.)

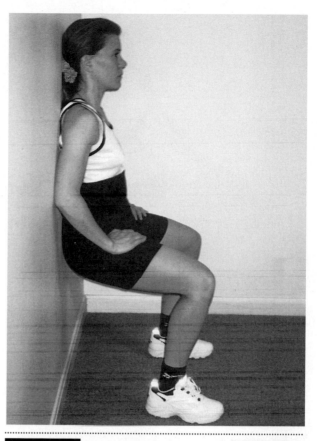

Figure 8-32 Wall squat; patient in a stable position with neutral spine.

almost invariably substitute knee flexion or trunk bend for motion that should take place around the hips and pelvis. Unfortunately, lumbopelvic hypomobility may be a causative factor in the development of low back dysfunction and chronic disability.

A functional squatting program begins with isometric wall squats (Figure 8-32). These exercises are ideally suited to patients in subacute care. The muscles of the lower limb, hip, and pelvis all contract; in addition, the abdominal and lower spinal muscles contract so that they statically contribute to maintaining this posture.

Next, to enhance flexibility, patients can begin to perform free-hand squats with no weight, or they may use a broom handle or stick to help maintain balance. This exercise can be done in conjunction with a myofascial care program (e.g., PNF) in the office and supplemented with a flexibility-stretching program for the home.

The focus of a functional squatting program should fall on form and volume (i.e., high number of repetitions and sets), since the subject will learn only through repetition (Figure 8-33). The following checklist on proper form emphasizes motion and rotation through the hips and pelvis and a vertical position of the lower leg (tibia):

1. Movements should be as deliberate and full as possible, with no jerky motion or swinging of the body or weight.
2. The amount lifted is not an important factor in rehabilitation; improving flexibility of the hips and spine is the primary goal.
3. The knees should never come forward, with the lower limb pivoting from the knee as the femur moves around a stationary tibia. The lower leg should have a vertical orientation at all times. The knees should never go past the toes!
4. The weight should feel flat on the foot throughout the movement.
5. The trunk should be inclined forward to activate the powerful hip extensor muscles as the hip and knee flex. The coordination of trunk, leg, and knee motion must be learned. To squat properly, the speed of movement at the hip and knee should be almost equal.

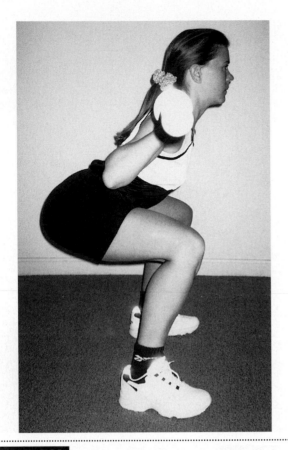

Figure 8-33 Proper form for squatting.

Repetitions of squats help patients with low back pain become more conditioned and flexible. Unlocking the hips and pelvis makes them feel less pressure at the lumbosacral joint and improves drastically their range of motion. Once they progress to weight, it should be kept light to encourage proper form and multiple repetitions. Spinal rehabilitation involves teaching patients to become more efficient and flexible in movement and to improve their capacity to perform work; lifting heavy weights is not task-oriented for most patients.

Mobility Training of the Lumbopelvic Spine

Once the patient with a low back problem has worked through the myofascial flexibility, spinal stabilization, and therapeutic squatting components of a spinal rehabilitation program, he or she can begin to perform more dynamic movements that require faster (ballistic) motion. The following are some generally accepted guidelines for dynamic exercise programs for the patient with low back pain:

1. Avoid isolated flexion and extension of the spine on a fixed pelvis.
2. Avoid trunk bending with both legs in the extended position.
3. Keep movement forces close to the limbs and spine.
4. In the beginning, limit the number of exercises performed to keep total spinal loading to a minimum.
5. Keep the exercises functional and task-specific.
6. Ensure that the patient has completed acute care treatment before recommending a mobility training program.
7. Use dynamic exercise programs in conjunction with a stretching and flexibility regimen.

Assuming that the individual is functional and has adequate strength, movements through an aquatic medium are often helpful. Straight swimming and turns in water promote dynamic function of the trunk. Walking or running in water, with or without a flack jacket or a weighted life preserver, may help the patient become stronger in a fairly safe environment.

Before the initiation of dynamic weight-bearing exercises, the patient can use a stationary bicycle or upper body ergometer. This type of exercise promotes fitness and weight control, both of which have a positive effect on the lumbar spine.

Running or ground-reactive force training should start carefully with jogging on grass. The subject can move up to harder surfaces, such as a cinder track, as long as the track has no great inclines. Treadmills, nordic climbers, and other weight-bearing aerobic equipment can be incorporated into the program as well. Hops, leaps, and other plyometric movements are not appropriate for the vast majority of patients in rehabilitation for spinal problems.

Lumbar Spine Surgery: A Reserved Procedure

Although spinal surgeons performed scores of procedures on patients with low back pain in the 1970s, the medical profession started to show more restraint in the 1980s. The number of poor clinical outcomes in lumbar spine surgery, the prospects for malpractice claims, and the narrowing field of "spinal surgical specialists" willing to accept these cases were all partly responsible for this trend. The increasing emphasis on spinal rehabilitation and alternatives to orthodox medical treatment were also contributing factors.

Clinicians in the 1990s are continuing to lean heavily on conservative care, including exercise rehabilitation, manipulative therapy, and life style changes. Managed care and the use of diagnosis-related groups (DRGs), both intending to help contain medical and hospital costs, place special emphasis on early intervention and ergonomic programs. Careful patient selection for surgery will continue to be the major reason that patients, whose conditions are refractory or not appropriate for conservative care, will have a greater chance for a successful outcome when surgery is indeed a necessity.

Overwhelming evidence points to the value of a conservative approach in the care of the lumbar spine:

- The scope of danger signs has narrowed for low back and leg impairment that require an immediate and aggressive surgical approach.
- Spontaneous regression of herniated nucleus pulposus has been documented on CT[196] and MRI scans.
- Some studies have shown, perhaps because of poor patient selection, that a large percentage of patients continue to have low back pain after lumbar surgery,[46] and some actually get worse.[223]
- Chiropractic adjustments may change the diameter of a sagittal canal compromised by a herniated nucleus pulposus.[47]
- Patients with free disk fragments have been shown to experience a reduction or loss of pain after conservative care.[174]
- Clinical findings on MRI and CT scans are often ambiguous and do not necessarily correlate with physical findings. For example, false positive results are not that unusual in asymptomatic patients.[130,213]
- Motor weakness, in and of itself, is not a mandate for an operative procedure.
- Sciatica in the absence of cauda equina syndrome must prove that it is recalcitrant to conservative therapy for a minimum of 3 to 6 months.
- The track record of such procedures as chemonucleolysis and percutaneous discectomy is quite tenuous.

It is estimated that only 1% of patients with low back pain will require surgery. Significant disk protrusions with no symptoms are noted incidentally in approximately 20% of the adult population. Most disk protrusions of the lumbar spine follow a self-limiting clinical course, however, and only rarely require surgical intervention. The risk, cost, and plethora of nonoperative options make a surgical procedure the last resort.

Patients who are the best candidates for surgery exhibit the following clinical signs and symptoms:

- Low back or leg pain lasting a minimum of 6 months
- Positive straight leg raise test (i.e., pain along the sciatic nerve) at an angle less than 45 degrees
- True nerve root compression signs
- Motor loss, weakness, or atrophy
- Progressive neurologic deficit or paralysis
- Loss of bowel or bladder function (cauda equina syndrome)
- Clinical correlation with advanced imaging procedures of the severely compromised patient.

PART THREE: CONDITIONS OF THE LUMBOSACRAL SPINE

It has often been said that acute conditions make it difficult to diagnose many cases of low back pain definitively. Acute pain and spasm can indeed blur the true origin of a lumbar spine problem, but the clinician can usually make a differential diagnosis. The application of proper biomechanical principles, together with a complete physical examination, should provide the greatest opportunity to make a thorough, workable diagnosis and to exclude the presence of organic pathology.

Lumbar Disk Disease

Unfortunately, even small disk lesions can cause significant spinal impairment. Central lesions may cause thecal sac displacement or lumbar spinal canal compromise. The level of disability associated with disk disease is usually dependent on the subject's ability to accommodate the lesion via the size of the spinal canal and the bony configuration of the space (Figure 8-34).

Two major types of low back abnormalities center around the intervertebral disk: acute impairment from herniated disks and chronic impairment from degenerative disk disease (Table 8-8). The practitioner approaches each patient with disk injuries from a different perspective, depending on the findings of the neurologic examination and the degree of impairment.

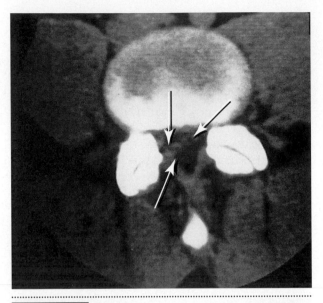

Figure 8-34 Computed tomography scan of a 36-year-old laborer, showing a large right paracentral herniated disk at the L4-L5 level. The patient has low back pain; right buttock, thigh, and leg pain; and L5-level motor weakness. He was treated with lumbar distraction for 4 to 6 weeks, followed by side posture, high-velocity manipulation. The patient successfully completed treatment and returned to work.

Herniated Nucleus Pulposus

The majority of patients with herniated lumbar disks are young adults, especially those in the third and fourth decades of life (Table 8-9). The relative avascularity of the intervertebral disk diminishes its potential for repair. The abnormal motion at the disk, combined with the lordotic posture, places unusual stresses at the lower lumbar region. Approximately 90% of all disk herniations occur at the L4 and L5 levels.[142]

A herniated disk typically signifies the migration of the nucleus of the intervertebral disk through the annulus (Figure 8-35, A-C). Unfortunately, the traditional nomenclature of disk lesions is often contradictory, especially when it comes to orthopedic and radiologic guidelines found in the literature (Figure 8-36). The following definitions of disk injuries, which can be confirmed on CT or MRI studies, are used here:

- DISK PROTRUSION. Nuclear material does not extend beyond the annulus in a contained HNP. This injury may be associated with radial tears of the annulus fibrosus. Stretching of the posterior longitudinal ligament irritates the sinuvertebral nerve.

The patient with a protruded lumbar disk usually has a provoking and palliative arc of movement in the absence of canal compromise, along with back pain and findings of increased intrathecal pressure (i.e., positive Valsalva's maneuver).

- DISK EXTRUSION. A focal herniation contained by the posterior longitudinal ligament extends into the spinal canal. The pathologic findings of the annular fibers are more abnormal than those associated with a protruded disk. The presence of a noncontained HNP in the epidural space may evoke a significant autoimmune-inflammatory response. An increasing number of authors have noted the presence of foreign proteins and phosphorylase A2 at this level, for example.[22,211]

- SEQUESTERED DISK. Also known as a prolapsed disk, a sequestered disk is a free fragment that has broken off or through the annular peripheral fibers in the vertebral canal. Leg pain may be worse than back pain, and the patient is often severely impaired. Many cases eventually require a surgical procedure to resolve the patient's disability.

The pathophysiology of disk injury is usually the result of mechanical trauma combined with the localized reaction of the individual's autoimmune system.

Signs and Symptoms of Herniated Nucleus Pulposus

Most patients with a HNP experience low back pain and some degree of peripheral pain. Typically, sagittal movement provokes pain in either flexion or extension. Individuals with large central herniations or vertebral canal compromise may develop limitations in both flexion and extension arcs. Radicular pain is common, with radiculopathy usually in the buttock, hip, or leg.

Paresthesia in a dermatomal distribution is usually the first sensory finding associated with herniation. Sciatic tension signs are usually present, with pain on the straight leg raise at 30 to 60 degrees the norm. Dorsiflexion of the foot (Bragard's sign), which further increases the tension on the nerve root, usually aggravates pain. A substantial central protrusion may refer pain down either or both legs.

In general, motor findings indicate the presence of nerve compression or extensive disk abnormalities, such as a sequestered (free-floating) fragment in the canal or a rupture. Spasm and an antalgic lean are also possible. Any movement that increases intrathecal pressure, such

Table 8-8	Major Types of Lumbar Disk Disease

	Lumbar Herniated Nucleus Pulposus	**Degenerative Disk Disease**

Physical examination findings	Back or leg pain
	Sciatic nerve tension signs:
	    Positive straight leg raise <60°
	    Positive Bragard's sign
	    Positive bowstring test
	    Positive Bechterew's test
	Painful arc of lumbar flexion, extension, or both
	True nerve root signs:
	    Radiculopathy
	    Motor or sensory deficit
	    Paresthesias
	    Diminished or absent deep tendon reflexes
	Possible antalgia, muscle spasm, instability
		Morning stiffness
		Lumbopelvic hypomobility
		Pain in lumbar flexion
		History consistent with spinal degeneration

X-ray findings	Need to rule out organic pathology Hypolordosis secondary to muscle spasm Possible loss of intervertebral disk height Possible diagnosis of degenerative arthritis	Radiologic signs in acute exacerbation Spur formation Loss of intervertebral disk height Discogenic spondylosis Compatible findings on CT or MRI scans
Treatment plan	CMT, ice, electrotherapy Exercises in palliative arc Short-term lumbosacral support for instability or spasm, if applicable	CMT, medication, or therapeutic modalities for acute flare-ups Exercise, spinal rehabilitation regimen for flexibility and functional strength Weight reduction, if applicable

CT, Computed tomography; **MRI,** magnetic resonance imaging; **CMT,** chiropractic manipulative therapy.

as Valsalva's maneuver, bothers most patients with a contained disk (intact annulus).

Hypomobility of the pelvis seems to be a common residual effect of lower lumbar disk disease. It is not at all rare to isolate a fixed sacroiliac articulation after an L5 disk herniation. It is important to examine the movement at the posterior joints of the level of the disk involved, as well as that above and below the segment.

The patient with acute sciatic neuropathy secondary to a lumbar herniated disk may report tenderness at different areas along the course of the sciatic nerve: the sciatic notch of the buttocks, posterior thigh, popliteal fossa, or calf. The patient with an inflamed sciatic nerve may even walk with a limp or with the knee held in flexion to keep from stretching the nerve. Paresthesias and dermatomal changes (i.e., sensory deficits) may be experienced first, with reflex and motor signs occurring next.

Testing Procedures for Herniated Nucleus Pulposus

Because therapy is initially worked into palliative arcs of motion, range-of-motion testing is critical. The findings of such tests are necessary both for exercise prescription and for chiropractic manipulative therapy. Arcs or posi-

Table 8-9	Age-Related Sites of Pathologic Impairment in the Functional Spinal Unit

Age Group	**Weak Structure**
Adolescence (10-19 years)	Pars interarticularis
Early adulthood (20-40 years)	Lumbar disk

tions that increase the peripheralization of pain are to be strictly avoided in the treatment regimen.

The sequence of imaging modalities is important to proper case management. Initial radiographic studies are appropriate for patients with abnormal neurologic findings, such as nerve root dysfunction (e.g., radiculopathy), motor and sensory disturbance, atrophy, and reflex changes; otherwise, the clinician can order radiographic films in 2 to 4 weeks if the patient does not make progress or regresses under care. Follow-up tests to confirm the nature or presence of a HNP include MRI and CT scans. Patients with suspected spinal canal or nerve root impairment should undergo MRI in the absence of organic disease and osseous pathologic conditions (Figure 8-37).

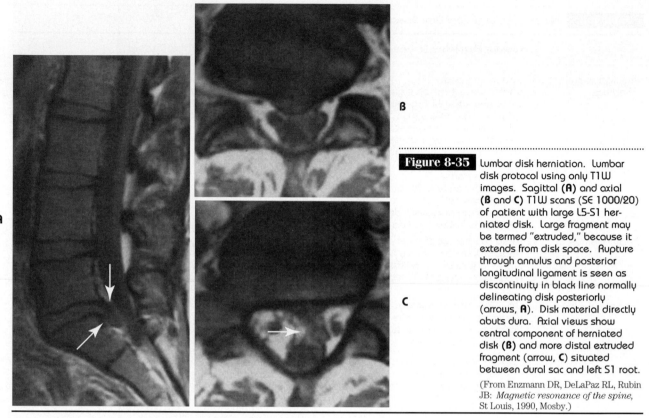

Figure 8-35 Lumbar disk herniation. Lumbar disk protocol using only T1W images. Sagittal (**A**) and axial (**B** and **C**) T1W scans (SE 1000/20) of patient with large L5-S1 herniated disk. Large fragment may be termed "extruded," because it extends from disk space. Rupture through annulus and posterior longitudinal ligament is seen as discontinuity in black line normally delineating disk posteriorly (arrows, **A**). Disk material directly abuts dura. Axial views show central component of herniated disk (**B**) and more distal extruded fragment (arrow, **C**) situated between dural sac and left S1 root.

(From Enzmann DR, DeLaPaz RL, Rubin JB: *Magnetic resonance of the spine,* St Louis, 1990, Mosby.)

Table 8-10 Imaging the Lumbar Spine

Modality	Purpose
Plain-film radiography	View the bony elements of the spine Rule out fracture, infection, arthritides Correlate case history with physical findings
Computed tomography	Delineate lumbar spine fractures Analyze posterior elements Differentiate lateral recess stenosis from facet arthrosis
Magnetic resonance imaging	Define intervertebral disk disease Evaluate neural elements, including the spinal canal and nerve roots
Technetium bone scan	Evaluate chronology of posterior spinal element disease Differentiate old and stable conditions from acute and healing conditions

CT can confirm bony disease, fracture, or lateral recess stenosis; it is also helpful for patients who have experienced gross trauma.

Electrodiagnostic testing should be saved for those patients who have exhibited lumbar nerve root dysfunction with clinical peripheral findings for at least 4 to 6 weeks. Nerve conduction velocity tests can rule out peripheral nerve entrapment of the lower extremity, and electromyography can confirm or rule out spinal nerve root disease.

Advanced diagnostic testing procedures should be reserved for those patients who have been debilitated for a significant period (i.e., a minimum of 4 weeks) and who have reproducible neurologic deficits that seem to have originated in a compromised lumbar spine (Table 8-10).

Treatment of Herniated Nucleus Pulposus

A three-pronged approach is appropriate for the treatment of a herniated disk. First, the patient should undergo a trial of spinal manipulation as indicated by the results of the orthopedic and neurologic examinations. Second, the patient may find supportive exercises and

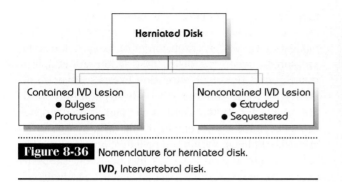

Figure 8-36 Nomenclature for herniated disk.
IVD, Intervertebral disk.

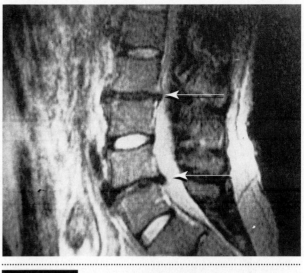

Figure 8-37 Magnetic resonance image of a 38-year-old man with right-sided low back, hip, leg, and calf and foot pain. He had been involved in a motor vehicle accident before this examination, and a previous injury to his back had been diagnosed as a sprain 2 years earlier. Advanced degenerative disk disease with bulging is evident at L2-L3 and L4-L5 (arrows).

rehabilitation methods helpful in the office or at home to restore function of the injured spine. Third, alterations in the patient's life style and daily living habits may be necessary to ensure that reinjury and exacerbations do not interfere with the patient's progress.

Chiropractic Manipulative Therapy. The profile of the patient determines the proper time to begin chiropractic manipulation therapy. Most patients with a herniated disk have both a provoking and palliative arc. Because the patient should be comfortable within the range of motion, rotational strain may not be appropriate initially. In these instances, distraction manipulation in the palliative arc may be useful until the patient's disk or nerve root is not as acutely inflamed (see Figure 8-20); it may be 1 week to 1 month before the inflammation subsides. At that time the clinician can decide whether side-posture adjusting is safe for the patient.

If a central or severely compromising disk herniation causes pain and greatly limits flexion and extension, gentle distraction can begin with the patient's spine in the neutral position. Ice and electrotherapy are helpful adjuncts as well. If spasm and pain make ambulation difficult, the temporary use of a lumbosacral support is advisable.

The patient may lie in the prone position with the spine in lateral flexion during distraction. The clinician should ask the patient repeatedly which postures are comfortable and which cause pain. When getting down from the table, the patient should use the following technique:

1. From the prone posture, roll onto one side with the sciatic leg *down* and the knees bent.
2. Push up with the arms to elevate the upper body *first.*
3. Flex the knees and hips toward the spine while swinging the legs to the side of the table.
4. Continue to push the arms and torso up as the legs clear the table.

These steps should enable the patient to get off the table with less pain and less tension on the sciatic nerve. This procedure is particularly helpful if the patient is experiencing low back instability with pain and spasm.

If the patient is experiencing less pain, less spasm, and greater freedom of movement after a short trial of distraction manipulation, the patient can more comfortably take the side posture (lateral recumbent) position for high-velocity manipulation. This type of therapy has many advantages, including aggressive restoration of joint play, stretching of the paraspinal musculature, motion directed at the functional spinal unit (especially the facet joints), and stimulation of mechanoreceptors. Again, while caution is essential in the treatment of the newly acute case of a HNP, randomized controlled trials have demonstrated the safety and effectiveness of most low-amplitude, high-velocity manipulations when properly applied.[36,38,112]

The clinician should be patient during the care process, using ancillary procedures and distraction, making certain that the side of leg pain and sciatica is always *down* during the initial stage of side posture adjusting, and monitoring patient improvement. Patients who show no positive response to conservative care in three to six treatments are likely candidates for medical intervention (e.g., medication), bracing, and diagnostic imaging procedures. Patients with cauda equina signs should be referred immediately out of primary care.

Those individuals who have a significant impairment that has lasted several months and whose lumbar disk or canal impairment is clearly documented may be candidates for a surgical consultation and, possibly, one of the following procedures:

● LAMINOTOMY. Protruded disk material is extracted mechanically through a small posterior incision of the spine. The particular side of the disk pathology and nerve root are exposed in this traditional operative approach.

● MICRODISCECTOMY. The procedure is similar to a laminotomy, but with minimal exposure and greater magnification via the microscope. Decreased morbidity, less soft-tissue insult, and shorter hospital stays (1 to 2 days average) are some advantages of this technique. The more narrow visual field may be a limiting factor of microdiscectomy in treating older patients with substantial degeneration.

● PERCUTANEOUS DISCECTOMY. This procedure does not involve dissection of muscle or bone removal. A special needle is inserted with fluoroscopic guidance into the disk space, and the nuclear material anterior to the disk herniation is removed by suction. A drawback from this procedure is that posterior fragments may not be accessible for removal.

Supportive Exercise. Listening carefully to a patient's complaints and descriptions of what makes him or her feel better helps the practitioner identify the dysfunction and provoking posture. The palliative arc is useful not only for manipulation, but also for mobilization and exercise methods.

Some patients report relief of pain in flexion, perhaps because of the stretching of the tight spinal musculature and the slackening of the psoas muscle. Many of these patients do well with simple knee-to-chest stretches (i.e., Williams' flexion exercises), which are fairly benign, as well as stretching the spinal erector muscles, gently mobilizing the lumbar facet joints, and stretching the gluteal muscles. Also, bending the knee, for example, by sleeping in the supine posture with pillows under the knee, helps take the pressure off the inflamed sciatic nerve.

In contrast, some patients with a herniated disk respond to gentle extension exercise early in their treatment. These patients experience pain early in the arc of lumbar flexion and have a range of 15 to 30 degrees of extension with which to work. They often state that arching

their backs and "tucking their hips underneath them" gives them relief while sitting or driving a car. This modest movement in extension most likely reduces the pressure between the disks. Distraction and mobilization through McKenzie extension exercises may be effective for these patients, since the hyperlordotic position in which patients perform the McKenzie exercises produces anterior movement of the disk.[40] Such exercises should begin within the palliative arc. At first, the patient is prone with the neck extended and the arms bent. The angles of the position should gradually be increased to the point that the arms are fully extended and the trunk arched in complete extension. Patient-generated end-range loading in extension is helpful in reaching functional status.

Once the patient can be placed in a position that is three fourths extended at the lumbar spine, it is usually safe to place the patient on the side for low-amplitude, high-velocity manipulation for any sacroiliac or posterior joint fixations. Eventually, all individuals with low back pain should be treated with the full range of spinal stabilization exercises geared toward spinal flexibility and strengthening of the hip and spinal extensor muscles.

Alterations in Life Style and Daily Living. To obtain the maximum benefits of a conservative treatment program for lumbar disk disease, the patient must follow certain instructions for home care. Not only does a home care program have obvious physical benefits, it gives the patient an active role in his or her spinal care. If using a lumbar support, the patient should put it on in the practitioner's office to ensure proper fitting of the orthosis. The practitioner should also review the proper use of any medication with the co-treated patient; for example, the patient must understand that nonsteroidal antiinflammatory medications are always taken with milk or food and that patients taking antispasmodic drugs should not drive. Prescribed exercises can be performed several times a day if the patient can tolerate it.

In addition to prescribed exercises, sleeping and postural corrections may be necessary.[45] Patients with sciatic nerve involvement and leg pain should sleep in a position that does not stretch the nerve or leg (e.g., with the hips and knees flexed). The two best sleeping postures are the supine position with pillows under the knees and the side-flexed fetal position. A small pillow placed between the patient's knees helps stabilize the pelvis and prevents the patient's spine from rotating. It is important to remind the patient to sleep with the side of leg pain *down* on the bed.

When traveling in a car, the patient should move the car seat forward so that the knees are bent; this avoids the extended posture of the legs and spine. Sneakers and shock-absorbing shoes should be worn as well. Aggravating activities, such as bending or lifting, should be avoided during the early stages of treatment.

Degenerative Lumbar Disk Disease

Biochemical and histologic changes are evident in the intervertebral disks of patients with degenerative lumbar disk disease. The correlation between back pain and the degenerative process is not yet clear. The pain may be the result of the chemical mediation of the spinal disk or from the biomechanical faults of the degenerated disk. Desiccation, combined with radial, peripheral, or circumferential tears of the annulus, provide for advanced disk deterioration.

The pain pattern associated with chronic intervertebral disk syndromes may be similar to that associated with arthritis—morning stiffness, changes in the severity of pain during sudden barometric changes in the weather,

---

Case History: Disk Herniation

A 37-year-old man complained of low back pain of 4 months' duration, numbness and tingling into the left shin, and pain in the right buttock, groin, and testicles. The findings of a urologic examination were normal. There were no motor or sensory deficits. Chiropractic examination revealed a fixed left sacroiliac joint with palpable tenderness. Because of chronic disability, an MRI scan was obtained (Figure 8-38 *A, B*), which revealed that the L4-L5 disk extended into the spinal canal centrally and to the left. The cauda equina was unremarkable.

The patient's condition was diagnosed as paracentral disk herniation at L4-L5 with thecal sac compression centrally and left. The treatment plan contained the following components:

- Application of ice several times daily
- Williams' flexion exercises (palliative arc)
- Proprioceptive neuromuscular facilitation patterns for contracted hamstring, quadriceps, and hip flexor muscles
- High-velocity chiropractic manipulative therapy for left sacroiliac fixation
- Flexion-distraction manipulation
- Avoidance of lifting

The patient showed increased spinal and pelvic mobility after three treatments. After 3 weeks of care, his low back pain was mild, with only occasional stiffness. Groin and buttock pain had vanished. He was fully functional after the fourth week and was discharged with recommendations for a static home stretching program and spinal strengthening exercises, as well as instructions to return if necessary.

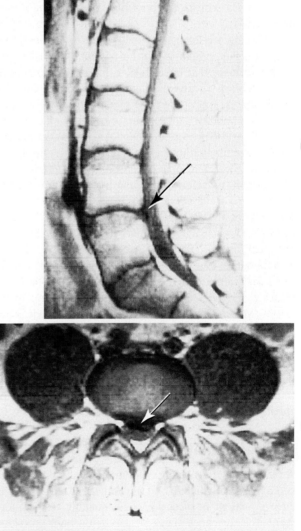

Figure 8-38 **A,** Paracentral disk herniation at L4-L5 in a 37-year-old man. **B,** Thecal sac compression centrally and left.

and secondary muscular complaints. Dull, achy pain over the midline of the spine that increases with lumbar flexion is the usual presentation. During acute flare-ups, the patient may have the same neurologic pattern of peripheralization as the patient with acute HNP (e.g., radiculopathy, antalgic gait). Correlation with prior pain patterns, radiographic studies, and other testing procedures are necessary.

Radiographic evidence of degenerative disk disease includes loss of intervertebral disk height, spur formation, and arthritic bone common to spondylosis. Loss of signal intensity on MRI indicates dehydration of the disk. Such changes in any imaging procedure are not always correlated with the presence of active symptoms, however.

Treatment for patients with signs of degenerative disk disease is similar to that for patients with HNP, except that the former has a shorter duration and is a little more aggressive at an earlier point in the treatment. Manipulation is appropriate for mechanical dysfunction, such as immobility, joint contracture, and mechanical fixation. Exercise prescription should complement manipulative treatment and focus on flexibility and muscle endurance. Stretching of the spinal erector, hamstring, and hip flexor muscles is of paramount importance. Strengthening the abductors and the hip and spine extensors is essential to restore everyday function. Weight reduction is crucial in obese patients who have degenerative disk disease. Smoking cessation is also essential. In a small percentage of patients with chronic disk impairment and nerve root disease, multiple attempts fail at treating the pain. Manipulation under epidural anesthesia (MUEA) with corticosteroid injection holds some promise. The focus on this form of chiropractic manipulative therapy is to change the status of adhesion formation and free spinal segment mobility, often times in difficult cases after unsuccessful surgery.[13] For cases of recalcitrant lumbar radiculopathy, manipulation under anesthesia may be a viable option.

Lumbar Spinal Stenosis

A particularly perplexing dilemma, spinal stenosis presents a special challenge to the clinician. Although it is clearly evident in most advanced imaging tests, spinal stenosis is the cause of many cases of low back problems that are refractory to conservative treatment.

Lumbar stenosis can occur at the central spinal canal or at the peripheral canal where the nerve root exits. Congenital factors such as malformation of poste-

rior elements, dysplastic changes in size and shape of structures, and achondroplastic dwarfism can all decrease the anteroposterior diameter of the canal. Acquired stenosis can result from trauma, infection, metabolic disorders, neoplasm, iatrogenic events, or degenerative spinal disease.[7] Degenerative joint disease of the facet or intervertebral disk or both may also lead to lumbar spinal stenosis.

Conditions That Compromise the Spinal Canal

Two major conditions, both of which compromise the vertebral canal and its neural contents, contribute to lumbar stenosis—facet disease and discogenic spondylosis. Facet disease may be the sequel of an abnormal biomechanical function of the spine, such as the loading of the apophyseal articulations with excessive weight. Posterior joint arthrosis can develop from synovial instability and recurrent sprains. Degenerative arthritis of the facets has the potential to cause stenosis by encroaching on the lateral recess of the spinal canal; not only do these patients usually have limitations in extension, but extension exacerbates their neurologic findings.

Patients with discogenic spondylosis usually have a long history of stiffness, intermittent radicular symptoms, and back pain that is aggravated by the environment (e.g., weather) and by exertion. If the disk disease produces enough degenerative arthritic changes, the patient develops multidirectional pain in addition to flexion discomfort.

Myofascial dysfunction and posterior joint dysfunction of the lumbar spine usually accompany both conditions. Activity may aggravate neurologic claudication, resulting in leg pain, but rest does not necessarily alleviate the pain. On the other hand, rest usually relieves the pain caused by vascular insufficiency of the lower limb after a period of exertion.

There are a variety of structural causes for central canal stenosis:

- Osseous: inferior facet arthrosis
- Discogenic: central disk herniation
- Ligamentous: ligamentum flavum buckling in degenerative spinal disease (Figure 8-39 *A, B*)

Patients with central lumbar canal stenosis exhibit neurogenic claudication with pain upon walking. Temperature changes and weakness of the legs are common, as are night pain and sciatic tension signs. These subjects report feeling that their "legs are giving way." It is necessary to examine both axial and sagittal planes during spinal imaging for central stenosis. Short pedicles

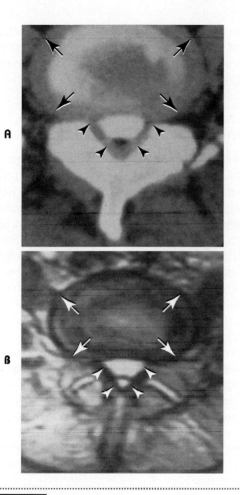

Figure 8-39 Central canal stenosis attributable to a diffusely bulging disk (arrows) and hypertrophy of the ligamentum flavum (arrowheads). Good correlation between **A,** axial computed tomography and **B,** magnetic resonance imaging.

(From Watkins RG: *The spine in sports,* St Louis, 1996, Mosby.)

can reduce anteroposterior canal dimensions (congenital stenosis); and hypertrophy of the facet points and ligamentum flavum, along with disk disorders, may lead to a trefoil-appearing canal (acquired stenosis).[111]

Patients with lateral lumbar canal stenosis have nerve root entrapment, which can be either recurrent or constant. Dynamic nerve root entrapment is more likely to respond to conservative manipulative care. Pain occurs intermittently over years, with occasional injury and flare-ups; it may not be present at the time of examination. Pain may be referred to the hips, buttocks, or pos-

terior thigh, but it is rarely referred to the foot or toes. Although the patient has no motor weakness, sensory changes at the calf are common. Sciatic pressure tests (sciatic notch, popliteal fossa) are usually positive (i.e., they produce pain). Single dermatomal findings are common. Flexion and extension of the lumbar spine may be limited by pain, and biomechanical findings are usually similar to those of degenerative disk disease, such as sacroiliac fixation, facet hypomobility, and myofascial tightness.

Diagnosis and Treatment of Lumbar Canal Stenosis

Computed tomography scans effectively visualize facet arthrosis, disk disease, and lumbar stenosis. X-ray findings of patterns of either heterotopic bone and spur formation or arthrosis of the posterior spinal unit are usually consistent with degenerative spinal arthritis. The neural contents, including nerve root, thecal sac, and spinal canal, as well as the lumbar disks, are best visualized through MRI, however.

Myelography has been used for several decades to diagnose neural compression. "Filling deficits" of intrathecal dye visualize the disk lesions (Figure 8-40 *A, B*). The test has two major disadvantages: it is invasive and requires hospitalization. Myelography is also unable to differentiate disk protrusions from bony encroachment of the spine. Even so, in cases of preoperative screening and multilevel stenotic symptomatology, myelography is still a useful diagnostic procedure.[209]

Specific treatment for individuals with spinal stenosis varies according to the presenting symptomatology and the patient's tolerance for the treatment modality in question (Table 8-11). Any manipulation or supportive exercise should usually avoid extension. If the patient can tolerate rotation, high-velocity manipulation in side posture aids in the restoration of spinal mobility and may provide relief from pain. Chiropractic manipulative therapy may not be successful in all patients, yet conservative treatment should be attempted for each patient for a specified period of time. The clinical trial of chiropractic manipulative therapy should be longer in patients with lateral canal disease, since it is usually a better treatment of choice than surgical correction for this condition.

Clinical findings must be carefully correlated with imaging and electrodiagnostic test results in the selection of a treatment regimen that will be the most effective for the patient. Individuals whose symptoms are infringing on their daily lives and who fail to show signs of

Table 8-11 Lumbar Spinal Stenosis

Physical examination findings	History of back, buttock, and leg pain Radicular signs in acute condition Painful sagittal motion, worse in extension Motor or sensory disturbances in lower extremity possible Need to correlate findings of lateral mass or central canal stenosis Secondary findings of facet or muscular dysfunction
X-ray findings	Degenerative disk disease, facet arthrosis
Treatment plan	Chiropractic manipulative therapy Monitoring neurologic (central canal) signs Physiotherapy and exercise, as indicated Surgical decompression, if unresponsive to conservative care

improvement during prolonged conservative treatment may opt for surgical treatment. For patients with severe canal compromise, surgical decompression of neural elements may be the most viable option.[100]

Posterior (Zygapophyseal) Joint Disorders

The posterior (facet) joints of the lumbar spine play a major role in mechanical back pain, both in the presence or absence of referred pain to the leg.[71,143,146] Not only are the facet joints responsible for coupled and sagittal movements, but they participate in checking or limiting rotation. Repetitive or excessive loading can injure the spinal joints, causing a kinetic disturbance in the joint, an inflammatory reaction in the fibrous capsule, or both. Neurologic compromise and the close relationship of the facet to the spinal canal can render the patient disabled. Osteoarthritis as a result of degenerative changes at the facet joint can also provoke pain.

Individuals with posterior joint disease can develop a myriad of symptoms, ranging from simple low back pain to lumbar spasm, thigh pain, and calf or ankle referral. Sagittal motion or clinical testing of paraphysiologic joint movement evokes pain in most cases. Pain usually occurs paravertebrally as well, with secondary soft-tissue changes a possibility. Manipulation has been shown to bring about a dramatic improvement in posterior joint dysfunction or injury.[35,116,197,199]

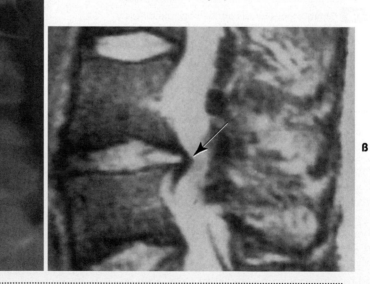

Figure 8-40 Severe spinal stenosis at the L4-L5 disk level on **(A)** the myelogram. **(B)** Central stenosis of the spinal cord, primarily attributable to a posteriorly bulging disk (arrow).
(From Watkins RG: *The spine in sports*, St Louis, 1996, Mosby.)

Facet Sprain

Traumatic injury to the lumbar spine many times involves the facets directly. High-speed impact events, such as motor vehicle accidents, can damage the facets, since the force of the impact may place the spine into rapid flexion and extension. Extension or lordotic loading of the lumbar spine, such as may occur when lifting a heavy object overhead, can also jam the zygapophyseal articulations, evoking an inflammatory response. Similarly, excessive twisting movements, such as those used in tennis or golf, can be the cause of facet sprains.

Lumbar sprains can produce localized pain over the vertebral segments with or without peripheralization of pain. Facet sprain can cause localized swelling, with paraspinal findings of hypertonicity, spasm, and referral of pain to the hip, buttock, or posterior thigh. Nerve root signs are conspicuously absent, and there are no motor or sensory deficits. Because the zygapophysis is innervated by the dorsal ramus, it is often the cause of somatic referral to distant sites. Irritation of the joint capsule, facet ligaments, or intrinsic muscles can all be painful.

On clinical examination, the individual with a facet sprain has pain over the posterior joint, with discomfort in joint play. Terminal flexion is painful, because it stretches the synovial capsule. Extension is painful initially, since the facet joints are imbricated. X-ray films may be taken at the discretion of the clinician, although the correlation of radiologic findings with subject impairment is tenuous at best.

The application of ice and electrotherapy in the office is helpful for acute pain. Flexion of the lumbar spine in a position of distraction or side-posture adjustment is often palliative as well (Table 8-12). Antilordotic exercises performed at home are helpful. Immobilization and medication are rarely necessary.

Posterior Joint Dysfunction (Facet Syndrome)

Postural changes, muscular weakness, and pathomechanical cycles of daily living may lead to posterior joint dysfunction. Clinically, orthopedic findings (other than spinal joint dyskinesia) are often vague or nonexistent. Posterior joint dysfunction can perpetuate lumbar impairment in time, since there is a close relationship between the facet and the intervertebral disk. Isolated single-level dysfunction may progress to degeneration of the functional spinal unit in the future. Chronic dysfunction at the zygapophysis may also be associated with degenerative disk disease, along with concomitant soft-tissue findings.

Examination may reveal swayback or exaggerated lumbar lordosis attributable to poor muscle tone or a protuberant abdomen. The pain is often poorly defined, may be described as "achy," and is commonly felt after exertion. If the dysfunction is chronic and a result of degenerative spinal disease, the patient may have significant morning stiffness. Not only may both passive and active motion produce discomfort, but gross motion may be somewhat limited. Joint play (e.g., paraphysiologic motion) is usually impaired significantly.

The patient may lack nerve root signs and sensorimotor deficits, but may have unusual pain patterns.

Table 8-12 Conditions of the Posterior Joint

	Facet Sprain	Facet Syndrome
Physical examination findings	History of recent trauma Painful sagittal motion, usually arcs of early extension and late flexion No nerve root signs Altered joint play with painful associated soft-tissue findings	Intersegmental dysfunction Altered paraspinal soft-tissue function No neurologic findings, except when advanced disease leads to spinal canal stenosis Sagittal motion and joint play impairment
X-ray findings	Not always applicable Poor correlation with dysfunction, osseous findings	Poor clinical correlation of plain films Degenerative disk disease or facet arthrosis possible in patients with chronic facet syndrome
Treatment plan	CMT Flexion exercises Ice, EMS for acute pain	CMT Flexion exercises Further testing for those with chronic disease and neurologic impairment

CMT, Chiropractic manipulative therapy; **EMS,** electrical muscle stimulation.

Patients with chronic facet syndrome develop adhesions of the synovial joint, which is innervated by the primary dorsal rami. Repeated episodes of hypomobility lead to the breakdown of facet cartilage and, ultimately, anatomic subluxation of the facet and degenerative arthritic changes.[70] When facet disease is advanced, bony encroachment on a susceptible spinal canal can occur (Figure 8-41). Lateral mass stenosis and neuroforaminal impingement can produce symptoms commonly seen in patients with lumbar stenosis. Thus the clinician should examine radiographic films to investigate suspected degenerative changes of the posterior joints for simultaneous lumbar disk disease.

Symptoms of low back and leg pain vary with frequent remissions and exacerbations, and the correlation between the level of impairment and radiographic changes is poor. Individuals with significant neurologic findings or intractable pain may require advanced spinal imaging. The best imaging modalities for these patients are CT and MRI. For ruling out osseous causes of impairment, CT is preferred; MRI is the procedure of choice for ruling out soft-tissue changes commonly associated with posterior joint dysfunction, such as vascular stasis, soft-tissue entrapment, and neural ischemia.

Normal biomechanics must be the goal of treatment. The focus should center not only on restoring joint motion, but on altering pathologic postural and muscular changes. Patients should be properly instructed in how to lift, sleep, and exercise. Weight reduction and improved fitness are often necessary for the patient to reach a satisfactory level of spinal health. Chiropractic adjustments, PNF, spinal stabilization and strengthening exercises, and a static home stretching program are all part of total care.

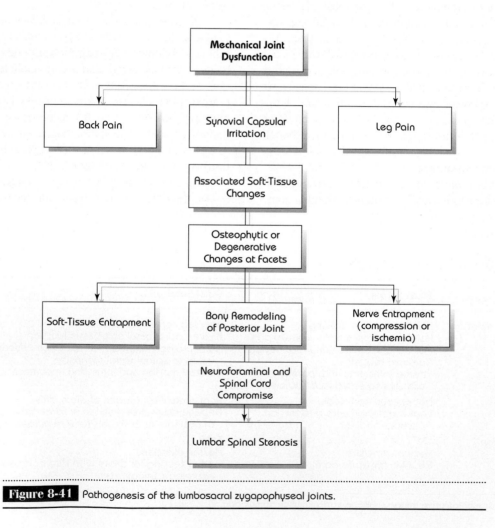

Figure 8-41 Pathogenesis of the lumbosacral zygapophyseal joints.

Pars Interarticularis

Etiologic factors of pars defects that lead to spondylolysis and spondylolisthesis are largely unknown, although there are several theories about the acquisition or development of such defects. Most orthopedic researchers have agreed that perhaps the most feasible of all theories is that a fatigue fracture may occur in segments of the population that are most vulnerable.[212,216]

The incidence of spondylolysis varies in different segments of the population, but it generally falls between 1% and 10%.[106] Acquired or congenital defects can provide the basis for anterior slipping (spondylolisthesis) of one vertebra over another. Although infants are not born with frank abnormalities at the neural arch or fractures of the pars segment, it is possible that dysplastic spinal segments or fibrocartilaginous weaknesses are present at the time of birth.

Repetitious sagittal movements can cause neural arch failure in the laboratory.[94] Thus cyclic loading onto the skeletally immature spinal unit may induce pathologic loads during the childhood years when the neural arch is most vulnerable. Constant lordotic loading in young athletes, such as female gymnasts and interior linemen in football, seems to increase drastically the incidence not only of spondylolysis, but also of eventual spondylolisthesis (Figure 8-42).

Even more unnerving to the academician than the lack of an identifiable major etiologic factor is the difficulty of correlating back pain with radiographic findings of pars pathology. Far too many cases of spondylolisthesis occur as incidental radiologic findings in both symptomatic and asymptomatic patients. Furthermore, findings of spondylolysis in certain individuals have very little, if any, clinical significance.

Chiropractic and biomechanical evaluation of the lumbar spine and pelvis is mandatory when pars pathology is suspected. Findings of sacral dyskinesia, muscle contractures, and abnormal dynamic function of the lumbopelvis and hip are common entities that need attention if the individual is to return to normal functional capacity.

Spondylolysis

A defect in the pars interarticularis with no forward displacement is termed spondylolysis. Defects can be dysplastic, isthmic, degenerative, traumatic, or pathologic.[192] In the Western world, spondylolysis is believed to occur in approximately 5% of the population, with 80% to 90% of these defects occurring at the L5 level.[105,220] No single factor has yet been proved to cause spondylolysis, and a combination of repetitive flexion-extension motion, inherent weakness or developmental defects, and fatigue or stress fracture appears most likely to be responsible for the pathologic process at the neural arch.

Certain segments of the population have an abnormally high incidence of spondylolysis, including American Eskimos and child athletes who participate in gymnastics and football. Several risk factors may be inherent in the growth status of child and adolescent athletes in particular. Rapid periods of growth place the child in a hyperlordotic position, for example, thereby increasing the vulnerability of the posterior spinal unit in extension loading. Because of the relatively immature osseous system of the spine with a fast turnover of bone, an increased remodeling of bone, and a large population of haversian canals, the bony structure may be vulnerable as well. Although spondylolysis may develop at the age of 5 to 7 years, the onset of symptoms may be delayed until the teenage years.

Stress fracture of the pars interarticularis can occur in sports that require extension, such as weight lifting, football, and gymnastics. Unilateral defects may heal more uneventfully than bilateral defects, which may also develop into spondylolisthesis.[121]

Lumbosacral spine films with additional oblique views help the clinician investigate or confirm defects of the pars interarticularis (Figure 8-43). A defect in the neural arch may be visualized on the lateral x-ray film, which should be obtained while the patient is standing. Larger defects or bilateral occurrences may be identified

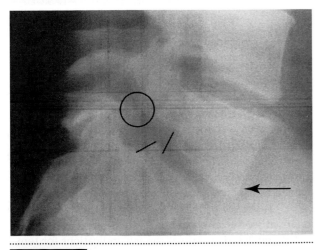

Figure 8-42 L5-S1 spot film depicting pars defect (circle) with a grade I spondylolisthesis at L5 (arrow, lines).

If the severity of symptoms limits the patient's tolerance for being moved, initial care should focus on pain reduction via the control of inflammation and joint swelling. Ice, electrotherapy, and the use of a lumbosacral brace are helpful for the first several treatments. Once the pain of the joint sprain subsides and the patient's range of motion improves, manipulation of the sacroiliac joint often provides dramatic results in mobility and relief from discomfort.

In some individuals with a history of recurrent sacroiliac sprains, capsular and ligamentous laxity may cause the afflicted joint to become hypermobile. Symptoms develop on the side of the unstable sacroiliac joint, but the contralateral hemipelvis often becomes fixated as a way to splint for the opposite sacroiliac joint sprain. The practitioner must carefully spring and palpate the sacroiliac joints on both sides to be certain of adjusting the hypomobile hemipelvis. Bilateral fixation occurs in a percentage of patients as well.

Although x-ray films are not very helpful in the diagnosis of sacroiliac sprain, they may be necessary in the rare case of a patient with leg pain that does not respond immediately to manipulation (Table 8-14). Further investigation may focus on the evaluation of the intervertebral disk spaces and the detection of possible degenerative arthritis. These factors may evoke the pain response; more likely, they are factors that delay recovery.

The goal of rehabilitation is the return to full strength of the spine and pelvis in all ranges of motion. The hip extensors need special attention, since they serve with the erector muscles of the spine to protect the sacroiliac joint. Although the sacroiliac articulation has no intrinsic musculature, proper lifting mechanics and fluid lumbopelvic motion protect the sacroiliac joints when the hip and spine extensors are strong enough. The patient can work on gluteal and hamstring strength with a series of straight leg raises while in the prone position. The practitioner should instruct the patient always to sleep either supine or on one side with the affected sacroiliac joint *down*. Initially, a pillow placed between the knees is helpful.

Sacroiliac Syndrome

Similar to the acute traumatic sprain, the sacroiliac syndrome commonly causes disability and associated mechanical problems. There may be little overt trauma involved in recurrent flare-ups of the sacroiliac syndrome, however, and with the exception of a serious acute exacerbation, swelling or spasm is rare. The patient has

---

Table 8-14   Disorders of the Sacroiliac Joint

	Acute Sacroiliac Sprain	Sacroiliac Syndrome	Hip/Spine Syndrome
Physical examination findings	History of trauma involving lifting or rotating in forward flexed position Palpable pain or swelling over sacroiliac joint Often signs of spinal instability, including an antalgic gait Fixed hemipelvis on motion analysis Referral of pain to buttocks, hips, or legs	Tenderness, hypomobility at sacroiliac joint Tight hamstring and spinal erector muscles Pain provoked by flexion, rotation Functional short leg, pelvic obliquity	Palpable tenderness at greater trochanter, sacrum, sciatic notch, and gluteal musculature Sacroiliac dysfunction Gluteal myofascitis Lumbopelvic inflexibility History of degenerative hip disease or lumbar disk disease
X-ray findings	Not helpful unless condition is unresponsive to treatment in 7-10 days	Possibly helpful in ruling out structural disturbance or metabolic pathologic defect	Need to rule out arthritic disorders of lumbosacral spine and hip joint
Treatment plan	Ice, electrotherapy, CMT Lumbosacral brace initially in cases of instability Sleep and sitting modifications	CMT, hip and pelvis stretching Flexibility, lumbopelvic strengthening	CMT Mobilization, stretching of lumbopelvis, lumbopelvic strengthening Therapeutic modalities as needed

CMT, Chiropractic manipulative therapy.

sacroiliac tenderness, various fixation patterns, and discomfort or limitation in lumbar flexion and rotation. Motion palpation of the pelvis is helpful in isolating the fixed sacroiliac articulation (see Figure 8-26).

Biomechanical findings include moderate-to-severe pelvic obliquity (tortipelvis) and a functional short leg. Subsequent changes in stride length and gait symmetry can lead to a secondary orthopedic problem at the hip, knee, ankle, or foot. Chronic fixation of the involved hemipelvis may lead to hamstring shortening, patellofemoral pain, and subtalar dysfunction. It is essential to rule out an anatomic leg length discrepancy.

X-ray films and clinical findings may be inconsistent, but there may be some useful information gathered from plain films in patients with sacroiliac syndrome. For example, x-ray films may help the practitioner recognize severe obliquity, determine joint asymmetry, and exclude metabolic and degenerative findings. The radiographic findings may do little to alter case management and manipulative treatment, however.

Chiropractic adjustment in side posture is extremely effective for alleviating sacroiliac joint fixation or dysfunction. The freedom of pelvic motion that comes from the restoration of proper joint mechanics at the sacroiliac level may in the long term end in a healthy relationship between the facet joints of the lumbar spine and the intervertebral disks. This change in sacroiliac motion patterns, combined with proper myofascial tension and strength, aids in intersegmental and lumbopelvic mechanics in moving and lifting, thereby improving the ergonomic profile of the individual with low back pain.

Adjunctive care should stress hip and pelvic flexibility by stretching the hamstring and spinal erector muscles. Spinal exercises in extension protect the joint as well. The practitioner should counsel the patient in proper lifting habits, proper footwear, and sleeping habits.

For example, the patient should be advised to avoid lifting objects far removed from the spine and to use the hip extensor muscles. Athletic footwear provide the best support for the human frame, and the patient should sleep in the supine posture or *on* the symptomatic side.

Hip/Spine Syndrome

Caused by a myriad of factors, the hip/spine syndrome affects the lumbopelvis and gluteal region (Figure 8-47). It differs from other sacroiliac syndromes in that pain and dysfunction are noted across the hip and pelvis and that pain does not always originate at the sacroiliac joint. It is commonly associated with gluteal myofascitis and degenerative joint disease at the hip or spine. Often, sacroiliac dysfunction secondary to an arthritic hip is chronic and has serious muscular components of pain and referral.

Palpable pain may emanate from the greater trochanter of the hip where the rotators of the pelvis attach, with pain radiating across the buttocks to the lumbosacral spine. Tenderness or fixation is observed at the sacroiliac joint, and pelvic rotation and lumbar flexion may be limited. There may be myofascial trigger points at the gluteal muscles and the piriformis, with referral to the thigh, hip, or leg. Many patients with hip/spine syndrome have advanced degenerative spinal disease with concomitant arthritis of the hip that causes severe problems in ambulation.

When the clinical findings in older patients suggest hip or spine degeneration, it is prudent to order radiographic studies to evaluate the extent of degenerative arthritic changes and the mineralization of bone before a trial of manipulation. Severe pelvic obliquity and joint arthrosis are seen. A complete orthopedic and neurologic examination of the spine and lower extremity is

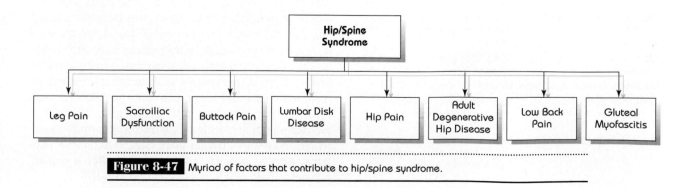

Figure 8-47 Myriad of factors that contribute to hip/spine syndrome.

necessary to rule out spinal cord compression syndromes and lumbar disk lesions that can cause nerve root compression.

A combination of chiropractic manipulative therapy of the sacroiliac joint and myofascial treatments can restore muscular function in the patient with hip or spine degeneration. Stretching and mobilization techniques are helpful, as are modalities such as trigger point ultrasonography and electrotherapy. It is important to monitor leg length and carefully scrutinize the patient's gait both before and after adjustment. The patient should perform static stretching movements at home and should avoid any aggravating activity in the workplace or home.

Lumbopelvic Myofascial Pain Syndromes

Unfortunately, many cases of acute low back pain that are not correctly identified and treated evolve into a chronic spinal problem with significant disability at the muscular level. Therefore, it is imperative that spinal dysfunction be addressed at multiple tissue levels and that all patients be thoroughly treated and rehabilitated to prevent future impairment (Table 8-15).

Patients with muscular dysfunction of the lumbar spine can have varying types of clinical findings and case histories. Although not all individuals have concomitant articular problems, spinal hypomobility is a common finding. Sites of pain and tenderness may vary, and some individuals with lumbar myofascitis have significant metabolic and/or arthritic conditions. Palpable findings of trigger points represent focal areas of inflammation and irritability in the muscle or fascia that refer pain to a distant site.

Muscular fixation alone can be the cause of spinal joint dysfunction. Shortened or contracted muscles of the hip flexors, for example, may affect spinal function in the following ways:

- Contracture of lumbodorsal fascia
- Anterior pelvic tilt
- Inappropriate transfer of loads to the lumbar spine
- Difficulty in attaining the proper biomechanical posture for lifting

In addition, muscle restriction in the presence of active trigger points can mask the proper diagnosis through peripheral referral of pain.[185] Myotogenous pain patterns may come about secondary to spinal trauma, lengthy immobilization, connective tissue disorders, ankylosing spondylitis, chronic low back dysfunction, and degenerative arthritis of the lumbar spine.[60]

Clinical findings that are commonly seen in muscle syndromes of the lumbopelvic spine include the following:

- Hip inflexibility, especially hamstring and psoas insufficiency
- Weakness of the hip and spine extensor mechanism
- Intersegmental lumbosacral fixation
- Myofascial trigger points in the spinal erector, quadratus lumborum, gluteal musculature, and psoas muscles
- Referred zones of pain to the hip, buttocks, thigh and lateral lower leg
- Severe tightness of the outward rotators of the hip
- Muscle hypertonicity
- Palpable tenderness with pressure or stretch
- Taut, tender, or ropelike muscle fibers

Histomorphologic changes in the thoracolumbar fascia of patients with chronic back pain can be extensive. Deficiencies in neural end organs and chronic tissue ischemia have serious clinical implications for patients with chronic back pain.[19] Treatment for myofascial conditions of the lumbopelvic region must be active and aggressive; the restoration of normal muscle length, tension, and strength should be the primary goal. Stretching and mobilization techniques, along with spinal manipulation and physiotherapeutic modalities, are helpful in restoring spinal and lower extremity mobilization and function. Spray-and-stretch technique with fluoromethane or ethyl chloride aids in restoring normal muscle length and reduces trigger point pain,[184] as do PNF patterns. Manual ischemic compression is often a helpful adjunct to therapeutic stretching (Table 8-16).

Table 8-15 Sites of Lumbopelvic Soft-Tissue Syndromes

Condition	Referral Zone or Site of Complaint
Quadratus lumborum syndrome	Gluteal region, anterior iliac spine, greater trochanter of femur
Gluteus maximus or medius syndrome	Sacral and gluteal region, lateral hip
Gluteus minimus syndrome	Lateral hip, thigh, and calf
Chronic lumbar strain (spinal erector muscles)	Laterally to ribs, caudally toward lumbosacral junction
Piriformis syndrome	Sacroiliac region; posterior hip, thigh, calf; possibly sole of foot

Quadratus Lumborum Syndrome

The most commonly overlooked source of lumbar muscle pain may be the quadratus lumborum.[186] This muscle—which not only contributes to the support of the lumbar spine and abdominal cavity, but also is a lateral flexor of the lumbopelvic spine—may be the most active muscle of the lumbar region during activities of daily living.[135] It may possess trigger points that cause localized and referred pain. Tenderness is usually 1 inch from the spine on the affected side, but there can be discomfort laterally over the ribs and flank to the iliac crest. Lateral bending to the opposite side exacerbates the symptoms. Concomitant findings of lumbar spinal fixation are common.

On palpation, the quadratus lumborum is usually tender, may be hypertonic, and may even have a ropelike consistency. Pain may radiate to the abdomen or downward to the iliac crest or greater trochanter. If the trigger points are located more medially toward the spine, the referral zone may be toward the buttocks. Concomitant trigger points may occur in the gluteus minimus muscle.[186]

Table 8-16   Lumbar Myofascial Pain Syndromes

Physical examination findings	Muscular hypertonicity and taut areas on palpation History of chronic low back pain and dysfunction Concomitant restriction of range of motion and joint subluxation, hypomobility Muscular restriction and fixation on stretch Active trigger points with distant referral zones
X-ray findings	Not applicable or not helpful
Treatment plan	Chiropractic manipulative therapy Mobilization, stretching therapy such as spray-and-stretch, proprioceptive neuromuscular facilitation Manual ischemic compression Therapeutic modalities for pain Ultrasound–high voltage trigger point combination therapy Strengthening exercises for postural muscles of trunk and pelvis

Gluteal Myofascitis

The three gluteal muscles can cause actual disability and dysfunction in the patient with low back pain. Often mimicking other types of lumbar spine disease, gluteal myofascial pain causes pelvic, hip, and leg pain.

Trigger points in the gluteus maximus refer pain medially to the gluteal and sacral areas. Gluteus medius trigger points refer pain to the gluteal and hip region, toward the attachment at the greater trochanter. The gluteus minimus refers pain primarily to the lower extremity, especially the lateral leg and calf. This symptom often mimics a disk lesion, but the findings of an orthopedic examination of the lumbar spine are unremarkable. Many of those who have chronic low back pain, however, have concomitant trigger points in the quadratus lumborum and spinal extensor muscles, as well as gluteal myofascitis.

Chronic Lumbar Strain

Patients with chronic postural or mechanical problems in the lumbar spine or those individuals who are vulnerable to repetitive injury may develop a chronic lumbar strain. The muscles of the thoracolumbar region that extend or aid in rotation of the vertebral column are injured, either the superficial or deep layer. Inhibition or endurance weakness of the multifidus, a primary intersegmental stabilizer of the spine, is often a predictor for mechanical low back injury.[131,165] Static flexion of the spine with or without rotation evokes pain. Palpable areas of inflammation often refer pain if active trigger points are present. Common pain referral zones include the ribs laterally and the lumbosacral junction caudally. Because of chronic muscular fixation, hypolordosis and vertebral subluxation and hypomobility are almost always present.

Piriformis Syndrome

One of the more common results of the peripheral entrapment of the sciatic nerve is the piriformis syndrome. A fairly perplexing diagnostic problem, patients with this syndrome have buttock pain in the region of the sciatic notch and down the back of the thigh and leg. *The lack of orthopedic and motion findings locally at the spine distinguishes this peripheral entrapment from a lumbar disk lesion.* In a small segment of the population, the sciatic nerve splits the piriformis muscle; strange and often confusing deficits in the lower extremity can highlight the neurologic examination in these individuals.

Reiter's Syn.
- *Conjunctivitis*
- *Urethritis*
- *Arthritis*
- *Dermatitis*

chlamydia ⟹ #1 venereal ds.

Hip flexion with rotation causes pain in an individual with this problem because it stretches the piriformis muscle, thereby compromising or irritating the sciatic nerve. Activities that externally rotate the thigh can strain the piriformis muscle, eventually leading to local swelling and irritation of the sciatic nerve sheath and, eventually, sciatic neuritis. Trigger points in the piriformis muscle refer pain to the buttocks; toward the hip, posterior thigh, and calf; and even to the sole of the foot, on occasion, as in typical cases of "sciatica" in radiculopathies. Palpation of myofascial trigger points leads to the diagnosis. Imaging and electromyography offer limited diagnostic value.[191] According to various cadaver studies, hypertonic bands of muscle fibers trap the nerve at the sciatic notch as it splits the muscle to varying degrees.[186]

Arthritic and Metabolic Disorders

In addition to the conditions that have already been discussed, arthritic and metabolic disorders can affect the lumbar spine. For example, inflammatory disease, degenerative spine disorders, rheumatoid conditions, and metabolic bone disease can all readily affect the lumbar spine and pelvis.

The seronegative spondyloarthropathies, a class of rheumatic disorders, have several factors in common: radiographic presentation, genetic predisposition, and certain clinical features. Included in this group are the so-called reactive arthritides (e.g., Reiter's syndrome) and inflammatory joint diseases (e.g., ankylosing spondylitis), along with the associated spondylitic disease psoriatic arthritis and inflammatory bowel disease.[39] Infectious components initiate certain conditions, such as reactive arthritis. In addition, there is a significant correlation between the presence of certain blood markers and the diagnosis of some of the spondylitic disorders, such as the strong association between the HLA-B27 antigen and ankylosing spondylitis.[124]

Paget's disease is the most common metabolic disorder that affects the lumbopelvic spine. The skull and lower limb may show clinical signs of the disease, and there may be assorted laboratory findings. Back pain and bony enlargement leading to neurogenic claudication may occur.

Ankylosing Spondylitis

The benchmark of ankylosing spondylitis, a common cause of low back pain and thoracolumbar stiffness, is the presence of sacroiliitis. Although it affects the axial skeleton, the disease may be seen in association with reactive arthritis, inflammatory bowel disease, or psoriasis. Like other seronegative spondyloarthropathies, ankylosing spondylitis has the unfortunate potential to affect several organ systems, such as the anterior ocular apparatus, the skin, tendon insertions, and the various connective tissue systems, such as large arteries.[108]

As noted earlier, there is a correlation between spondyloarthropathies such as ankylosing spondylitis and the histocompatibility antigen HLA-B27. Patients with ankylosing spondylitis lack IgM rheumatoid factor, however.[152] An elevated erythrocyte sedimentation rate (ESR) is found in 75% of the patients with ankylosing spondylitis. The relationship of the ESR to ankylosing spondylitis symptoms or activity is not always clear.[109] Approximately 80% to 98% of Caucasian patients with ankylosing spondylitis have the HLA-B27 genetic marker, whereas it is present in only 8% of the general population.[109] Therefore there seems to be a genetic predisposition for the disease. It is more prevalent in men than in women; furthermore, radiographic evidence of the disease often appears later in women.[110] In spite of all this information, the precise etiology of ankylosing spondylitis remains relatively obscure.

The typical patient is a man 35 to 55 years of age who is experiencing spinal immobility, loss of chest expansion, multiple sites of inflammation at tendinous attachments to bone (enthesitis), and chronic low back pain. The latter is a common and early symptom. The onset of back pain usually occurs before the age of 40 years, which is an important consideration in making the distinction between ankylosing spondylitis and noninflammatory back pain. Morning stiffness and spinal symptoms have generally lasted longer than 3 months.

Lateral bending is found to be extremely limited. Multiple musculotendinous tender points and extra-articular bony tenderness are also common. "Girdle" tenderness at the hips and shoulders often occurs early in the disease, even before spinal symptoms.[108,169] Posture deteriorates, leading to such conditions as thoracic kyphosis and lumbar hypolordosis, later in the disease (Figure 8-48). Peripheral arthropathy is not often associated with ankylosing spondylitis.

The most common extraskeletal problem in ankylosing spondylitis is acute anterior uveitis; 25% to 30% of patients develop this condition during the course of their disease.[107,108] Connective tissue disorders can also occur in patients with ankylosing spondylitis, although they are less frequent than uveitis. Cardiovascular involvement, skin lesions, amyloidosis, and pulmonary involvement may occur late in the disease.[108]

Radiographic findings are evident primarily at the axial skeleton, especially at the sacroiliac joints. The costotransverse, apophyseal, discovertebral, and costovertebral articulations are also affected, however. The "bamboo" spine is not always so typical in the patient with ankylosing spondylitis, although ankylosis may occur later in the disorder.

On the x-ray film, sacroiliac involvement is usually bilateral, and there are signs of progressive sclerosis and erosion.[210] Reactive sclerosis and bony erosions may also be seen at the site of osseous attachment of ligaments and tendons, especially at the ischial tuberosity, greater trochanter of the femur, iliac crest, and vertebral spinous processes. Syndesmophytes and bony remodeling is often apparent in the vertebral column of the older patient with ankylosing spondylitis.

Mechanical back pain from intervertebral disk, facet, or canal involvement is usually aggravated by activity and ameliorated by rest. Generally, lateral flexion of the thoracolumbar spine and chest expansion is not drastically limited. Radiographic confusion with diffuse idiopathic skeletal hyperostosis (DISH, also known as ankylosing hyperostosis or Forestier's disease), is common. *The most characteristic feature of ankylosing hyperostosis radiographically is the flowing ossification of the anterior longitudinal ligament with sparing of the intervertebral disk spaces.*

Treatment for ankylosing spondylitis centers on symptomatic relief, maintenance of spinal mobility, and the preservation of functional capacity (Table 8-17). Although manipulation may be difficult or seemingly futile in the advanced cases involving bony ankyloses, the patient who is younger or whose condition is diagnosed in an earlier stage may benefit from these techniques. Spinal mobilization, including various stretching and muscle techniques, should be employed along with traditional physiotherapeutic modalities to aid in symptomatic relief in any phase of the disease process.

Rheumatoid arthritis affects the spine less frequently than ankylosing spondylitis, especially in regard to the sacroiliac, apophyseal, or costovertebral joints. Typically, rheumatoid arthritis affects the cervical spine first, whereas ankylosing spondylitis affects the lumbosacral region initially. Inflammation and destruction are seen with rheumatoid disease, and extraspinal joint lesions are the norm.

Osteoarthritis

Degenerative joint disease affects weight-bearing articulations, and the lumbar spine is no exception. As a non-inflammatory arthritis, osteoarthritis (also termed degenerative spondylosis) differs from the inflammatory spondyloarthropathies in many ways: age at onset, presentation, systemic disease, laboratory profile, and radiographic appearance.

Osteoarthritis of the lumbar spine follows patterns of aging similar to those of other weight-bearing joints. It may have its basis in a myriad of factors, such as genetic traits, obesity, and trauma. For example, patients with osteoarthritis may have had previous trauma to the spine, such as disk herniation, contact sports injury, or multiple motor vehicle accidents (Figure 8-49). Aggravating factors (e.g., endocrine-metabolic disease and inherent hypermobility) may also play an important role.[50,182] Spinal osteoarthritis can affect the articular facets and intervertebral joints. Degenerative changes at the intervertebral disk usually accelerate any degenerative changes at the vertebral apophyseal joints. Motion disturbance, such as repetitive microtrauma in sagittal loading and chronic joint dysfunction, leads to osteoarthritic changes at these joints.[208]

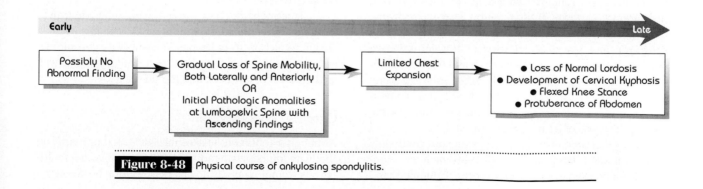

Figure 8-48 Physical course of ankylosing spondylitis.

Table 8-17 Arthritic and Metabolic Disorders

	Ankylosing Spondylitis	Osteoarthritis	Osteitis Condensans Ilii	Paget's Disease
Physical examination findings	Loss of thoracolumbar lateral bending History of spinal stiffness and back pain (longer than 3 months in duration) Impedance of chest expansion Concomitant organ system involvement, usually anterior uveitis Early hip and shoulder discomfort HLA-B27 antigen compatibility on serologic testing Elevated ESR in 75% of patients Enthesopathies at tendon-bone interface	History of back pain and morning stiffness Muscular, soft-tissue hypomobility Painful and limited lumbar flexion	Findings possibly consistent with mechanical low back pain Dull, achy lumbopelvic pain with palpable tenderness over sacroiliac joints	History of bone, back, appendicular skeletal pain, or signs of nerve compression Skeletal enlargement, especially skull, lumbar vertebrae, and femoral head Bowing of long bones
X-ray findings	Sacroiliitis Thoracolumbar syndesmophytes Bamboo spine or ankylosis in later stages	Typical findings of degenerative arthritis: joint space narrowing, osteophytes, marginal sclerosis, bony spurs	Sclerosis of iliac side of sacroiliac joints	Focal areas of radiolucency and osteoblastic activity Cortical thickening Pseudofractures (transverse) or cortical stress fractures Lumbopelvis, skull, and lower leg involvement
Treatment plan	CMT, spinal mobilization Therapeutic stretching program to maintain mobility Physiotherapy modalities for symptomatic relief Deep breathing exercises to maintain rib mobility	CMT, stretching, mobilization Life-style changes (e.g., weight loss)	CMT, spinal exercise Physiotherapy for acute pain	CMT, gentle mobilization in advanced cases Monitoring of alkaline phosphatase levels in patients with active symptoms Medical or pharmacologic therapy for aggravated symptoms or advanced disease

ESR, Erythrocyte sedimentation rate; **CMT,** chiropractic manipulative therapy.

Osteoarthritis of the spine has typical patterns on x-ray films. Age-related changes at the intervertebral disk are well-known; intervertebral space narrowing, bony spurs at the vertebral body margins (lipping, spurring), and marginal sclerosis of the vertebra are common radiographic findings. Claw and traction osteophytes common to osteoarthritis differ from the bony bridges seen as syndesmophytes in ankylosing spondylitis. Early changes indicative of degenerative disk disease such as loss of hydration appear on MRI.

Degenerative changes of the spine are commonly seen with age-related skeletal changes such as osteoporosis. Increased radiolucency, cortical thinning, and altered trabecular patterns are all evident in patients with senile osteoporosis.[176]

Treatment centers around pain relief, improvements in spinal mobility, and life style changes such as weight reduction, if applicable. Patients with chronic disability must improve their level of overall fitness, as well as their level of low back and hip flexibility.

Osteitis Condensans Ilii

Although osteitis condensans ilii is detected primarily on the plain lumbopelvic radiographic films of young multiparous women, there is no clear correlation between the radiologic diagnosis and physical impairment. The condition is often asymptomatic. On the other hand, it is sometimes associated with mechanical low back pain.

The articular instability of osteitis condensans ilii may be present secondarily to the hormonal changes and stress associated with pregnancy. It is thought that the hormonal influx of relaxing, which relaxes the spinal and pelvic ligaments during pregnancy, may contribute to instability in the vertebral column.[159] This fact, along with the theory of pelvic expansion in association with birth trauma, may be enough to cause osteitis condensans ilii.[61]

The typical finding of this condition is marginal sclerosis of the iliac side of the sacroiliac articulation, while the sacrum is spared. Involvement at the sacroiliac joints is usually bilateral. Typically, there are no erosive arthropathic findings, but the reactive sclerosis can be quite extensive. Resolution of radiologic abnormalities may occur over time.[187]

The patient usually has diffuse, achy low back pain over the lower lumbar region and pelvis. Palpable tenderness at the sacroiliac joints is common. Leg pain is unusual, and the results of a neurologic evaluation are usually unremarkable.

Conservative care consisting of exercise, manipulation, and therapies for acute pain is usually effective. Rehabilitation exercises should center around strengthening of the low back and pelvic musculature.

Paget's Disease of Bone

A disorder of osseous architecture resulting from altered bone metabolism, Paget's disease (also called osteitis deformans) is marked by early osteoclastic activity followed by osteoblastic bony formation. Etiologic factors are largely unknown. There is a variable occurrence of family traits; only 17% of patients have a family history of the disease.[188] European populations have a much higher incidence of Paget's than do Asian or African populations.

Men predominate 3:2 over women among patients with Paget's disease, and the usual age of discovery is 50 years or older. At least 10% to 20% of patients with the disorder are totally asymptomatic. Those who are symptomatic frequently have skeletal deformities and skeletal-related complaints, the most frequent being bone and back pain.[139] Common areas of involvement include the spine, skull, hip, and lower leg. There may even be an increase in hat size because of calvarium enlargement. In addition, there may be signs and symptoms of nerve compression as a result of bony enlargement and vertebral canal compromise.

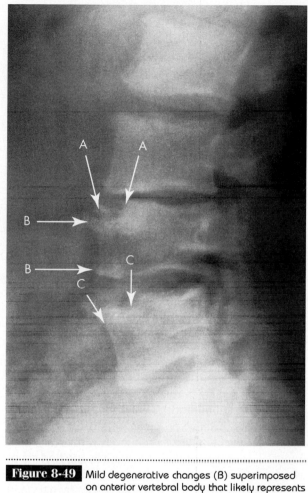

Figure 8-49 Mild degenerative changes (B) superimposed on anterior vertebral body that likely represents an old vertebral apophysitis and end-plate fracture (A) in a 26-year-old man with dull, achy low back pain and a 10-year history of participation in contact sports and weight lifting. Note the superior end-plate irregularity at L5 (C).

Generally, the diagnosis follows incidental radiographic findings that are almost pathognomonic of the disease. Typical plain-film findings include focal areas of resorption and disturbed trabecular patterns. Bony enlargement, cortical thickening, and sclerosis are common. Late disease findings include transverse pseudofractures, arthritis-induced changes, and small cortical stress fractures, which are often seen on the convex side of a bowed long bone, such as the tibia.[5]

The spine is frequently involved in Paget's disease, and the patient with back pain often has the radiographic finding of a single dense lumbar vertebra. Vertebral enlargement can cause neurogenic claudication of the lower extremity as well. The femoral head, neck, and proximal femur are often involved, as well as the pelvis. Areas of increased density may be mixed with lytic areas of bone. "Cross-hatchings" of the pelvic brim and proximal hip are typical. Patients with hip or pelvic findings may be asymptomatic, but may have a decreased range of motion. Pseudofractures frequently occur in the hip and pelvic region, whereas complete fractures (pathologic) are more common and clinically significant at the femoral neck.

Bone scanning is helpful if the diagnosis remains uncertain after plain-film analysis, since it can aid in differentiating metastatic carcinoma from Paget's disease. MRI and CT are helpful in assessing bony changes such as osteolytic and osteoblastic activity. Because of its unique capacity for detecting altered skeletal physiology, MRI will most likely be a great help in diagnosing the stage of Paget's disease.

Routine laboratory tests may indicate an elevated alkaline phosphatase level in patients with an unremarkable history, which can help confirm the presence of Paget's disease. In patients with advanced and more complicated disease, the alkaline phosphatase level may be 25 to 30 times the normal. Other blood laboratory findings are usually normal. The urine hydroxyproline level rises in patients with an active disease state and often parallels alkaline phosphatase activity. Follow-up studies of alkaline phosphatase levels can be procured from the isoenzyme isolation if there is question about liver versus bone disease. Patients with an elevated serum calcium level should have their parathyroid gland evaluated.

Many patients with asymptomatic Paget's disease need only observation and a baseline assessment. Individuals with back or hip pain can be treated conservatively as long as the practitioner checks periodically for fractures, neurologic deficits, or advanced systemic illness (e.g., cardiac insufficiency). Physiotherapy, gentle mobilization, and spinal manipulation may be beneficial.

Pharmacologic agents have been used with varying degrees of success. The primary agents that have been used include the calcitonins (e.g., porcine, salmon, human) and diphosphonates (e.g., disodium etidronate). Severe polyostotic disease has also been treated with pamidronate disodium.[133]

Some patients may require co-treatment with orthopedic surgeons or hematologists. Laboratory monitoring of alkaline phosphatase levels is routine in advanced stages of the disease. Concomitant fracture management or elective surgery, such as joint replacement

for arthritic complications secondary to Paget's disease, is also a possibility in these patients. Neoplastic development from Pagetic bone occurs in less than 2% to 4% of all symptomatic patients. The incidence is substantially lower if all patients with the disease are taken into consideration.[139]

Conclusion

The first 75 years of the twentieth century produced great bodies of research in clinical anatomy, supportive and surgical medical care, and pharmacology. As the cost of health care has dramatically risen since the 1970s, the business of providing patient treatment has sharply changed. The purchasers of health care policies are increasingly seeking effective and fiscally efficient treatments for low back pain, one of the more common maladies known to modern humankind.

Research in the area of lumbar spine treatment methods has intensified, and both exercise and spinal manipulation show great promise. Passive therapies such as bed rest and medication have only limited use in reducing long-term morbidity from low back pain. Health care providers should continue to educate the public about methods to promote each individual's overall health and fitness, self-determination, and self-reliance. This approach, in turn, will have a positive impact on the national economy, thus improving the quality of all our lives.

Review Questions

1. The devastating economic and social effects of low back pain are far-reaching, encompassing both the private and public sectors of American businesses. (a) Name some of the direct and indirect costs to American companies and local and state governments from the back pain crush. (b) What are some current biomechanical issues for occupational health to the spine in the workplace? (c) What are some current trends in the delivery and treatment choices in care for the patient with low back pain?

2. (a) Describe the general factors in spinal degeneration that may ultimately lead to lumbar spine disability. (b) Name two broad categories of pathologic abnormalities that can directly cause lumbar pain.

3. Discuss an optimal ergonomic model of lumbar kinetics during lifting tasks.

4. Your history and physical examination are the foundation of your assessment of the patient with low back pain. (a) State some warning signs and symptoms of organic disease. (b) Standard x-rays films should be ordered before instituting manual treatment for which patients?

5. (a) What are the differences between radicular and somatic-referred pain? Give examples of each. (b) What are the differences between dermatomal patterns and myotogenous referral? Give examples of each.

6. (a) State the mechanical and neurohormonal influences of chiropractic manipulative therapy on the spine. (b) What are some examples of spinal rehabilitation exercises?

7. A 40-year-old man with a 10-year history of intermittent back pain has an antalgic gait, limited lumbar flexion, and a palliative arc of extension, as well as a unilateral hip, buttock, and leg pain in a radicular pattern. Sciatic tension signs are positive, and heel walking is difficult on the side of pain. (a) What is your initial diagnosis? (b) Your initial conservative care may include what? (c) What type of injury may cause bilateral symptomatology and great disability? (d) What is the advanced imaging modality of choice to evaluate and confirm this diagnosis?

8. (a) What are some of the signs and symptoms of spondylolysis? (b) What is visualized on x-ray films? (c) What types of defect exist in spondylolysis? (d) What are appropriate conservative measures to treat a Grade I or II spondylolisthesis?

References

1. Adams MH: The effect of fatigue on the lumbar IVD, *J Bone Joint Surg* 65B:199, 1983.
2. Agency for Health Care Policy and Research, Public Health Service, US Department of Health and Human Services: Diagnostic imaging for low back pain gets mixed review, *Research Activities* 126:3, 1990.
3. Agency for Health Care Policy and Research, Public Health Services, US Department of Health and Human Services: *Acute low back pain in adults,* Clinical Practice Guideline, Number 14. Rockville, MD, 1994, AHCPR Publication No. 95-0642, The Agency.
4. Alan G: *High voltage stimulation,* Chattanooga, Tenn, 1984, Chattanooga Corporation.
5. Altman RD: Musculoskeletal questions and answers, *J Musculoskeletal Med* 7(11):10, 1990.
6. American Chiropractic Association: Vital signs, *J Am Chiropractic Assoc* 28(7):10, 1991.
7. Amundsen T: Lumbar spinal stenosis: clinical and radiologic features, *Spine* 20(10):1178, 1995.
8. Andersson GBJ: Epidemiological aspects of low back pain in industry, *Spine* 6:53, 1981.
9. Andersson GBJ: The epidemiology of spinal disorders. In Frymoyer JW, editor: *The adult spine: principles and practice,* New York, 1990, Raven Press.
10. Andersson GBJ: Occupational biomechanics. In Weinstein J, Wiesel SW, editors: *The lumbar spine,* Philadelphia, 1990, WB Saunders.
11. Andersson GBJ, Chaffin DB, Pope MH: Occupational biomechanics of the lumbar spine. In Pope MH, Andersson GBJ, Frymoyer JW, Chaffin DB, editors: *Occupational low back pain,* St Louis, 1991, Mosby.
12. Andersson GBJ, Ortengren R, Nachemson A: Quantitative studies of back loads in lifting, *Spine* 1:178, 1976.
13. Aspegren DD, Wright RE, Hemler DE: Manipulation under epidural anesthesia (MUEA) with corticosteroid injection: two case reports, *J Manipulative Physiol Ther* 20:618, 1997.
14. Asserdelft WJJ, Koes BW, Knipschild PG, Bouter LM: The relationship between methodological quality and conclusions in reviews of spinal manipulation, *JAMA* 274:1942, 1995.
15. Bartol KM: *Long and short lever-specific/nonspecific contact procedures.* Proceedings of the 7th Annual Conference on Research and Education, St Louis, 1992, Mosby.
16. Bartol KM: Osseous manual thrust techniques. In Gatterman MI, editor: *Foundations of chiropractic subluxation,* St Louis, 1995, Mosby.
17. Battie MC, Bigos SJ: Industrial back pain complaints, *Orthop Clin North Am* 22(2):273, 1991.
18. Bednar DA, Orr FW, Simon GT: Observations on the pathomorphology of the thoracolumbar fascia in chronic mechanical back pain: a microscopic study, 20(1):38, 1995.
19. Bergmann TF, Jongeward BV: Manipulative therapy in low back pain with leg pain and neurological deficits, *J Manipulative Physiol Ther* 21:288, 1998.
20. Biering-Sorensen F, Thomsen C: Medical, social and occupational history as risk indicators for low back trouble in a general population, *Spine* 11:720, 1986.
21. Boden SD, Wiesel SW, Laws ER, Rothman RH: *The aging spine,* Philadelphia, 1991, WB Saunders.
22. Bogduk N: *Autoimmune response in lumbar disc disease,* Toronto, 1991, American Back Society.
23. Bogduk N: *Pathogenesis of degenerative disc disease,* Toronto, 1991, American Back Society.
24. Bogduk N, McIntosh J: The applied anatomy of the thoracolumbar fascia, *Spine* 9:164, 1984.
25. Bogduk N, Twomey LT: *Clinical anatomy of the lumbar spine,* ed 2, New York, 1991, Churchill Livingstone.
26. Bower V, Cassidy JD: Macroscopic and microscopic anatomy of the sacroiliac joint from embryonic life until the eighth decade, *Spine* 6:620, 1981.
27. Breen A: The reliability of palpation and other diagnostic methods, *J Manipulative Physiol Ther* 15:54, 1992.
28. Breen A: *The reliability of palpation and other diagnostic methods,* Proceedings of the Scientific Symposium, Toronto, 1991, World Chiropractic Congress.
29. Brennan PC, McGregor M, Hondras MA, Kokjohn K: Enhanced neutrophil respiratory burst as a biological marker for manipulative forces, *J Manipulative Physiol Ther* 15:83, 1992.

211. White AA: *The disc as a possible source of chemical mediators in the production of low back and radicular pain,* East Rutherford, NJ, 1990, NYCC Second Multidisciplinary Symposium..

212. White AA, Panjabi MM: *Clinical biomechanics of the spine,* ed 2, Philadelphia, 1988, JB Lippincott.

213. Wiesel SW, Tsourmas N, Feffer HL: A study of CAT: the incidence of positive CAT scans in an asymptomatic group of patients, *Spine* 9:549, 1984.

214. Wiltse L, Jackson D: Treatment of spondylolysis and spondylolisthesis in children, *Clin Orthop* 117:92, 1976.

215. Wiltse LL, Newman PH, McNab I: Classification of spondylolysis and spondylolisthesis, *Clin Orthop* 117:23, 1976.

216. Wiltse LL, Widell EH, Jackson DW: Fatigue fracture: the basic lesion in isthmic spondylolisthesis, *J Bone Joint Surg* 57A:178, 1975.

217. Wycke BD: Articular neurology and manipulative therapy. In: Glasgow EF, Twomey LT, Seull ER, Kleynhans AM, editors: *Aspects of manipulation therapy,* New York, 1985, Churchill Livingstone.

218. Wycke BD: Neurology of low back pain. In Jayson MIV, editor: *The lumbar spine and back pain,* ed 3, London, 1987, Churchill Livingstone.

219. Yochum TR: *A closer look at spondylolisthesis,* East Rutherford, NJ, 1990, NYCC Second Multidisciplinary Symposium.

220. Yochum TR, Rowe LJ: *Essentials of skeletal radiology,* vol 1, Baltimore, 1987, Williams & Wilkins.

221. Yong KH, King AI: Mechanisms of facet load transmission as a hypothesis for low back pain, *Spine* 9:557, 1984.

222. Yoshizawa H, Kobayashi S, Hachiya Y: Blood supply of nerve roots and dorsal root ganglia, *Orthop Clin North Am* 22(2):195, 1991.

223. Zucherman J, Schofferman J: Pathology of failed back surgery syndrome, *Spine: State of the Art Reviews* 1(1):1, 1986.

Chapter 9

Hip, Thigh, and Pelvis

Steven R. Brier and Patrick J. DeRosa

Chapter Highlights

Physical Examination
Adult Disorders of the Hip, Thigh, and Pelvis
Childhood Hip Disorders

Hip disorders are not the most common medical problems; however, their effects can be severe if the disorder is not diagnosed and treated promptly. The most frequently seen hip problems are fractures, arthritis, contusions, tendonitis, bursitis, and muscle strains. Less often, epiphyseal injuries and apophysitis may occur. Symptoms of hip dysfunction include pain, loss of range of motion or strength, abnormal gait, and inability to bear weight.

The pain patterns of lumbosacral spine disorders and degenerative arthritis of the knee may mimic that of hip ailments. Herniated lumbar disks, spinal stenosis, sacroiliac sprains, lumbopelvic myofascitis, and internal derangements of the knee joint may all contribute to hip pain. Thus when a patient complains of hip pain, it is essential to perform range-of-motion testing at the knee and lumbosacral spine to rule out local mechanical pathologic conditions that refer to the hip.

Physical Examination

The two most common examination findings with hip pathology are alterations in gait and range of motion. The examination begins therefore with an analysis of the patient's gait and an assessment of the patient's ability to bear weight symmetrically.

With the patient supine on the examination table in shorts or in a gown, the practitioner can evaluate all ranges of hip motion, including flexion and extension. To check hip extension, the practitioner slides the patient to the near side of the table and hangs the leg being tested off the table, gently placing the hip into extension. Adduction, abduction, flexion, and internal and external rotation can all be tested with the subject lying supine. It is important to check bilaterally for any difference in fullness of mobility and for pain. If pain is present, palpation can help determine whether the problem is over a muscle-tendon unit or the joint capsule itself. Bony landmarks of the hip and pelvis, including the iliac spines, should be palpated for tenderness (Figure 9-1). Most internal derangements of the hip, such as the onset of adult degenerative diseases and childhood disorders, affect internal rotation and flexion of the hip joint most severely.

The Patrick's test may reproduce pain in internal degeneration and synovitis of the hip (Figure 9-2 *A-C*). Sometimes this test reveals a painful sacroiliac lesion as well (i.e., hip or spine syndromes). The examination continues with an evaluation of active hip flexion, extension, adduction, abduction, and rotation. With the patient in the weight-bearing position, the Trendelenburg's test should reveal any hip joint or gluteus medius lesion. Anatomic and functional length measurements should be taken of each leg and compared. It is important to determine whether the patient is febrile to rule out infection.

The Thomas test, conducted with the patient in the supine position, indicates any tightness in the psoas muscle (Figure 9-3 *A, B*), although its status may be evident while the patient is in the prone position with the affected leg in knee flexion and hip extension. A tightened or shortened psoas muscle may contribute not only to anterior thigh and hip discomfort, but also to low back pain and an altered gait.

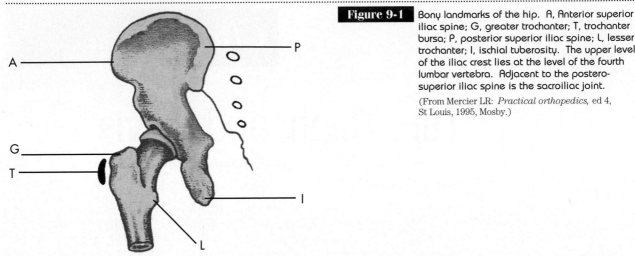

Figure 9-1 Bony landmarks of the hip. A, Anterior superior iliac spine; G, greater trochanter; T, trochanter bursa; P, posterior superior iliac spine; L, lesser trochanter; I, ischial tuberosity. The upper level of the iliac crest lies at the level of the fourth lumbar vertebra. Adjacent to the postero-superior iliac spine is the sacroiliac joint.

(From Mercier LR: *Practical orthopedics*, ed 4, St Louis, 1995, Mosby.)

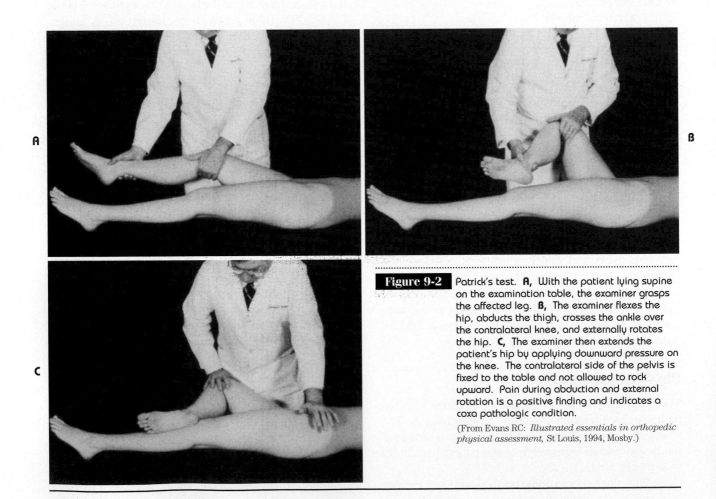

Figure 9-2 Patrick's test. **A,** With the patient lying supine on the examination table, the examiner grasps the affected leg. **B,** The examiner flexes the hip, abducts the thigh, crosses the ankle over the contralateral knee, and externally rotates the hip. **C,** The examiner then extends the patient's hip by applying downward pressure on the knee. The contralateral side of the pelvis is fixed to the table and not allowed to rock upward. Pain during abduction and external rotation is a positive finding and indicates a coxa pathologic condition.

(From Evans RC: *Illustrated essentials in orthopedic physical assessment*, St Louis, 1994, Mosby.)

Adults with hip pain and a history of systemic illness, long-term degenerative processes, or a history of infection should undergo x-ray studies (Figure 9-4). Magnetic resonance imaging (MRI) is often used for the early detection of avascular necrosis.

Children with a remarkable history (e.g., hip trauma) and presentation usually require plain radiographic films for diagnosis. Ultrasonography is helpful for detecting small effusions, for guiding arthrocentesis, and for diagnosing dislocated, subluxed, or congenitally dysplastic hips in young children.[20,22] Ultrasound has the added advantage of being an imaging modality that can be used on a moving child.[12]

Adult Disorders of the Hip, Thigh, and Pelvis

Fractures

Hip Fractures

Traumatic or metabolic in origin, hip fractures may be subcapital, cervical, intertrochanteric, subtrochanteric, or stress fractures. Elderly patients commonly fracture the hip in a fall, often as a result of visual impairment, Parkinson's disease, a previous stroke, or lower limb dysfunction.[9] Physical examination and radiographic studies of the hip are the basis of diagnosis. Physical examination indicates pain with range of motion and may reveal shortening and external rotation in those fractures that are displaced. Standard radiographic views are usually anteroposterior and lateral projections (Figure 9-5), although frog projections may also be ordered in cases of suspected stress fractures. For some purposes, such as preoperative planning or rehabilitation planning for a patient after multiple trauma, computed tomography (CT) may be appropriate.[6]

Fractures of the hip may occur at the greater trochanter, lesser trochanter, and femoral neck. They may be classified as nondisplaced, displaced, or comminuted. Nondisplaced fractures, such as stress fractures and impacted cervical fractures, do not require surgical intervention. All remaining types of hip fractures require closed reduction or open reduction and internal fixation with compression screws (Table 9-1).

The prognosis for a full recovery from a hip fracture is generally good. A cervical fracture in which the blood supply is compromised has a less favorable prognosis, however. In this condition, early reduction and internal fixation are imperative.

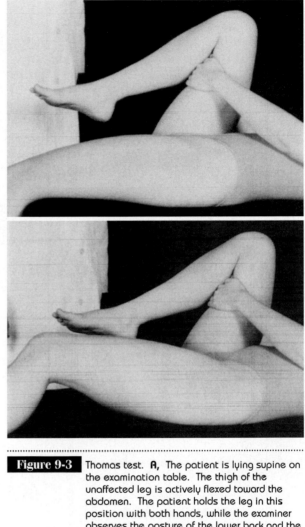

Figure 9-3 Thomas test. **A,** The patient is lying supine on the examination table. The thigh of the unaffected leg is actively flexed toward the abdomen. The patient holds the leg in this position with both hands, while the examiner observes the posture of the lower back and the affected leg. The lumbar spine should flatten, and the opposite leg should remain flat on the table. **B,** If the lumbar spine maintains a lordosis and the affected leg flexes and if the patient is unable to lay the leg flat on the table, the test is positive. A positive test indicates a shortened Iliopsoas muscle.

(From Evans RC: *Illustrated essentials in orthopedic physical assessment,* St Louis, 1994, Mosby.)

Femur Fractures

In the femoral shaft, fractures may be proximal, midshaft, or distal. They may be classified as simple, compound, or stress fractures. Generally, stress fractures occur in the proximal third aspect of the shaft. Nondisplaced fractures occur primarily in the distal third aspect of the shaft.

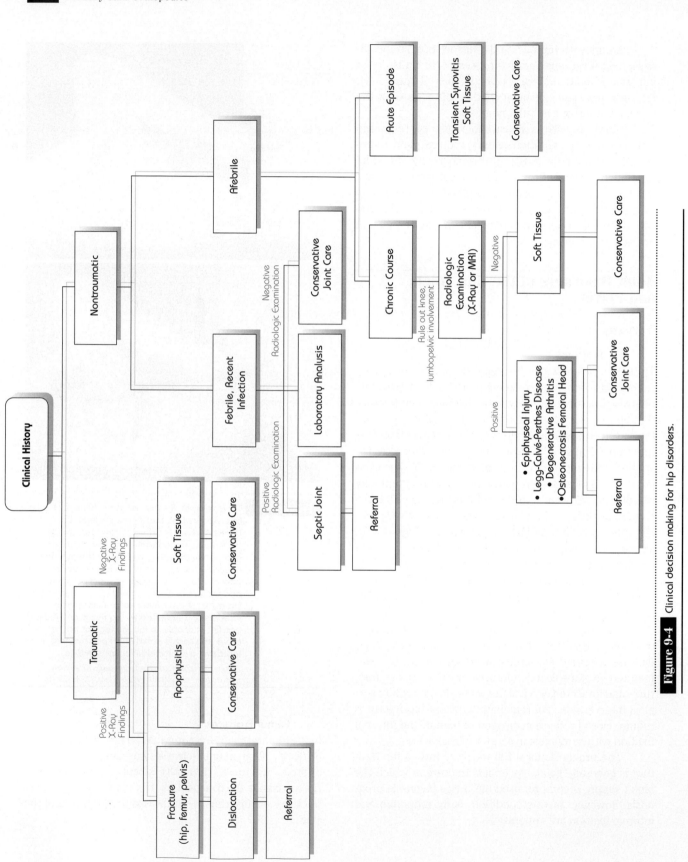

Figure 9-4 Clinical decision making for hip disorders.

	Hip	Femur	Pelvis
Table 9-1	Fractures of the Hip, Femur, and Pelvis		
Physical examination findings	History of significant trauma Severe hip pain and swelling Altered limb length or angular deformity Inability to bear weight Possibly metabolic disease in older populations	History of significant trauma Acute pain and swelling of thigh Leg deformity Inability to bear weight	History of blunt trauma Pelvic pain and swelling Possible bony deformity of pelvis Possible difficulty to bear weight
X-ray findings	At minimum, anteroposterior and lateral projections Need to rule out displacement or comminution	At minimum, antero-posterior and lateral projections Shortening of femoral neck and angulation	Anteroposterior, lateral, and oblique projections
Treatment plan	Immobilization Orthopedic surgical referral Possible need for follow-up with CT	Immobilization Orthopedic surgical referral Evaluation, monitoring of distal neuromuscular status	Immobilization or use of crutches to avoid bearing weight Orthopedic surgical referral Possible need for follow up with CT

CT, Computed tomography.

Physical examination shows acute pain, swelling, and deformity. It is important to check the neurovascular status of the lower extremity. All femoral fractures require immediate immobilization. If there is a physician present when a displaced fracture occurs, the physician may attempt gentle manipulation and immobilization until the injured person can be taken to a hospital.

In the hospital the treatment of nondisplaced fractures includes cast immobilization. Most femoral fractures in the skeletally mature individual require skeletal traction and closed reduction, or open reduction and internal fixation. Problems with delayed union and nonunion may develop in compound and comminuted fractures; if so, bone graft and internal fixation may be necessary.

The prognosis of femoral fractures is good, especially for those in young age groups. Young patients usually heal within 6 to 8 weeks. Those in older age groups heal within 3 months.

Pelvic Fractures

Injuries to the pelvic ring may result in bony fracture, as in high-speed trauma caused by a motor vehicle accident or skiing. Cyclists and pedestrians are at particular risk of pelvic fracture through the direct impact of a motor vehicle, and such a fracture may or may not be stable.[14] Treatment depends on the site, severity of the injury, stability, and required weight-bearing function of the fracture area (Figure 9-6).

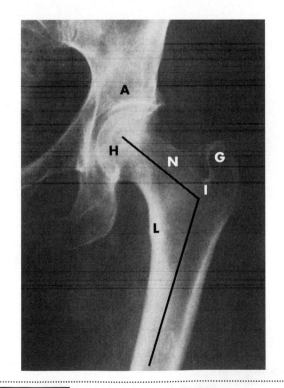

Figure 9-5 Anteroposterior roentgenogram of the normal hip. A, Rim of the acetabulum; H, head of the femur; N, neck of the femur; L, lesser trochanter; G, greater trochanter; I, intertrochanteric region. The angle of inclination is marked.

(From Mercier LR: *Practical orthopedics,* ed 4, St Louis, 1995, Mosby.)

Greater Trochanteric Bursitis

In most cases, greater trochanteric bursitis is traumatic in origin. It occurs more commonly among individuals in young age groups and may result from a direct blow or from exertion in such sports as running, golf, or tennis. Older individuals may develop the condition because of the formation of calcium in the bursae through normal activity.

The diagnosis is based on the physical examination and, in rare instances, on radiographic films that reveal calcification over the greater trochanter. Among the physical findings may be palpable pain over the greater trochanter that sometimes radiates down the leg along the tensor fascia latae (Table 9-2).

Differential diagnosis includes lumbopelvic myofascial referral and meralgia paresthetica. Because the latter condition causes lateral leg pain and paresthesia along the course of the lateral femoral cutaneous nerve, it is often confused with hip or low back pathologic impairment. It occurs rarely, except in patients who are pregnant, those who are obese, or those who wear tight undergarments.

During the acute stages, treatment focuses on control of pain and swelling through rest, ice, compression, and elevation (RICE). In some instances, antiinflammatory medication or physical therapy is appropriate. Proper footwear is important to absorb shock. In resistant cases, injections of antiinflammatory medication or surgical excision of the bursa may be required. The prognosis for a full recovery is good.

Myositis Ossificans

Trauma may lead to myositis ossificans, the formation of calcium in a muscle belly. The quadriceps or biceps muscle is the most commonly involved. Frequently, the condition develops after a direct blow in a contact or collision sport.

In the initial stages the patient experiences pain and swelling in the muscle belly. Other symptoms include a decrease in the range of motion and an inability to contract the muscle. Radiographic studies are often normal in the first 4 to 6 weeks, although MRI may reveal early hematoma formation. As the condition progresses and the body does not reabsorb the blood and fluid collected in the area because of the injury, a thickening begins that may develop into a calcification at 3 to 4 weeks (Figure 9-7).

The calcification of a myositis ossificans begins at the periphery of a hematoma and progresses inward in a centripetal maturation pattern.[4] The calcification con-

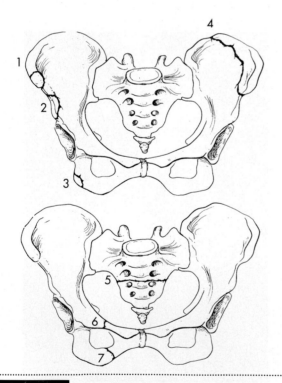

Figure 9-6 Stable fracture of pelvis ring; numbers 1 through 7 indicate fracture sites. 1, Anterior superior iliac spine; 2, anterior inferior iliac spine; 3, ischium; 4, iliac wing; 5, sacrum; 6, superior pubic ramus; 7, inferior pubic ramus.

(From Berquist TH, Coventry MM: The pelvis and hips. In Berquist TH, editor: *Orthopaedic radiology: imaging of orthopedic trauma and surgery,* Philadelphia, 1986, WB Saunders.)

Table 9-2	Greater Trochanteric Bursitis
Physical examination findings	Palpable tenderness or swelling over affected bursa Lateral thigh pain Pain from long-standing weight bearing
X-ray findings	Often normal Need to rule out calcification of bursa
Treatment plan	Ice with EMS or ultrasound Proper footwear

EMS, Electrical muscle stimulation.

tinues to develop over a period of months and then gradually resolves. Some calcification may remain permanently, however.

Early treatment focuses on controlling the swelling with ice and compression so that the contusion does not go through the phases of hematoma formation and calcification. The treatment also includes active rest and elevation. Most practitioners prescribe physical therapy to achieve the goals of the initial treatment. When the swelling is under control, it is imperative to begin gentle range-of-motion and strengthening activities (Table 9-3).

The prognosis depends on early and aggressive treatment. If the contusion is over the quadriceps muscle, the patient should have full knee flexion and at least 80% to 90% of the muscle's strength restored before returning to normal activities; otherwise, he or she is vulnerable to reinjury or a new injury, particularly to

the knee. If an effusion is present in the knee joint after a quadriceps contusion, this signifies that treatment is lacking or the patient has not been compliant.

Strains

Quadriceps Strain

Those who begin an activity or sport without prior warm-up, stretching, or conditioning often strain the quadriceps muscle. This injury is particularly common in those who participate in running activities. They may complain of the sudden onset of pain that stops their activity, or they may develop pain and soreness several hours later.

The physical examination reveals swelling and sometimes a palpable defect in the muscle belly. The patient is generally very apprehensive about contracting the quadriceps muscle because of the pain, or he or she may even be unable to contract it. Radiographic findings, if films seem necessary, are normal.

Grading may be performed to categorize and describe the strain according to the severity of the findings. A grade I strain is mild, grade II is moderate, and grade III is severe with a complete rupture or defect.

Treatment is RICE (Table 9-4). The clinician may prescribe physical therapy, depending on the severity of the tear. Crutches are not usually necessary, except for those patients with a grade III strain. Stretching and strengthening should begin once the pain and swelling are under control. Again, these patients should not return to their normal activity until the symptoms have subsided and they have regained their flexibility, strength, and functional capacity.

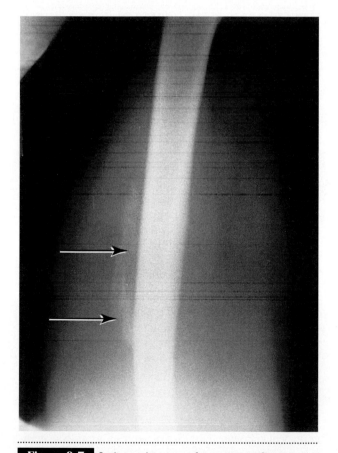

Figure 9-7 Radiographic signs of myositis ossificans in a 16-year-old lacrosse player 6 weeks after sustaining a quadriceps contusion.

Table 9-3 Myositis Ossificans

Physical examination findings	History of anterior thigh contusion
	Common participation in contact sports
	Painful knee flexion
	Swelling or tightness in anterior thigh
X-ray findings	Possibly normal, especially early in course of treatment
	Rule out calcific mass in thigh
Treatment plan	Aggressive cryotherapy
	Pulsed ultrasound
	EMS to sensory level only
	Gentle restoration of range of motion
	Protection of area in sports when patient returns to full activity or contact

EMS, Electrical muscle stimulation.

Table 9-4 Muscle Strains

	Quadriceps	Hamstring	Adductor
Physical examination findings	History of overuse or sudden stretch, contraction of extensor mechanism Palpable pain and swelling over muscle Possible deficit in muscle belly Discomfort on stretching Ecchymosis in moderate-to-severe injuries	Palpable tenderness at midbelly, origin, or insertion Swelling and ecchymosis in moderate-to-severe strains History of ground-based sports or chronic dysfunction; tightness Need to rule out short leg syndrome, pelvic tilt, or lumbosacral joint dysfunction	Palpable pain over adductors or pubic attachments Discomfort with hip abduction and active adduction against resistance
X-ray findings	Usually not applicable	Normal	Need to rule out pubic symphysitis
Treatment plan	RICE, electrotherapy, and ultrasound Flexibility program, including PNF, static stretches, and strengthening activities	RICE, electrotherapy, and ultrasound Hip flexibility program, strengthening of thigh CMT to lumbopelvic spine to treat concomitant dysfunction Monitoring of pelvic tilt and asymmetry in stride or gait	Ice, ultrasound, gentle stretching Follow-up films or bone scan to rule out stress fracture

RICE, Rest, ice, compression, and elevation; **PNF,** proprioceptive neuromuscular facilitation; **CMT,** chiropractic manipulative therapy.

Hamstring Strain

Similar to the onset of a quadriceps strain, the onset of a hamstring strain can be sudden or gradual. Acute tears often occur in athletes during moments of rapid deceleration or at a sudden change of direction. Pain and disability can be significant. The individual usually holds the knee in flexion and, in severe strains, is unable to bear weight on the leg.

The physical examination reveals pain on palpation, generally at the origin, insertion, or mid-muscle belly. Grading the tear is the same as that with a quadriceps strain. Ecchymosis is a sign of intramuscular bleeding and may be significant. Again, radiographic findings, if applicable, are normal.

Hamstring strains can become chronic pulls, and initial treatment is imperative to prevent complications. The treatment is basically the same as that for a quadriceps strain. It is important that the initiation of RICE be immediate, and the injured individual should use crutches in the immediate period after injury and should continue to use them until the pain and swelling disappear. Rehabilitation includes aggressive strengthening and stretching of the hamstring mechanism. As part of follow-up care, the clinician should rule out pelvic tilt, lumbosacral joint dysfunction, and short leg syndrome.

Adductor Strain

Often chronically incapacitating, adductor strains may be the result of either overuse or single-episode injuries. Aerobic athletes (e.g., runners), hockey and football players, and soccer players commonly develop such injuries. Pain may occur in the adductor mass or at the pelvic attachment. In individuals with a history of chronic strain, pelvic radiographic studies are helpful to rule out a stress fracture of the pubic symphysis (Figure 9-8).

Treatment includes the application of ice, ultrasound, and rest. Runners and other athletes who develop symphysitis as a result of ground-based sports (i.e., activities that require weight bearing in the upright position) will heal only with a protracted period of rest. Once pain, swelling, and gait problems dissipate, it may be advisable for the individual to participate in an active flexibility program for the hip, thigh, and lower back.

Follow-up films may be needed 4 to 12 weeks after the injury for patients whose initial radiographic studies were normal. Athletes whose radiographic findings are equivocal and whose injuries are refractory to conservative treatment may require a bone scan to rule out a stress fracture. Sclerosing of the pubis on plain films confirms pubic symphysitis.

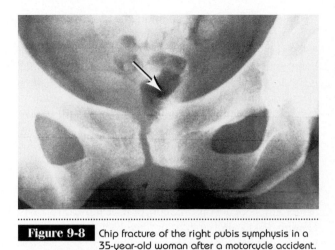

Figure 9-8 Chip fracture of the right pubis symphysis in a 35-year-old woman after a motorcycle accident.

Degenerative Arthritis of the Hip

Adults may develop degenerative arthritis of the hip as a result of earlier hip impairment. Childhood disorders such as hip dysplasia or undiagnosed slipped capital epiphysis can cause problems later in life, for example. Trauma and aging can also contribute to the degenerative process.

Physical examination findings include loss of motion, especially internal rotation and flexion. The patient may complain of knee or groin pain. Bursitis, tendonitis, and gluteal myofascitis often accompany arthritis, and the clinician should be careful to rule out lumbar spine disease as well. Radiographic findings include heterotopic bone formation and joint space narrowing (Figure 9-9). In severe cases, bony remodeling may occur. Patients with advanced disease may be unable to perform everyday tasks and may experience night pain.

Treatment depends on the severity of the symptoms, the expectations of the patient, and the degree of the patient's dysfunction. Weight reduction, medication, and therapeutic modalities may all be helpful. It is important to maintain range of motion and strength (Table 9-5). Older and more debilitated individuals may find a cane useful. Patients who do not respond to oral medications can be referred to an orthopedic surgeon, who may administer steroids to reduce inflammation.

Joint replacement surgery (total hip arthroplasty) is performed for relief of pain only. Although this procedure can have remarkable results, it can also have serious side effects, such as thrombophlebitis, fracture, loosening, infection, and a toxic reaction to metal.[5] Thus the treating surgeon, patient, and family should all partici-

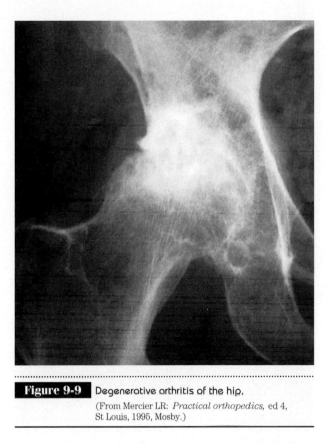

Figure 9-9 Degenerative arthritis of the hip.

(From Mercier LR: *Practical orthopedics,* ed 4, St Louis, 1995, Mosby.)

pate in the process of deciding to perform a total hip replacement procedure (Figure 9-10). Crucial factors to be considered in planning surgery are the patient's health status and age.

Osteonecrosis of the Femoral Head

Childhood hip disorders, such as slipped capital femoral epiphysis, may lead to osteonecrosis of the femoral head in the adult.[11] (The terms *osteonecrosis, avascular necrosis,* and *ischemic necrosis* all describe the same syndrome of cell death, bone proliferation, and revascularization.) An increase in venous pressure, prolonged use of steroids, prior trauma (i.e., fracture or dislocation), and the abuse of alcohol may also be causative factors. There is a 50% bilateral incidence.

The patient with osteonecrosis of the femoral head may have a history of hip pain and disability. Some have an anatomic short leg; others may suffer concomitant low back pain. A synovitis with a painful loss of motion may also be present. Internal rotation and hip flexion are most severely affected. Groin, proximal thigh, and buttock pain may occur as well.[19]

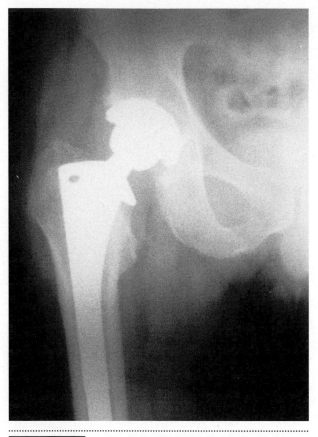

Figure 9-10 Total hip arthroplasty for degenerative arthritis in a 58-year-old man.

Osteonecrosis of the femoral head has four stages of progression: (1) bony ischemia with bone and marrow cell death, (2) cell proliferation, (3) revascularization of bone, and, finally, (4) reossification.[8] Bone scan or MRI is best for early detection. Plain radiographic films clearly document the staging of the disease.

Chiropractic care should center around the consequences of altered gait, pelvic tilt, short leg syndrome, and joint dysfunction. Lumbopelvic derangements warrant manipulation and orthopedic follow-up to the hip (Table 9-6). Debilitated patients should be referred to an orthopedic surgeon for consultation on the need for osteotomy, core decompression, or total hip arthroplasty (Figure 9-11). Rehabilitation involves restoration of healthy gait patterns and hip mobility.

Childhood Hip Disorders

Acute and subacute physeal injury is unique in the pediatric patient. Presentations and etiology may vary, but most cases of hip pain in a child involve a limp, hip-pelvis-leg pain, and painful and limited internal rotation. Several causes of a childhood limp directly involve the hip joint. The age of involvement is a critical clinical clue. For example, congenital dislocation, transient synovitis, and trauma are common causes of limping in children aged 1 to 3 years. In older children (i.e., 4 to 10 years of age), Legg-Calvé-Perthes disease or a slipped capital femoral epiphysis is a common cause of limping.[15]

Table 9-5 Degenerative Arthritis of the Hip

Physical examination findings	History of chronic pain and disability Painful loss of range of motion, especially internal rotation and flexion of hip Associated gluteal myofascial pain Need to rule out lumbar disk disease and degenerative arthritis of knee
X-ray findings	Bony remodeling Loss of joint space
Treatment plan	Maintenance of range of motion Physiotherapy modalities for pain control Weight control and loss, if applicable Referral for medication, if necessary CMT, if concomitant lumbopelvic problem Total hip arthroplasty in advanced cases

CMT, Chiropractic manipulative therapy.

Table 9-6 Osteonecrosis of the Femoral Head

Physical examination findings	Synovitis of affected hip Limp with altered weight bearing Pelvic tilt: need to rule out short leg syndrome Painful range of motion, especially limited internal rotation and hip flexion
X-ray findings	Whitening, fragmentation, and remolding of femoral head Need to monitor for containment of femoral head within acetabulum
Treatment plan	CMT to lumbopelvic spine Referral to orthopedic surgeon

CMT, Chiropractic manipulative therapy.

Osteonecrosis and infection both may affect the vascular supply of the femoral head. Tumors (e.g., Ewing's sarcoma, neuroblastoma, osteoid osteoma), infection (e.g., osteomyelitis, septic hip), and transient synovitis with a recent history of upper respiratory infection may also cause childhood hip pain (Tables 9-7 and 9-8). Apophyseal avulsion occurs exclusively during late childhood and adolescence. Clearly, disorders of the hip, including traumatic and idiopathic conditions, that occur during the developmental years are serious and deserve careful attention (Table 9-9). The key to satisfactory outcomes in hip joint abnormalities is prompt recognition.

Slipped Capital Femoral Epiphysis

Those in the preadolescent and adolescent age groups may displace the capital femoral epiphysis. If the cause is nontraumatic, the symptoms may be insidious in onset, and the etiology is often unknown.[2] The condition is frequently associated with a specific body type (i.e., the somewhat endomorphic phenotype), such as that seen in an overweight adolescent. It occurs more commonly in male African-American children. If the condition affects one hip, there is a 25% probability that it will affect the opposite hip as well.[3]

If the cause of the condition is traumatic, it may be difficult to diagnose in the early stages. Most cases of physeal injury occur in a child with a chronic progressive problem.[13] Patients generally complain of knee or groin

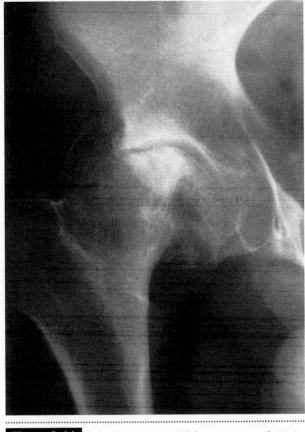

Figure 9-11 Avascular necrosis and degenerative arthritis in a 46-year-old man.

Table 9-7 Diagnosis of Diseases of the Developing Hip Joint

	Synovitis	Legg-Calvé-Perthes	Septic Hip	Slip Epiphysis	Snap Hip
Age	2-12 yr	4-10 yr	Any	8-16 yr	Birth-6 mo
Sex (M:F)	3:2	5:1	1:1	2.2:1	1:5
Trauma	±	±	±	±	0
Infection elsewhere	0	0	+	0	0
Height	Norm	↓	Norm	↑	Norm
Weight	Norm	↓	Norm	↑	Norm
Temperature	Norm	Norm	↑	Norm	Norm
X-ray hip	—	+	+	+	Norm
Bone age	Norm	↓	Norm	↓	Norm
CBC	Norm	Norm	± WBC ↑	Norm	Norm
ESR	Norm	Norm	↑	Norm	Norm
Technetium bone scan	+	+	+	+	Norm

CBC, Complete blood count; **ESR,** erythrocyte sedimentation rate; **WBC,** white blood cells.

(From Chung SMK: Diseases of the developing hip joint, *J Pediatr Clin North Am* 33(6):1458, 1986.)

pain, which in the active child may be interpreted as a muscle strain. The physical examination can indicate pain in the knee, the groin, or both.[18] The range of motion may be limited, and pain may be associated with flexion and internal rotation (Figure 9-12). In cases that are not diagnosed promptly, the range of motion may become fixed or a flexion contracture of the hip may develop.

The history and physical examination findings are the basis for the initial diagnosis. An x-ray film that resembles the slipping of an ice cream cone confirms the diagnosis. The degrees of the slip are used to classify the condition. A grade I capital femoral epiphysis slip may be as great as 25% of the circumference of the head; a grade II slip may be as great as 50%; a grade III slip may be as great as 75%; and a grade IV slip may be greater than 75%.

One of the primary goals of treatment in the early stages of a slipped capital femoral epiphysis is to prevent the progression of the slip. Treatment for synovitis of the hip, which occurs in the preslip period, is the avoidance of weight bearing, Buck's traction, and observation. Once slippage has occurred, the grade of the slip determines the treatment approach (Table 9-10). Grade I warrants pin fixation to prevent progression. Grades II through IV necessitate closed reduction and pin fixation. In rare instances, open reduction and fixation are necessary.

The prognosis associated with a slipped capital femoral epiphysis depends on the time of both diagnosis and initial treatment. In general, the prognosis is favorable if treatment begins in the preslip or grade I period. It becomes poorer as the disease progresses. Conditions that go undetected until they require reduction have the worst prognosis. The end result in these cases will be degenerative arthritis of the hip. Thus early and accurate diagnosis is essential.

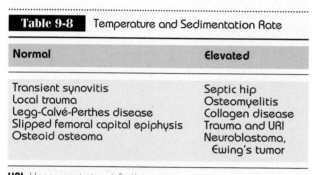

| **Table 9-8** | Temperature and Sedimentation Rate |

Normal	Elevated
Transient synovitis	Septic hip
Local trauma	Osteomyelitis
Legg-Calvé-Perthes disease	Collagen disease
Slipped femoral capital epiphysis	Trauma and URI
Osteoid osteoma	Neuroblastoma, Ewing's tumor

URI, Upper respiratory infection.

(From Chung SMK: Diseases of the developing hip joint, *J Pediatr Clin North Am* 33(6):1458, 1986.)

| **Table 9-9** | Developmental Hip Problems in Children |

	Slipped Capital Femoral Epiphysis	Legg-Calvé-Perthes Disease	Infection	Congenital Dysplastic Hip
Occurrence	Puberty	4-9 years of age	Newborn, young children	Female > male Left > right Breech > normal birth
Etiology	Familial (obese minority children)	Unknown hormonal possibilities	Infectious organism	Cerebral palsy, birth process Associated with metatarsus adductus, club foot, torticollis
Presentation	Limp, synovitis, decreased range of motion X-ray examination diagnostic	Limp, synovitis, decreased range of motion X-ray examination helpful to rule out infection and CDH	Fever, abnormal CBC, decreased range of motion Possibly normal bone scan	Barlow test for subluxation, Ortolani test for reduction
Treatment	Avoidance of weight bearing, pinning, traction	Avoidance of weight bearing, traction, immobilization	Medication, surgery, drainage	Maintenance of congruity, immobilization, traction
Consequences	Osteonecrosis, chondrolysis, short leg syndrome	Degenerative arthritis	Vascular insult	Contracture, limp

CDH, Congenital dysplastic hip; **CBC,** Complete blood count.

Apophyseal Avulsion (Iliac Apophysitis)

The avulsion of the iliac apophysis is an inferior displacement of the anterior superior iliac spine. Apophyseal pain occurs at the insertion of the sartorius muscle (Figure 9-13). Associated with a burst of quadriceps extension and hip flexion, apophyseal avulsion most commonly occurs suddenly in adolescents during athletic activities that require running and jumping, such as hurdling, sprinting, or playing basketball (Figure 9-14). Overuse injuries in child athletes can also produce pain over the iliac crest and, to a lesser extent, the ischial apophysis of the hamstring insertion. In its initial stages, apophyseal avulsion appears to be a serious injury because it is immediately disabling. The athlete commonly falls to the ground and is generally unable to bear weight on the affected side. Flexion is the most comfortable position.

During the physical examination, palpation over the anterior superior iliac spine demonstrates the exquisite tenderness of the area. The lowering (slipping) of the anterior superior iliac spine is frequently clear on an oblique x-ray film, although it may at times be evident on the anteroposterior projection.

Treatment is symptomatic with the use of ice directed at controlling the swelling and pain. The patient should use crutches to avoid placing any weight on the affected side. In cases of severe pain, bed rest in Buck's traction may be necessary. When tolerated, electrical modalities may be added to control the swelling. Antiinflammatory or analgesic medication is warranted only on rare occasions.

When the condition improves, the patient should begin with range-of-motion exercises and progress to weight-bearing and strengthening exercises for the lower extremity. Recovery may take 2 to 6 weeks, depending on the severity of the injury. Although the injury appears to be severe, it resolves completely and leaves no disability.

Legg-Calvé-Perthes Disease

Osteonecrosis of the femoral head is known as Legg-Calvé-Perthes disease in children. Although the cause is largely unknown, there may be a hormonal component to the pathologic process.[1] The lack of growth hormone (i.e., metabolic somatomedin) has been implicated.[10,21] Interruption of the blood supply to the femoral head also remains a generally well-accepted theory.[17] The condition often affects children who are short in stature and most commonly appears between the ages of 4 and 9 years. Male children predominate by a ratio of 4:1 or 5:1, and the condition is bilateral in 20% of affected children.[16]

The child's most prominent symptoms are a loss of hip motion and a painful limp. A synovitis of the hip as a result of osteonecrosis must be differentially diagnosed

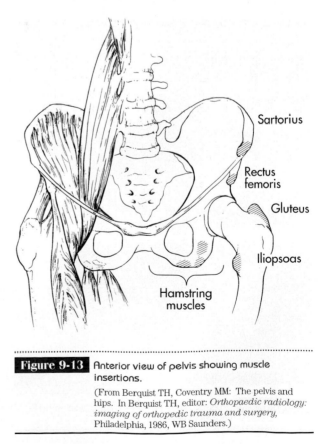

Figure 9-13 Anterior view of pelvis showing muscle insertions.

(From Berquist TH, Coventry MM: The pelvis and hips. In Berquist TH, editor: *Orthopaedic radiology: imaging of orthopedic trauma and surgery*, Philadelphia, 1986, WB Saunders.)

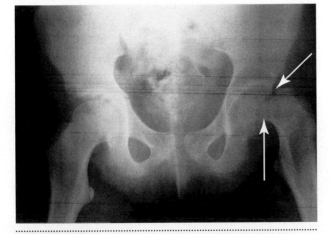

Figure 9-12 Slipped capital femoral epiphysis in an 11-year-old adolescent, who had experienced knee pain for 1 year. The hip lacks flexion and internal rotation.

Table 9-10 Disorders of the Hip in Children

	Slipped Capital Femoral Epiphysis	Apophyseal Avulsion	Legg-Calvé-Perthes Disease
Physical examination findings	Altered gait with limp Complaint of knee or groin pain Limited internal rotation, flexion of hip Possible flexion contracture with externally rotated foot	History of ballistic athletic activities Immediately painful on weight bearing Affected hip held in flexion Exquisite tenderness over anterior iliac apophysis	Synovitis of affected hip Limp with altered weight bearing Pelvic tilt, need to rule out short leg syndrome Painful range of motion, especially limited internal rotation and hip flexion
X-ray findings	Best visualization on anteroposterior view Slipping of "ice cream cone" Grade slippage 25% to greater than 75%	Anteroposterior and oblique projections Slipping of iliac apophysis best seen on oblique view	Whitening, fragmentation, and remodeling of femoral head Need to monitor radiologically for containment of head within acetabulum
Treatment plan	Use of crutches to eliminate weight bearing Referral to orthopedic surgeon	Ice, EMS Use of crutches to eliminate weight bearing	CMT to lumbopelvic spine Referral to orthopedic surgeon

EMS, Electrical muscle stimulation; **CMT,** chiropractic manipulative therapy.

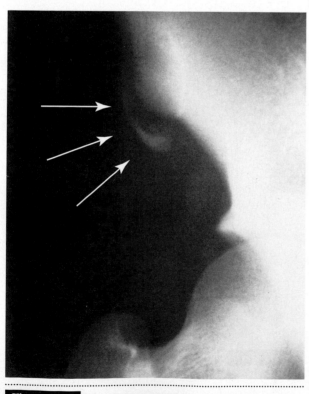

Figure 9-14 Avulsion (slip) of the iliac apophysis in a 12-year-old female sprinter.

from an acute infection.[7,11] Sepsis of the hip joint, of course, requires immediate treatment with antibiotics. Diagnostic x-ray films are helpful in excluding other pathologic conditions, such as congenital hip dysplasia.

Children with Legg-Calvé-Perthes disease should use crutches to avoid further joint destruction. It is imperative to contain the femoral head, and taking weight off the joint may prevent fragmentation, chondrolysis, and flattening of the head (Figure 9-15, *A-C*). Follow-up films are necessary to monitor the child's condition. Referral to an orthopedic surgeon for care is advisable, since neovascularization via surgery may be a treatment option.

Review Questions

1. (a) What is a common examination finding in patients with internal derangements of the hip joint? (b) What populations of patients with hip disorders are candidates for radiographic studies?
2. (a) Hip fractures are commonly seen in what segment of the population? (b) What are some etiologic factors involved in this injury? (c) What are common sites for fractures of the hip?

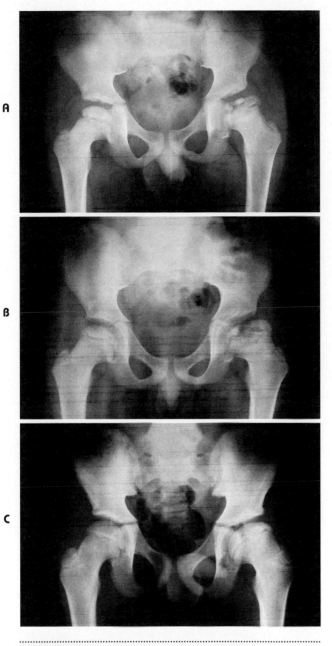

Figure 9-15 Legg-Calvé-Perthes disease of the hip.
A, Radiographic signs of fragmentation and chondrolysis. **B,** Remodeling and healing 1 year later. Note that the femoral head is fairly well contained. **C,** Complete remodeling and healing 3 years later.

3. A football player sustains a blow to the anterior thigh. He has pain, limited knee flexion, and swelling and redness over the site. (a) What is your initial diagnosis? (b) When should you apply heat? (c) When should you use aggressive therapy? (d) Cryotherapy, pulsed ultrasound, gentle range-of-motion movements, and pad protection during return to play are all aimed at avoiding what medical condition?

4. (a) What clinical presentation in a pediatric patient should alert the examiner to a serious hip problem? (b) What afflictions affect children 1 to 3 and 4 to 10 years of age?

5. A 12-year-old basketball player experiences pain over the anterior hip while running and jumping. When she can no longer bear weight, she is seen in your office. Physical examination findings include a hip in mild flexion, tenderness over the iliac crest with mild swelling. (a) What is your initial diagnosis? (b) What diagnostic tests should be ordered? (c) What is considered appropriate care for this condition?

References

1. Bennett EL: Legg-Calvé-Perthes disease, *Adv Orthop Surg* 11(1):108, 1987.
2. Busch MT, Morrissy RT: Slipped capital femoral epiphysis, *Orthop Clin North Am* 18(4):637, 1987.
3. Chung SMK: Diseases of the developing hip joint, *Pediatr Clin North Am* 33(6):1457, 1986.
4. Estwanik JJ, McAlister JH Jr: Contusions and the formation of myositis ossificans, *Physician Sports Med* 18(4):52, 1990.
5. Evans BG, Salvati EA, Huo MH, Huk OL: The rationale for cemented total hip arthroplasty, *Orthop Clin North Am* 24(4):599, 1993.
6. Feldman D, Zuckerman JD, Frontel VH: Geriatric hip fractures: preoperative decision making, *J Musculoskel Med* 7(9):69, 1990.
7. Gerberg LF, Micheli LJ: Nontraumatic hip pain in active children: a critical differential, *Physician Sports Med* 24:1, 1996.
8. Glimcher MJ, Kenzora JE: The biology of osteonecrosis of the human femoral head and its clinical implications, *Clin Orthop* 140:273, 1979.
9. Grisso JA, Kelsey JL, Stram BL: Risk factors for falls as a cause of hip fracture in women, *N Engl J Med* 324:1326, 1991.
10. Harrison MHM, Burwell RG, Kristmindsdotir F: Delayed skeletal maturation in Perthes disease, *Acta Orthop Scand* 58:277, 1987.
11. Kallio P, Ryoppy S, Kunnamo V: Transient synovitis and Perthes disease, *J Bone Joint Surg* 68B(5), 1986.
12. Mayekawa DS, Ralls PW, Kerr RM, Lee KP, Boswell WD, Halls JM: Sonographically guided arthrocentesis of the hip, *J Ultrasound Med* 8:665, 1989.

13. Micheli LJ: Injuries to the hip and pelvis. In Sullivan JA, Grana WA, editors: *The pediatric athlete,* Park Ridge, IL, 1990, American Academy of Orthopedic Surgeons.

14. Nicholas JA, Hershman EB: *The lower extremity and spine in sports medicine,* ed 2, vol 2, St Louis, 1995, Mosby.

15. Rose CD, Doughty RA: Zeroing in on the cause of a child's limp, *J Musculoskeletal Med* 8(7):22, 1991.

16. Thompson GH, Salter RB: Legg-Calvé-Perthes disease, *Orthop Clin North Am* 18(4):617, 1983.

17. Weinstein SL: Legg-Calvé-Perthes disease, *Orthop Clin North Am,* 32:272, 1983.

18. Waters PM, Millis MB: Hip and pelvic injuries in the young athlete, *Clin Sports Med* 7:513, 1988.

19. Weissman BN, Sledge CB: *Orthopedic radiology,* Philadelphia, 1986, WB Saunders.

20. Wilson DJ, Green DJ, MacLarnon J: Arthrography of the painful hip, *Clin Radiol* 35:17, 1984.

21. Wynn-Davies R: Some etiological factors in Perthes disease, *Clin Orthop* 150:12, 1980.

22. Ziegler MM, Dorr V, Schultz RD: Ultrasonography of the hip joint effusions, *Skeletal Radiol* 16:607, 1987.

Chapter 10

Knee

PART ONE: EVALUATION OF THE KNEE JOINT

The knee is a critically important joint in the lower extremity, strong enough to serve as an anchor in weight bearing, yet flexible enough to provide dynamic function. The joint remains one of the most complex and vulnerable articulations.[113]

Applied Anatomy and Biomechanics

At first glance, the knee looks simple, with the nature of its movement primarily flexion and extension. Knee flexion increases the forces transmitted to the patellofemoral joint, which affects compressive loading. Movements involving knee flexion, such as bending and stair walking, magnify this effect. A significant amount of rotation takes place at the knee, however, in the last 15 degrees of terminal extension; this is termed the *screw-home mechanism*. The lack of stability via the bony structures around the knee, combined with the shearing forces that are introduced by the rotational element, explains in large part the potential for traumatic injuries of the knee.

The knee joint has three separate compartments: (1) the medial compartment, which consists of the articulation between the medial femoral condyle and the tibia; (2) the lateral compartment, which consists of the articulation between the lateral femoral condyle and the tibia; and (3) the patellofemoral articulation (Figure 10-1 *A*, *B*). The synovial membrane that envelops these three chambers is continuous and extends into the suprapatellar pouch.[113]

In addition to the medial and lateral compartments, the knee joint includes the patellofemoral joint. The patella sits on top of the trochlear groove of the femur, where the synovial capsule of the knee forms around the joint in a continuous fashion.[36] The patella is the largest sesamoid bone in the human body and acts as a fulcrum to increase the moment arm of the quadriceps muscle.[36]

The quadriceps tendon inserts into the top of the patella and gives off branches to either side. Referred to as the patellar retinaculum, this tendon is often a site for inflammation in malalignment and mechanical disturbances. This broad fibrous expansion aids in extending the knee joint even when the patellar tendon is ruptured. Fibers of the medial retinaculum include the aponeurosis of the vastus medialis obliquus muscle, plus part of the vastus itself. These fibers insert directly onto the medial aspect of the patella, where they form a depression and medial restraint to the kneecap that helps prevent lateral displacement of the patella.

Ligamentous stiffness and anatomic attachment limit the motion of the tibia. The tibial and femoral attachments of the medial collateral ligament limit the direction of stretch.[49] Although both rotation and translation take place at the knee, manual stress tests are designed to test one motion and one structure at a time.

A

B

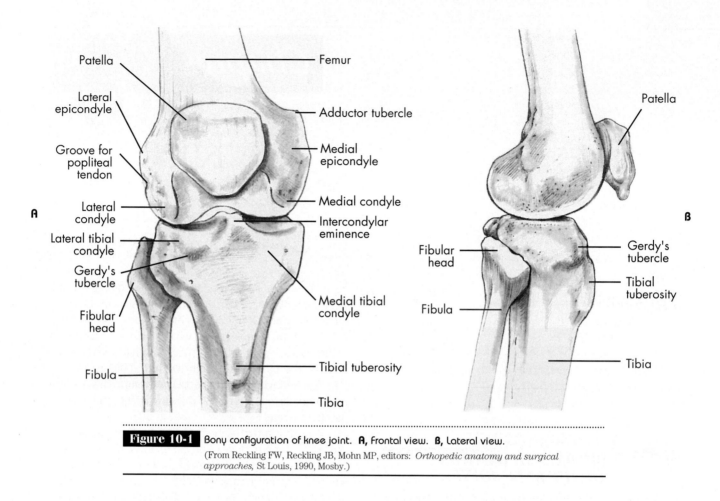

Patella

Lateral epicondyle

Groove for popliteal tendon

Lateral condyle

Lateral tibial condyle

Gerdy's tubercle

Fibular head

Fibula

Femur

Adductor tubercle

Medial epicondyle

Medial condyle

Intercondylar eminence

Medial tibial condyle

Tibial tuberosity

Tibia

Patella

Fibular head

Fibula

Gerdy's tubercle

Tibial tuberosity

Tibia

Figure 10-1 Bony configuration of knee joint. **A,** Frontal view. **B,** Lateral view.

(From Reckling FW, Reckling JB, Mohn MP, editors: *Orthopedic anatomy and surgical approaches*, St Louis, 1990, Mosby.)

Obviously, multiple movement trauma occurs at times, and the clinician must understand the implications of physically complex trauma at the knee joint.

Secondary Restraints

Although the knee joint does not have good bony stability, it does have a strong system of secondary restraints (Figure 10-2). An intricate network of ligamentous and musculotendinous structures acts as a barrier to injury. The tibiofemoral (or medial collateral) ligament and the fibulofemoral (or lateral collateral) ligament prevent excess adduction or abduction of the knee joint, respectively. The cruciate or "crucial" ligaments form the central pivot of the knee joint. The anterior cruciate ligament (ACL) provides a secondary restraint to excessive extension of the tibia on the femur; the posterior cruciate ligament (PCL) provides a secondary restraint to excessive flexion of the tibia on the femur. Both cruciate liga-

ments contribute to the rotatory stability of the joint. Thus the cruciate ligaments often aid the meniscus in shear resistance.

The cruciate ligaments pass each other in a criss-cross pattern between the tibia and femur. The ACL attaches to the posterior aspect of the medial surface of the lateral femoral condyle. The PCL, on the other hand, attaches to the posterior aspect of the lateral surface of the medial femoral condyle. Whereas the ACL attaches to the anterior tibial spine, the PCL attaches to the tibia in a depression posterior to the articulating tibial surface.[10]

The meniscofemoral ligament is an accessory ligament that extends from the posterior horn of the lateral meniscus to the lateral aspect of the medial femoral condyle near the attachment of the PCL. It may be divided into an anterior portion (Humphry's ligament) and a posterior portion (Wrisberg's ligament). The function of the meniscofemoral ligament is variable and quite questionable. During flexion it pulls the posterior horn

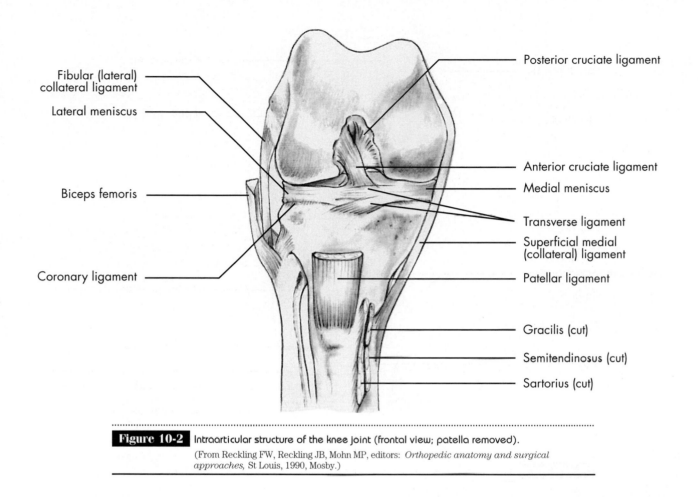

Fibular (lateral) collateral ligament

Lateral meniscus

Biceps femoris

Coronary ligament

Posterior cruciate ligament

Anterior cruciate ligament

Medial meniscus

Transverse ligament

Superficial medial (collateral) ligament

Patellar ligament

Gracilis (cut)

Semitendinosus (cut)

Sartorius (cut)

Figure 10-2 Intraarticular structure of the knee joint (frontal view; patella removed).

(From Reckling FW, Reckling JB, Mohn MP, editors: *Orthopedic anatomy and surgical approaches*, St Louis, 1990, Mosby.)

of the lateral meniscus anteriorly, which increases joint congruity between the meniscotibial pouch and lateral femoral condyle.[50]

Large muscle groups around the thigh contribute to stability and play a major role in proper knee function. Because the quadriceps muscle group is the anchor of the extensor mechanism of the knee joint, the prevention of injury to the knee and its rehabilitation after trauma depend on the proper alignment and strength of this group (Figure 10-3). The hamstring muscle group in the posterior thigh not only provides gravitational assistance in the postural mechanism, but it also participates in knee flexion. The biceps femoris, semitendinosus, and semimembranosus that make up the hamstring group together act as shock absorbers and secondary restraints. This particular group of posterior thigh muscles is especially sensitive to insult, as exhibited by the hamstring spasm or contracture that frequently develops as a protective measure after internal derangement of the knee. The upper head of the gastrocnemius muscle also

aids in knee flexion and posterior protection. Flexibility of the flexors and proper strength, alignment, and tone of the extensors are necessary to ensure patellofemoral joint function and prevent injury to the knee as a unit. Knee rehabilitation centers around these fundamental elements of dynamic movement.

Role of the Menisci

The proximal tibia expands into two spherical flat surfaces, called plateaus, that articulate with the distal femur. An intercondylar eminence separates the two plateaus and provides attachment sites for the cruciate ligaments and menisci.[36]

The role of the menisci is multifaceted. For example, the menisci

- Serve as important secondary restraints;
- Contribute to the overall stability of the knee joint;
- Help in load transmission;
- Aid in the lubrication process;

Terrible Triad of the Knee
medial meniscus
medial collateral lig.
Ant. cruciate lig.

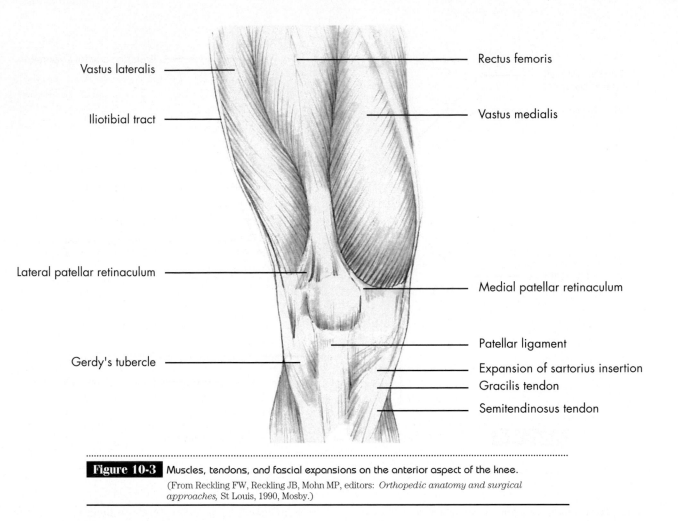

Vastus lateralis

Iliotibial tract

Lateral patellar retinaculum

Gerdy's tubercle

Rectus femoris

Vastus medialis

Medial patellar retinaculum

Patellar ligament

Expansion of sartorius insertion

Gracilis tendon

Semitendinosus tendon

Figure 10-3 Muscles, tendons, and fascial expansions on the anterior aspect of the knee.
(From Reckling FW, Reckling JB, Mohn MP, editors: *Orthopedic anatomy and surgical approaches*, St Louis, 1990, Mosby.)

- Function as major shock absorbers;
- Help control joint motion (especially extremes);
- Aid in nutrition of the joint.

The menisci play a significant role in the stability of the knee joint. For example, the medial meniscus has a stabilizing effect with the knee in 90 degrees of flexion.[85] In addition, the menisci limit motion as they move back and forth during flexion and extension. Thus the cartilage plays a role in blocking excessive translation in the sagittal plane. In the ACL–deficient knee, the menisci assume even greater importance as secondary restraints.

The menisci also have an impact on the distribution of load at the knee joint. Although contact force transmission is high on both sides of the knee, several investigators have documented a higher percentage of load in the lateral compartment.[84,115,131] It has also been gen-

erally accepted for the past 20 years that removal of the meniscus (as little as 16% to 34%) can increase joint contact surface forces by 350%.[51] This, in turn, places the knee severely at risk for early degenerative arthritis.

The articular surface of the knee functions smoothly with proper lubrication, and the movement of the menisci aids in distributing lubricants and nutrients throughout the joint. The menisci also provide a greater degree of compliance and serve to transfer stresses.[82]

It is essential that the primary care practitioner who is providing conservative care to a patient with a knee problem understands the peculiar anatomy of the vascular supply to the menisci. A working knowledge of the indications for arthroscopic repair of the fibrocartilage is also crucial. After studying both human and dog menisci, Arnoczky mapped out vascular zones of the cartilage. He discovered a capillary network at the peripheral border of the meniscus near the attachment of the joint capsule.[8,9] The primary care practitioner can apply these anatomic findings to apparent small peripheral tears of the menisci in deciding whether these tears are best treated with conservative, nonsurgical treatment.

Kinematics of the Knee Joint

The basic mechanism of joint movement at the knee is a combination of rolling and gliding.[60,74,91,94] Automatic rotation during the initial and end stages of movement, in addition to voluntary rotation, is superimposed on the basic knee motions of flexion and extension. The ratio of rolling to gliding often changes during the different phases of flexion. Hyperextension halts the rolling-gliding mechanism, however, because of the angulation in the terminal sulcus of the femoral condyle between the femorotibial and femoropatellar articular surfaces.[94,125]

Joint laxity with insufficiency of the ACL leaves the knee without a ligamentous restraint to hyperextension. Chronic ACL deficiency is potentially devastating, which can compromise activities, cause secondary changes in associated structures, and lead to arthritis.[120] This mechanical aberration often produces an impression or ridge on the lateral femoral condyle (termed *impressio terminalis*), resulting in an osseous pathologic abnormality.[96] Disintegration of the rolling-gliding mechanism can also harm the menisci in the ACL-deficient knee by causing the femoral condyle to roll excessively before it glides. Thus there may be a potential for degenerative changes at the joint line.

Biomechanics of the Patellofemoral Joint

Damage may occur at the articulating surface of the patellofemoral joint because of either intrinsic or extrinsic factors. Possible intrinsic factors include osseous alignment of the lower extremity, shape of the patella, and structural abnormalities of the trochlear groove of the femur. Extrinsic factors such as postural habitus, certain activities, and extensor mechanism strength also play a major role in patellar pain. Through their effect on the patella's pathomechanical track, these factors may cause damage that leads to articular surface abnormalities, dysfunction, or pain.[48]

The major active stabilizer of the patella is the vastus medialis obliquus muscle, which contributes to both patella positioning and optimum knee function.[36] Secondary stabilizers of the patellofemoral joint include the pes anserine muscle group: the sartorius, gracilis, and semitendinosus. Flexibility of the hamstring muscle group, along with a strong extensor mechanism at the posterior thigh, is important in patellofemoral health.

The particular shape of the patella determines patellofemoral joint congruity. Wiberg defined several types of patellae that are classified according to the shape and width of each facet.[134] Several authors have noted that a small medial facet is more likely to be associated with articular surface abnormality and patellofemoral instability.[26,134]

Joint congruity is greater on the lateral side of the patellofemoral joint, because the lateral facet is concave in both planes and fits well with the lateral femoral condyle.[48] The medial facet, however, is convex and touches the medial femoral condyle over only a small part of its surface. As a result of this and the tendency for lateral tracking during the first 20 degrees of knee flexion, the load increases on the lateral facet, but not on the medial side. A high-riding patella or "patella alta" is also associated with a lateral tracking mechanism, since such a patella fails to sit in the trochlear groove early in flexion and then it continues to ride over the lateral femoral condyle.[48]

Bony alignment of the lower extremity plays a large role as a determinant of patellar tracking. The alignment creates the Q angle, which determines the lateral insertion of the patellar tendon. The Q angle is calculated by drawing one line from the center of the patella through the center of the tibial tuberosity and a second line from the middle of the patella through the center of the anterior superior iliac spine at the pelvis.[36] The greater this angle, the greater the valgus vector. This in itself is not pathologic malalignment. An excessive Q angle (i.e., greater than 15 to 20 degrees) must be evaluated, along with strength faults at the extensor mechanism. Other cases of lower extremity malalignments, such as excessive femoral anteversion, genu valgum (knock-knee), and external tibial torsion, can also increase the Q angle.[77]

Malalignment, weakness, or trauma can all lead to irritation of the articular cartilage at the patellofemoral joint. Not all cases of anterior knee pain or even patellofemoral pain are attributable to chondromalacia, however. Retropatellar pain may accompany damage to the subchondral bone as well. It is well-documented that the healing of articular cartilage is imperfect.[11,88] Thus it is in the best interest of the clinician to understand both the mechanism of mechanical insult and the path to patellofemoral health.

Pathologic Movement

Five peripheral ligaments and two central ligaments act passively in concert to stabilize the knee. The peripheral ligaments are the lateral collateral ligament, the medial collateral ligament, the posterior oblique ligament (semi-membranosus-posteromedial capsular complex), the arcuate-popliteal complex, and the lateral capsule ligament. The rupture of *one* of these structures does not result in a large deficiency. However, the loss of one of the two central ligaments (i.e., ACLs and PCLs) in addition to the loss of one of the peripheral restraints may result in a gross insufficiency.

Pathologic motions that may result from a combined lesion of the knee's stabilizing system include the following:

- Increased rotation, as in anterior-rotatory instability
- Increased gapping, as in the varus or valgus deformation associated with lesions of the medial and lateral collateral ligaments
- Increased translation, primarily in the antero-posterior direction, as in lesions of the ACL and PCL

The ACLs and PCLs make up the centerpiece of knee stability. If there exists a large gapping of the knee joint under valgus or varus stresses, it is necessary to rule out a central joint lesion as well.

In total, there are six knee motions (6 degrees of freedom) at the knee.[49] Therefore there are six different types of laxities involved. If opposite movements are taken into consideration, there are then twelve possible limits of knee motion (Table 10-1). Although the clinician examines several structures individually, the overall accumulation of injury to restraints usually involves more than a single structure. Thus the diagnosis of internal derangements of the knee is a challenge. To reach an accurate diagnosis, the practitioner must be able to apply individual stability tests to the multiplicity of joint trauma. The ability to isolate a particular structure and test that structure accurately is clearly the key to differentially diagnosing knee injuries.

Components of a Case History

When evaluating the knee joint's condition, the old axiom, "listen, look, and feel," is a good guideline. Because of the complexity of this joint, a systematic approach to patient evaluation and care is crucial (Figure 10-4); thus organization is a high priority from the beginning. Certain patterns evolve throughout the evaluation of knee com-

Table 10-1	Twelve Limits of Joint Motion
Motion Limit	**Structures Limiting Motion**
Flexion	Ligaments, leg and thigh shape
Extension	Ligaments and joint compression
Abduction	Ligaments and lateral joint compression
Adduction	Ligaments and medial joint compression
Internal rotation	Ligaments and menisci
External rotation	Ligaments and menisci
Medial translation	Bone (spines interlocking with femoral condyles) and ligaments (to prevent distraction)
Lateral translation	Bone (spines interlocking with femoral condyles) and ligaments (to prevent distraction)
Anterior translation	Ligaments
Posterior translation	Ligaments
Joint distraction	Ligaments
Joint compression	Bone, menisci, and cartilage

(From Feagin JA, editor: *The crucial ligaments*, New York, 1988, Churchill Livingstone.)

plaints; such a pattern becomes evident both in the questioning process and during the actual examination.

The first rule in taking a case history is to listen to the patient. Using key terms such as "pop" or "twist," the patient will relay all the details of the injury. These details may provide a fundamental clue as to which anatomic structure is compromised and what the actual mechanism of injury is.

Prior Injuries

The clinician needs information about preceding trauma or prior complaints of knee pain leading up to the initial visit. Because patients often try to minimize their plight, direct questioning about prior injuries may be necessary. For example, the clinician needs to know about any prior difficulty in stair walking in patients with patellofemoral disease or any dysfunction and recurrent swelling in those with prior meniscal tears. It is common to see a patient who has symptomatology consistent with patello-femoral syndrome, but who reports a history of internal derangement with a lengthy period of immobilization. The atrophy and weakness that often follows a long period of immobilization may, in turn, lead to an insult to the extension mechanism and patella.

Previous Care

If the patient experienced a prior incident or painful episode in the knee, it is essential to determine whether the patient sought professional evaluation and treatment. A review of previous care is valuable for several reasons.

First, it serves as an indication of the clinical picture according to the first practitioner on the scene. What did the physician or therapist say? Was he or she concerned about the appearance of the knee? Did he or she recommend a specialist or suggest further testing procedures? If the patient reports that the knee was swollen and if the treating clinician ordered an arthrogram, for example, then the chances are great that the previous practitioner suspected a torn meniscus.

Second, a review of prior treatment provides patient feedback about the success or failure of the care received—whether it was professional treatment or self-treatment. Did the treatment provide relief? How long did it take? What was the method of treatment (e.g., ice, heat, aspirin)? This information may suggest the severity of the prior injury. If the patient received primary care during the previous episode, the clinician should ask if the patient received proper follow-up care after rehabilitation.

Third, a pattern of dysfunction or reinjury may become apparent, directing attention to certain internal structures in the knee joint. If the questioning suggests possible internal derangement, for example, the subsequent line of questioning should center around signs and symptoms of cartilage and ligamentous damage. For example:

Physician: Mrs. Jones, has your knee ever swelled up like this before?

Mrs. Jones: Oh, yes, several times. The last time, I was playing golf. I twisted my leg in a hole, and the next morning the knee blew up like a balloon.

Physician: Did you do something about it?

Mrs. Jones: Well, I put ice on once for 20 minutes, took two aspirin, then wrapped it with an Ace bandage.

Physician: How long did it take for the swelling to reduce?

Mrs. Jones: Oh, I'd say a few days.

Physician: Did you see your doctor?

Mrs. Jones: No, actually. I didn't show this to anyone except my husband. He told me not to play golf for a while.

At this juncture, depending on the age of the patient, the clinician may suspect a degenerative process inside the knee joint, a ligamentous insufficiency, or meniscal damage. In each case, both listening and a proper line of questioning help make the clinician's job as detective easier.

Extent of Trauma

While listening to the patient's story and expressions, the clinician begins to understand the extent of injury to the patient's knee and the impact of the injury on the patient's life style. If the injury resulted from an external force, such as a tackle in a football game or a table's fall on the leg, it is helpful to attempt to determine the magnitude of the blow. High-speed, ballistic trauma, such as occurs in skiing accidents or basketball game collisions, tends to cause an enormous amount of damage to the internal structures of the knee, especially the ligaments. Damage to these secondary restraints not only causes exquisite pain and joint effusion, but it also makes it clearly impossible for the person to bear weight fully.

Smaller amounts of self-imposed trauma, such as twisting a knee while walking, can and often do produce significant injury. Indeed, it takes only moderate force to sprain the ACL if the vectors of force are in place. Football and basketball players rapidly accelerate and decelerate as they sprint, cut, and change direction; many times they slip or fall, hyperextending the knee joint and causing damage to the ACL, which can be quite debilitating. Normally, however, a smaller force is likely to cause a simpler injury, such as a partially torn meniscus or a mild sprain to one of the collateral ligaments. Higher speed and higher impact movements tend to cause more severe, complex injuries to the knee, such as compound derangements that involve cartilage, ligaments, and joint capsule. These patients often require immediate surgical repair of the knee.

Mechanism of Injury

Of all the questions asked during the taking of the patient's history, perhaps those related to the exact mechanism of injury are the most important to the diagnostic process. In fact, experienced practitioners often say that this information alone gives them an idea as to the structures damaged, even before they actually examine the patient's knee.

be an ACL tear. In this case a traumatically induced hemarthrosis forms in the knee within 12 hours. In other cases a "snap" or "pop" may indicate a fracture or dislocation of the patellofemoral joint. Again, this is a clue that requires further investigation.

If there is swelling after an injury to the knee, it is important to ask the patient whether the swelling occurred immediately or was delayed in onset. Acutely injured ligaments always cause swelling at the knee, and the swelling is usually immediate. Joints affected by arthritis and other chronic conditions may take 1 or 2 days to swell because there are no broken blood vessels to cause a hemorrhage.

The presence of an effusion is a key factor and an often ominous clinical sign of an internal derangement. Usually, a *tense* effusion that expands the joint capsule causes a painful response. This is indicative of a hemarthrosis, which follows an injury to the knee ligaments or joint capsule. A torn ACL is one of the most common causes of an acute hemarthrosis. Meniscal tears evoke a synovial reaction that culminates in a knee effusion, but this response may not be apparent for 24 hours or more. Moreover, a torn meniscus causes a synovial effusion that is more *serous* in nature than the hemarthrosis. If this effusion is drained via arthrocentesis, the fluid appears straw colored. This effusion is not tense, is less painful than a hemarthrosis, and may take a shorter time to eliminate.

Physical Examination of the Knee

Observation: Gait and Attitude of the Knee

The visual scan begins the physical evaluation of the knee joint. (The patient must wear shorts or a gown so that the clinician can observe the entire lower extremity for comparison.) Observation of gait and attitude of the knee is important to assess the severity of injury. Many patients hold their injured knee in flexion because of the protective spasm of the hamstring muscle. A flexion contracture is a sign of a neglected knee injury, and the achievement of terminal extension in an injury is the key to returning the patient to proper function.

The clinician then compares the injured side with the "good" side—after ruling out any prior injury on the good side—to identify a proper baseline. A comparison of the two sides facilitates the recognition of knee displacement, swelling, and deformity. The alignment of the lower extremity can be evaluated simply by looking for an acute valgus angulation at the knee joint (excessive Q angle), torsion at the tibia, and malposition of the patella.

In comparing the affected side with the unaffected side once again, the clinician checks for atrophy and inspects carefully above the patella and at the medial aspect of the patella for vastus medialis size and tone. A weak extensor mechanism (quadriceps muscle) and vastus medialis atrophy may signify a lengthy period of immobilization, lack of proper muscular rehabilitation, or the beginning of a patellofemoral tracking problem. When the patient is seated, the clinician watches as the patella tracks during flexion and extension of the knee joint. Slight lateralization of the patella with extension of the knee is normal.[89] A marked lateral excursion may indicate pathologic misalignment or a faulty tracking mechanism, however.

As the patient lies down with the legs out straight, contraction of the quadriceps muscles, one leg at a time, should reveal any muscle inhibition, lack of tone, or inability to achieve terminal extension of the knee (0 degrees via a proper contraction). If the patient cannot contract the muscle, the clinician inspects the knee for signs of an internal derangement or severe neuromuscular dysfunction (e.g., prolonged disuse). Terminal extension is necessary to rule out a cartilage block in the knee joint of a patient with a suspected tear of the meniscus. Thus patients who have a hypermobile knee joint (i.e., exhibit genu recurvatum) at the knee should be examined to determine if they can achieve the same amount of extension bilaterally.

If the patient cannot achieve terminal extension through contraction of the extensor mechanism, placing a hand under the knee in the popliteal space is helpful to determine whether there is indeed a difference between one side and the other. The clinician should feel the knee against the hand equally on both sides, as the posterior knee approximates the table in extension. If terminal extension is not clearly possible, having the patient take the prone position and slide down on the examining table so that the knees are at the table's edge can make it easier for the clinician to determine whether the knees are extended equally. If they are not, the clinician checks for visible hamstrings spasm and palpates the musculature for hypertonicity and spasm. Most cases of flexion contracture in the posttraumatic knee are attributable to hamstrings spasm. The larger the contracture or shortening, the longer it will take the attending clinician to break the cycle and restore the knee to a healthy state of extension.

Palpation: Symmetry

Beginning with the unaffected side, the examining clinician palpates both the patient's legs for muscular tone, bogginess of the patellofemoral joint, and any tender structures. The clinician then asks the patient to contract the quadriceps muscle and feels for extension at the knee. It is important to determine whether the knee on the dominant side is stronger than the knee on the nondominant side. A knee that is weaker or exhibits muscle atrophy on the dominant side is certainly an injured joint in need of rehabilitation.

One of the most important aspects of palpation is to rule out the presence of a joint effusion, since an effusion is indicative of a pathologic abnormality at the knee. After trauma or injury, an effusion signifies a fracture, torn cartilage, or ligamentous sprain. An effusion of a nontraumatic origin can signify infection, systemic illness, or arthritide. Extraarticular swelling is less ominous, but the clinician still needs to evaluate thoroughly the periarticular soft-tissue structures.

The most efficient way to test for effusion requires the use of both of the examiner's hands. While standing beside the supine patient, the examiner uses the superior hand to seal off the suprapatellar pouch (see Figure 1-2); this milks any fluid down from the pouch into the knee joint proper. Then the examiner uses the finger tips of the inferior hand for ballottement, a palpation technique in which the clinician moves the patella up and down to ascertain whether it is swimming in a sea of fluid underneath it. If the patella is ballottable, an effusion is present in the knee joint. Swelling on top of the patella with no ballottement suggests that the swelling is superficial and does not involve the joint itself. This is usually caused by a traumatic bursitis of the prepatellar bursa, commonly termed *housemaid's knee*. Traumatic bursitis is the result of a blow on top of the kneecap, whereas a joint effusion from an internal derangement involves more complex joint loading.

Next, the examiner palpates the joint lines for symmetry, deformity, and pain. The sides of the finger pads provide sensitivity as the examiner feels for the contour at the joint line. Bending the knee to 90 degrees, if possible, can open up the joint space and make it easier for the clinician to find the tibial plateau and place the finger pad there. Joint line tenderness usually signifies a torn meniscus in an acutely injured patient, but older patients may have degenerative changes that cause them to feel pain upon palpation at the joint line. Usually plain films are helpful to rule out degenerative arthritis.

While the patient keeps the knees flexed at 90 degrees, the clinician palpates bilaterally over the collateral ligaments from their origin on the femur to the proximal lower leg. These areas are painful after a collateral ligament sprain from varus or valgus loading.

Other soft-tissue structures that are palpable at the knee include the patellar tendon and retinaculum, the hamstring tendon, the quadriceps and hamstring muscles, the gastrocnemius muscle (upper head), the iliotibial band, and the popliteal tendon. Osseous structures that should be palpated include the tibial plateau, fibular head, patella, and medial and lateral femoral condyles.

Stability Testing

The hallmark of a good orthopedic evaluation is careful stability testing. During the stability testing portion of the physical examination, answers to important questions begin to appear:

- Is ligamentous or capsular integrity compromised?
- How much laxity is present in the joint?
- Should the patient ambulate?
- Does the injured joint require bracing or immobilization?
- Is the knee joint unstable; if so, is the knee joint unstable on two planes (i.e., anteroposterior and lateral planes)?

The secondary restraints of the knee joint must be checked bilaterally, and any apparent physical changes documented in the chart (Table 10-2). The first step is to obtain a good baseline value of joint mobility and ligamentous integrity through a manual examination of the unaffected knee joint. Because many individuals have inherent joint laxity in their ligamentous system—not only at the knee joint, but also in other articulations—care is essential to avoid mistaking an inherently lax joint for an acutely compromised joint. Patellofemoral hypermobility, genu recurvatum, and capsular laxity occur in many women, for example, and do not automatically imply a traumatic injury.

Although several devices are available in the clinical laboratory for documenting the degree of gapping in a ligament, the experienced examiner is capable of manually discerning the presence of instability at the knee. Adhering to certain guidelines makes the testing easier, however. First, testing the supporting structures of the knee *before* swelling, spasm, and severe guarding provides a truer value of joint stability, although testing may not be possible unless the examiner is present at the time

Table 10-2 Stability Tests for Ligaments at the Knee

Type of Stability	Test	Structures Involved
Uniplanar: medial/lateral	Abduction (valgus) test (30°, 0°)	Medial collateral ligament, posteromedial capsule
	Adduction (varus) test (30°, 0°)	Lateral collateral ligament, posterolateral capsule
Uniplanar: anterior/posterior	Lachman's test (20°)	Anterior cruciate ligament
	Anterior draw test (sign)	Anterior cruciate ligament
	Posterior draw or sag sign	Posterior cruciate ligament
Anterolateral rotatory: anterior/lateral rotation	Pivot shift test	Anterior cruciate ligament, anterolateral capsule, possible arcuate complex
	Flexion-rotation draw test (Slocum test)	Anterior cruciate ligament, lateral or medial secondary restraints
Biplanar: anterior/medial	Lachman's test	Anterior cruciate ligament
	Abduction (valgus) test (at 0°)	Posteromedial capsule, posteromedial compartment
	Abduction (valgus) test (at 30°)	Medial collateral ligament

of the traumatic injury (e.g., at the athletic event involved). Second, if the patient does not seek treatment until several weeks after the injury, the application of ice and electrotherapy in the office can remove some muscular guarding and patient inhibition during the examination. Third, when testing joint stability, the examiner may need to begin by reassuring the patient to help him or her relax and counteract the factors that can block an accurate recording of ligamentous instability, such as patient guarding, hamstring contracture, and pain.

Collateral Ligament Testing

Because both the medial and lateral collateral ligaments aid in the overall stability of the knee joint, it is necessary to test them to clarify the presence of valgus or varus instability. The medial (tibial) collateral ligament attaches to the medial meniscus in its deepest layers and is contiguous with the joint capsule.[87] The lateral (fibular) collateral ligament does not attach to the lateral meniscus. The examiner tests both structures for uniplanar lateral instability at the knee.

Abduction Test (Valgus Stress Test). To assess medial instability in one plane, the examiner performs the abduction test, sometimes called the valgus stress test. Pushing the knee medially, the examiner slightly rotates the ankle externally and stabilizes it. As shown in Figure 10-5 A, B, this test should be performed with the knee both in terminal extension (0 degrees) and in flexion (30 degrees). Performing this procedure in full extension tests the integrity of the posteromedial joint capsule and the medial collateral ligament. If the knee joint gaps or opens up in the medial aspect at 0 degrees of extension,

the examiner must determine whether there is any damage to other structures, such as the cruciate ligaments, medial meniscus, or soft-tissue structures adjacent to the knee joint.

At 30 degrees of flexion, the examiner is carrying out a truer test of medial collateral ligament laxity because the capsule is markedly relaxed in flexion. Thus the test is the true procedure to screen for uniplanar medial joint stability of the medial collateral ligament. Gapping or medial joint opening of up to 5 mm is usually seen in grade I sprains, whereas up to 10 mm is seen in grade II sprains; grade III sprains evoke gapping of more than 10 mm.[95] Thus both grade I and grade II sprains have a definite end-point of movement, but grade III sprains do not.[31] An alternative instability rating scale uses 0, 1+, 2+, or 3+ to describe degrees of laxity in centimeters (Figure 10-6).

Adduction Test (Varus Stress Test). To assess the integrity of the lateral stabilizers of the knee joint, the examiner pushes the knee joint laterally while stabilizing the ankle. Similar to the abduction test, this procedure, called the adduction test or varus stress test, is performed at both 0 degrees (i.e., terminal extension) and 30 degrees of flexion. Also, similar to the abduction test, the adduction test is positive if the joint gaps (opens); this time, however, any laxity is evident at the lateral joint complex.

A positive test in full extension indicates damage to the posterolateral capsule and lateral collateral ligament. In addition, the examiner should check for damage at the arcuate-popliteal junction, cruciate ligament, and biceps tendon.

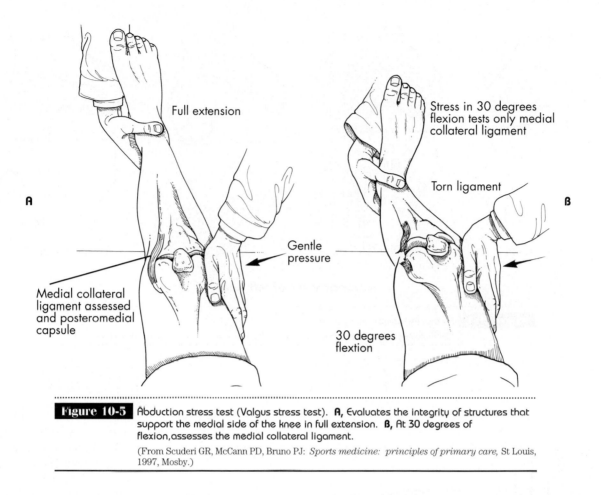

Full extension

Stress in 30 degrees flexion tests only medial collateral ligament

Torn ligament

A

B

Gentle pressure

Medial collateral ligament assessed and posteromedial capsule

30 degrees flextion

Figure 10-5 Abduction stress test (Valgus stress test). **A,** Evaluates the integrity of structures that support the medial side of the knee in full extension. **B,** At 30 degrees of flexion, assesses the medial collateral ligament.

(From Scuderi GR, McCann PD, Bruno PJ: *Sports medicine: principles of primary care,* St Louis, 1997, Mosby.)

At 30 degrees of flexion, the examiner can obtain an accurate test of the lateral collateral ligament, because this position relaxes the posterolateral capsule. A grade I sprain usually exhibits 5 mm of gapping with a firm end-point; a grade II sprain gaps approximately 8 mm with a soft end-point; a grade III sprain is greater than 10 mm.

Cruciate Ligament Testing

Lachman's Test. The examiner holds the patient's knee in approximately 20 degrees of flexion for the Lachman's test. While the patient is supine, the examiner stabilizes the femur with the superior hand and grasps the proximal tibia with the inferior hand (see Figure 1-3). The examiner attempts to draw the tibia forward on the femur, thus testing for ACL laxity.

Because bending the knee neutralizes the hamstring muscle, the Lachman's test is the most accurate test for the ACL.[33] It is the most reliable test in detecting the increased anterior tibial translation attributable to an ACL injury, since it can elicit even small amounts of tibial

excursion.[99] Moreover, even a few millimeters may be indicative of a complete ACL disruption. On the other hand, a definite end-point or "hardness" does not always mean that the ligament is intact; secondary restraints can contribute to this sensation. Experienced examiners may rate laxity as 0, 1+, 2+, or 3+ with either a soft or firm end-point (Figure 10-7), and they can usually diagnose a disruption of the ACL because of changes in end-point stiffness. Thus the Lachman's test is sensitive to even partial tears of the ACL, whereas other tests (e.g., the anterior draw) are not.

Anterior Draw Test. The examiner places the patient's knee in 90 degrees of flexion for the anterior draw test. The examiner usually holds the patient's foot down or sits on it and, with both hands placed around the tibia, attempts to draw the tibia forward on the femur (Figure 10-8). The tibia must remain in a neutral position (i.e., not rotated). An internally rotated tibia produces a taut iliotibial band that will block anterior translation of the tibia.

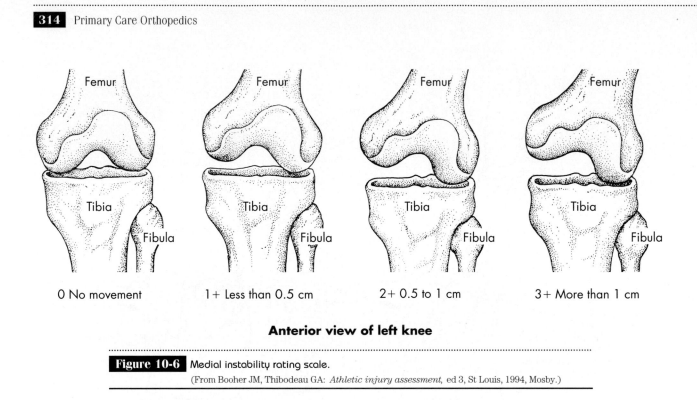

0 No movement   1+ Less than 0.5 cm   2+ 0.5 to 1 cm   3+ More than 1 cm

Anterior view of left knee

Figure 10-6 Medial instability rating scale.

(From Booher JM, Thibodeau GA: *Athletic injury assessment,* ed 3, St Louis, 1994, Mosby.)

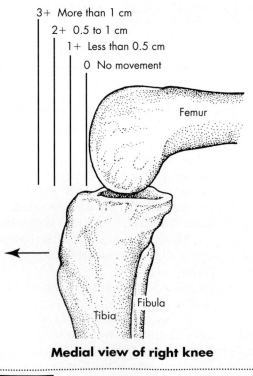

Medial view of right knee

Figure 10-7 Anterior instability rating scale.

(From Booher JM, Thibodeau GA: *Athletic injury assessment,* ed 3, St Louis, 1994, Mosby.)

Although similar to the Lachman's test for ACL stability, this test is not as accurate; the hamstring muscles tend to pull back on the tibia in the acutely injured knee, neutralizing the draw to a certain extent.[69] Thus the results of the anterior draw test may be negative in the presence of partial tears, although the Lachman's test will detect such tears. Demonstrable laxity in the anterior draw test may help confirm a complete tear of the ACL, however.

An average of 6 mm of tibial translation, side to side, is common in KT-1000 arthrometer testing for complete disruptions of the ACL.[29] Also, it is important to check the PCL; damage to this ligament allows the tibia to be displaced back on the femur, causing the result of the anterior draw test to be false positive. In addition to the ACL, the posteromedial and posterolateral capsules are tested.

Posterior Draw Test. For the posterior draw test (e.g., "sag" sign), the patient lies supine with the knees flexed to 90 degrees. The examiner looks for a "sag" of the tibia on a PCL–deficient knee. The examiner also can push down on the tibia, attempting to push the tibia back on the femur. Laxity or posterior draw is evident, if the patient has a torn PCL. If the patient does have such a tear, it is wise to investigate the possibility that the ACL is torn as well.

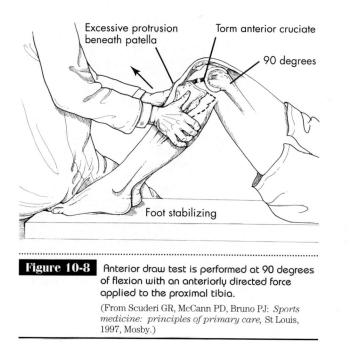

Excessive protrusion beneath patella

Torm anterior cruciate

90 degrees

Foot stabilizing

Figure 10-8 Anterior draw test is performed at 90 degrees of flexion with an anteriorly directed force applied to the proximal tibia.

(From Scuderi GR, McCann PD, Bruno PJ: *Sports medicine: principles of primary care*, St Louis, 1997, Mosby.)

Anterolateral Rotatory Instability

The most commonly encountered rotatory instability at the knee is anterolateral rotatory instability. It is the abnormal or pathologic anterior subluxation of the lateral tibial plateau in relation to the lateral femoral condyle as the knee approaches terminal extension.[24] In the healthy knee joint, the intact ACL guides the knee through its screw-home mechanism. The ligament becomes progressively tighter as the knee begins to extend from a flexed position. The ACL also aids in external rotation as the knee approaches full extension and then helps lock the knee in its stable, closed-packed position for weight bearing.[24] A deficiency in the ACL eliminates or reduces the effectiveness of this guiding mechanism and allows the anterolateral portion of the tibia to rotate internally and sublux anteriorly.[24] Tests for anterolateral instability are designed to elicit the pivot shift action.

Pivot Shift Test. Used to detect cruciate ligament–deficient knees with anterolateral capsular instability patterns, the pivot shift maneuver can have positive results in both acute and chronic ACL injuries. Also known as the McIntosh test, this procedure documents a "shift" in the knee joint by a subluxing tibia.[109] The knee is in full extension for the examination with the tibia internally rotated (Figure 10-9). Grasping the patient's foot with the inferior hand, the examiner uses the superior hand to apply a mild valgus stress force at the level of the knee

joint. As the examiner flexes the knee 20 to 30 degrees, he or she can usually feel a sudden jerk at the anterolateral aspect of the proximal tibia. When the knee approaches 30 to 40 degrees of flexion, there is a sudden reduction of the tibia that may be quite visible and painful. The reduction is believed to be the result of a pull of the iliotibial band,[46] and it signifies to the clinician that both the ACL and its secondary restraints are damaged.

If the patient is relaxed and the hamstring muscles are not contracted, this maneuver can provide a great deal of information. It is easier, however, to document a chronic case of ACL insufficiency with rotatory instability by means of the pivot shift procedure, rather than with an acute knee injury with swelling and muscle spasm.[69] Also, signs of anterolateral rotatory instability in other procedures may appear, even when the pivot shift test is normal. These cases are usually quite mild and result in subtle orthopedic findings.

Flexion-Rotation Draw (Slocum Anterolateral-Anteromedial Rotatory Instability Test). The examiner may perform the flexion-rotation draw test to check both medial and lateral rotatory instability. With the patient in the supine position, the patient's hip is flexed to 45 degrees, and the knee is first tested at 90 degrees of flexion. The foot of the side being tested rests on the table, and the examiner sits on that side of the table, trapping the patient's foot. Placing both hands on the upper tibia as in the anterior draw test for ACL tears, the examiner palpates the hamstring muscles to be certain they are relaxed. He or she then records the degree of anterior draw with the tibia in the neutral position, and checks the medial and lateral tibial plateaus to see if there is any asymmetric rotational movement. With the patient's foot in the neutral position, the examiner applies a rotational force to the lateral tibial plateau and notes the anterolateral rotational motion. The examiner then repeats the procedure for the medial tibial plateau. Next, the examiner brings the patient's knee to about 20 degrees of flexion and repeats the rotatory stability tests (Table 10-3).

The extent of ACL damage and the length of time between any trauma and its subsequent treatment play a role in the overall stability of the knee. In moderate knee instability after an ACL disruption, both the ligament and secondary restraints (medial and lateral compartments) exhibit laxity. Grossly unstable (subluxed) knee joints show associated laxity of medial and lateral extra-articular restraints as well. The gross subluxation of both the medial and lateral tibial plateaus is quite apparent during the Lachman's test and the flexion-rotation

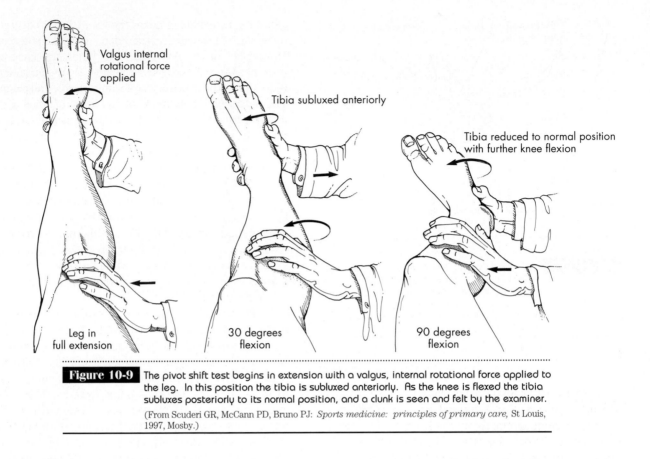

Valgus internal rotational force applied

Tibia subluxed anteriorly

Tibia reduced to normal position with further knee flexion

Leg in full extension

30 degrees flexion

90 degrees flexion

Figure 10-9 The pivot shift test begins in extension with a valgus, internal rotational force applied to the leg. In this position the tibia is subluxed anteriorly. As the knee is flexed the tibia subluxes posteriorly to its normal position, and a clunk is seen and felt by the examiner.

(From Scuderi GR, McCann PD, Bruno PJ: *Sports medicine: principles of primary care*, St Louis, 1997, Mosby.)

draw procedures. In such cases the midcapsular ligament, ACL, and iliotibial band, along with the arcuate complex, are likely to be damaged.[5]

Posterior and Posterolateral Instability

The importance of the PCL and the incidence of posterolateral instability are greatly debated. There do not appear to be as many patients with PCL deficiency and posterolateral instability as compared those with ACL deficiency of the knee. In rare cases a patient experiences an isolated tear during hyperflexion loading as a result of, for example, squatting improperly while trying to lift too much weight in power lifting or "Olympic style" weight lifting. In another scenario a patient may damage the knee beyond the scope of conservative care by tearing the capsule, medial capsule, and both cruciates as a result of a severe valgus load in a planted and rotated leg, such as in football. Severe traumatic hyperextension can damage the PCL, as well as the ACL.[73] A direct blow to the anterior knee, such as slamming the knee against the dashboard in a motor vehicle accident, is a classic injury to the PCL.

In the presence of posterolateral instability, the lateral tibial plateau rotates posteriorly on the femur, which can damage not only the PCL, but also the lateral compartment. The arcuate complex, lateral collateral ligament, popliteus tendon, and posterolateral capsule may all be affected. Stability testing shows that the fibular head has excessive excursion posteriorly.

Meniscal Injuries

Tears of the meniscus have deleterious effects on the overall stability of the knee. The natural course of patients with such an injury is consistent with degeneration of the joint.

Bounce Home Test. To check the ability of the injured knee joint to achieve terminal extension, the examiner may use the bounce home test to screen for a mechanical block in the joint. For example, a torn piece of fibrocartilage can cause the joint to fall short of 0 degrees of extension. (Hamstring spasm and contracture can also cause the knee joint to maintain flexion.)

The examiner supports the popliteal aspect of the patient's knee joint with the superior hand as the patient

Table 10-3 Primary and Secondary Ligamentous Restraints to Laxity Tests

Laxity Test	Primary Restraint				Secondary Restraint		
	Medial	Central	Lateral		Medial	Central	Lateral
A. Anterior drawer	—	ACL	—	20°/90°	TCL+MM	—	ALS
B. Anterior drawer plus internal rotation	—	ACL	ALS	20°/90°	—	—	FCL+PLS
C. Anterior drawer plus external rotation	TCL+MM	ACL	—	20°/90°	PMS	—	—
D. FRD, pivot shift	—	ACL	—	15°	MM+TCL+PMS	—	ALS+FCL
E. Posterior drawer	—	PCL	—	20°/90°	PMS+TCL	—	FCL+PLS
F. Posterior drawer plus external rotation	—	—	FCL+PLS	30°	—	PCL	—
	—	PCL	FCL+PLS	90°	—	—	—
G. Posterior drawer plus internal rotation	TCL+PMS	—	—	20°	—	ACL+PCL	—
	TCL+POL	PCL	—	90°	—	ACL	—
H. Valgus	TCL+PMS	—	Bone	5°	—	PCL+ACL	—
	TCL	—	Bone	20°	PMS	PCL	—
I. Varus	Bone	—	FCL+PLS	5°	—	ACL+PCL	—
	Bone	—	FCL	20°	—	ACL	PLS
J. External rotation	PMS+TCL	—	FCL+PLS	30°	MM	PCL	—
	MM+TCL	PCL	FCL+PLS	90°	PMS	—	—
K. Internal rotation	TCL+PMS	ACL	ALS	20°	—	PCL	FCL
	TCL+POL	ACL+PCL	ALS	90°	—	—	FCL

ACL, Anterior cruciate ligament; **ALS**, Iliotibial band plus anterior plus midlateral capsule; **FCL**, fibular collateral ligament; **FRD**, flexion rotation drawer; **MM**, medial meniscus; **PCL**, posterior cruciate ligament; **PLS**, popliteus, posterolateral capsule; **PMS**, posterior oblique ligament plus posteromedial capsule; **POL**, posterior oblique ligament; **TCL**, tibial collateral ligament.
(From Noyes FR, Grood ES: Classification of ligament injury. In Griffin PP, editor: *Instructional testing,* vol 36, 1987, Rosemont, Ill, AAOS.)

lies supine. Instructing the patient to let the knee drop in the examiner's hands helps eliminate muscle guarding. Gently grasping the affected leg under the heel or ankle with the inferior hand, the examiner attempts to bring the injured knee into a gentle "bounce" of terminal extension. This test should not be a forceful ballistic and painful maneuver; it can and should be performed gently and effectively.

McMurray Test and Sign. Through the years the McMurray test has become a standard screening tool for meniscal tears. It has a fairly high degree of specificity for posterior horn tears.[1] The test attempts to pinch the fibrocartilage tag that a meniscal tear may leave between adjacent articular surfaces; the reproduction of pain by this maneuver confirms the diagnosis. The test is performed as follows:

1. Have the patient recumbent in the supine position.
2. Bring the knee of the affected leg into flexion until the heel reaches the buttock.

3. Rotate the tibia on the femur, first laterally then medially.
4. Extend the knee while still rotating the tibia, internally for the lateral meniscus and externally for the medial meniscus.
5. Listen and feel for a click, which may indicate a reduction of the meniscal tag that is being disengaged.

The examiner must distinguish common clicks heard from the patellofemoral joint from the click of a torn cartilage inside the joint. The test is not specific for diagnosing tears in the anterior one third of the meniscus.

Apley Test. Although not as practical as other testing procedures, the Apley test can help the beginning practitioner differentiate cartilage tears from ligament sprains. The test has two parts. The first part is an attempt to confirm or rule out a ligament or joint capsule sprain; the second is an attempt to detect the presence of a meniscal tear.

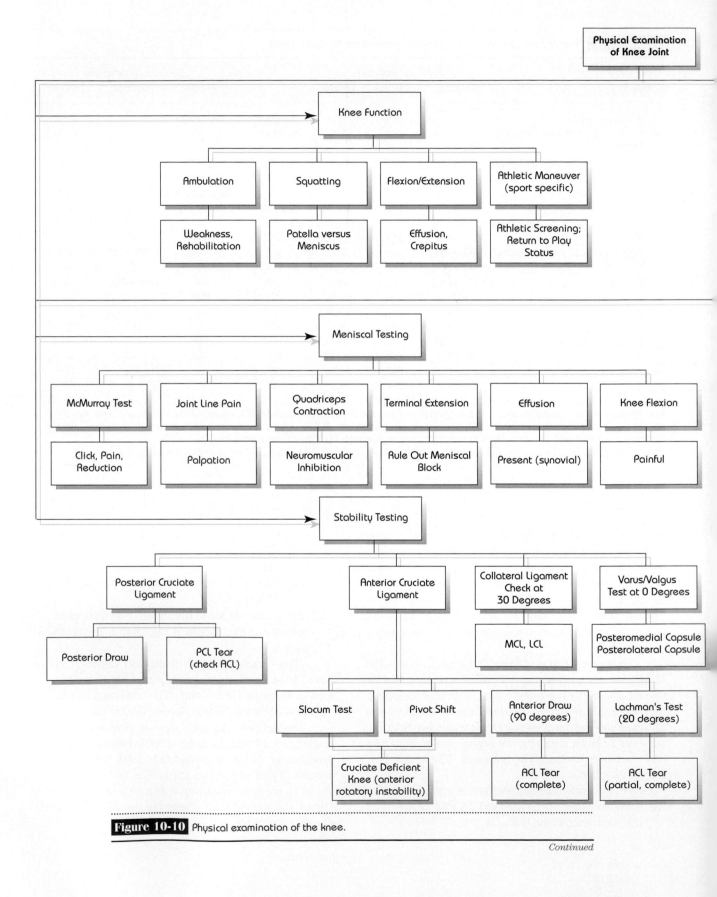

Figure 10-10 Physical examination of the knee.

Continued

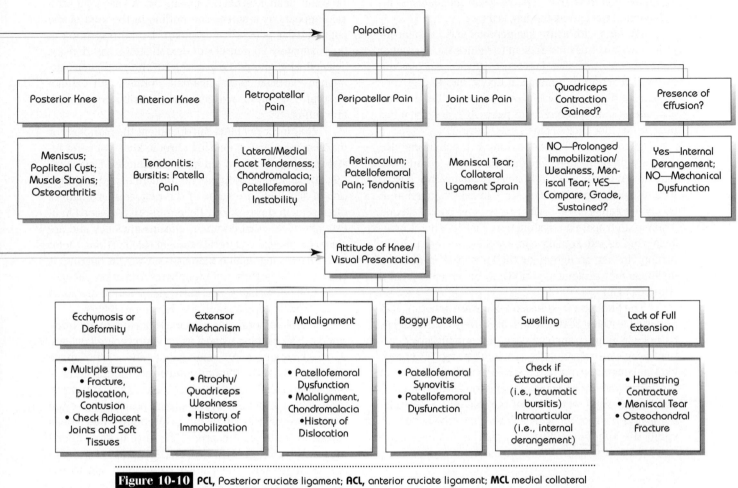

Figure 10-10 PCL, Posterior cruciate ligament; **ACL,** anterior cruciate ligament; **MCL** medial collateral ligament; **LCL,** lateral collateral ligament.

1. With the patient prone, the examiner flexes the affected knee to 90 degrees. Grabbing below the ankle and rotating the injured leg, the examiner applies upward traction to the knee via the lower leg. If the patient feels pain in the knee, there may be a ligamentous or capsular injury.
2. With the patient in the same position, the examiner rotates the leg with the knee bent and applies downward pressure. If the maneuver causes a pain or a click, there may be a meniscal tear.[21]

Testing Functional Status

Although the case history, palpation, and stability testing portion of the knee examination is critically important, it is also essential to assess the functional capabilities (i.e., range of motion) of the patient (Figure 10-10). Some injuries may appear worse than they really are. In cases of acute trauma, the following is a checklist of functional procedures that should be performed during assessment:

1. Ask the patient to go through the ranges of motion to determine, for example, if the knee can be flexed and to what extent.
2. Have the patient attempt to lock the knee into terminal extension. If the patient cannot fully extend the knee, rule out either an internal block or muscle spasm as the cause.
3. Check the patient's weight-bearing ability, starting with the ability to stand on both feet, balance on one foot, and walking.
4. Determine whether the patient can contract the extensor mechanism. This indicates the patient's ability to maintain neuromuscular integrity at the knee.
5. Ask the patient to lift the leg 6 inches off the table

after contracting the quadriceps group. This procedure confirms that the extensor mechanism, including the patella tendon, is intact.

Patients with acute ligamentous and capsular injuries have an effusion sufficient to reduce the amount of knee flexion. A smaller, less tense effusion, such as the synovial reaction to a meniscal injury, allows a greater amount of flexion. In both cases, however, flexion usually causes some discomfort or pain. ACL abnormalities may or may not evoke pain in knee flexion.

Inflammation of the extensor mechanism also evokes pain on flexion. Quadriceps strains, contusions, patella tendonitis, and retinaculitis all involve partial flexion loading at the knee. Mechanical dysfunction at the patellofemoral joint also presents as partial flexion loading. Retropatellar dysfunction, such as chondromalacia patellae, can actually cause locking at some point in flexion. In fact, straightening the knee after it has been in flexion for a prolonged period may be the most painful stimulus of all.

The findings of extension testing are generally less remarkable than flexion findings. Severe retropatellar pathologic injuries, such as a fracture or avulsion of cartilage, can cause a patient to inhibit extension. Posterior joint inflammation, such as a strain of the upper head of the gastrocnemius muscle, or a hamstring strain and tendonitis, can make extension of the knee discomforting. Lumbar nerve root tension can also cause the patient to splint the knee in slight flexion and avoid extension to prevent stretching of the sciatic nerve.

Radiologic Examination of the Knee

Because of its location in the lower extremity and its complex biomechanical makeup, the knee joint is often significantly injured in acute trauma. Conventional radiography should always be the first radiologic examination performed. Plain films are easy to obtain, rather inexpensive, and useful in the detection of fractures, joint effusions, metabolic disturbances, and old pathologic conditions.

Any acute knee injury warrants careful examination. Obviously, if a fracture or dislocation is suspected, such as in the patient who is unable to perform a straight leg raise, conventional radiography should immediately follow the examination. Stress and osteochondral fractures, calcification of ligaments, and acute fractures produce effusions that are identifiable on routine radiographic films.

The clinician who has any suspicion of an internal derangement should order plain films promptly, as radiographic evidence of a joint effusion aids in confirming the presence of an internal derangement. A knee joint effusion appears as a soft-tissue outline in the area of the suprapatellar pouch.[75] A standard lateral projection at approximately 20 degrees of flexion shows this density. This effusion should be palpable to the meticulous examiner. Cartilage tears, ligament sprains, and patellofemoral dislocation are common contributors to such knee effusions.

Routine x-ray films can document the pathology or malalignment that is causing chronic knee pain and instability. Patella views aid in the diagnosis. Degenerative arthritis, heterotopic bone formation, and calcification of ligaments are some of the radiographic changes often seen in these cases. Pellegrini-Stieda lesions indicate chronic medial compartment insufficiency and are evident as medial collateral ligament calcifications. Joint space narrowing, which increases on weight bearing, is seen in osteoarthritis. Osteophyte formation, irregularity of joint surfaces, and varus deformation are some of the sequelae apparent in the degenerated knee.

Patellofemoral disease can be documented on the standard lateral film, as well as on various patella views. Spur formation, bony remodeling, and mirror-image osteophytosis at the femoral condyle are routine findings that occur at the patellofemoral joint. Merchant views, taken with the patient in the supine position, are often used; however, the Hughston projection of the patella (taken with the patient prone, the knee in flexion, and the central ray angled through the tibial tubercle) shows the examiner how the patella structurally sits in the trochlear groove and thus makes it possible to view patella malalignment and tilt (Figure 10-11).

Patients with recurring knee pain who have previously received care, but who have not had a thorough assessment of their condition for a period of time should undergo x-ray examination as a screening procedure for more extensive abnormalities. Only the soft-tissue injuries to extraarticular structures for which the diagnosis is easily made require no x-ray examination. If a structured and well-planned treatment program does not resolve such a condition within a reasonable amount of time, conventional radiographic films, or even advanced imaging techniques, may be used to ensure that a disease entity is not present (Table 10-4).

Initial Radiographic Views

Practitioners order standard films as required by the individual patient and the disease entity. Routinely, however, there are three standard views. The lateral projection taken in slight flexion at 20 degrees is commonly agreed upon as a standard film (Figure 10-12 *A, B*). Although some clinicians prefer a tunnel view to the anteroposterior view, the anteroposterior projection in neutral is generally sufficient as the second standard view (Figure 10-13 *A, B*). A tunnel view in flexion can be ordered as an additional view when intraarticular pathologic variations are suggested or when the patient has experienced severe, complex trauma. The third and final standard view should be a patella view, such as a Hughston film of the patellofemoral joint taken in knee flexion.

In addition to the three routine x-ray films, several other views are available to the orthopedic clinician. Stress radiographic studies are usually taken in both the valgus and varus positions on an anteroposterior film. Such films usually provide some insight into the status of

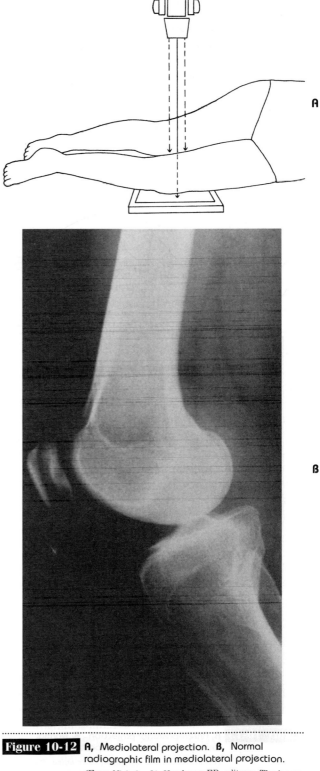

Figure 10-12 **A,** Mediolateral projection. **B,** Normal radiographic film in mediolateral projection.

(From Nicholas JA, Hershman EB, editors: *The lower extremity and spine in sports and medicine,* ed 2, vol 1, St Louis, 1995, Mosby.)

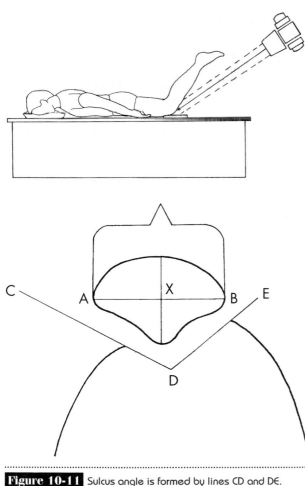

Figure 10-11 Sulcus angle is formed by lines CD and DE. Patellar index is the width of patella (AB) divided by difference of lateral facet (AX) and medial facet (XB).

(Modified from Hughston JC: Subluxation of the patella, *J Bone Joint Surg* 50A:4003, 1968.)

Recent studies have shown MRI to be quite accurate in detecting tears of the ACL.[54,111] Complete tears appear as discontinuity in the ligament, with fluid filling the defect.[15] Thin-section sagittal images are most useful in diagnosing ACL tears; coronal and perhaps axial images augment the sagittal study to evaluate partial tears. In chronic tears there is a distinct lack of hemorrhage and edema.[129] The collateral ligaments, as well as the extensor mechanism (e.g., quadriceps tendon, patella ligament), are also well-imaged.[45]

Additional Studies. Arteriography is not often used to image the knee. Its primary value is in the examination of an acutely traumatized knee that shows signs of vascular insufficiency. The most common reason for this clinical scenario is a total knee dislocation, which stretches and lacerates vascular structures.[68] After such an injury, the presence of pulses may mask arterial compromise. Magnetic resonance angiography is an additional clinical option. Obviously, this would be a surgical emergency that would require a vascular consultation.

Bone scans are valuable in the early stages of knee symptomatology, before plain radiographic films demonstrate osteoblastic activity.[90] Subtle stress fractures, osteoblastic diseases, and neoplasm are instances in which scintigraphy may be helpful.

PART TWO: DISORDERS OF THE KNEE

Pathologic disorders of the knee can be divided into two broad categories: extraarticular and intraarticular. Most extraarticular problems are mechanical and dysfunctional in nature and are caused by either pathomechanical forces or simply overuse. They are usually less serious and far less disabling than their internal counterparts.

Mechanical Dysfunction of the Knee

The diagnosis of extraarticular problems is largely based on the mechanism of injury and surface anatomy. Effusion of the knee joint is rare, and the history is usually that of repetitive microtrauma. Contraction and stretching of periarticular structures usually provoke pain. Malalignment of the pelvis and lower extremity must be considered in the examination, as well as any change in activity or work habits before the injury.

Tendonitis

Because there are large supporting muscle groups around the knee joint, there are many possible sites for injury and inflammation (Figure 10-18). Most cases require the clinician to inspect the anatomy of the knee, pinpoint the area of palpable tenderness, and review the activities that caused the injury.

The goals of treatment are to reduce the inflammation of the associated tendon, change the habits or activities that caused the problem, and rehabilitate the affected tendon unit with therapeutic exercises and gradual stretching. Ice massage is excellent for most cases of superficial tendonitis. Ultrasound should be used for chronic cases where scarring and fibrosing may have occurred in the tendon sheath. Electrotherapy may reduce pain or swelling.

Superior Pole-Patellar Tendonitis

Some patients develop tendonitis just proximal to the patella or at the tendon-bone interface at the superior pole of the patella. Repetitive flexion such as going up and down stairs, squatting improperly, or lifting heavy weights can cause this problem. Diagnosis is made after the results of all other tests are negative. Swelling is

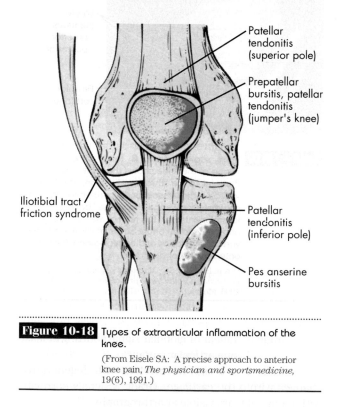

Figure 10-18 Types of extraarticular inflammation of the knee.

(From Eisele SA: A precise approach to anterior knee pain, *The physician and sportsmedicine,* 19(6), 1991.)

rarely present, and bracing is usually not necessary. Altering the biomechanics of the patella is usually the most helpful step in patient care. Cryotherapy in the form of ice massage and avoidance of painful positions are the keys to a successful outcome (Table 10-6). Gradual strengthening of the extensor mechanism and deep transverse friction massage are also helpful in treatment.

Inferior Pole-Patellar Tendonitis

In the mature knee, repetitive overuse can cause the inferior pole to become inflamed and tender. Flexion is painful, and stair climbing or jumping makes it worse. Individuals with this condition should avoid high-heeled shoes; sneakers are a better choice. Hyperflexion of the knee should be avoided. Sometimes, swelling is evident

Table 10-6   Types of Tendonitis of the Knee

	Superior Pole-Patellar Tendonitis	Inferior Pole-Patellar Tendonitis	Patellar Tendonitis (Jumper's Knee)	Iliotibial Band Friction Syndrome	Popliteal Tendonitis	Biceps Tendonitis
Physical examination findings	Painful knee flexion at extreme range of motion No instability; no effusion Palpable tenderness at superior pole of patellar tendon Possible crepitus, if condition is chronic	Painful arc of knee flexion No instability; no effusion Palpable tenderness over inferior pole of patellar tendon superior to insertion into tibia Bogginess over infrapatellar fat pad Possibly, mild swelling in tendon sheath	Anterior knee pain over patella tendon Insidious onset of discomfort Exacerbation of pain with running and jumping Pain evoked by sustained flexion of knee or eccentric loading of quadriceps muscle Need to rule out malalignment and short leg syndrome	Palpable tenderness over lateral femoral condyle Possible hip/abductor tightness, sacro-iliac fixation Lower extremity malalignment Pain evoked by repetitive flexion of knee Radiation of pain over lateral joint line Need to rule out pes planus	Lateral knee pain (extra-articular) Exacerbation during running, especially downhill running Palpable tenderness between lateral collateral ligament and biceps tendon Reproduction of pain with affected leg crossed over opposite knee	Posterolateral knee pain Painful Hardy position Discomfort with resisted knee flexion Need to differentiate from popliteal tendonitis
X-ray findings	Usually normal Possibly calcific deposits in tendon in chronic cases	Usually normal Old calcium deposit possible in cases of chronic traction apophysitis (Osgood-Schlatter disease)	Normal	Normal	Normal	Normal
Treatment plan	Ice massage; electro-therapy; ultrasound, if chronic Deep transverse friction massage Gradual strengthening exercises	Ice massage; electrotherapy; ultrasound, if chronic Gradual strengthening exercises	Rest; application of ice; ultrasound Concentric/eccentric strengthening program CMT to lumbo-pelvic spine, if applicable	Rest; application of ice; stretching; electrotherapy Gradual strengthening program for abductor muscles CMT to lumbo-pelvic spine, if applicable	Rest; application of ice; ultrasound; electrotherapy Alterations in running surfaces Gradual strengthening program for calf, knee flexors	Application of ice; rest; ultrasound Activity modification Gentle stretching and gradual strengthening program for hamstring muscle

CMT, Chiropractic manipulative therapy.

in the tendon sheath. Bogginess over the infrapatellar fat pad is palpable at times. An effusion is usually not present in these cases. The counterpart of inferior pole-patellar tendonitis in the young knee is a traction apophysitis.

Patellar Tendonitis

An overload at the tendinous portion of the extensor mechanism may lead to patellar tendonitis. Excessive loading on hard surfaces is usually the reason for a painful episode, which occurs as palpable tenderness over the patella. Sports such as basketball and cross-country running are often associated with patellar tendonitis. Because eccentric loads and absorption of shock at the extensor tendon may result from the athlete's landing of a jump, many clinicians refer to the condition as "jumper's knee."

High tensile forces and eccentric strain are avoided initially to reduce pain and inflammation.[41,97] Malalignment and structural asymmetry of the lower extremity, including leg length discrepancy, should be ruled out as the source of the problem.[6] A strengthening program aimed at both eccentric and concentric recruitment of the extensor mechanism is efficiently accomplished through a program of proper therapeutic squatting.

Iliotibial Band Friction Syndrome

Considered a form of tendonitis, iliotibial band friction syndrome may develop where the fibrous mass of this band rubs over the lateral femoral condyle. Although the extension of the tensor fascia lata attaches distally at the lateral proximal tibia (Gerdy's tubercle), most of the stress from movements such as running occurs above the joint line.[78] Repetitive flexion of the knee from running long distances or running on embanked roads and other sloped terrain, for example, all add to lateral distal thigh pain. Chronic pelvic obliquity, gluteal myofascitis, and hip contracture are contributing factors in iliotibial band friction syndrome.

A snapping motion causes friction and inflammation at the lateral aspect of the knee. The anatomic fact that the iliotibial band is free to glide in an anterior and posterior fashion often leads to a synovitis of the tendinous mass. With the knee in flexion, the band drops posteriorly and rubs against the femoral condyle.[36]

Careful examination of the patient should include testing for leg length discrepancy, pelvic obliquity, and iliotibial band tightness. Anatomic considerations such as lower extremity malalignment may predispose certain athletes and individuals to the injury. Internal tibial torsion, genu varum (bowleggedness), and pronation of the subtalar joint may all be causative anatomic factors. Rest is usually quite palliative. Ancillary procedures, including the application of ice and stretching, can facilitate healing.

Popliteal Tendonitis

Another common cause of lateral knee pain is popliteal tendonitis. Often ignored or misunderstood in clinical practice, this inflammatory condition can become chronic and quite painful. It is common in young, active patients who may report an increased intensity of recreational or competitive running or sprinting. Downhill running aggravates the condition.

The patient with popliteal tendonitis complains of pain at the lateral joint line of the knee. The condition must be differentially diagnosed from iliotibial band friction syndrome, hamstring tendonitis (e.g., biceps tendonitis), and lateral compartment degeneration. The fact that no effusion is present can be helpful in ruling out internal derangements of the knee.

The popliteus is responsible for the internal rotation of the tibia on the femur when the leg is flexed. Sprinting causes high-level torque at the lower leg, thus increasing activity at the popliteus. On examination, the clinician finds the knee to be palpably tender just posterior to the lateral collateral ligament and in front of the biceps tendon. Rotation of the leg, such as crossing the affected leg over the opposite knee (i.e., Hardy position), reproduces the discomfort. This position of flexion, abduction, and external rotation of the hip allows better palpation of the popliteus tendon.

Treatment includes cessation of running or aggravating activities, exercises to strengthen the knee flexors, and the application of ice. Activities that require running up or down hill should cease. Adjuncts to treatment include ultrasound, electrotherapy, and antiinflammatory medication in recalcitrant cases.

Biceps Tendonitis

The most common tendon injury of the hamstring group is tendonitis of the biceps femoris. The primary basis for the diagnosis is surface anatomy, and the examiner must differentially diagnose biceps tendonitis from popliteal tendonitis. Not only does biceps tendonitis produce pain in an area near that in which popliteal tendonitis causes pain (i.e., posterolateral joint pain), but crossing the affected leg over the opposite knee in the Hardy position also exacerbates both conditions. It is important to attempt to reproduce pain with these movements, because straight stretching of the hamstring muscle may not evoke pain in the case of biceps tendonitis. Rotation is necessary to elicit this symptom.

Patients with biceps tendonitis must refrain from crossing the affected leg when sitting. Running and bicycle riding to the point of pain should also be avoided.

Chronic cases can be quite troublesome to both practitioner and patient. In some instances, fibrosis can occur. Often the examiner can roll palpable nodules or "rice bodies" over the biceps tendon sheath with the fingertips. When chronic changes in the sheath occur, therapeutic ultrasound can be a helpful adjunct in care; rest and the application of ice should also be part of the patient's treatment. Rehabilitation includes gradual strengthening and stretching of the hamstring muscle. The patient should avoid high-heeled shoes and will find sneakers most comfortable.

Bursitis

The novice examiner may find the diagnosis of bursitis around the knee a bit confusing because the bursae lie in close proximity to tendons and ligaments. The function of the bursae is to provide a lubricating medium to reduce friction between adjacent tissues, such as tendon and bone. Bursae are closed, fluid-filled sacs lined with synovium. Although there are many bursae around the knee joint, problems occur with only a few.

In acute traumatic bursitis, the sac fills with fluid, distends, and causes pain and deformity. In chronic bursitis, the repeated inflammation causes the bursa to thicken and the fluid to distend. Chronic bursitis may also be associated with crepitus. Most cases of traumatic bursitis are treated with the application of ice, compression, and protection from external blows (Table 10-7).

Infrapatellar Bursitis
Either the deep or the superficial infrapatellar bursa may become inflamed (Figure 10-19). The examiner usually finds a tender area just beneath the inferior pole of the patellar tendon above the tibial tubercle. In the adolescent, infrapatellar bursitis is usually indistinguishable from a traction apophysitis of the proximal tibia. In the adult it is clinically similar to inferior pole-patellar tendonitis and patellofemoral synovitis. Because the deep infrapatellar bursa lies in front of the infrapatellar fat pad, hypertrophy of this fat pad in patients with chronic anterior knee pain can make this type of bursitis anonymous in causing the patient's pain.

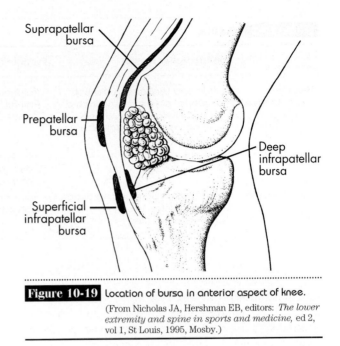

Figure 10-19 Location of bursa in anterior aspect of knee.
(From Nicholas JA, Hershman EB, editors: *The lower extremity and spine in sports and medicine,* ed 2, vol 1, St Louis, 1995, Mosby.)

Localized pain and tenderness over the affected area is the usual presentation. Sometimes the infrapatellar region takes on a boggy appearance that makes the condition resemble patellofemoral synovitis. The superficial bursa may experience direct trauma, but only rarely is the deep bursal area injured through a direct external force. Treatment usually centers around the application of ice, compression, and ultrasound. Surgical excision is not a treatment option.

Prepatellar Bursitis
Superficially located over the patella and under the skin, the prepatellar bursa is commonly injured. In cases of acute trauma it is necessary to distinguish superficial swelling from a true joint effusion. After palpating the knee for swelling, the examiner uses the ballottement maneuver to determine whether the fluid is over the patella as in a traumatic bursitis or whether the patella rests in a true joint effusion. If the latter condition exists, the swelling is intraarticular and the patient has an internal derangement of the knee.

Chronic prepatellar bursitis is common in those people who are often in the kneeling posture. Thus it is sometimes called "housemaid's knee." Infection is a concern in both acute and chronic prepatellar bursitis. The distended, swollen bursa makes flexion quite painful. Point tenderness can be exquisite, especially if there is a superficial skin wound over the bursa.

Table 10-7 Bursitis

	Infrapatellar Bursitis	Prepatellar Bursitis	Pes Anserine Bursitis
Physical examination findings	Pain and tenderness beneath inferior pole of patellar tendon Boggy discomfort over anterior knee between tibial tubercle and patella	Palpable tenderness over patella Painful knee flexion Superficial swelling over patella	Palpable tenderness over pes anserine bursa Anteromedial tibia pain Congestion and bogginess over bursa
X-ray findings	Normal	Usually normal Need to rule out fractured patella or internal derangement	Normal
Treatment plan	Application of ice, compression, ultrasound Protection of area	Application of ice, compression Protection of area	Application of ice, ultrasound Avoidance of aggravating activities

Ice and compression should be applied to the area. Protective measures should be taken to avoid further injury (e.g., bumping into an object) and irritation. Aspiration is reserved for cases of extreme distension. Surgical excision is rare, because even if the bursa is removed, the body eventually forms another synovial sac in its place.

Pes Anserine Bursitis

The pes anserine muscle group consists of the gracilis, sartorius, and semitendinosus. Lying between the tendons and inferior portion of the medial collateral ligament at the proximal tibia, the pes anserine bursa is palpable only when it has undergone direct trauma or excessive friction. In fact, palpable tenderness and crepitus are the distinguishing features of pes anserine bursitis.

Although it is essential to rule out medial knee compartment pathology, physical examination of the involved knee joint reveals no positive orthopedic findings and no effusion. The patient may complain of pain just underneath the joint line, but the point tenderness associated with pes anserine bursitis is most severe over the bursa approximately 2 cm distal to the joint.

Identification of the aggravating activity is paramount for swift, successful treatment. Ice applications are helpful in alleviating symptoms; ultrasound can also be beneficial if the problem persists.

Patellofemoral Dysfunction

The most common type of knee complaint in the general population is patellofemoral pain. This type of mechanical knee pain can affect anyone. Athletes develop patella pain as a result of intense workouts and overuse. Sedentary people develop patella pain as a result of weakness and disuse. Women frequently experience patellofemoral pain because of the combination of malalignment, muscle weakness, and high-heeled shoes.[61] Clearly, a variety of risk factors contribute to the development of patellofemoral dysfunction:

- Weak quadriceps muscle
- Faulty tracking mechanism
- Repetitive flexion loading
- Direct blows
- History of instability, such as subluxing or dislocating patella
- Dysplastic or poorly developed vastus medialis obliquus muscle
- Malalignment, including femoral anteversion, external tibial torsion, foot pronation, and excessive varus or valgus orientation at the knee[59]
- Tight hamstring muscles

In addition, a myriad of disorders in a variety of other sites can produce anterior knee pain:

- Lumbar spine
  1. Herniated nucleus pulposus
  2. Spinal stenosis
  3. Neoplasm
  4. Somatic-referred (sclerotogenous) pain
- Hip joint
  1. Degenerative arthritis
  2. Legg-Calvé-Perthes disease
  3. Slipped capital femoral epiphysis
  4. Avascular necrosis of the femoral head
- Soft-tissue overuse syndromes
  1. Patellar tendonitis (jumper's knee)
  2. Inferior pole-patellar tendonitis
  3. Superior pole-patellar tendonitis
  4. Infrapatellar bursitis
  5. Quadriceps muscular strain

- Synovial joint disorders
  1. Synovitis
  2. Plica syndrome
  3. Infection
  4. Osteochondral loose bodies
- Ligamentous injuries
  1. Medial collateral ligament sprain
  2. Lateral collateral ligament sprain
  3. Anterior cruciate–deficient knee
  4. Posterior cruciate ligament sprain
- Meniscal tears
  1. Lateral meniscus
  2. Medial meniscus
  3. Discoid meniscus
  4. Meniscal cyst
- Traction apophysitis
- Reflex sympathetic dystrophy

Acute onset of patella pain suggests that a sudden, single traumatic event may have taken place. In motor vehicle accidents, for example, it is common for front seat passengers to hit their knees on the dashboard and injure their patella. Traumatic chondromalacia patellae is usually the outcome of this injury. Dislocation and subluxation of the patella, as well as plica syndrome, are also traumatic causes of patellofemoral pain. Causes described as insidious in nature are often the result of mechanical soft-tissue syndromes. Malalignment, overuse, and repetitive flexion loading are common precipitatory events. Diagnoses of this nature include patellofemoral syndrome, patella malalignment syndrome, and chondromalacia patellae.

Orthopedic Aspects of Patellofemoral Dysfunction

Although the etiology of patellofemoral pain varies in different individuals, certain signs and symptoms seem to be somewhat consistent in these patients. For instance, most patients report a feeling of discomfort in two distinct regions: the retropatellar region and peripatellar region. Retropatellar pain is indicative of irritation at the articular surface of the patella; patients point "through the joint" and describe the pain as "inside the knee." When the pain is in the peripatellar area (i.e., around the sides of the patella), patients circle their kneecap along the retinaculum with their hands as they point to the site of pain.

Another hallmark of patellofemoral dysfunction is painful flexion loading, which can become evident in a variety of ways. The most common is pain while walking up or down stairs. Walking down stairs forces the extensor mechanism to contract eccentrically, which increases the tensile loading forces at the patella. In fact, body weight is distributed to the knee threefold in the form of the patellofemoral joint reaction force.[67] Therefore any weakness in the quadriceps muscle exacerbates pain when the patient is going down stairs to a greater extent than when going up. Squatting down and wearing high-heeled shoes also increase flexion at the patellofemoral joint.

Sitting in a car or the theater with the knee in a flexed position for a long period also causes moderate-to-severe irritation at the patella. When attempting to straighten the leg after a period of prolonged flexion, the individual may experience locking, crepitus, and pain (sometimes called "cinema sign").

The principles of biomechanics explain why flexion loading is detrimental to the patellofemoral joint. Flexion causes the patella to track in the trochlear groove of the femur.[128] The articular surface of the patella approximates the femur when the knee bends. Although the patella tracks from 30 to 110 degrees of flexion, the maximum force across the patella through the femoral surface occurs at 30 to 60 degrees of flexion.[127] Therefore the potential for both retropatellar and peripatellar pain is great during repetitive flexion loading.

Examination of the Patient with Patellofemoral Dysfunction

In addition to the pattern of pain, some visual clues point to the patellofemoral joint as the focus of pathologic anomalies in patients with patellofemoral dysfunction. Nonoptimal alignment of the lower limb involves several features of anatomy that contribute to patellar pain, including a widened pelvis, acute Q angle (Figure 10-20), femoral anteversion, tibia varum, genu valgum, genu recurvatum, lateral-riding patella, and subtalar pronation (Figure 10-21).

If the patient is gowned appropriately, the examiner can visually screen the patient for all these factors. While the patient stands and walks, the examiner should view him or her from both the back and front. Finally, the examiner places the patient supine on the examination table and views the alignment of the patient's legs from the base of the table. Do both legs lock out at the knee? Does the tibial tubercle line up directly below the patella, or is there gross malalignment? If the knee is flexed and extended, does the patella track laterally? Is the Q angle acute?

The radiologic examination of the patient with mechanical patellofemoral dysfunction should include the standard anteroposterior, lateral, and patella views. The anteroposterior and lateral films do not always show abnormalities, except in older individuals who may have

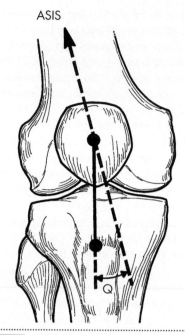

Figure 10-20 The Q angle, which may indicate patellar tracking problems, is formed by two lines, one drawn from the anterior superior iliac spine (ASIS) through the center of the patella, and the second line drawn from the tibial tubercle to the center of the patella.

(From Scott WN: *The knee*, vol 1, St Louis, 1994, Mosby.)

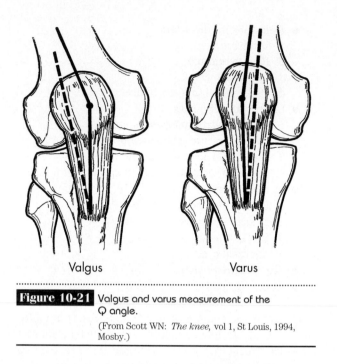

Figure 10-21 Valgus and varus measurement of the Q angle.

(From Scott WN: *The knee*, vol 1, St Louis, 1994, Mosby.)

signs of patellofemoral disease or degenerative arthritis on routine radiographic films.

The Hughston projection (i.e., infrapatellar view) visualizes the patella in its orientation at the trochlear groove. It demonstrates the femoral condyles and retropatellar surfaces as well. For example, the Hughston film can clearly show a laterally tilted patella. The lateral facet of the patella approximates the lateral condyle of the femur. If malalignment is severe, the poor patellofemoral tracking produces a bony override of these two osseous structures. Advanced cases can be documented on x-ray films as mirror image osteophytosis involving the lateral facet of the patella and lateral femoral condyle. Acute or repetitive trauma to the extensor mechanism can also be documented on the standard lateral x-ray film at 20 degrees of knee flexion.

In some instances of retropatellar dysfunction, the degree of inflammation is so great that even the slightest amount of knee flexion may be difficult for the patient. Patients with such conditions as acutely inflamed chondromalacia, patellar dislocation or subluxation, or acute traumatic chondromalacia patellae may find it more comfortable to flex their knee as much as possible in the prone position and then lay their painful leg on the table. The Hughston projection can be sufficiently and more comfortably taken in this fashion.

Treatment of Patellofemoral Dysfunction

Although the causes of patellofemoral dysfunction are varied, treatment is similar for all patients with this condition. An active program of treatment includes both patient participation and moderate forms of exercise. At the same time the patient must avoid all forms of aggravating activities (e.g., running, riding a bicycle, aerobics) and poor positions of the knee joint (e.g., riding in a car or a plane for a long trip with the knee in a prolonged stance of flexion, climbing stairs repeatedly, wearing high-heeled shoes, sitting on the floor with the legs crossed).

In this treatment approach, which can be called "active rest," the patient refrains from flexion loading while maintaining a regimen of isometric quadriceps exercise at home. Isometric exercises are performed with the leg at 0 degrees of extension to reduce irritation of the patellofemoral joint. Once the patient has a reduction of pain, crepitus, retropatellar and peripatellar discomfort, or bogginess (synovitis), the practitioner can add more activities to the regimen, such as isotonic short arc knee extension with or without ankle weights. Ice can be applied as a precautionary measure after exercise. In patients with severe dysfunction and pain, the application of ice both before and after exercise is helpful. A towel can be rolled up and placed at the popliteal space during the first stage of isometric (quadriceps) exercises for comfort in patients who experience pain associated with isometric exercise.

The use of a patellofemoral brace can be an excellent ancillary strategy in addition to standard primary care for anterior knee pain. Caution is essential in the use of this strategy, however, since some patients become dependent on the brace and subsequently develop functional weakness. Because quadriceps weakness or atrophy is a major contributor to patellofemoral dysfunction, a brace should be used only in conjunction with a program of adjunctive therapeutic exercises that includes hamstring stretching and quadriceps strengthening.

There are two groups of patients with patellofemoral dysfunction for which the use of a brace is appropriate: those who have patellofemoral instability and those who are competitive athletes. Patients with a history of patellofemoral instability (e.g., subluxation, dislocation) are likely to require some immobilization after any new trauma. If they have experienced multiple episodes of trauma, they have probably used a posterior immobilizer (full length). Multiple subluxations are usually less traumatic after the initial injury, and many of these individuals can use a patellofemoral sleeve with a horseshoe cutout to stabilize the patella. Patients who experience minor-to-moderate degrees of pain and swelling at the site of injury and are able to ambulate may find a patellofemoral brace beneficial.

Athletes who compete on a fairly high level can reap the benefits of a patellofemoral brace in conjunction with a strengthening program. These patients must be highly disciplined and compliant with instructions for care. The brace must be used as an aid during games or meets, not as a crutch in practice sessions. It is not a substitute for exercise. Graded therapeutic exercise is always the cornerstone of a sound patellofemoral rehabilitation program.

Conditions Associated with Patellofemoral Pain

Several types of injuries and disorders may first appear as patellar pain:

- *Patellofemoral syndrome* encompasses short-term insult and overuse of the joint. It is mostly a vague, repetitious diagnostic entity with few orthopedic findings, except a dull, achy pain that is either retropatellar or peripatellar.

- In *patellar malalignment syndrome,* there are usually several malaligned structures that result in poor patella tracking. Pain generally persists longer in patients with patellar malalignment syndrome than in those with patellofemoral syndrome, and signs of inflammation are more common at physical presentation.

- *Chondromalacia patellae* is a histopathologic diagnosis that may be either the culmination of multiple traumatic episodes or the end stage of a chronic patella problem. such as patellofemoral syndrome and patella malalignment.

- *Patellofemoral instability* is characterized by frequent episodes of patellar subluxation or dislocation.

- The symptoms of *synovial plica syndrome* arise insidiously over the anterior knee; flexion aggravates these symptoms. The cause is an embryonic fold that extends under the quadriceps tendon in the suprapatellar region and attaches to the lateral retinaculum.

Patellofemoral Syndrome. More or less a negative diagnosis that is made as other causes of anterior knee pain are ruled out, patellofemoral syndrome is the most benign of the patellar diagnoses. Individuals with this syndrome generally complain of patella pain on and off for several weeks or months, yet possess few clinical orthopedic findings. Unlike patients with an internal derangement of the knee, for example, those with patellofemoral syndrome have no effusion, no instability, and no joint line pain (Figure 10-22).

Typically associated with patellofemoral syndrome are complaints of retropatellar and peripatellar pain. The most objective finding on examination is a bogginess around the patella. Sometimes the area around the kneecap appears bluish or purplish as a result of inflammation. These are all indications of the presence of patellofemoral synovitis. Sometimes crepitus or clicking may be evident during flexion in patients who have been experiencing patellofemoral problems for at least 1 month or longer. Palpation of the medial facet usually reproduces some of the patient's discomfort.

Repetitive flexion loading on a weak extensor mechanism is usually the cause in patellofemoral syndrome. Thus the key to successful treatment is to avoid repetitive flexion loading while strengthening the quadriceps muscles. Electrotherapy and the application of ice can help abate inflammation and pain (Table 10-8).

Anterior Knee Pain

Question: One of my patients has been complaining of anterior knee pain around the kneecap area. She is a 15-year-old girl who participates in aerobics and stationary bicycle riding. Should she be taken out of aerobic classes? I was also thinking of referring her for antiinflammatory medication. Is this prudent?

Answer: A large percentage of the hundreds of patients in orthopedic clinics who have experienced an insidious onset of knee pain that cannot be traced to a single episode of trauma are adolescent girls. Complaints may start during the beginning or middle teenage years, when their hips are widening and their hormone levels are rising, but the pain may taper off as these patients enter young adulthood.

Orthopedically, the etiology of patellofemoral pain includes obesity, a weak extensor mechanism, a lateral-riding patella, and patellar malalignment syndrome. The faulty patellar "tracking" mechanism in the trochlear groove of the femur that is the result of patellar malalignment syndrome is secondary to a host of factors: an acute Q angle set up from a wide pelvis, excessive genu valgum at the knee joint, femoral anteversion, and tibial varum. The result of these features, which are typical in the adolescent girl, includes painful flexion loading of the patellofemoral joint, a boggy presentation of the anterior knee, and, finally, retropatellar and peripatellar tenderness.

Treatment should center around strengthening the extensor mechanism, because a strong quadriceps muscle offers some protection against anterior knee pain. The vastus medialis muscle, which works primarily from 30 degrees to terminal extension (i.e., 0 degrees), is an important factor in neutralizing the inherent lateral pull of the patella during tracking. Thus beginning a rehabilitative exercise program with isometrics for the quadriceps will enable this patient to strengthen her thigh muscle at full extension without producing the retropatellar pain experienced in flexion-arc exercises.

Quadriceps setting, which serves as an isometric first-step exercise, entails tightening the quadriceps muscle with the leg in extension for a count of 5 to 10 seconds. Initially the patient should perform this exercise several times during the day, bilaterally, for four sets of ten repetitions. The patient can progress to performing straight leg raises 6 inches off the floor in approximately 1 week to 10 days after the implementation of the quadriceps setting. Patients should achieve full strength in the isometric program before graduating to short arc isotonic exercises.

The application of ice and electrotherapy may be important ancillary procedures to control pain and inflammation, and antiinflammatory drugs, both over-the-counter and prescription, should be used *sparingly.* Only acute orthopedic trauma warrants the use of such medications.

Treatment by means of the application of ice, isometric exercise, and electrotherapy is successful in 99% of patellar pain in adolescents. The cornerstone of treatment, however, is the quadriceps strengthening program. If this 15-year-old patient is not strong enough to withstand the stress-loading of aerobics class or the flexion loading from bicycle riding, she should reduce her activity level in these areas until she gains enough strength from her exercise program. Approximately 4 to 6 weeks of rehabilitation may be required before the patient begins to make strides in her ability to withstand patellofemoral loading.

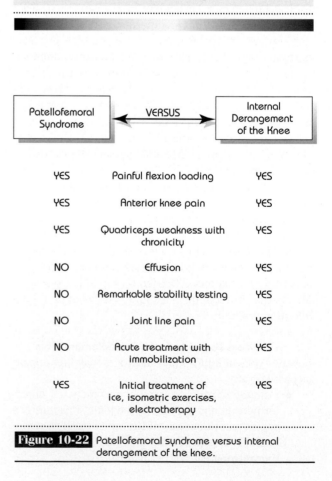

Patellofemoral Syndrome	VERSUS	Internal Derangement of the Knee
YES	Painful flexion loading	YES
YES	Anterior knee pain	YES
YES	Quadriceps weakness with chronicity	YES
NO	Effusion	YES
NO	Remarkable stability testing	YES
NO	Joint line pain	YES
NO	Acute treatment with immobilization	YES
YES	Initial treatment of ice, isometric exercises, electrotherapy	YES

Figure 10-22 Patellofemoral syndrome versus internal derangement of the knee.

| **Table 10-8** | Causes of Patellofemoral (Anterior) Knee Pain |

	Patellofemoral Syndrome	Patellar Malalignment Syndrome	Traumatic Chondromalacia Patellae	End-Stage Patellofemoral Dysfunction	Patellofemoral Instability	Plica Syndrome
Physical examination findings	Negative effusion Peripatellar discomfort Retropatellar discomfort Patellofemoral synovitis No instability History of painful flexion locking	Genu valgum or tibial varum Lateral patella tracking Weak or dysplastic vastus medialis obliquus Possible patello-femoral hypermobility Possible subtalar pronation	Synovitis Crepitus Retropatellar pain Positive patellar grinding test Painful flexion loading Possible peripatellar discomfort	Synovitis Crepitus Retropatellar pain Positive patellar grinding test Painful flexion loading Peripatellar tenderness Lateral tracking Possible patellar malalignment Weakness of extensor mechanism	Patellofemoral synovitis Retropatellar, peripatellar pain Positive patella apprehension test Positive patella grinding test Possible quadriceps weakness (atrophy) Possible malalignment	Swelling and pain Clicking Locking Weakness or sense of "giving way"
X-ray findings	Normal	Lateral patellar tilt (Hughston projection)	Three views usually normal Need to rule out fracture	Possible spurring of patella and/or lateral femoral condyle Lateral tilted patella (Hughston view)	Need to rule out gross patellar malalignment Need to rule out patellofemoral arthritis	Usually normal
Treatment plan	Application of ice Isometrics Electrotherapy	Application of ice Isometrics Electrotherapy	Application of ice Isometric exercise Electrotherapy	Application of ice Isometric exercise Electrotherapy Arthroscopy (lateral release only if refractory to rehabilitation)	Application of ice Isometric exercise Electrotherapy Patellar brace, if necessary	Application of ice Isometric exercise Avoidance of flexion loading Arthroscopy in recalcitrant cases

Patellar Malalignment Syndrome. Several possible features of lower extremity malalignment can be severe enough to have a pathologic effect on the extensor mechanism. As a result of nonoptimal mechanics, the patellar tracking mechanism functions poorly, and the patient develops symptoms of patellar pain, sometimes chronic and quite severe.

When the patient describes all the common features of mechanical anterior knee pain during the case history, the practitioner should begin to suspect a particular type of patellar dysfunction. On examination, however, the visible features of malalignment are quite obvious: wide hips; poorly defined extensor mechanism, especially vastus medialis obliquus; laterally tilted patella;

and faulty attitude of the knee joint, including genu valgum and tibial varum. The practitioner should also check for bogginess, retropatellar pain, subtalar pronation, and hypermobility of the patellofemoral joint.

The treatment for patellar malalignment syndrome is *nonoperative.* The purpose of treatment is not to realign the bony alignment of the knee, but to strengthen the extensor mechanism so as to effect more efficient tracking. Palliative treatment includes changing the habits of daily living in a way that will alleviate symptoms, such as instructing the patient to sit with the affected leg straight out, to avoid deep squatting, and not to wear high-heeled shoes. Patients with this syndrome should be placed on a program that includes the application of ice, isometric strengthening exercises, and electrotherapy for pain for at least 4 to 6 weeks before they return to a full spectrum of their normal physical and recreational activities.

Chondromalacia Patellae. When Koenig first described chondromalacia patellae in 1924, he had an idea that his subject was complex.[89] Since that time there have been many theories and controversies regarding the genesis, pain-producing capability, and diagnosis of this condition. The ultimate question is, "Does chondromalacia patellae stand alone as a primary disease of the patellofemoral joint, or is it simply the sequela of some other syndrome or abnormality?"

To answer this question, the clinician must combine the results of research with personal experience. Bentley and Dowd explained chondromalacia patellae as a clear-cut syndrome complete with retropatellar pain and crepitus.[14] Insall and colleagues felt that chondromalacia was a vague diagnosis, yet the findings of compression testing were consistent in their subjects with this diagnosis.[62] Dugdale and Barnett,[35] similar to Wiberg,[134] and Outerbridge and Dunlop,[102] seemed to believe that pressure and patellofemoral loading are associated with chondromalacia. Fulkerson, Schutzer, and Stougard noted that the existence of chondromalacia was poorly correlated with the presence of anterior knee pain.[114,124]

In chondromalacia, histopathologic changes occur at the articular surface of the patellofemoral joint. The pathologic changes begin at the basilar layer, move to the surface cartilage, and finally lead to the exposure of bare bone.[89] Outerbridge described four stages of change, which range from initial softening of articular cartilage to advanced fibrillation and eburnation of bony surfaces (Figure 10-23).[101]

The articular cartilage of the patella is not the source of pain in chondromalacia patellae, since there are no nerve fibers within it. It is difficult to detect histopathologic changes of the articular cartilage, and such changes are often incidental findings at the time of surgery.[58] Acute or chronic trauma, however, can cause a synovitis to occur at the patellofemoral joint. The release of destructive enzymes in response to the breakdown of articular cartilage can cause additional damage. Aberrant patellofemoral biomechanics can cause the individual to experience peripatellar pain over the retinaculum.

There is some controversy regarding the diagnosis of chondromalacia patellae without diagnostic imaging (e.g., CT) or arthroscopy.[126] Because surgical procedures are both inefficient and risky for patellofemoral

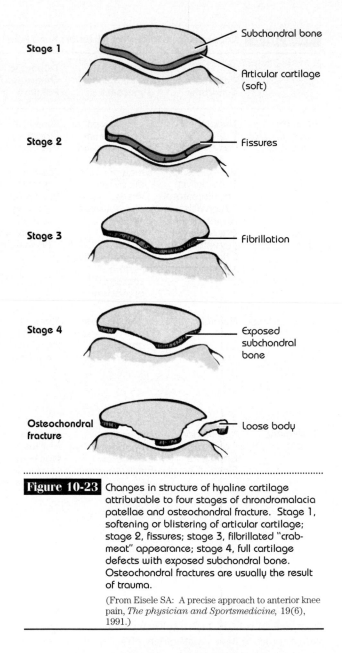

Figure 10-23 Changes in structure of hyaline cartilage attributable to four stages of chondromalacia patellae and osteochondral fracture. Stage 1, softening or blistering of articular cartilage; stage 2, fissures; stage 3, filbrillated "crab-meat" appearance; stage 4, full cartilage defects with exposed subchondral bone. Osteochondral fractures are usually the result of trauma.

(From Eisele SA: A precise approach to anterior knee pain, *The physician and Sportsmedicine,* 19(6), 1991.)

complaints, it is best to rely on a combination of physical examination findings and a proper history to distinguish simple patellofemoral dysfunction from more advanced articular cartilage anomalies, such as chondromalacia patellae.

There are two types of chondromalacic complaints (Figure 10-24). Patients with the first type have no prior problems with knee pain, but they have sustained an external blow to a flexed knee. For example, a patient may have hit the knee against the dashboard during a motor

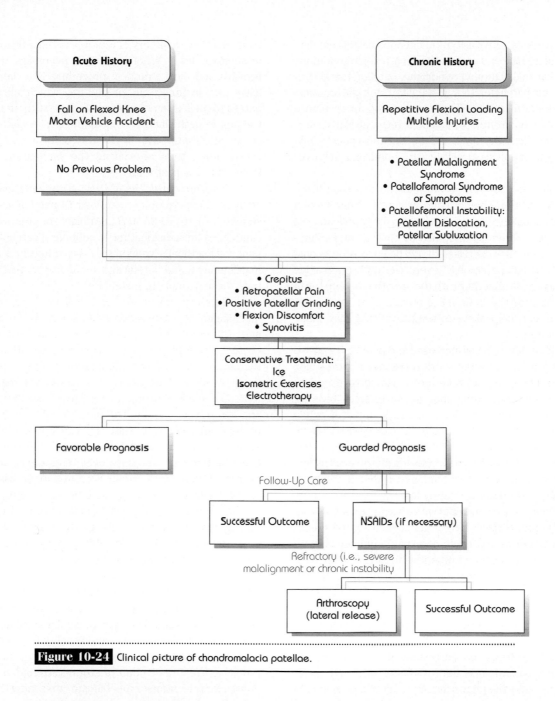

Figure 10-24 Clinical picture of chondromalacia patellae.

vehicle accident or may have banged the knee against the sidewalk as a result of a fall on a wet surface. In both cases, acute flexion loading with compression forces the patella against the femur. The patient develops retropatellar pain, possible crepitus, and synovitis. Flexion evokes pain, and compression tests aggravate the patellofemoral joint.

The second type of chondromalacia typically involves an individual with a history of patellofemoral pain. The problem usually starts gradually and builds over time until the person can no longer participate in activities such as bicycle riding or aerobics. Generally these individuals have previously experienced patellar pain that prompted a different patellofemoral diagnosis. In other words, patients with this type of chondromalacia patellae have reached the *end-stage* of such pathologic conditions as patellar malalignment syndrome, patellofemoral syndrome, or patellofemoral instability. Multiple injuries, poor attention to rehabilitative measures, or recurrent subluxation have often damaged the retropatellar surface beyond repair. Aberrant malalignment and a poor patella tracking mechanism can also lead to chondromalacia over time.

Patients with chondromalacia who have signs of active inflammation should avoid prolonged knee flexion and wear sneakers for better support. The application of ice and electrotherapy are palliative for pain and inflammation. Isometric exercises should begin as soon as possible. If the inflammation is severe, the application of ice before exercise, together with the use of a rolled up towel in the back of the knee for gentle support during the exercise, can help alleviate symptoms that may block rehabilitation.

Once strength has increased and pain has begun to subside, the patient should perform isometric straight leg raises in sets of 10 to 15 repetitions. Isometric exercises must precede any isotonic short arc movements, because isometrics strengthen the quadriceps muscles while sparing the retropatellar surface. All exercises should be performed bilaterally, since many patients unconsciously distribute their weight and workloads on the healthy leg. It is not uncommon for these individuals then to complain about the contralateral, healthy leg.

In most cases, patients with an acute onset of traumatic chondromalacia have a faster recovery time than those with chronic patellofemoral pain. Individuals with a long course of pain and repetitive injuries usually have a longer course of inflammation and retropatellar dysfunction. They have to be quite compliant with exercises and must avoid reinjury at all costs to achieve a complete recovery. Those individuals who are experiencing prolonged bouts of pain and disability may need an oral anti-inflammatory drug in the early stage of rehabilitation. In fact, these patients may improve faster with such medication, because the pharmaceutic reduction of their pain and inflammation allows them to take a more proactive role in the rehabilitation process. The application of ice and electrotherapy are helpful adjuncts to treatment.[20]

Only in rare cases is surgical treatment advisable, since most patients with patellofemoral pain are treated successfully with conservative care. For that rare patient who experiences chronic, disabling symptoms, a surgical consultation may be necessary, but the patient must show a recalcitrance to rehabilitative therapy for at least 6

months or have a history of multiple patellar dislocations or subluxations.[20] When surgery is necessary, the least invasive and most practical procedure is a "lateral release" via arthroscopic procedure, which allows the patella to track in a more normal fashion without the typical pull from the lateral musculature. The vastus lateralis sheath is splayed along the lines of the lateral patellar retinaculum, thus alleviating the inclination of the kneecap to track laterally.

Patellofemoral Instability. Traumatic events or congenital hypermobility can lead to patellofemoral instability (Figure 10-25 *A, B*). Adolescent girls are prime candidates for a dislocating or subluxing patellofemoral joint.[63] Quadriceps weakness, a laterally tilted patella, malalignment, and patella alta are all factors that predispose these patients to instability.[57]

Rotatory movement of the knee is usually the mechanism of a traumatic dislocation. Young women and athletes of both sexes are commonly injured. The initial trauma may produce a significant effusion, although any subsequent subluxation may not cause as much swelling. The patella dislocates over the lateral femoral condyle, causing the medial retinaculum to tear and stretch at the medial patellar attachments.[38] A positive apprehension sign (i.e., an apprehensive response to manual lateral displacement of the patella over the femoral condyle), facet tenderness, and pain over the retinaculum are all signs of patella dislocation or chronic instability. Repetitive flexion loading further insults an already poor tracking mechanism. Feelings of "giving way" at the knee may signal extreme weakness or patellofemoral joint instability. Functional patella bracing may in fact become necessary as an adjunct to exercise in an active population.[20]

Chronic instability can lead to severe retropatellar pain and dysfunction. The combination of patellar malalignment, subluxability, and muscular weakness may lead to an articular cartilage abnormality (e.g., chondromalacia patellae) and may become a disabling orthopedic problem. Treatment centers around strengthening exercises for the extensor mechanism, stretching the hamstring muscle, alleviating pain and inflammation with the application of ice and electrotherapy, and the possible use of a patellofemoral brace for certain recreational and work-related activities.

Synovial Plica Syndrome. Some individuals have folds or vestiges of embryonic pouches in the synovial membranes of their knee joints. These pieces of extra tissue, called plicae, come in three varieties. The infrapatellar plica is the most common type and is usually

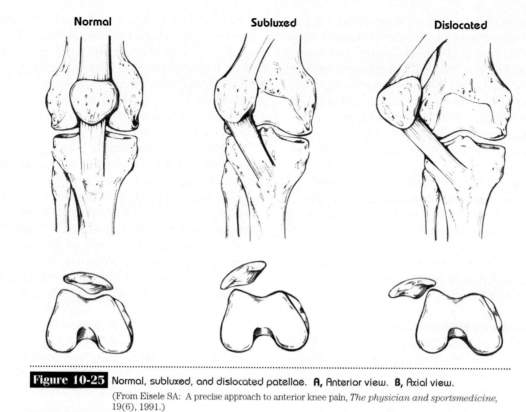

Normal **Subluxed** **Dislocated**

A

B

Figure 10-25 Normal, subluxed, and dislocated patellae. **A,** Anterior view. **B,** Axial view.
(From Eisele SA: A precise approach to anterior knee pain, *The physician and sportsmedicine,* 19(6), 1991.)

asymptomatic.[22] The medial plica may cause pain of a mechanical origin similar to patellofemoral pain in flexion and may be seen in as many as 20% of knees examined for internal pathologic abnormalities.[22] The suprapatellar plica is found in approximately 20% of all knees and, similar to the infrapatellar plica, is usually asymptomatic.

Some authors suggest that a traumatic event may trigger synovial plica pain syndrome.[16,103] Blunt trauma can also start the inflammatory process. Symptoms may include recurrent swelling, clicking, locking, and a feeling of "giving way." There may be a correlation between active symptomatic medial plica syndrome and findings of chondromalacia.

The result of an active plica syndrome is a synovitis. Conservative care should begin as soon as the clinician has ruled out more ominous diagnoses. The application of ice, compression, and quadriceps strengthening should be the foundation of treatment, with oral nonsteroidal antiinflammatory medication used if the thickened plicae require it. If conservative care is unsuccessful and the patient's life style is compromised, an arthroscopic surgical procedure may be warranted.

Internal Derangements of the Knee

Meniscal Tears

Injuries to the menisci of the knee constitute a large percentage of internal derangements at the knee joint and, as such, pose a tremendous challenge to the clinician. Injuries occur from rotational stress during weight bearing. Because the medial meniscus is attached at its periphery and therefore is less mobile than its lateral counterpart, tears to the medial meniscus are more common than similar injuries to the lateral meniscus; in fact, they are three times as common. Both conservative and nonconservative care have a place in the care of the meniscus.

The orthopedic approach to meniscal tears has changed dramatically over the past 2 decades. The advent of arthroscopy has forever altered the treatment of these injuries. Until the 1970s, the old adage, "When in doubt, take it out," applied to the menisci. Several authors of that time noted that the meniscus appeared to have no important role, and the number of total meniscectomies performed in those years reflected this opinion.[66] Postoperative degenerative changes were not fully recognized until the completion of extensive follow-up studies into the 1970s. Many investigators have since shown that the meniscus serves an important function and that the knee joint degenerates after removal of the cartilage.[3] With the advent of partial meniscectomy and meniscal repair by means of arthroscopic techniques, the morbidity of the injured knee joint has decreased drastically.

Barring exacerbated pathologic changes, meniscal tears do not require immediate treatment. Peripheral tears may actually heal spontaneously, partly because of the peripheral vascularity of the meniscus. Arnoczky's extensive work in the canine and human meniscus has led to the adoption of a fairly conservative stance regarding the treatment of small, peripheral tears in an otherwise healthy knee.[7]

Examination for Meniscal Tears

Acute joint line tenderness, painful knee flexion, and effusion usually accompany a meniscal tear. A normal knee contains approximately 5 to 10 cc of synovial fluid under usual conditions. The knee with a torn meniscus, however, contains approximately 50 cc of viscous inflammatory fluid. This synovial effusion is yellow in color.

McMurray test may be positive in a patient with a meniscal tear, and hamstring spasm is common if the knee has been acutely injured and treatment has been delayed for several days. Locking, clicking, dysfunction, weakness, and recurrent effusions suggest chronic tears. The examiner should be careful to check the quality of the patient's quadriceps contracture and the patient's ability to reach terminal extension. The patient with a meniscal tear may find squatting difficult (i.e., positive Childress test) and may lean on the unaffected leg to alleviate pressure on the damaged meniscus.

The differential diagnosis of meniscal lesions includes patellofemoral conditions. Patellofemoral pain syndromes rarely yield an effusion like that associated with a meniscal tear; usually, only a dislocated or subluxed patella produces such a knee effusion. In general, most of the tenderness associated with a dislocation or subluxation of the patella occurs at the retinaculum (peripatellar) or under the kneecap at the facets (retropatellar). Surface anatomy considerations during palpation (e.g., joint line pain) are the deciding factors.

Conservative Care: A Common Sense Approach

Certain types of meniscal injuries respond to a systematic, progressive, and intelligent program of care when it is instituted within a safe and protected environment (i.e., with a full-length knee immobilizer). The application of ice, electrotherapy, and quadriceps setting (isometric) exercises should begin immediately to reduce pain, swelling, atrophy, and joint dysfunction. The patient must avoid aggravating movements while attempting to heal without surgery. Medication is rarely necessary for these patients.

Nonoperative treatment is appropriate for small tears that do not cause great pain and swelling or that cause only moderate joint line pain; for meniscal lesions that are incidental findings in diagnostic reports; and for stable, vertical, longitudinal tears that cover the peripheral vascular aspect of the meniscus.[133] Tears of less than 1 cm in the peripheral vascular zone heal spontaneously, even in a knee with multiple-structure damage.[43,116] Traumatic full-substance tears in the vascular zone have healing rates of approximately 90%.[30] In fact, a trial of conservative care may be advisable for any borderline meniscal lesion, provided that a response to nonsurgical treatment is at least possible and the patient does not show signs of decompensation. Prolonged pain, swelling that continues after 2 weeks of care, muscle weakness and atrophy, inability to achieve a terminal extension or a contraction of the quadriceps mechanism—all signs of decompensation—warrant an orthopedic surgical consultation and diagnostic imaging studies.

Patients who are unable to bear weight on their knee should use a full-length knee immobilizer (posterior splint) with crutches. Ice should be applied consistently throughout the treatment program (Table 10-9). Electrotherapy is helpful to alleviate pain and reduce swelling. Isometric quadriceps setting can begin immediately, and the patient can then progress to straight leg raises. When able to maintain stability at 0 degrees of extension, the patient can gradually introduce arcs of flexion as long as they are free of pain. The patient who has a large knee effusion or who cannot achieve terminal extension should try to achieve these goals for 10 to 14 days. If the patient does not make progress under this conservative care, the practitioner should order an orthopedic surgical referral and an MRI (or arthrogram) to determine the extent of the injury (Figure 10-26 A, B).

Indications for Surgical Treatment: A New Look

Meniscal tears that may require surgical repair are long lesions (i.e., 7 mm or greater) in the vascular zone, peripheral detachment, and vertical longitudinal tears in the substance of the vascular third of the meniscus.[13] Surgical repair of meniscal tears at the peripheral zone is con-

Table 10-9	Meniscal Tears
Physical examination findings	Positive effusion Discomfort in flexion Positive McMurray test possible Hamstring tightness, contracture possible Joint line pain Difficulty in squatting Evaluation of terminal extension necessary
X-ray findings	Normal in acute tears Possibly joint space narrowing in chronic, degenerative tears
Treatment plan	Application of ice, isometrics, electrotherapy to achieve terminal extension Immobilization, use of crutches, if necessary Follow-up magnetic resonance imaging (or arthrography), if recalcitrant in 10-14 days

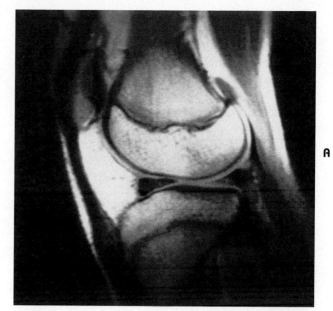

Anterior   **Posterior**

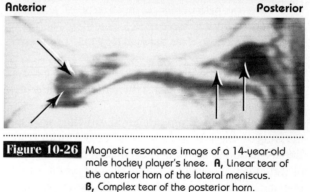

Figure 10-26 Magnetic resonance image of a 14-year-old male hockey player's knee. **A,** Linear tear of the anterior horn of the lateral meniscus. **B,** Complex tear of the posterior horn.

sidered logical for a dysfunctional knee in young, active patients. The presence of otherwise healthy tissue and an acute repair aid in successful treatment.[56]

Tears in the avascular zone, which is beyond 5 mm from the periphery, are more likely to be treated by partial meniscectomy. The indications for this arthroscopic procedure include the following:

- Significant size and instability of the tear
- Injury to the body of the meniscus
- Prolonged locking, clicking, and weakness
- Inability to gain terminal extension for a prolonged period
- Interference with normal everyday function
- Continued pain and effusion

Partial meniscectomy is a prudent option for most patients. Because it is now a principle of the standard of care to spare as much meniscal tissue as possible, total meniscectomy is recommended only if the meniscus has been damaged extensively.

All patients whose conditions are recalcitrant to a conservative protocol must undergo a diagnostic imaging study of the damaged cartilage. MRI or double-contrast arthrography makes it possible for the practitioner to assess the location and extent of meniscal damage before recommending surgical treatment. Although the cost is high, MRI is noninvasive, efficient, and accurate; furthermore, it does not involve ionizing radiation. The cost of arthrography is approximately one half the cost of MRI, but arthrography is invasive and perhaps not as sensitive for imaging conditions of the fibrocartilage. Arthrography is accurate in the diagnosis and evaluation of meniscal lesions, however, and still has a place in orthopedic medicine.

Ligament Sprains

Because the ligaments of the knee are largely responsible for the gross stability of the knee joint, any injury (e.g., a sprain) to the ligamentous structures of the knee has a great potential for disability. The key to restoring the knee's functional capacity lies in muscular rehabilitation after immobilization to promote healing of connective tissues. Ligament injuries can be anterior, posterior, medial, or lateral, or any combination of these.

Positive results of orthopedic stability tests are the hallmark signs of knee sprains. Ligament stress tests are not always easy to perform, however, since swelling, pain, and spasm sometimes inhibit the proper examination of a ligament sprain. In certain cases of an acute sprain, it may be wise to test the injured knee before severe inflammation develops, when possible. A large, tense effusion, which is also a telltale sign of a ligament sprain, may trigger muscle guarding; when this occurs the results of stability testing may be false-negative.

The following guidelines ensure accurate stability testing:

- Make certain the patient is in unrestrictive clothing, such as shorts or gown; the patient's knee and thigh must be clearly visible.
- Gain the patient's confidence by explaining everything that will happen during the examination.
- Be gentle and reassure the patient that the affected ligaments will be checked only a few times.
- Have the patient relax as much as possible, and release the leg to avoid muscle guarding; instructing the patient to close the eyes may help promote relaxation.
- Examine the unaffected knee first for inherent laxity and gapping; ask if there have been any prior injuries.

If a ligament is torn or injured, any fluid aspirated from inside the joint is commonly "tinged" with blood. The formation of such a bloody effusion within 12 hours of the injury is usually a sign of an ACL tear. A tense hematoma can also indicate a multiple-structure injury, such as collateral ligament– capsule insult with an ACL sprain.

Whenever a ligament is sprained, there is a chance that there was enough rotational stress at the time of injury to tear the meniscus as well. Therefore the wise practitioner always rules out a torn cartilage when examining a patient with a ligament injury. This is important because most ligament sprains are treated conservatively with immobilization as needed; only a torn meniscus may require arthroscopic surgery.

Medial Collateral Ligament Sprains

Isolated medial collateral ligament sprains are fairly common. The mechanism of such a sprain is a valgus force that stresses the medial compartment. Examination reveals palpable tenderness along the medial collateral ligament. An effusion is seen with most of the swelling over the medial aspect of the joint. Valgus instability and pain on stress testing is classic in these injuries.

The medial collateral ligament should be tested at 30 degrees of flexion for an isolated injury and at 0 degrees of extension for a tear with concomitant injuries. A gap at 0 degrees of extension indicates a serious injury. Usually the posteromedial capsule and ACL are injured as well. The medial meniscus, PCL, and posterior oblique ligament are also at risk.[68]

Conservative treatment with the application of ice, compression, elevation, and isometrics is appropriate for any medial collateral ligament sprain, except possibly a grade III sprain. In general, the collateral ligaments are excellent healers and do not often require invasive treatment.

A grade I sprain of the medial collateral ligament may necessitate placement in a posterior splint for a few days or at night to reduce valgus stresses to the knee caused by such actions as rolling over in bed. Grade II sprains may require a longer period of immobilization, from 2 to 4 weeks. The application of ice, isometrics, and electrotherapy are helpful in reducing pain and edema, as well as in combating weakness and atrophy. Grade III tears, which are caused by a large valgus force, are usually associated with concomitant injuries to the ACL, posteromedial capsule, or medial meniscus. Follow-up referral and surgery may be necessary (Table 10-10).

Follow-up mobilization and range-of-motion exercises are important in returning the patient to normal function. Also, the practitioner should check the lumbopelvic region for postural deformity and dyskinesia attributable to improper gait mechanics during convalescence. When medial collateral ligament sprains are chronic, calcific infiltrates over the medial joint line can appear on plain x-ray films. Pellegrini-Stieda disease occurs in patients with chronic medial knee pain and medial compartment instability.

Lateral Collateral Ligament Sprains

A varus force that causes an opening stress at the lateral compartment of the knee is necessary to damage the lateral collateral ligament. Because most recreational and sporting events cause valgus stresses on the knee, the lateral collateral ligament is not injured nearly as often as its medial counterpart.

If there is sufficient force in the direction of varus to injure the ligament, adjacent structures at the lateral knee joint can also be injured. Thus the iliotibial band, popliteus, posterolateral capsule, and fibular head should all be examined thoroughly (Table 10-11). The patient with a lateral collateral ligament sprain may exhibit signs of a peroneal nerve injury. A peroneal neurapraxia may

Table 10-10	Collateral Ligament Sprains	
	Medial Collateral Ligament Sprain	**Lateral Collateral Ligament Sprain**
Physical examination findings	Effusion Valgus instability Palpable tenderness	Effusion Varus instability Palpable tenderness
X-ray findings	Normal except in chronic medial compartment instability (Pellegrini-Stieda lesion)	Normal
Treatment plan	Immobilization Application of ice Electrotherapy Isometrics Use of crutches in some cases	Immobilization Application of ice Electrotherapy Isometrics Use of crutches in some cases

Table 10-11	Differential Diagnosis of Lateral Knee Pain		
Diagnosis	**Stability Testing**	**Presence of an Effusion**	**Site**
Lateral meniscus tear	Painful flexion Positive McMurray test	Yes	Lateral joint line
Lateral collateral ligament sprain	Positive	Yes	Across fibular collateral ligament
Popliteal tenderness	Negative	No	Pain on palpation between biceps tendon and lateral collateral ligament
Iliotibial band friction syndrome	Negative	No	Tenderness over lateral femoral condyle
Biceps tendonitis	Negative	No	Pain posteriorly on biceps femoris tendon
Anterolateral rotatory instability	Positive	Usually	Most commonly seen in lateral joint line pain

show signs of foot drop that improves with time. Complete disruption of the nerve is uncommon.

For stability testing, the examiner places the patient's knee under a varus stress at 30 degrees of flexion to evaluate the lateral collateral ligament and at 0 degrees of extension to evaluate the posterolateral capsule and the lateral collateral ligament. The treatment protocol follows that for an isolated medial collateral ligament injury (see Table 10-10).

Anterior Cruciate Ligament Sprains

In the maintenance of knee stability and function, the ACL plays several roles. It resists anterior displacement of the tibia, prevents hyperextension of the knee, resists excessive internal rotation of the tibia and femur, aids in the locking mechanism of the knee, and acts as an important secondary restraint against varus or valgus loading. The primary role of the ACL is to prevent internal rotation of the tibia on the femur in a flexed knee.[79] The ACL–deficient knee has been the source of controversy in orthopedics and sports medicine. As new techniques for knee reconstruction became prominent in the 1980s, the debate intensified. Although it is true that an injury to the ACL poses a greater challenge to the clinician than does an isolated collateral ligament sprain, it is important for the clinician to examine all the facts before recommending either conservative or surgical treatment for ACL deficiencies.

The frequency of ACL injuries is nine times that of injuries to the PCL.[69] A combination of extension and valgus-rotational forces generally causes an ACL sprain. Such sprains are commonplace in active individuals. Typically the individual was participating in an athletic event and reports that he or she either twisted the knee while cutting away from someone or slipped and hyperextended the knee. There is usually an audible pop at the time of injury, and swelling occurs within 12 hours. It has been estimated that 75% of individuals with a bloody effusion have an ACL tear.[89]

Both partial and complete tears of the ACL can occur. A total rupture can occur at three different sites: at the tibial attachment, in the midsubstance of the ligament, or at the femur. Tears that occur in the midsubstance are difficult to treat surgically, often requiring a patellar tendon graft.

The patient with an acute sprain usually has significant pain and holds the leg in an attitude of slight flexion. Stress testing reveals anteroposterior instability. In the case of partial ACL tears (sprains), the result of the Lachman's test is generally positive, and the result of the anterior draw test is negative at 90 degrees (Table 10-12). These findings occur because (1) the Lachman's test at approximately 20 to 30 degrees of knee flexion makes it impossible for the muscular restraints to produce false-negative results during stability testing, and (2) the hamstrings splint causes the anterior draw test to be unremarkable. In contrast, because of the amount of anterior tibial translation that occurs, the results of both tests are positive when the rupture of the ACL is complete. A large hemarthrosis will also be present. In addition, whereas partial tears have a soft, yet definite, end-point on stress testing, complete tears have no identifiable end-point.

Positive results related to ACL tests are graded as trace, 1+, 2+, or 3+ laxity. Stability testing can be classified via the following guidelines:

    1+ laxity   Up to 5 mm of tibial excursion
    2+ laxity   6 to 10 mm of tibial excursion
    3+ laxity   More than 10 mm of tibial excursion

The first two grades of laxity are commonly seen with a definite end-point in partial ACL tears. Complete tears have 3+ laxity and no definite end-point evident during anteroposterior stress testing maneuvers.

Instrumented knee arthrometry (KT-1000) is used to quantify knee-joint laxity in millimeters after an ACL injury; greater sensitivity has been demonstrated for concluding anterior tibial displacement at 20 to 30 degrees of knee flexion (Lachman's test) compared with 90 degrees of knee flexion (anterior draw test).[132]

The practitioner should screen the patient for joint line tenderness and for the McMurray sign to rule out a concomitant meniscal tear. Plain films should be ordered first to rule out an avulsion fracture, and an MRI scan can be ordered to confirm the diagnosis. It is also important to check for any inherent laxity in the opposite knee and to screen for any prior traumatic injury to the ACL.

Profile of an ACL Injury. Although the forces of trauma are important, the position of the knee at the time of the trauma and the specific mechanism of the injury are the keys to understanding injuries to the ACL. In athletic events such as skiing and football, fast changes of direction or deceleration of movement with a planted or fixed foot is the classic mechanism of injury. External contact does not necessarily have to occur. If an individual generates enough force on a vulnerable knee in a compromising position, ballistic movements are sufficient to cause an injury to the ACL.

One grave concern about these injuries is that they are easily overlooked in primary care. In many cases, ACL laxity is an incidental finding during a knee examination. Most of these patients do not complain about

---

Table 10-12   Anterior Cruciate Ligament Injury

	Acute Injury	Chronic Injury
Physical examination findings	Effusion (tense) Hemarthrosis (upon arthrocentesis) Abnormal Lachman's test Possibly, remarkable anterior draw test Need to check for collateral instability and joint line pain	Possibly, recurrent effusion Instability, subluxation on pivot shift or Slocum tests Abnormal Lachman's test Concomitant meniscal damage Latent joint line pain
X-ray findings	Plain films (i.e., three views) to rule out avulsion fractures, gross instability Sometimes, magnetic resonance imaging to rule out concomitant injury to meniscus and to confirm diagnosis	Need to rule out degenerative changes Need to rule out damage to secondary restraint, menisci
Treatment plan	Application of ice, electrotherapy Immobilization of knee in 20 degrees of flexion for 4 to 6 weeks (i.e., Bledsoe brace) Isometrics for hamstring and quadriceps muscles Follow-up examination in 7 days Follow-up supervised physical therapy according to extent of injury	Hamstring muscle strengthening exercises Derotation bracing for athletic events

their knee giving way or exhibit signs and symptoms of chronic instability. They have adapted in one way or another, most likely through muscular restraints. There are, in fact, many competitive and recreational athletes who have performed well without a fully functional ACL.

There are several critical considerations in determining the type of care that is appropriate for an ACL injury. The severity of the tear, including the laxity of the ligament, is very important. Disruption of the ligament is the key contributing factor to rotary instability that can lead to arcuate ligament complex damage or posterior oblique ligament injury.[47] The possibility of concomitant chondral and meniscal damage should be assessed. In addition, stability testing must be thorough to rule out damage to secondary restraints at the knee. Clearly the clinician has the unenviable task of piecing together all aspects of injury assessment and determining the next step in orthopedic care.

Appropriateness of Nonsurgical Care: The Case Against Surgery. Various factors are important in determining who will have a good chance of returning to function via conservative care for ACL sprain. Age, occupation, recreational activities, compliance, willingness to modify activities, and expectations are all pertinent factors that will help determine the success of ACL rehabilitation.[79] Patients with ACL tears whose collateral ligaments remain intact *generally* do well with conservative care.

A diligent, supervised physical therapy program is the key to a successful outcome. Early motion, progressive weight-bearing and closed kinetic-chain exercises, and functional activities represent a more modern, aggressive approach to ACL rehabilitation.[135,136]

Obviously, patients with biplanar instability (e.g., complete rupture of both the ACL and a collateral ligament) with capsular tearing require surgical treatment, usually immediately after injury. These are usually skiing, automobile, or football injuries. Not all patients with a hemarthrosis require arthroscopic evaluation, however. The deciding factor is always the degree to which any instability interferes with the individual's life style.

Occasionally a patient has a large avulsion fragment from the tibial plateau. Although such an injury usually requires an open reduction, treatment with a non–weight-bearing cast for 6 to 8 weeks can be successful for small, nondisplaced fragments.[98] These types of chondral injuries occur primarily in the adolescent, who should avoid or delay surgery on the ACL, if at all possible. In the child with open physes, intraarticular re-

constructive procedures (i.e., arthroscopy) may interfere with the growth plate (Figure 10-27). Thus open physes all but preclude reconstruction in the skeletally immature patient with chronic laxity of the ACL.[93] If the condition of a young, highly competitive athlete does not respond to conservative treatment and the athlete is not satisfied with his or her ability or competitive level, then surgery can be a last resort when the child reaches skeletal maturity. Until then, it is essential to rule out any associated meniscal injuries that can be managed successfully via either arthroscopy or physical therapy.

Conservative versus Surgical Care for Injury to the Anterior Cruciate Ligament: The Great Debate

Certain orthopedic surgical procedures have been efficiently documented for efficacy, mobility, and long-term follow-up. The probability of success and the consequences of not undergoing one of these procedures when conditions warrant it are well understood. Other procedures, such as those used in the treatment of an isolated anterior cruciate ligament tear or an anterior cruciate ligament–deficient knee with a partial

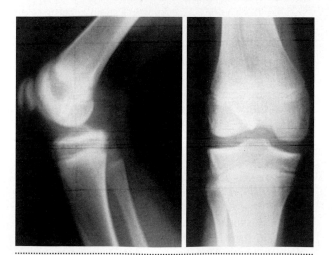

Figure 10-27 Open epiphyseal plates in a 14-year-old soccer player. The screw at the lateral femoral condyles is indicative of anterior cruciate reconstructive surgery. Despite operative treatment, this patient still exhibited moderate laxity 2 years after reconstruction.

collateral ligament injury (sprain), have not been proven empirically to produce above-average results.[42] These operative events have not had proper long-term follow-up and have not been shown to provide better results than conservative care.[65]

Surgical procedures for knee reconstruction after injury to the anterior cruciate ligament generally use the gracilis, semitendinosus, iliotibial tract, or patellar tendon for augmentation of the ligament. Patellar tendon transfer is the preferred procedure in patients with healthy joint surfaces.[44] Extraarticular reconstruction of the anterior cruciate ligament is inadvisable, however, because it may lead to chronic ligamentous laxity.[130,137] In contrast, extraarticular augmentation may be beneficial in a reconstructive procedure on the lateral side of the knee, because this procedure may reduce the possibility of recurrent laxity later.[80] Prosthetic ligaments (e.g., Gore-Tex) have been tested in recent years with results that are fair at best[106]; extraarticular procedures such as the Ellison or Slocum methods have also been studied.

Although many researchers have reported good results, their follow-up periods have generally been too short for their results to be considered reliable.[71,81] Many studies with follow-up periods of 5 years or longer do not support the theory that surgical treatment is the best treatment for the restoration of stability.[42,70,81,100,105] Repair of the anterior cruciate ligament without augmentation has not withstood the test of time.

In *The Crucial Ligaments,* Feagin's classic text on clinical decision making, knee kinematics, and biomechanics of trauma, he stated the following regarding isolated anterior cruciate ligament tears:

> There certainly is not a consensus that operative care is either the best choice or the accepted standard for the "isolated ACL [anterior cruciate ligament]." This lack of unanimity, perhaps more than any other factor, was the impetus for this book.[39]

He described a case of a young athlete with an anterior cruciate ligament tear:

> If this patient had declined surgery, I would consider immobilizing the knee in 20 degrees of flexion for 4 to 6 weeks. This course at least would have allowed the secondary restraints to begin healing and might have allowed the ACL to fall upon the PCL [posterior cruciate ligament] and gain a secondary source of attachment and blood supply. I believe this is why the natural history of ACL injury was not quite so unsatisfactory

in the past as today: Immobilization after injury, formerly the usual recommendation, gave opportunity for the secondary restraints to heal, as well as for the ACL to join with the PCL, somewhat as described in the surgical work of Wittek.[39]

Highly active or athletically competitive patients with nonisolated tears of the anterior cruciate ligament or chronic debilitating laxity of the ligament are candidates for intraarticular reconstruction. Successful intraarticular reconstruction of the knee joint has the following essential requirements:

- Proper selection of a graft substitute for augmentation
- Reliable method of fixation
- Proper graft positioning
- Proper preparation of the intercondylar notch region
- Proper tension or isometricity of the graft
- Proper revascularization of the graft after reconstruction
- Extended time for rehabilitation to ensure functional knee capacity
- Amelioration of concomitant meniscal pathologic deficiencies

Treatment of combined disruptions of the anterior cruciate and medial collateral ligaments usually involve surgical repair. Nonoperative results are poor in patients with biplanar instability.[2] Those who experience acute gross knee trauma, as occurs in football injuries, generally undergo surgical treatment immediately.

Personal experience indicates that reconstructive grafts loosen over a period of a few years. Even patellar tendon-bone grafts that have been shown to stabilize the anterior cruciate ligament continue to exhibit potential morbidity with limitation of motion.[37] Synthetic materials do not possess the same tensile strength as human ligaments. Furthermore, both natural and synthetic grafts require approximately 12 months of intense rehabilitation before a full-scale return to athletic events is possible.

Some orthopedic specialists argue that young patients with high levels of athletic activity will fare poorly in a nonoptimum spectrum of treatment, but it is precisely this type of active patient who may benefit the most from conservative rehabilitation (Table 10-13). The patient begins with a series of isometric exercises, focusing first on the hamstring muscle and then progressing to the abductor, adductor, and hip flexor muscles. Once through the initial stage of rehabilitation, when swelling has been reduced and normal range of motion has been established, the patient can begin functional multijoint closed kinetic chain movements,[64] such as therapeutic squats (see Figure 8-33). The use of progressive isotonic movements that encompass eccentric loading have a dramatic effect on hamstring strength.[72] They should be a part of the rehabilitation protocol for knee injuries. Barring biplanar gross instability, these exercises, together with functional bracing and physical therapy after immobilization of the acutely injured anterior cruciate ligament, make up prudent conservative treatment.

Posterior Cruciate Ligament Sprains

PCL sprains or tears make up only 16% to 23% of all ligamentous injuries to the knee.[55] PCL-deficit knees exhibit posterior laxity (tibial translation) with or without excessive external or varus rotation. Injuries are either isolated or involve the posterolateral structures of the knee, such as the lateral collateral ligament, popliteus muscle, arcuate complex, and posterior horn of the lateral meniscus.[18,55] Sequelae of PCL injury is consistent with *disability* rather than gross *instability*. Pain and stiffness are common. An effusion is present in acute cases; laxity is graded on stability testing with the posterior drawer test, and an ACL injury is graded with the Lachman's and anterior drawer tests. MRI is diagnostic

Table 10-13 Rehabilitation Exercise Programs for Common Knee Problems

Diagnosis	Rehabilitation Areas to Stress	Method	Cybex
Chondromalacia patella Subluxating patella Postsurgical status for chronic dislocations or chronic irritative processes	1. Strengthening the quadriceps and, particularly, VMO muscles without placing additional stress on patellofemoral surface 2. Achieve or maintain full ROM 3. General strengthening of hamstring, abductor, adductor, and lower leg muscles	1. Quadriceps setting, straight leg lifts, short arcs with progressive resistance 2. ROM and strengthening of hamstring, abductor, adductor muscles can be done conventionally	Only for strength testing
Anterior cruciate deficient knees, chronic or acute; postsurgical casting and postsurgical reconstruction, intraarticular or extraarticular	1. Achieve full ROM 2. Emphasis is placed on strengthening secondary stabilizers to anterior cruciate ligament	1. Active ROM exercises 2. Hamstring strength aims to equal quadriceps strength of nonaffected leg, done with exercise programs of isometrics; isotonic with concentric and eccentric contractions (closed kinetic chain); isokinetics 3. Quadriceps strength to be elevated by use of isometrics at 90°, 60°, 30° and full extension; isotonic resistance done only in 90°-45° flexion	1. For strength 2. For hamstring strengthening 3. For quadriceps strengthening 90°-45° only
Medial collateral ligament sprains, chronic or acute, postsurgical reconstruction; postsurgical immobilization	1. Special emphasis should be placed on strengthening quadriceps and adductor muscles 2. General ROM 3. General strengthening of hamstring, adductor, and lower leg muscles	1. Achieve or maintain full ROM 2. Quadriceps muscle sets 3. Straight leg lifts with progressive resistance in hip flexion and adduction 4. Isotonics for quadriceps and hamstring muscles (closed kinetic chain) 5. Isokinetics for quadriceps and hamstring muscles	For testing and workouts

VMO, Vastus medialis obliquus muscle; **ROM,** range of motion.

(Adapted from Ellison AE, editor: *Athletic training and sportsmedicine,* ed 2, Chicago, 1989, American Academy of Orthopaedic Surgeons.)

of ligament and associated structural tears, such as a torn lateral meniscus.

Limited studies have shown that less posterior laxity results in fewer symptoms and better function of the knee joint. Patients with excessive posterior tibial translation have more pain, swelling, and arthrosis over time than their mildly injured counterparts. As in ACL insufficiency, PCL laxity leads to a decrease in meniscal load bearing capabilities.[76]

Isolated injuries that occur in sporting activities have a good prognosis with conservative treatment.[18,76,119] In patients with combined PCL and posterolateral structural damage, anatomic repair or reconstruction may become necessary. PCL rehabilitation focuses on early control of pain and swelling with aggressive quadriceps exercises. In the early stages, resisted knee flexion is avoided in open kenetic chain exercises to prevent posterior shear forces on the knee.[19] Sensorimotor control, strength, and full range of motion and function are the long-term goals of treatment (Table 10-14).

Injuries to the Patella

Patellar Dislocation

Years ago, it was thought that only young girls with severe lower extremity malalignment dislocated their patellofemoral joints. As more people engaged in athletic endeavors and as orthopedic diagnostic capabilities expanded, however, the diagnosis of patellar dislocation became more common in both sexes. It is now well-known that men and women athletes dislocate the patella, although women probably still account for the majority of patellofemoral injuries in the sedentary population.

Patellar dislocation is common in ground-based sports that involve ballistic-type movements. Forceful deceleration of the leg with simultaneous twisting or cutting movements causes a dislocation. Nonathletes may be subject to similar forces.

Weakness in the extensor mechanism may be associated with a vastus medialis defect. A dysplastic, high-attaching vastus medialis obliquus muscle further highlights the quadriceps weakness. It is important to evaluate the opposite knee for patellar hypermobility, since individuals with sufficient anatomic weakness or muscular insufficiency may sustain multiple dislocations or subluxations and develop chronic patellar insufficiency.

The patella dislocates in a lateral direction, thereby damaging the medial aspect of the joint. The patient often hears an audible "pop" when the injury occurs, which signifies the tearing of the medial restraints. A rent then develops at the damaged medial retinaculum and attachment of the vastus medialis.[36] Tenderness is palpable over the lateral femoral condyle during examination, but it may be most exquisite over the damaged medial patellofemoral joint. It is important to rule out true medial joint line tenderness seen in a torn meniscus.

Standard plain radiographic films, including an axial patellar view (Hughston projection), are useful in ruling out a fracture.[57] Articular cartilage damage at the patellofemoral joint may occur in association with patellar dislocation, which can lead eventually to chondromalacic changes if the patient experiences multiple episodes of trauma. Excessive weakness and malalignment facilitate this process.

The patient with a first-time dislocation develops a moderate effusion that is usually serosanguinous. The knee should be immobilized in a splint for approximately 3 weeks, and crutches should be used for at least the first 2 weeks to make certain that the patient places no weight on the leg. The use of plaster casts or patellar bandages leads to excessive morbidity, because they restrain mobility.[86] The application of ice, electrotherapy, and isometrics can begin as soon as tolerated (Table 10-15). The key to preventing recurrence is to strengthen the stabilizers of the patellofemoral joint.[52]

Table 10-14 Posterior Cruciate Ligament Injury	
Physical examination findings	Effusion Hemarthrosis (on arthrocentesis) Abnormal posterior draw test Need to check posterolateral instability, lateral joint line pain, and lateral structures
X-ray findings	Plain films to rule out fractures, gross instability MRI may be necessary to confirm diagnosis and to rule out lateral meniscus tear
Treatment plan	Application of ice, electrotherapy Immobilization of knee in posterior splint (terminal extension) for acute stage Aggressive quadriceps exercises, avoidance of early knee flexion loads Follow-up supervised physical therapy according to extent of injury

MRI, Magnetic resonance imaging.

Once the swelling and pain decrease with therapy and immobilization, the patient can begin to attempt small amounts of flexion. This can be achieved by sitting at the edge of a table and slowly bending the affected leg. To ensure safety and increase confidence, the patient can hook the ankle of the "good" leg under the affected limb and gently guide the injured knee into flexion.

Patellofemoral Subluxation

Although neither as dramatic nor as severe an injury as a dislocation, a patellar subluxation may be more common and often leads to chronic dysfunction. The mechanism of injury of an acute patellofemoral subluxation is similar to that of a patellar dislocation; however, the joint usually reduces spontaneously to its normal resting position. The medial restraints sustain less extensive damage than in a full dislocation. Patellofemoral subluxation can become chronic after a dislocation that was not properly treated or rehabilitated. Athletes involved in ballistic sports or individuals with weakness and malalignment are prone to injury.

Symptoms include a positive patella apprehension sign, pain and crepitus with flexion, tightness in the hamstring muscles, and a history of locking or giving way at the patellofemoral joint. Swelling, Fairbanks sign at 30 degrees of flexion, and pain upon quadriceps loading are all common.[53] In addition, the patient may experience pain or discomfort going up and down stairs, the patella may appear to be hypermobile malaligned, and there may be evidence of dysplasia in the vastus medialis muscle. Only acute subluxations accompanied by pain and swelling should undergo a short period (i.e., a few days) of immobilization. The application of ice, electrotherapy, and strengthening of the quadriceps muscle are key features for rehabilitation.[34]

Chronic subluxability can lead to patellofemoral degeneration, chondromalacia, and progressive pain or dysfunction. In most patients with chronic subluxability, there is evidence of extensive quadriceps weakness or patellar malalignment.[34] Tibial varum, genu valgum, excessive femoral anteversion, subtalar pronation, and genu recurvatum all contribute to excessive patellofemoral stress and subluxability. For most of those with chronic patellar subluxation or dislocation, the treatment of choice is nonoperative. Only a handful of chronic subluxers may need an arthroscopy or lateral release to regain function and reduce pain. Most realignment procedures are unwarranted.

Patellar Fractures

An external blow to the anterior knee is generally the mechanism of a fractured patella. The superior aspect of the patella is most commonly fractured without gross displacement. Sometimes, the tendon is severed, although

---

Table 10-15 Patellar Injuries

	Patellar Dislocation	Patellar Subluxation	Patellar Fracture
Physical examination findings	Moderate effusion Peripatellar pain Medial retinaculum tenderness Limited flexion Possible quadriceps weakness Need to rule out patellar malalignment Need to differentiate patellar injury from meniscal injury	Medial patellar pain Retropatellar, peripatellar pain Swelling, bogginess Locking, weakness Painful flexion loading (stairs) Fairbanks sign at 30° flexion Positive apprehension test Need to rule out malalignment, chondromalacia patellae	Effusion Palpable tenderness over patella Inability to achieve a straight leg raise Lack of knee flexion Weak or absent quadriceps contraction
X-ray findings	Anteroposterior, lateral, Hughston views Need to rule out patellar fracture	Anteroposterior, lateral, Hughston views Lateral patellar position seen on Hughston view	Most often seen on anteroposterior view
Treatment plan	Use of crutches, application of ice, isometrics Immobilization for approximately 3 weeks Posterior splint	Application of ice, isometrics, electrotherapy Short immobilization period, if acute and incapacitating Patellofemoral bracing for athletes, if subluxability becomes chronic	Application of ice, electrotherapy Immobilization, use of crutches Follow-up isometric exercises for quadriceps

this is not common. Severed tendons can be sutured in a figure of eight.

A fractured patella should be confirmed radiographically (Figure 10-28). The differential diagnosis includes a bipartate patella, which is visible on an x-ray film as well. If the patient not only has a hematoma from a contusion, but also cannot complete an active straight leg raise, the clinician should suspect damage to the extensor mechanism. The patient should be placed in a posterior knee immobilizer. Treatment centers around non–weight bearing activities with the use of crutches for 2 to 4 weeks, the application of ice, and electrotherapy—followed by rehabilitation exercises for the quadriceps muscle.

Degenerative Arthritis (Osteoarthritis)

Being the largest of the weight-bearing joints, the knee is a common site for degenerative arthritis. This condition is seen in individuals with long-term complaints and previous traumatic episodes. It is confirmed on radiographic

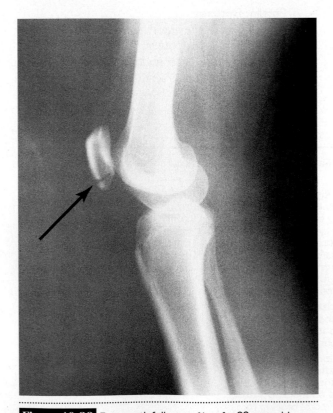

Figure 10-28 Two-month follow-up film of a 22-year-old woman's fractured patella. Fibrous defect appears at the fracture site.

films and treated according to life style, age, and patient expectations.

There are several mechanisms for developing osteoarthritic changes at the knee. Years of trauma, wear and tear, disease processes, and anatomic factors (e.g., a neglected mechanical or internal derangement) can all lead to osteoarthritis. Chronic, recurrent ligamentous instability has been biomechanically proven to be a causative factor in the development of degenerative arthritis. In addition, prior surgery (e.g., a total meniscectomy), a history of infectious disease, or severe malalignment (e.g., advanced genu varum) can all predispose the patient to osteoarthritis.

The patellofemoral joint is often a site for arthritis as well. Recurrent patellofemoral instability, quadriceps weakness, and malalignment of the extensor mechanism may ultimately lead to arthritic changes. Patellofemoral disease causes a potential host of problems in flexion movements at the knee. Retropatellar spurs have a great potential for being symptomatic and causing disability in older patients.

The first symptom can be discomfort after activity, such as stair climbing or distance walking, or achiness in the morning. Later the patient may report recurrent joint swellings, which mandate further investigation. Effusions of a mild-to-moderate size are commonplace. Some individuals have such advanced arthritis that bony deformity is obvious just on physical examination. Most active athletes, either recreational or competitive, who are over the age of 40 years show some radiographic sign of degenerative arthritis on an x-ray film.

Bony enlargement, medial joint line pain, crepitus, and painful flexion are all signs and symptoms of this disease. The joint becomes boggy or effused during flare-ups. The pain is sometimes referred to the back of the knee joint, causing posterior knee pain over the hamstring and gastrocnemius muscles, or up the anterior thigh over the quadriceps muscle. If physical examination findings at the knee are normal, the examiner should also rule out referred pain from an arthritic hip joint.

Radiographic studies usually show joint space narrowing, sclerosis, marginal osteophytes at the femoral condyle and proximal tibia, spurring of the tibial eminence, and heterotopic bone at the patellofemoral joint. It is common to see an arthritic spur at the inferior or superior aspect of the patella. This may cause the most pain, especially when the individual is walking up and down stairs. Advanced degenerative arthritis exhibits the common varus malalignment on a plain film (Figure 10-29). On an MRI of the osteoarthritic knee, large amounts of water are seen in menisci with degeneration. This condition is not to be confused with acute tears of the cartilage.

Treatment consists primarily of controlling the pain and swelling (if present) with cryotherapy and electrotherapy; isometric exercises for the extensors; supportive footwear (good sneakers are best); and the administration of oral medication for acute, disabling flare-ups (Table 10-16). Older individuals with severe problems may benefit from an orthopedic surgical consultation. Arthroplasty is appropriate for individuals debilitated by advanced degenerative arthritis if they meet certain criteria:

- In general, patients should be at least 60 years of age, because the life span of the implant averages only 10 or 15 years.
- The patient must be in pain that is sufficient to hamper their lives.
- The patient should find it difficult to participate in everyday tasks or activities such as walking or shopping.

People with advanced arthritis may find themselves wondering if they are a candidate for a joint replacement. Although arthroplasty of the knee can add quality to the life of some of these individuals, not all patients are candidates for the procedure. Because a joint replacement is usually good for a limited number of years, the patient who is younger than 60 years may be wise to delay surgery for a few years, if at all possible.

Essentially, all the options must be discussed with the patient, his or her family, the primary care physician, and the specialist. The following list of questions is helpful as a checklist in screening patients for a surgical consultation:

- How far can you walk at any one time?
- Do you have difficulty performing everyday chores, such as walking up and down stairs and going food shopping?
- How often do you experience severe pain that disables you for at least 1 day?
- Are there any recreational activities that you once enjoyed that you can no longer participate in because of your knee pain?
- Have you previously tried physical therapy, exercise, braces, and various medications for your arthritis to no avail?

The practitioner should ask many questions, show empathy, and involve the spouse and children in the decision-making process. This makes it easier to reach an accurate and reasonable decision about joint replacement. The patient who remains debilitated despite activity modification, oral medication, and a brace may consider surgery the only recourse, however.

Pediatric Knee Problems

Knee pain in young people can be quite alarming to parent and practitioner alike. Thankfully, most knee pain in youngsters is self-limiting with no complicating factors. There are, however, certain patterns of pain that relate to periods and stages of growth in the developing adolescent.

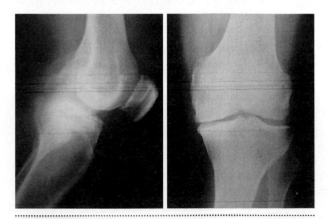

Figure 10-29 Osteoarthritis of the right knee in a 67-year-old man. Note varus deformity secondary to degenerative joint disease and patellofemoral arthritis.

Table 10-16	Osteoarthritis of the Knee
Physical examination findings	Recurrent effusions and pain Crepitus and bony irregularity Medial joint line pain Referral of pain to posterior knee or anterior thigh
X-ray findings	Varus deformity Osteophytes and marginal spurring Medial joint space narrowing
Treatment plan	Ice, electrotherapy, isometrics, administration of nonsteroidal anti-inflammatory drugs, if necessary Activity modification Bracing or orthopedic consultation for knee arthroplasty, if needed

Children younger than 8 or 9 years of age who develop knee pain usually have a precipitatory factor, such as trauma or a gait problem. Falls from bicycles and skateboards typically produce fractures of the tibial spine. Subtalar pathologic changes or arch deficits may create an aberrant lower extremity or biomechanical fault that transmits forces awkwardly to the knee joint itself.

Children above the age of 10 years usually have mechanical knee pain that is a direct result of rapid growth. Traction apophysitis culminates from the tightness around muscle-tendon units. This physiologic phenomenon arises from the fact that the long bones grow at a faster rate than the accompanying tendons. Thus during periods of rapid growth, children experience a loss of flexibility that increases their chances of developing pain and dysfunction.

Other causes of knee pain in the child include severe patellofemoral malalignment and subluxability, as discussed earlier, as well as tumors. Screening for metabolic or neoplastic disease is essential for children who complain of knee pain, but have no physical findings and an unremarkable history. Fortunately, these conditions are not common, but a thorough diagnostic evaluation should take them into account.

Physical Examination of the Child's Knee

To examine the knee of a patient at any age, the practitioner must evaluate the entire lower extremity as a whole. In youngsters this principle is particularly important, since their lower extremity is a dynamically changing entity. When examining a child, the practitioner should be sure to

- Look for signs of tibial torsion, pronation, and general laxity in the joints;
- Check for functional ability by watching the child walk, run, and hop;
- Determine what does and does not cause pain;
- Inspect the child's footwear, looking for irregular wearing of soles and asking if the child has always worn those types of shoes;
- Question the parents about periods of rapid growth in the child; and,
- Ask about a prior lower extremity complaint, such as foot or shoe pain.

For the most part, however, the examination procedures are the same as those used for adult patients.

Large stress forces on the young knee usually injure the developing bones and growth centers well before the ligaments yield to overload. For example, a knee injury that involves a sufficient amount of twisting force in the presence of an open physis culminates in an epiphyseal fracture at the distal femur before any ligament injury results.[122] Therefore the general diagnosis of a ligamentous "sprain" in a child should be approached with caution. Although ligament injuries do occur in children, plain radiographic films should be used in cases of trauma to exclude epiphyseal plate changes or fracture.

A fact of practice that involves pediatric injuries is that the children usually do just fine with care; it is the parents who may need some nurturing.

Pathologic Conditions of the Knee in the Child

Several clinical entities seen in the pediatric or adolescent patient are specific in nature to a population of developing youngsters: osteochondritis dissecans, tibial spine fractures, epiphyseal fractures, and traction - apophysitis.

Osteochondritis Dissecans

Classified as one of the osteochondroses, osteochondritis dissecans is a significant clinical pathologic condition in adolescents. It involves a defect of subchondral bone and articular cartilage, which may become separated from the joint surface. Etiologic factors may include an anomaly of ossification in the maturing child or an episode of trauma to the anterior knee.[21]

The medial femoral condyle, particularly the lateral portion, is the most common site for osteochondritis dissecans. The lateral femoral condyle is the second most common site, with the undersurface of the patella involved only infrequently.

Osteochondritis dissecans occurs in boys more often than girls, and the youngsters are athletically active in many cases. Twenty percent of the cases are bilateral[32]; occasionally, the condition afflicts both knees simultaneously. The onset of pain is usually somewhat insidious. The youngster usually begins to limp and complains of a feeling of the knee giving way. Intermittent locking and swelling are usually the other presenting symptoms. True locking of the knee joint is possible in cases involving a loose body, which is generally osteocartilaginous in nature and may be much larger than its radiographic appearance because of a large cartilaginous cap surrounding the fragment.

Symptoms are nonspecific, and a careful radiographic examination is necessary for an accurate diagnosis. Any child or adolescent with suspected osteochondritis dissecans should immediately undergo x-ray studies that include anteroposterior, lateral, Hughston, and tunnel projections. Radionuclide bone scans can provide additional information, because uptake is increased at the site of the abnormality (Figure 10-30 *A-C*).

The tunnel or intercondylar film is important to obtain an image of the femoral condyles and trochlear notch of the femur. Taking the tunnel projections with the knee flexed and the x-ray tube angled to visualize the intercondylar notch prevents the tibia or patella from blocking the view. In particular, the posterior surfaces of the femoral condyle are brought into profile. The intercondyloid projection taken in the bent knee or prone position is recommended.

As is the case with many diseases of musculoskeletal development, treatment for osteochondritis dissecans centers around alleviating the symptoms while protecting the immature and rapidly growing structures. The application of ice, rest, and time are all important components of treatment (Table 10-17). Immobilization or crutches are used only when weight bearing is painful for the youngster. Quadriceps exercises can begin as soon as the patient can tolerate them and will contribute to the overall stability of the joint.[121]

Surgery is rarely necessary. It is reserved for those cases in which a loose body in the joint requires surgical excision (Figure 10-31) or a displaced osteochondral fracture requires open reduction and internal fixation.

Tibial Spine Fractures

Although fractures around the knee are rare in comparison with the overall rate of other knee injuries that are the result of trauma and overuse syndromes in the general population, fractures of the tibial spine are fairly common in childhood and early adolescence. One typical mechanism of injury is a fall, usually from a bicycle. The child develops a tense hemarthrosis after a fall and is brought into the clinician's office or emergency room. The practitioner should order radiographic studies immediately after the history taking, since they clearly reveal a tibial spine fracture. The patient should be referred to an orthopedic surgeon, who usually attempts a closed reduction and cast immobilization in extension.[108] If it is impossible to achieve a satisfactory closed reduction, the child may require surgical care.

A second mechanism of injury involves an ACL injury. Trauma that ruptures the ligament in an adult causes an avulsion fracture of the tibial spine in a youngster.[108] In a child, the ACL rarely tears at its midportion, because the immature bone at the growth plate is generally the weaker point and thus gives way earlier than the ligament. An avulsion fracture of the spine of the tibia holds a more promising prognosis for healing than does a torn ACL, however. It is important to rule out

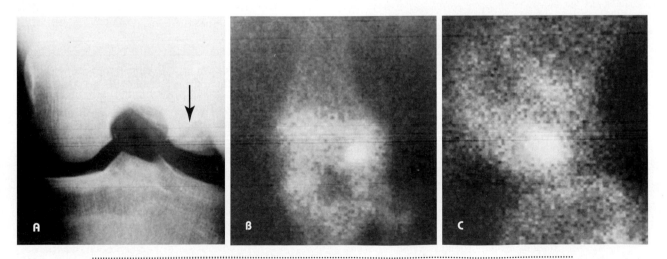

Figure 10-30 Osteochondritis dissecans. **A,** Tunnel view showing lesion involving lateral femoral condyle (arrow). **B,** Frontal and **C,** lateral views on radionuclide bone scan, revealing increased uptake in lateral femoral condyle corresponding to lesion in the tunnel view.

(From Nicholas JA, Hershman EB, editors: *The lower extremity and spine in sports and medicine,* ed 2, vol 1, St Louis, 1995, Mosby.)

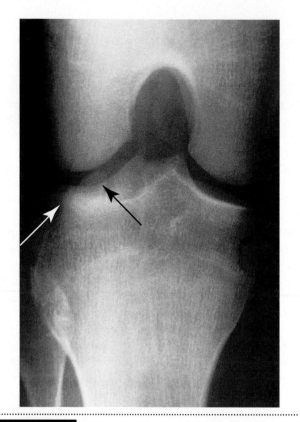

Figure 10-31 Tunnel projection revealing a loose body in the lateral compartment of the knee joint in a 21-year-old man.

any other type of internal structural damage that may have occurred at the time of the injury. An orthopedic surgeon should also be consulted in this type of case.

Epiphyseal Injuries

As noted previously, the growth plate is the weak link in the pediatric musculoskeletal system. Thus the imposition of angular forces at the knee can cause a fracture across the cartilaginous growth plate. Tenderness over the epiphysis and pain with varus or valgus stress lead the clinician to suspect a growth plate injury. Plain films should be taken; however, if the presence of an effusion and the findings of stress testing strongly suggest an epiphyseal injury, a referral to an orthopedist for possible additional stress films is necessary.

An epiphyseal injury may jeopardize the growth of the child's lower extremity because the distal femur growth center is responsible for 40% of this longitudinal growth.[36] Closed reduction, cast immobilization, and instructions to avoid placing weight on the involved leg for 6 to 8 weeks are usually in order. The medial collateral ligament may be sprained in many children with such an injury, but it is rarely torn. Like ligamentous injuries, meniscal injuries are fairly rare in children.

Termed Salter-Harris fractures, these types of fractures are classified according to site and displacement. They are fairly stable and common among adolescent athletes.[25] Some injuries ultimately cause leg length in-

Table 10-17 Pediatric Knee Problems

	Osteochondritis Dissecans	Tibial Spine Fracture	Epiphyseal Fracture (Distal Femur)	Traction Apophysitis (Proximal Tibia)
Physical examination findings	Anterior knee pain Swelling Limp Locking possible Sensation of knee giving way, quadriceps weakness	Painful motion around knee Tense hemarthrosis Difficulty walking and with knee flexion	Hemarthrosis Difficulty in ambulation History of sports-related trauma Abnormal stress, stability test findings	Point tenderness and swelling over tibial apophysis Pain in extreme knee flexion Possible callus formation at tibial tubercle Symptomatic during period of rapid growth
X-ray findings	Standard three views plus intercondylar (tunnel) projection Area of rarefaction or fragmentation, usually medial femoral condyle	Standard three views at a minimum Possibly, better visualization of fragments via oblique projection	Possibly normal routine films Abnormal varus-valgus stress films	Open growth plate evident on standard views Need to rule out apophyseal irregularity or fragmentation (avulsion fracture)
Treatment plan	Application of ice Rest, immobilization, avoidance of weight bearing, if necessary	Application of ice Immobilization Referral to orthopedic surgeon	Application of ice, immobilization Referral to orthopedic surgeon	Rest, application of ice Isometric exercises when tolerated

equality, however, and require careful follow-up, especially in regard to lower back pain. If deformity and extensive shortening occur, a more invasive approach to orthopedic care may become necessary.

Traction Apophysitis (Osgood-Schlatter Disease)

The growth plate represents a cartilaginous weak link in the growing child's musculoskeletal system. The proximal tibial apophysis is a common area of injury in this age group. Traction apophysitis, often called Osgood-Schlatter disease, results from the pull of the patellar tendon on the growth plate. An avulsion fracture type of injury may also occur at the apophysis, but microtears at the patellar tendon insertion into the apophysis, with subsequent fragmentation of the secondary ossification center, are more likely (Figure 10-32 *A-C*).

Children who are experiencing a rapid growth spurt are more susceptible to traction apophysitis than are others because, as noted earlier, these children can lose flexibility in the muscle-tendon unit around rapidly growing long bones. When this occurs, such activities as jumping, bending, and running cause an eccentric load on the quadriceps mechanism and pull on the tendinous-cartilaginous junction at the proximal aspect of the tibia. Boys predominate over girls, and the average ages of involvement are 12 to 18 years.[107]

The youngster with traction apophysitis usually has a palpable tenderness at the attachment of the patellar tendon on the tibial tubercle over the apophysis,[112] as well as discomfort in extreme knee flexion. Contraction of the knee extensor on a flexed knee causes pain because the quadriceps muscle is being prestretched. Ballistic, eccentric loading of the extensor mechanism will cause pain, and some localized swelling is usually apparent over the growth plate.

Many of these children are quite active. They may even participate in two or three organized sports, which can pose a potential problem for the clinician who is attempting to formulate a time-efficient treatment program. It may be necessary for the child who is in the ac-

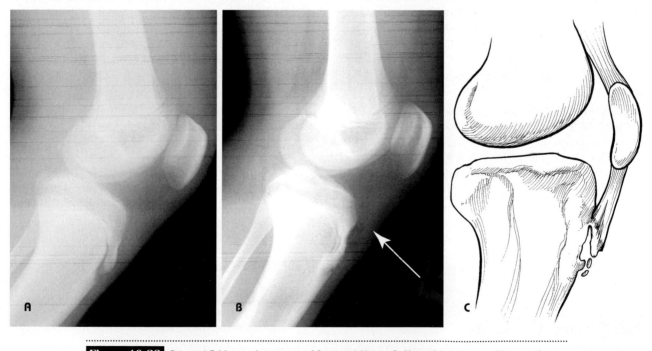

Figure 10-32 Osgood-Schlatter disease in a 12-year-old boy. **A,** Normal right knee. Observe the normal secondary ossification center of the tibial tuberosity. Although it has not yet completely fused, it has a smooth and regular contour. **B,** Affected left knee. Fragmentation of the secondary ossification center is evident. Soft-tissue edema (arrow) is observed over the tuberosity. **C,** This diagram depicts the classic fragmentation and avulsion of the tibial tuberosity.

(Part B. Courtesy of Brian Kleinberg, DC, Concord, Ontario. Part A and C. From Deltoff MN, Kogon PL: *The portable skeletal x-ray library,* St Louis, 1998, Mosby.)

tive growth stage and has acute symptomatology to stop participating in competitive sports until the inflammation resolves. This condition is a mechanical problem of development and overuse, and fortunately it is quite self-limiting. Therefore patiently waiting out the growth period and protecting the area from further overuse greatly decrease the chances of calcification and deformity.

Plain films serve a multitude of purposes for the orthopedic care of youngsters with traction apophysitis. These include the following:

- Assessment of the apophysis for the status of plate closure and the prognosis for future skeletal growth
- Evaluation of the growth plate for any resultant damage from overuse, such as fragmentation, ossicle formation, and loose body displacement
- Elimination of any other pathologic anomaly of the knee as a cause for pain and dysfunction
- Formulation of a timetable for prognosis and recovery based on the status and maturation of the tibial apophysis

Timing is an important factor in the treatment of these individuals. Most authorities agree that rest is the key to alleviating the symptoms of traction apophysitis, since the young, rapidly growing body cannot overcome the constant stress across the growth plate.[4,23] Because the patient usually appears with a tightened and weakened leg, most reasonable clinicians no longer advocate casting.[92] A tight muscle is usually a weak muscle; therefore, the patient can begin a straight leg raise–isometric exercise program once the performance of such a program is pain-free.

Once knee pain and swelling have subsided, a period of active rest can be inserted into the program. Bicycle riding with the seat placed high to avoid excessive knee flexion should provide more protection than running or jumping events. The patient should also continue to strengthen the quadriceps muscles and avoid extreme flexion. Excision of a symptomatic fragment of an avulsed tibial tubercle is a rare necessity.

Review Questions

1. (a) Name the movements of the knee joint. (b) What are the major secondary restraints that lend stability to the joint and motions they prevent?
2. (a) Name four functions of the menisci. (b) What are four clinical orthopedic findings in patients with a torn meniscus? (c) Name two imaging modalities used to confirm a tear in the meniscus.
3. What are nine signs and symptoms associated with patellofemoral pain?
4. A 21-year-old male basketball player sustained a blow to the lateral side of the knee joint. He was examined in your office several hours after taken out of the game, and he was unable to walk. Orthopedic findings included moderate, nontense effusion; medial joint-line pain; limited flexion; moderate gapping medially at 30 degrees on stability testing; and mild gapping medially at terminal extension. A Lachman's test and an anterior draw were unremarkable. (a) What is your tentative diagnosis? (b) What does your initial treatment include?
5. A 14-year-old football player is referred to you for a second opinion. He twisted his knee while running away from a defender and hyperextended the joint. The injured joint swelled within 1 day of the injury. X-ray films at the hospital provided negative findings, except for some swelling around the knee, and the epiphyseal plates were almost closed. Physical examination findings included mild effusion, discomfort in flexion, positive Lachman's test (1+ laxity) at 25 degrees, unremarkable anterior draw at 90 degrees, medial joint-line pain, and positive McMurray test. (a) What is your initial diagnosis? (b) If this patient continues to exhibit pain and swelling, what is your next step?
6. What is the proper sequence regarding graded therapeutic exercise for patients with internal derangements (postsurgical, immobilized) and patellofemoral pain?
7. A 13-year-old girl active in gymnastics and dance complains of anterior knee pain toward the insertion of the patella tendon, swelling over the tibial tubercle, and difficulty achieving full knee flexion. What is your diagnosis?

References

1. Adams JC, Hambler DL: The thigh and knee. In *Outline of orthopedics*, ed 11, New York, 1980, Churchill Livingstone.
2. Adams M, Boyle JJ: Simultaneous tears of the anterior cruciate and medial collateral ligaments, *Orthop Consult* 8(1):6, 1987.
3. Allen PR, Denham RA, Swan AV: Late degenerative changes after meniscectomy, *J Bone Joint Surg* 66B:666, 1984.
4. Andersen SJ: Overuse knee injuries in young athletes, *The Physician and Sportsmedicine* 19(12):69, 1991.
5. Andrews JR, Baker CL, Curl WW, Gidumal R: Surgical repair of acute and chronic lesions of the lateral capsular ligamentous complex of the knee. In Feagin JA, editor: *The crucial ligaments*, New York, 1988, Churchill Livingstone.

6. Arnheim DD, Prentice WE: *Principles of athletic training,* ed 8, St Louis, 1993, Mosby.

7. Arnoczky SP: Cellular repopulation of deep-frozen meniscal autografts: an experimental study in the dog, *Arthroscopy* 8:428, 1992.

8. Arnoczky SP: Microvasculature of the human meniscus, *Am J Sports Med* 10(2):90, 1982.

9. Arnoczky SP: Vascularity of the meniscus, *Am J Sports Med* 11(3):131, 1983.

10. Arnoczky SP, Warren RF: Anatomy of the cruciate ligaments. In Feagin JA, editor: *The crucial ligaments,* New York, 1988, Churchill Livingstone.

11. Assimakopoulos A, Katonis PG, Agapitos MV et al: The innervation of the human meniscus, *Clin Orthop* 275:232, 1992.

12. Bach BR, Warren RF: Radiographic indicators of anterior cruciate ligament injury. In Feagin JA, editor: *The crucial ligaments,* New York, 1988, Churchill Livingstone.

13. Baum JA, Fu F, Rosenberg TD, Harner C: Arthroscopic meniscal repair, *Orthop Consultation* 8(2):1, 1987.

14. Bentley G, Dowd G: Current concepts of etiology and treatment of chondromalacia patellae, *Clin Orthop* 189:209, 1984.

15. Boerce NR, Watkinson AF, Ackroyd CE et al: MRI of meniscal and cruciate injuries of the knee, *J Bone Joint Surg* 73B:452, 1991.

16. Boland ML, Hulstya MJ: Soft tissue injuries of the knee. In Nicholas JA, Hershman E, editors: *The lower extremity and spine in sports medicine,* ed 2, St Louis, 1995, Mosby.

17. Booher JM, Thibodeau GA: *Athletic injury assessment,* ed 3, St Louis, 1994, Mosby.

18. Boynton MD, Tietjens BR: Long-term follow-up of the untreated isolated posterior cruciate ligament–deficient knee, *Am J Sports Med* 24:306, 1996.

19. Borsa PA: *Current concepts in PCL rehabilitation,* Proceedings from the 49th Annual Meeting and Clinical Symposium, Baltimore, 1998, NATA.

20. Brier SR: Patella malalignment syndrome, *J Chiropractic* 27(2):73, 1990.

21. Cailliet R: *Knee pain and disability,* ed 2, Philadelphia, 1989, FA Davis.

22. Calvo RD et al: Managing plica syndrome of the knee, *The Physician and Sportsmedicine* 18(7):64, 1990.

23. Carrick JG, Webb DR: *Sports injuries: diagnosis and management,* Philadelphia, 1990, WB Saunders.

24. Carson WC Jr: The role of lateral extra-articular procedures, *Clin Sports Med* 7(4):754, 1988.

25. Cohn SL, Sotta RP, Bergfield JH: Fractures about the knee in sports, *Clin Sports Med* 9(1):136, 1990.

26. Cross MJ, Waldrup J: The patella index as a guide to the understanding and diagnosis of patellofemoral instability, *Clin Orthop* 110:174, 1975.

27. Crues JV III: MR imaging of the bone injuries of the knee, *Radiol* 176:296, 1990.

28. Crues JV III, Mink JH, Levy TL et al: Meniscal tears of the knee: accuracy of MR imaging, *Radiol* 164:445, 1987.

29. Daniels DM, Stone ML: KT-1000 anterior-posterior displacement measurements. In Daniels DM, Akeson WH, O'Connor JJ, editors: *Knee ligaments: structure, function, injury, and repair,* New York, 1990, Raven Press.

30. DeHaven KE: Decision-making factors in the treatment of meniscal lesions, *Clin Orthop* 252:49, 1990.

31. DeLee JC, Riles MB, Rockwood CA: Acute straight lateral instability of the knee, *Am J Sports Med* 11:404, 1983.

32. Deltoff MN, Kogon PL: *The portable skeletal x-ray library,* St Louis, 1998, Mosby.

33. Donaldson WF, Warren RF, Wickiewicz T: A comparison of acute anterior cruciate ligament examinations, *Am J Sports Med* 10:100, 1992.

34. Doucette SA, Goble EM: The effect of exercise on patellar tracking in lateral patellar compression syndrome, *Am J Sports Med* 20(4):434, 1992.

35. Dugdale TW, Barnett PR: Historical background: patellofemoral pain in young people, *Orthop Clin North Am* 17:211, 1986.

36. Ellison AE, editor: *Athletic training and sports medicine,* ed 2, Chicago, 1989, American Academy of Orthopaedic Surgeons.

37. Emerson RJ: Basketball knee injuries and the anterior cruciate ligament, *Clin Sports Med* 12(2):320, 1993.

38. Fairbank JCT, Pynset PB, Van Poortvliet JA et al: Mechanical factors in the incidence of knee pain in adolescents and young adults, *J Bone Joint Surg* 66B:685, 1984.

39. Feagin JA, editor: *The crucial ligaments,* New York, 1988, Churchill Livingstone.

40. Feagin JA Jr: Principles of diagnosis and treatment. In Feagin JA, editor: *The crucial ligaments,* New York, 1988, Churchill Livingstone.

41. Fry RW, Morton AR, Keast D: Periodization and the prevention of overtraining, *Can J Sports Sci* 17(3):241, 1992.

42. Fu FH: *Current concepts in anterior cruciate ligament reconstruction,* Proceedings from the 49th Annual Meeting and Clinical Symposium, Baltimore, 1998, NATA.

43. Fu FH: Severe injury in a gymnast, *Orthop Consultation* 9(6):10, 1988.

44. Funk DA: Anterior cruciate instability, *Orthop Consultation* 9(9):3, 1988.

45. Gallimore GW, Harms SE: Knee injuries: high resolution MR imaging, *Radiol* 160:457, 1986.

46. Gersoff WK, Clancy WG Jr: Diagnosis of anterior cruciate ligament tears, *Clin Sports Med* 7(4):727, 1988.

47. Giattini JG, Dowd AJ: Anterolateral rotary instability in the knee, *Orthop Consultation* 8(6):8, 1987.

48. Grana WA, Kriegshauser LA: Scientific basis of extensor mechanism disorders, *Clin Sports Med* 4(2):247, 1985.

49. Grood ES, Noyes FR: Diagnosis of knee ligament injuries: biomechanical precepts. In Feagin JA, editor: *The crucial ligaments,* New York, 1988, Churchill Livingstone.

50. Heller L, Langman T: The menisco-femoral ligaments of the human knee, *J Bone Joint Surg* 46B:307, 1964.

51. Henning CE, Lynch MA: Current concepts of meniscal function and pathology, *Clin Sports Med* 4(2):259, 1985.

52. Henry JH: The patellofemoral joint. In Nicholas JA, Hershman ED, editors: *The lower extremity and spine in sports medicine,* ed 2, St Louis, 1995, Mosby.

53. Henry JH: Patellofemoral problems: conservative treatment of patellofemoral subluxation, *Clin Sports Med* 8(2):261, 1989.

54. Höher J, Haghighi P, Trudell D et al: The cruciate ligaments of the knee: correlation between MR appearance and gross and histologic findings in cadaveric specimens, *Am J Roentgenol* 159:357, 1992.

55. Höher J, Harner CD, Vogrin TM, Carlin GJ et al: In situ forces in the posterolateral structures under posterior tibial loading in the intact and PCL-deficient knee, *J Orthop Res* 2, 1998.

56. Horibe S, Shino K, Nakata K et al: Results of isolated meniscal repair evaluated by second-look arthroscopy, *Arthroscopy* 12(2):150, 1996.

57. Hughston JC: Patellar subluxation: a recent history, *Clin Sports Med* 8(2):158, 1989.

58. Hughston JC: Patellofemoral problems: patellar subluxations, *Clin Sports Med* 8(2):153, 1989.

59. Hughston JC, Walsh WM, Puddu G: *Patellar subluxation and dislocation,* Philadelphia, 1984, WB Saunders.

60. Huson A: Biomechanische probleme des kniegelenkes, *Orthop* 3:119, 1974.

61. Hutchinson MR, Ireland ML: Knee injuries in female athletes, *Sports Med* 19(4):288, 1995.

62. Insall J, Falvo KA, Wise DW: Chondromalacia patellae, *J Bone Joint Surg* 58A:1, 1976.

63. Ireland ML: *Injury epidemiology in female athletes,* Proceedings from the 49th Annual Meeting and Clinical Symposium, Baltimore, 1998, NATA.

64. Irrgang JJ: Modern trends in anterior cruciate ligament rehabilitation: nonoperative and postoperative management, *Clin Sports Med* 12(4):797, 1993.

65. Ishibashi Y, Rudy TW, Livesay GA, Stone JD, Fu FH, Woo SLY: A robotic evaluation of the effect of anterior cruciate ligament graft fixation site at the tibia on knee stability, *J Arthroscopy and Related Surg* 13:177, 1997.

66. Jackson JP: Degenerative changes in the knee after meniscectomy, *Br Med J* 2:525, 1968.

67. Jacobson KE, Flandry FC: Diagnosis of anterior knee pain, *Clin Sports Med* 8(2):180, 1989.

68. Jensen JE, Conn RR, Hazelrigg G, Hewett JE: Evaluation of acute injuries of the knee, *Clin Sports Med* 4(2):304, 1985.

69. Johnson DL, Warner JJ: Diagnosis for anterior cruciate ligament surgery, *Clin Sports Med* 12(4):671, 1993.

70. Johnson RJ, Beynnon BD, Nichols CE et al: Current concepts review: the treatment of injuries of the anterior cruciate ligament, *J Bone Joint Surg* 74A:140, 1992.

71. Johnson RJ, Eriksson E, Haggmark T et al: Five to ten year follow up evaluation after reconstruction of the anterior cruciate ligament, *Clin Orthop* 183:122, 1984.

72. Kaminski TW, Wabbersen CV, Murphy RM: Concentric versus enhanced eccentric hamstring strength training, *J Athletic Training* 33(3):216, 1998.

73. Kannus P, Johnson RJ: Downhill skiing injuries: trends to watch for this season, *J Musculoskel Med* 8:13, 1991.

74. Kapandji IA: *The physiology of joints,* vol 2, New York, 1970, Churchill Livingstone.

75. Kaye JJ, Nance EP Jr: Pain in the athlete's knee: radiological diagnosis of pain in the athlete, *Clin Sports Med* 6(4):873, 1987.

76. Keller PM, Shelborne KD, McCarroll JR et al: Nonoperatively treated isolated posterior cruciate ligament injuries, *Am J Sports Med* 21:132, 1993.

77. Kettlekamp DB: Current concepts review: patella malalignment, *J Bone Joint Surg* 63A:1344, 1981.

78. Kijala UM, Kvist M, Österman K: Knee injuries in athletes, *Sports Med* 3:447, 1986.

79. King JB, Aitker M: Treatment of the torn anterior cruciate ligament, *Sports Med* 5:203, 1988.

80. Kohn D: Arthroscopic evaluation of anterior cruciate ligament reconstruction using a free patellar tendon autograft: a prospective, randomized study, *Clin Orthop* 254:220, 1990.

81. Kriegsman J, Berg D, Smith M: Conservative treatment of the torn anterior cruciate ligament, *Contemp Orthop* 16(5):35, 1988.

82. Kurosawa M, Yoshiya S, Andrish JT: A biomechanical comparison of different surgical techniques of graft fixation in anterior cruciate ligament reconstruction, *Am J Sports Med* 15:225, 1987.

83. Kursinoglu-Brahme S, Resnick D: Magnetic resonance imaging of the knee, *Orthop Clin North Am* 21(3):561, 1990.

84. Levy IM, Torzilli PA, Gould JD et al: The effect of lateral meniscectomy on motion of the knee, *J Bone Joint Surg* 71A:401, 1989.

85. Levy IM, Torzilli PA, Warren RF: The effect of medial meniscectomy on anterior-posterior motion of the knee, *J Bone Joint Surg* 64A:883, 1982.

86. Maenpaa H, Lehto MU: Patellar dislocations: the long-term results of nonoperative management in 100 patients, *Am J Sports Med* 25(2):213, 1997.

87. MaGee J: *Orthopedic physical assessment,* Philadelphia, 1987, WB Saunders.

88. Markin HJ: The reaction of articular cartilage to injury and osteoarthritis, *N Engl J Med* 291:1285-1292, 1974.

89. Marone PJ: Causes and treatment of anterior knee pain. In Zawadsky JP, editor: *Post-graduate advances in sports medicine,* (Course II), Berryville, Vir, 1988, Forum Medicum.

90. Martin P: Bone scanning of trauma and benign conditions. In Freeman LM, Weissmann HS, editors: *Nuclear medicine annual,* New York, 1982, Raven Press.

91. Menschik A: Mechanik des kniegelerkes, Te:11.2, *Orthop* 112:481, 1978.

92. Micheli LT, O'Neill DB: Overuse injuries in the young athlete, *Clin Sports Med* 7(3):604, 1988.

93. Minkoff J: Chronic anterior instability, *Orthop Consultation* 8(9):3, 1987.

94. Müller W: Kinematics of the crucial ligaments. In Feagin JA, editor: *The crucial ligaments,* New York, 1988, Churchill Livingstone.

95. Müller W: *The knee: form, function and ligament reconstruction,* New York, 1983, Springer-Verlag.

96. Nicholas JA, Hershman EB: *The lower extremity and spine in sports medicine,* ed 2, St Louis, 1995, Mosby.

97. Nike, Inc: Common running injuries, *Sport Research Review,* 1989.

98. Nisonson B: Acute hemarthrosis of the adolescent knee, *The Physician and Sportsmedicine* 17(4):83, 1989.

99. Noyes FR, Grood ES: Diagnosis of knee ligament injuries: clinical concepts. In Feagin JA, editor: *The crucial ligaments,* New York, 1988, Churchill Livingstone.

100. Oderstein M, Sysholm J, Gillquist J: Long-term follow-up study of a distal iliotibial band transfer, *Clin Orthop* 176:129, 1983.

101. Outerbridge RE: The etiology of chondromalacia patellae, *J Bone Joint Surg* 43B:752, 1961.

102. Outerbridge RE, Dunlop J: The problem of chondromalacia patellae, *Clin Orthop* 110:177, 1975.

103. Patel D: Plica as a cause of anterior knee pain, *Orthop Clin North Am* 17(2):273, 1986.

104. Pattee G, Fox J, Del Pizzo W et al: Four to ten year follow-up of unreconstructed anterior cruciate ligament tears, *Am J Sports Med* 17:430, 1989.

105. Paulos LE, Cherf J, Rosenberg TD et al: Anterior cruciate ligament reconstruction with autografts, *Clin Sports Med* 10:469, 1991.

106. Paulos LE, Rosenberg TD, Grewe SR et al: The Gore-Text anterior cruciate ligament prosthesis: a long-term followup, *Am J Sports Med* 20:246, 1992.

107. Pizzutillo PD: Osteochondroses. In Sullivan JA, Grana WA, editors: *The pediatric athlete,* Park Ridge, Ill, 1990, American Academy of Orthopaedic Surgeons.

108. Rang M: *Children's fractures,* ed 2, Philadelphia, 1983, JB Lippincott.

109. Ray JM: Proposed natural history of anterior cruciate ligament injuries, *Clin Sports Med* 7(4):700, 1988.

110. Reikeras O, Hoiseth A: Patellofemoral relationships in normal subjects determined by computed tomography, *Skeletal Radiol* 19:591, 1990.

111. Remer EM, Fitzgerald SW, Friedman H et al: Anterior cruciate ligament injury: MR imaging diagnosis and patterns of injury, *Radiographics* 12:901, 1992.

112. Schmidt DR, Henry JH: Stress injuries of the adolescent extensor mechanism, *Clin Sports Med* 8(2):343, 1989.

113. Schousboe JT, Chang RW: Diagnosis and management of non-traumatic knee pain, *Occupational Problems in Medical Practice* 2(2):1, 1989.

114. Schutzer SF, Ramsby GR, Fulkerson JP: CT classification of patellofemoral pain patients, *Orthop Clin North Am* 17:235, 1986.

115. Seedholm BB, Hargreaves DJ: Transmission of the load in the knee joint with special reference to the role of the menisci: II. *Eng Med* 8:220, 1979.

116. Shelbourne KD: *Rehabilitation after meniscal repair: current concepts,* Proceedings from the 49th Annual Meeting and Clinical Symposium, Baltimore, 1998, NATA.

117. Shellock FC: MR imaging of the metallic implants and materials: a compilation of the literature, *Am J Roentgenology* 151:811, 1988.

118. Sherman M, Warren RF, Marshall J, Savatsky GJ: A clinical and radiographic analysis of 127 anterior cruciate insufficient knees, *Clin Orthop* 227:229, 1988.

119. Shino K, Horibe S, Nakata K et al: Conservative treatment of isolated injuries to the PCL in athletes, *J Bone Joint Surg* 77B:895, 1995.

120. Smith BA, Livesay GA, Woo SLY: Biology and biomechanics of the anterior cruciate ligament, *Clin Sports Med* 12(4):637, 1993.

121. Smith JB: Knee problems in children, *Pediatr Clin North Am* 33(6):1454, 1986.

122. Steiner ME, Grace WA: The young athletic knee: recent advances, *Clin Sports Med* 7(3):527, 1988.

123. Stoller DW, Martin C, Crues JV III et al: Meniscal tears: pathologic correlation with MR imaging, *Radiol* 163:731, 1987.

124. Stougard J: Chondromalacia of the patella, *Acta Orthop Scand* 46:309, 1975.

125. Strasser H: *Lehre der Muskel-und Gelerkmechanik,* Berlin, 1917, Springer.

126. Swerson ET, Hough DO, McKeany DB: Patellofemoral dysfunction, *Postgrad Med* 82(6):125, 1987.

127. Terry GC: The anatomy of the extensor mechanism: patellofemoral problems, *Clin Sports Med* 8(2):167, 1989.

128. Tyson AD: Patellofemoral pain (part II), *Strength and Conditioning* 20(5):54, 1998.

129. Vahey TN, Broome DR, Kayes KJ et al: Acute and chronic tears of the anterior cruciate ligament: differential features of MR imaging, *Radiol* 181:251, 1991.

130. Vail TP, Malone TR, Besset FH: Long-term functional results in patients with anterolateral rotatory instability treated by iliotibial band transfer, *Am J Sports Med* 20:274, 1992.

131. Walker PS, Erkmann MT: The role of the meniscus in force transmission across the knee, *Clin Orthop* 109:184, 1975.

132. Webright WG, Perrin DH, Gansneder BM: Effect of trunk position on anterior tibial displacement measured by the KT-1000 in uninjured subjects, *J Athletic Training* 33(3):233, 1998.

133. Weiss C, Lindberg M, Hamberg P et al: Non-operative treatment of meniscal tears, *J Bone Joint Surg* 71A:811, 1989.

134. Wiberg G: Roentgenographic and anatomic studies on the femoropatellar joint, *Acta Orthop Scand* 12:319, 1941.

135. Wilk KE, Escamilla RF, Flesig GS: A comparison of the tibiofemoral joint forces and EMG activity during open and closed kinetic chain exercises, *Am J Sports Med* 24(4):518, 1996.

136. Wilk KE, Zheng N, Flesig GS et al: Kinetic chain exercises: implications for the anterior cruciate ligament patient, *J Sports Rehabil* 6(2):125, 1997.

137. Zarins B, Fish DN: Knee ligament injury. In Nicholas JA, Hershman EB, editors: *The lower extremity and spine in sports medicine,* ed 2, St Louis, 1995, Mosby.

Lower Leg, Ankle, and Foot

PART ONE: LOWER LEG

During ambulation, the lower leg serves as a conduit that transfers load from the trunk and hips to the foot. The act of weight bearing may have clinical implications during repetitive motions in persons with malalignment and deformity of the lower extremity.

Applied Anatomy and Biomechanics of the Lower Leg

There are three distinct anatomic compartments in the lower leg: posterior, anterior, and lateral. A fascial plane and an intermuscular septum separate each compartment. The posterior compartment is composed of the plantar flexors of the foot, namely the soleus and gastrocnemius, which control subtalar inversion and flexion of the toes. The structures of the posterior compartment are innervated by the posterior tibial nerve. This region has the most mass in the lower leg (Figure 11-1, A, B).

The anterior compartment contains the tibia, which lies in an almost subcutaneous position and thus is vulnerable to external forces. The major weight-bearing forces of the lower leg travel through the tibia (Figure 11-2). Therefore fractures of this bone are serious and require a lengthy period of care. The tibia is a common site for musculoskeletal overload, and typical overuse injuries include tibial stress fractures, tibial periostitis, and muscular strains.

Described as a long and slender bone, the fibula is not a major weight-bearing structure. The proximal aspect of the fibula is involved in an arthrodial joint below the knee, and the distal fibula is the site of a syndesmosis. Strong ligaments and an interosseous membrane hold the fibula in position. The primary function of the fibula is to complete the mortise joint at the ankle and to serve as an attachment base for muscles of the lower leg.[62]

In addition, the anterior compartment contains the structures that provide for ankle dorsiflexion and extension of the foot and toes: the tibialis anterior, extensor hallucis longus, and extensor digitorum longus muscles, as well as the deep peroneal nerve and tibial artery (Figure 11-3, page 365). A tight fascial covering envelops the muscles of the anterior compartment. Because of the anatomic tightness, there is little room for expansion if fluid or blood accumulates in this compartment. Blows to the anterior shin or chronic exertional overload may produce a hematoma or enough fluid in the compartment to evoke a neurovascular insufficiency.[63]

The lateral compartment of the lower leg is made up of the muscle group that everts the foot and aids in plantar flexion: peroneus longus and brevis. The superficial branch of the peroneal nerve is found in the lateral compartment as well..

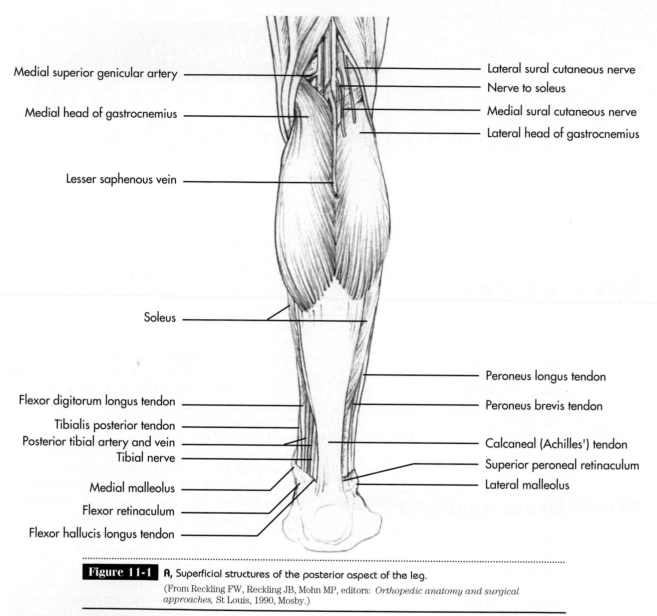

Medial superior genicular artery

Medial head of gastrocnemius

Lesser saphenous vein

Soleus

Flexor digitorum longus tendon

Tibialis posterior tendon

Posterior tibial artery and vein

Tibial nerve

Medial malleolus

Flexor retinaculum

Flexor hallucis longus tendon

Lateral sural cutaneous nerve

Nerve to soleus

Medial sural cutaneous nerve

Lateral head of gastrocnemius

Peroneus longus tendon

Peroneus brevis tendon

Calcaneal (Achilles') tendon

Superior peroneal retinaculum

Lateral malleolus

Figure 11-1 **A,** Superficial structures of the posterior aspect of the leg.

(From Reckling FW, Reckling JB, Mohn MP, editors: *Orthopedic anatomy and surgical approaches*, St Louis, 1990, Mosby.)

Continued

The distal lateral portion of the lower leg is the site of many musculoskeletal injuries. Some individuals with recurrent lateral ankle sprains or hypermobility may also develop recurrent subluxation of the peroneal tendons. This area is also the site for herniation through the fascial sheath of the lateral compartment over the same peroneal muscles. Usually benign, this condition may appear as a cosmetic deformity.

The midportion to dorsal portion of the medial leg is the region for tendonitis and tibial abnormalities. Periostitis, posterior tibial tendonitis, and stress fractures are all commonly seen here, especially in active and athletic populations.

Pathomechanics of the Lower Leg

Aberrant mechanics can adversely affect the lower leg from either above or below. For example, patellofemoral dysfunction may cause pain below the knee at the lower leg. Patellar malalignment syndrome with tibial varus can cause local knee and shin pain. Exaggerated foot pathomechanics can come from shin or knee pain. Sub-

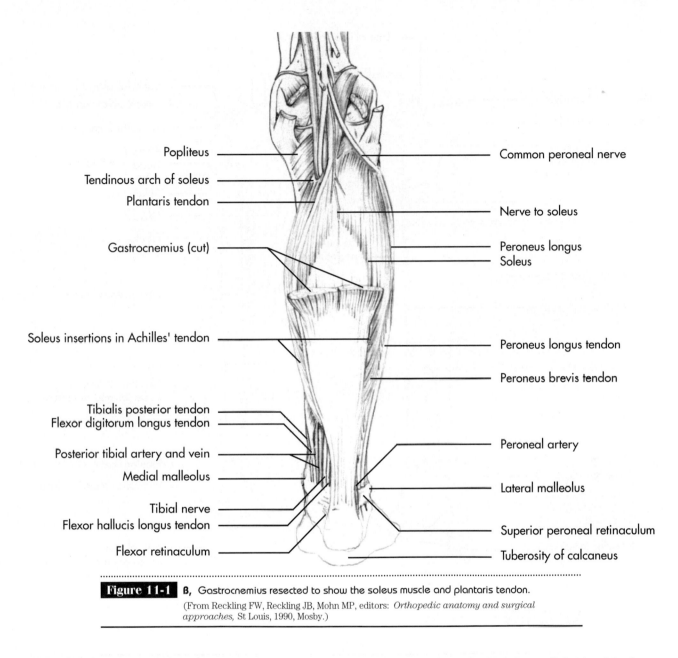

Popliteus

Tendinous arch of soleus

Plantaris tendon

Gastrocnemius (cut)

Soleus insertions in Achilles' tendon

Tibialis posterior tendon
Flexor digitorum longus tendon

Posterior tibial artery and vein

Medial malleolus

Tibial nerve
Flexor hallucis longus tendon

Flexor retinaculum

Common peroneal nerve

Nerve to soleus

Peroneus longus
Soleus

Peroneus longus tendon

Peroneus brevis tendon

Peroneal artery

Lateral malleolus

Superior peroneal retinaculum

Tuberosity of calcaneus

Figure 11-1 B, Gastrocnemius resected to show the soleus muscle and plantaris tendon.
(From Reckling FW, Reckling JB, Mohn MP, editors: *Orthopedic anatomy and surgical approaches*, St Louis, 1990, Mosby.)

talar problems and arch insufficiency can also contribute to lower leg problems.

Conditions that frequently occur in association with patellofemoral pain syndromes (e.g., subtalar pronation, pes planus, tibial rotation) can cause anterior lower leg pain. Individuals with foot supination place enormous amounts of stress on the lateral muscular compartment of the lower leg, causing peroneal strain.

Foot and ankle problems may originate at the knee, but the complaint that generally brings the patient into a primary care office is anterior leg pain. Genu varum (i.e.,

bowleggedness) localizes on the medial side of the knee and lateral leg. In children this deformity can result in Blount's disease, a condition in obese, male African-American adolescents. It is indicative of severe tibial torsion and lower extremity malalignment.

Patients with medial leg pain often have a poorly developed longitudinal arch of the foot. The relationship between pes planus and posterior tibial tendonitis is almost cause and effect. Ligamentous laxity, compensated forefoot varus, limb length discrepancy, and malinsertion of the posterior tibial tendon are all etio-

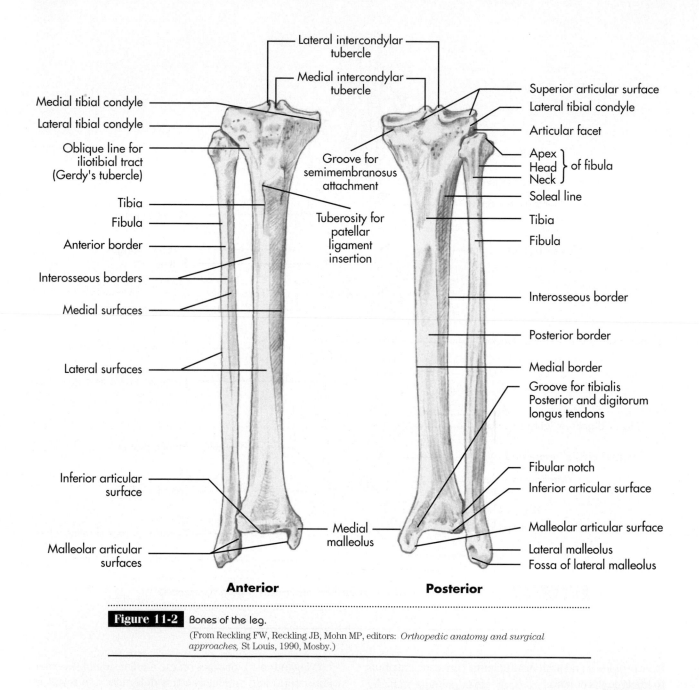

Lateral intercondylar tubercle

Medial intercondylar tubercle

Medial tibial condyle

Lateral tibial condyle

Oblique line for iliotibial tract (Gerdy's tubercle)

Tibia

Fibula

Anterior border

Interosseous borders

Medial surfaces

Lateral surfaces

Inferior articular surface

Malleolar articular surfaces

Groove for semimembranosus attachment

Tuberosity for patellar ligament insertion

Medial malleolus

Anterior

Superior articular surface

Lateral tibial condyle

Articular facet

Apex ⎫
Head ⎬ of fibula
Neck ⎭

Soleal line

Tibia

Fibula

Interosseous border

Posterior border

Medial border

Groove for tibialis Posterior and digitorum longus tendons

Fibular notch

Inferior articular surface

Malleolar articular surface

Lateral malleolus

Fossa of lateral malleolus

Posterior

Figure 11-2   Bones of the leg.

(From Reckling FW, Reckling JB, Mohn MP, editors: *Orthopedic anatomy and surgical approaches,* St Louis, 1990, Mosby.)

logic factors in pes planus.[75] Athletes who participate in several sports and runners who log many miles are at risk for periostitis and, ultimately, tibial stress fractures. These injuries are especially prevalent in the presence of poor alignment or foot abnormalities. The role of aberrant lower extremity mechanics and nonoptimal anatomic variations in lower leg pathologic conditions cannot be overestimated.

History and Examination of the Lower Leg

The first objective of the history and examination is to determine whether the condition is in the lower leg or the result of compensation for a mechanical problem at another site. It is important to ask about pain in the foot, ankle, knee, or lower back—or a previous injury to those

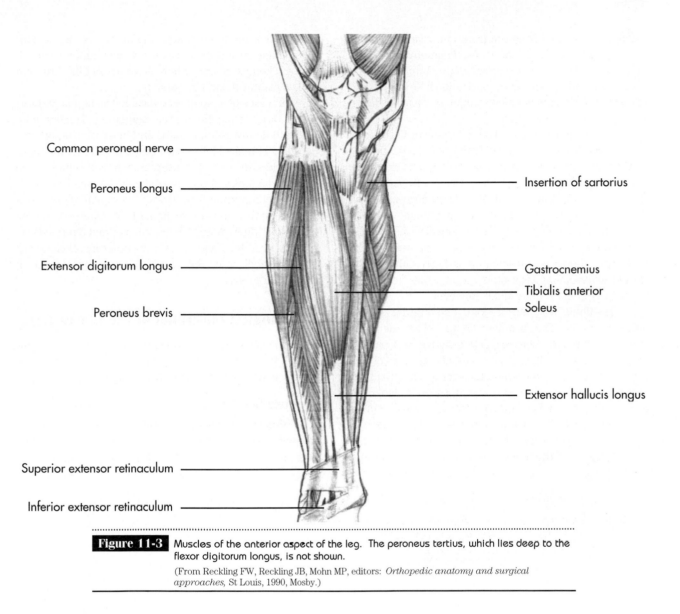

Figure 11-3 Muscles of the anterior aspect of the leg. The peroneus tertius, which lies deep to the flexor digitorum longus, is not shown.

(From Reckling FW, Reckling JB, Mohn MP, editors: *Orthopedic anatomy and surgical approaches,* St Louis, 1990, Mosby.)

areas. If direct trauma is involved, the nature, severity, and exact mechanism of impact must be investigated. If there was no trauma, the injury may be the result of overuse; the practitioner should ask about changes in habits or training (i.e., if athletic-related activities) that may suggest a tentative diagnosis. Hard surfaces, hills, or uneven terrain can all contribute to overuse injuries of the lower leg in runners.

If the history does not indicate trauma or an overuse pattern, the identification of the underlying problem may be difficult. The reason for the pain may be distal to the site; therefore the practitioner should examine the entire lower kinetic chain in a search for a patho-

mechanical reason for the patient's leg pain. Practitioners should ask patients to bring in their usual footwear or running shoes, if applicable, and they should look for exaggerated patterns of wear and tear. Good footwear may play a major role in helping alleviate the patient's pain and keeping it from returning.

An important part of the leg examination is a thorough analysis of gait-and-static stature, including the lumbopelvic region, thigh, hip, knee, lower leg, ankle, and foot. The practitioner should check for arch sufficiency, subtalar motion, tibial torsion, patellar tilt and aberrant tracking, excessive femoral anteversion, and lumbopelvic dysfunction or hypomobility. While watching the patient stand and ambulate from the front and rear, the examiner checks for heel strike and toe-off maneuvers (Figure 11-4), searches for poor excursion of the Achilles' tendon in cases of heel cord tightness and ankle inflexibility, and visually inspects for heel-foot valgus or varus, a fallen arch, and subtalar movement.

The examiner then palpates the lower leg over all three compartments. It is essential to palpate the leg meticulously for muscle tightness, herniations or bulges, swelling, and asymmetry in comparison with the opposite leg. The examiner should place both legs supine on the examination table and compare alignment.

The muscle-bone interface along the shaft of the tibia should receive particular attention. In cases of tibial periostitis, the area of discomfort is fairly diffuse. The area of involvement associated with a stress fracture of the tibia or fibula is quite small, however.

The fibula head, mortise joint, and anterior shin require palpation. The examiner should place the ankle and knee through their respective active and passive ranges of motion. It is also necessary to inspect the patellofemoral joint for lateral tracking, to feel the bulk of the posterior musculature for atrophy or swelling, and to palpate the Achilles' tendon-gastrocnemius junction for tenderness. The Thompson test, which involves squeezing the posterior calf and making certain that full plantar flexion of the foot is possible, indicates whether the Achilles' tendon is intact (Figure 11-5 *A, B*). A ruptured plantaris muscles evokes a weak plantar response to the Thompson test, whereas a torn Achilles' tendon makes plantar flexion impossible.

In cases of suspected exertional ischemia, hemorrhage, or systemic illness, the examining clinician must evaluate neurovascular status and dermatomal patterns carefully (Figure 11-6 *A, B*). Distal pulses, motor capability, and skin and hair texture may provide clues to the correct diagnosis. Foot drop should be ruled out with anterior compartment pathology. Peroneal neurapraxia secondary to contusion or fibula head subluxation may also occur after trauma. Venous stasis and lymphedema may occur in localized cases of vascular insufficiency or cardiorenal disease. Patency of pulses is important in all these conditions.

Pathologic Conditions of the Lower Leg

Specific pathologic conditions of the lower leg are generally the result of overuse syndromes, direct trauma, or anatomic deformities and malalignment.

Overuse Syndromes

Posterior Tibialis Strain and Tendonitis
Runners and basketball players commonly experience posterior tibialis tendonitis. Physical findings include

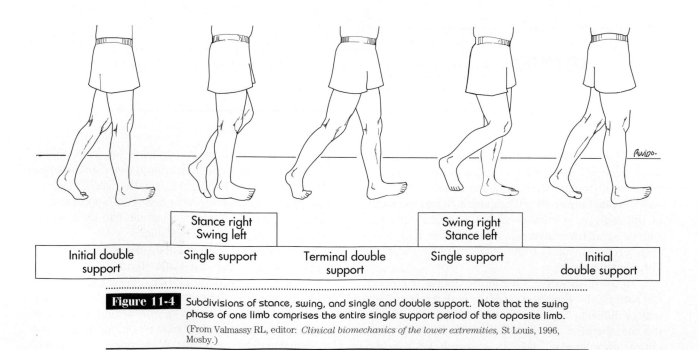

Stance right Swing left		Swing right Stance left	

Initial double support	Single support	Terminal double support	Single support	Initial double support

Figure 11-4 Subdivisions of stance, swing, and single and double support. Note that the swing phase of one limb comprises the entire single support period of the opposite limb.

(From Valmassy RL, editor: *Clinical biomechanics of the lower extremities*, St Louis, 1996, Mosby.)

palpable tenderness along the medial tibia at the muscle-bone interface at the distal one third of the lower leg. Sometimes the pain distribution may follow the posterior tibialis tendon as it wraps around the posterior aspect of the medial malleolus. Arch pain may, in fact, be found concomitantly with anterior leg pain. Bogginess may be palpated along the distal medial leg.

The differential diagnosis includes a tibial stress fracture and tibial periostitis. Pain caused by a posterior tibialis strain is more diffuse than that of a stress fracture. The pattern of diffuse pain along the anterior lower leg associated with posterior tibialis strain is more distal than that associated with tibial periostitis.

Some authors refer to posterior tibialis strain as "medial stress syndrome," because they are not certain whether the pain stems from the tibial attachments of the posterior tibialis or the attachment of the medial one half of the soleus muscle to the posterior medial tibia.[35] For several reasons the soleus theory of anterior leg pain seems unlikely, however. First, a fairly large percentage of patients have pain not only at the most proximal portion of the distal one third of the tibia, but also along the distal course of the tibialis posterior tendon at the rear of the medial malleolus and at the navicular insertion.[75] Second, many of these patients are flatfooted, which ultimately leads to pathomechanical problems, especially in runners. Third, as Subotnick stated, subtalar pronation often leads to lower leg pain.[72]

It seems logical that pes planus, pronation, and various malalignment maladies may indirectly lead to posterior tibialis strain. Because of overuse and errors in athletic training, many individuals develop chronic tendonitis, and some may develop periostitis. Their orthopedic problems may be exacerbated from the foot on up through the lower leg.

Physical findings of foot and lower extremity conditions, combined with normal radiologic findings, are the basis for a diagnosis of posterior tibialis strain (Table 11-1). Treatment revolves around rest, the application of ice, electrotherapy, and a gradual increase in activities on soft surfaces. Individuals with severe foot and ankle deformities (e.g., excessive calcaneal eversion and forefoot abduction) may need orthotics. Patients whose pain is recalcitrant to active treatment or orthotics may take over-the-counter nonsteroidal antiinflammatory drugs (NSAIDs) to reduce the inflammation and discomfort. If the over-the-counter medication does not alleviate the symptoms, the use of a prescription-strength NSAID may be necessary.

Tibial Periostitis

Although tibial periostitis is a common condition among endurance athletes, general practitioners may not see many patients with this condition. Without extreme care to prevent further aggravation of such an injury, however, the patient may develop a stress fracture of the tibia.

Tibial periostitis results from an overload at the lower leg. Pounding and overuse affect the tibia and the muscular attachments at the periosteal interface. As inflammation increases, small microhemorrhages develop and blood accumulates underneath the periosteum, producing pain; even simple walking on hard sur-

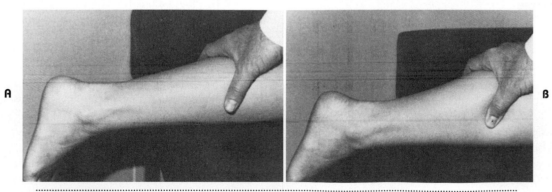

Figure 11-5 Thompson test. **A,** No pressure on gastrocnemius. **B,** Pressure on gastrocnemius and associated plantar flexion. If Achilles' tendon is torn, plantar flexion does not accompany pressure.

(From Nicholas JA, Hershman EB, editors: *The lower extremity and spine in sports medicine,* ed 2, vol 1, St Louis, 1995, Mosby.)

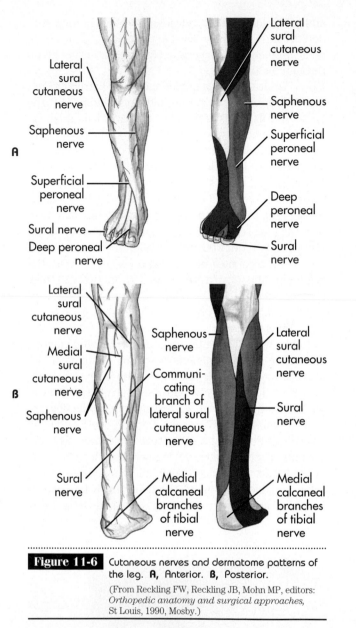

Figure 11-6 Cutaneous nerves and dermatome patterns of the leg. **A,** Anterior. **B,** Posterior.

(From Reckling FW, Reckling JB, Mohn MP, editors: *Orthopedic anatomy and surgical approaches,* St Louis, 1990, Mosby.)

such as grass or a cinder track. In addition, avid runners should get new shoes every few months.

Examination of the patient with tibial periostitis reveals an area of diffuse tenderness along the shaft of the tibia. This tender region is usually below the midshaft level of the tibia. Some patients describe pain distally, along the anterior margin of the lower leg, but most report a feeling of discomfort at the anteromedial aspect of the bone. The pain may be described as deep and burning (i.e., muscle tearing away from the bone), because of the periosteal reaction and resorption associated with repetitive microtrauma.

The first step in providing care is to rule out a stress fracture. The practitioner should also determine whether there is any joint fixation in the lumbopelvic spine, paying careful attention to sacroiliac function and hip flexor tightness.

Rest is the initial treatment. To reduce shock to the lower leg, the patient should wear proper footwear. Sneakers or walking shoes are the best shock absorbers. Ice should be generously applied to the lower leg, and electrotherapy may help reduce pain and inflammation.

Most likely, athletes develop a stress fracture of the lower leg by running excessively on weakened and fatigued anterior leg muscles, particularly since these muscles are weaker than those in the calf. The key to maintaining a pain-free environment and preventing further complications is to strengthen the dorsiflexors of the foot and ankle. Repetitive dorsiflexion in the standing position helps strengthen this muscle group. It is also beneficial to use a leg curl machine in a reverse manner; the patient simply sits facing the rollers and places the foot under the roller while performing dorsiflexion movements.

If the shin pain is not resolved by these interventions, the patient may be fitted with a shoe insert to absorb shock or an orthotic appliance to resolve rear foot pathomechanics or arch problems. Generally, it is preferable to try the shoe insert first, since it is less expensive than an orthosis. Most patients respond to an improvement in footwear and a simple and inexpensive insert in their shoe.

Tibial Stress Fracture

Severe pelvic obliquity, short leg syndrome, sudden changes in athletic routine, or overuse can all exert stress on the lower leg. Repetitive stress causes microfractures of the bone, eventually leading to interruption of the osseous structure. Also known as fatigue or insufficiency fracture, a stress fracture represents the bone's inability to repair itself during times of chronic stress.[20]

faces may prompt symptoms. If an athlete continues to run with tibial periostitis, the next tissue to be affected is the cortex of the tibia itself; thus a stress fracture occurs within the bone.

Any athlete who performs on a hard surface (e.g., roadway, gymnasium floor) can develop periostitis. Cross-country runners and basketball players are prime candidates. In fact, runners often develop periostitis bilaterally. It is helpful if they can run on a softer surface,

Table 11-1 Overuse Syndromes of the Lower Leg

	Posterior Tibialis Strain or Tendonitis	Tibial Periostitis	Tibial Stress Fracture	Chronic Exertional Anterior Compartment Syndrome	Achilles' Tendonitis
Physical examination findings	Palpable tenderness over distal one third of medial tibia Pain down course of posterior tibial tendon Possible discomfort posterior to medial malleolus and navicular insertion Often, pes planus and subtalar pronation	Diffuse tenderness along the antero-medial tibial shaft Possible pain during walking and running Sometimes, feeling of warmth along tibial spine Possible pes planus and excessive pronation Need to rule out lumbopelvic, sacroiliac dysfunction	Pinpoint pain 1-2 cm on shaft of tibia Swelling and undulation at site History of shin pain or periostitis Pain on weight bearing or running Need to rule out pelvic obliquity or short leg	Pain at anterior compartment musculature Classic history of pain on exertion Pain on running that is alleviated by rest Tenderness and possible bogginess from increased muscle volume Neurovascular examination normal; pedal pulses intact	Palpable pain over Achilles' tendon Discomfort on excessive dorsiflexion Swelling and thickening in chronic cases Ankle or heel cord inflexibility
X-ray findings	Usually normal Need to rule out tibial stress fracture	Usually normal Need to rule out tibial stress fracture	Plain films initially normal Possible cortical thickening or callous formation on follow-up radiographic films Bone scan, if plain films are equivocal while signs and symptoms persist	Normal	Usually normal; sometimes calcific deposits
Treatment plan	Application of ice, rest Electrotherapy Orthotics, if moderate-to-severe deformity exists	Application of ice, rest Electrotherapy Dorsiflexion strengthening exercises Inserts or orthotics, if necessary Chiropractic manipulative therapy to lumbopelvic spine, if necessary	Application of ice, total rest, air splint, electrotherapy	Application of ice, rest, electrotherapy	Application of ice, ultrasound Heel pad Stretching of Achilles' tendon and hindfoot Iontophoresis, phonophoresis

In most cases, a period of inflammation precedes a tibial stress fracture. For example, a bout of extended tibial periostitis is the common pathway to a stress fracture. Repetitive microtrauma at the bone-periosteum interface causes small hemorrhages and weakens the cortex. If the trauma continues, localized metabolic changes, including osteoblastic activity, appear on x-ray films or bone scans (Figure 11-7 *A, B*).

Physical findings include tenderness over a 1- to 2-cm area on the tibial shaft, swelling, and undulation. Loading the leg causes pain, and continuing to pursue any athletic activity may subject the patient to injury at removed areas, secondary to altered biomechanics.

If the initial plain x-ray films are normal, but the patient has not responded to a diverse array of therapy, the practitioner should order follow-up radiographic films to exclude the presence of a fracture. Radiographic studies do not usually show signs of a stress fracture until 2 weeks after the onset of problems. Many times, however, the only finding in a follow-up set of plain films is cortical hypertrophy. Diphosphanate scintigraphy is the diagnostic test of choice to confirm the presence of a

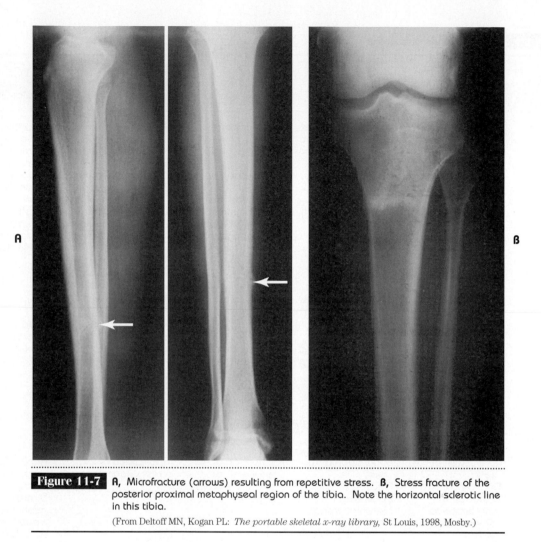

A

B

Figure 11-7 **A,** Microfracture (arrows) resulting from repetitive stress. **B,** Stress fracture of the posterior proximal metaphyseal region of the tibia. Note the horizontal sclerotic line in this tibia.

(From Deltoff MN, Kogan PL: *The portable skeletal x-ray library,* St Louis, 1998, Mosby.)

stress fracture (Figure 11-8 *A, B*). If the bone scan confirms a stress fracture, even the most volatile and active athlete requires total rest. Otherwise, healing may not be complete.

Initially, treatment of tibial stress fractures centers around complete rest and avoidance of athletic activity. The application of ice helps reduce swelling and pain. An air splint can support the lower leg for ambulation, and proper footwear is helpful for shock absorption. Electrotherapy may aid in healing and is helpful in alleviating pain.

Athletes in sprinting and jumping sports must discontinue their sports activities for a minimum of 10 to 12 weeks. They cannot resume their activities until all pain and swelling have disappeared and their dorsiflexor muscles have been strengthened through a rehabilitation exercise program. Riding a bicycle and swimming are two non–weight-bearing activities that can help patients maintain cardiovascular health during the required rest period. If they have undergone 10 to 12 weeks of treatment or if they have been pain-free for 2 weeks, they can begin to jog gently on grass while continuing to strengthen the muscles of the lower leg.[27] When the injury has shown signs of healing, they can progress to jogging on harder surfaces and performing more of the movements that typify their activities.

Chronic Exertional Anterior Compartment Syndrome
Tissue edema and hemorrhage may develop in the anterior, lateral, or posterior compartments of the leg after chronic exertional stress. Without immediate attention to this problem, the possibility of myoneural ischemia is

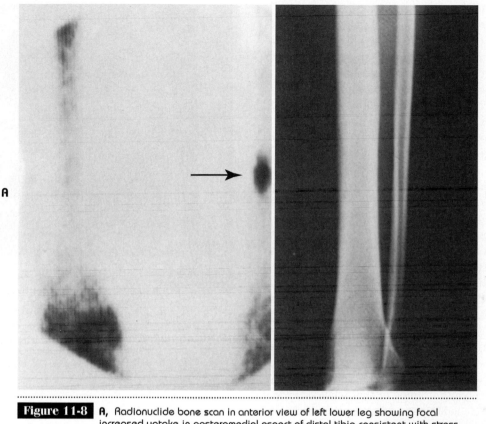

Figure 11-8 **A,** Radionuclide bone scan in anterior view of left lower leg showing focal increased uptake in posteromedial aspect of distal tibia consistent with stress fracture (arrow). **B,** Frontal views obtained at the same time shows no abnormality.

(From Nicholas JA, Hershman EB, editors: *The lower extremity and spine in sports medicine,* ed 2, vol 1, St Louis, 1995, Mosby.)

real, particularly in the anterior compartment. As a result, deformity, tissue death, and permanent impairment may occur in the lower leg.[6]

The typical presentation of chronic exertional anterior compartment syndrome involves the four *P*s of compartment syndromes: (1) pain, (2) painful passive stretch, (3) pallor, and (4) pulselessness. Occurring primarily in runners, this condition is the result of excessive exercise that increases muscle volume and thus intracompartmental pressure and cramplike pain. Individuals with signs of exertional anterior compartment syndrome may be running an enormous number of miles during a typical training week. They describe their pain as dull and achy, often adding that it develops within the first 10 to 20 minutes of running. It continues during rest with a feeling of "fullness" at the anterior leg,[9] but eases after 5 to 10 minutes of rest. Although the nature of the pain resembles that associated with vascular claudication, examination and history aid in the ultimate diagnosis.

The practitioner reviews the terrain, footwear, and possible training errors with the runner. Rest is the most important feature of the treatment plan. The athlete not only must allow enough recuperation time to heal, but he or she must gradually ease back into training once symptoms abate. Cross-training with non–weight-bearing modes of exercise is helpful in active treatment with ambulatory populations. The treatment of chronic exertional anterior compartment syndrome differs from that of acute traumatic anterior compartment syndrome in that decompression is not usually a component of treatment for chronic exertional anterior compartment syndrome.

Achilles' Tendonitis

The largest tendon in the body, the Achilles' tendon plays a major role in the attachment of the calf musculature to the os calcis and a stabilizing role in ankle and foot function. Therefore a chronic and disabling injury of the Achilles' tendon can be devastating, especially to those who lead active lives. Achilles' tendonitis is common among athletes, especially endurance runners. Individuals who lack heel-cord flexibility or who have ankle problems are susceptible to this condition as well.

In these patients, overuse leads to tenosynovitis and swelling. Pain may be diffuse, extending over the entire tendon into the gastrocnemius muscle, or localized over 1 to 2 cm of the tendon sheath. If the tenosynovitis becomes chronic, attenuation and weakening of the tendon sheath make the Achilles' tendon vulnerable to rupture. Scarring may occur with thickening of the tendon. Some patients develop Haglund's disease, a particularly disabling condition that involves chronic tendonitis and calcific calcaneal bursitis; the resulting deformity is palpable and may require surgical debridement.

Rest and the use of a soft, thin heel pad help relieve the pressure over the Achilles' tendon in most patients. Because high-heeled shoes tend to promote hindfoot inflexibility through a shortening of the Achilles' tendon, patients with this condition should wear flat-heeled, comfortable footwear. The application of ice, ultrasound, and gentle stretching exercises should be the primary components of treatment. Patients whose condition does not respond to initial therapy may need oral antiinflammatory medication or local iontophoresis or phonophoresis to reduce pain and swelling.

Complete rehabilitation and injury prevention must include active exercises, such as heel-calf raises on a stair or platform, to promote gastrocnemius–Achilles' tendon strengthening (Figure 11-9 *A, B*) and stretching with proprioception.

Trauma

Acute Traumatic Anterior Compartment Syndrome

Although venous disease secondary to diabetes, cellulitis, and arterial occlusion all simulate findings of anterior compartment syndrome, trauma is the most common cause of this condition. A severe blow to the tibia with a hard object, as frequently occurs in football, lacrosse, baseball, softball, and field hockey, is typically the precipitating event for compartmental bleeding. As the pressure increases, localized pain at the anterior lower leg develops; distal numbness or a loss of feeling in the

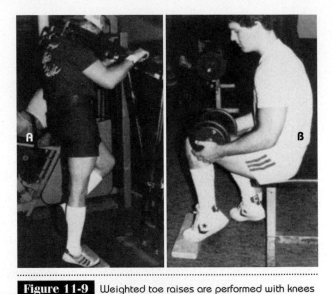

Figure 11-9 Weighted toe raises are performed with knees straight (gastrocnemius activated) and flexed (soleus activated). Eccentric exercise can be done lifting weight with (**A**) both legs and lowering it with only the injured limb, or (**B**) using hands to help lift weight before lowering it with only the injured limb.

(From Nicholas JA, Hershman EB, editors: *The lower extremity and spine in sports medicine,* ed 2, vol 1, St Louis, 1995, Mosby.)

foot may accompany this pain (Figure 11-10). The toes may turn blue or purple, and a foot drop may develop. If the patient cannot ambulate or heel-walk, the situation is serious and warrants a surgical referral. Intrafascial catheterization may become necessary to check compartmental pressure, and a fasciotomy may ultimately be necessary (Table 11-2).[6]

An early sign of anterior compartment syndrome is the presence of exquisite pain on passive stretch. A patient with this symptom requires close observation. Severe muscular necrosis occurs after approximately 8 hours of tissue pressurization at 30 mm Hg, and nerve conduction losses may follow. Thus careful examination for any pathologic signs or symptoms is essential after direct trauma to the lower leg. In general, pallor and pulselessness are not present at the initial examination; their subsequent appearance may signify that permanent myoneural damage has already occurred.

Fibula Head Subluxation

Although not commonplace in a general practice, a subluxed fibular head sometimes appears in a practice that focuses on sports such as wrestling. Occasionally, an individual who is doing a mechanical task in the squatting position or with a bent knee on the floor makes a twisting motion that causes such an injury. The synovial joint stretches at the proximal fibula, and there is an audible "pop" as the head of the fibula subluxes.

At first the individual believes that the injury is at the knee joint. A close physical examination and inspection of the affected leg reveals that the site of trauma is inferior and lateral to the actual knee joint, however. The distinguishing symptom of the fibular head subluxation is paresthesia or referred pain down the lateral leg or calf. This is secondary to contusion or swelling around the common peroneal nerve as it envelops the fibular head.

The mechanism of injury indicates a peripheral nerve injury rather than a spinal nerve injury. A positive Tinel's sign shows peroneal nerve inflammation. There may be some swelling over the proximal fibula. Sitting with the affected leg crossed or squatting down evokes discomfort, but the results of all stability and effusion tests at the knee are normal. A popping sensation or a local click may be present on passive flexion and extension. This may, in fact, release the fibular head.

The presence of clinical findings of neurologic insult to the common peroneal nerve determines the treatment of this injury. Persistent paresthesia or lower leg weakness and foot drop are indications for electrophysiologic testing. Manipulation of the fibular head may be helpful if joint incongruency or fixation is present. The application of ice and avoidance of knee hyperflexion should alleviate pain and swelling. If myofascitis develops secondary to the injury, soft-tissue work (e.g., acupressure, massage) provides palliative care.

Subluxation of the Peroneal Tendons

The retinaculum of the distal leg holds the tendons of the peronei in a track behind the lateral malleolus (Figure 11-11). This track is a groove that allows the tendons to slide gently up and down. Instead of following a course behind the malleolus, subluxed tendons lie over the lateral malleolus (Figure 11-12).

Subluxation of the peroneal tendons can be either acute or chronic. Most cases of acute subluxation are the result of sudden or violent dorsiflexion of the foot.[49] Chronic subluxation may result from repeated ankle sprains and lateral instability that lead to tears in the lateral retinaculum of the leg over time. Either type of injury should be referred to an orthopedic surgeon for evaluation.

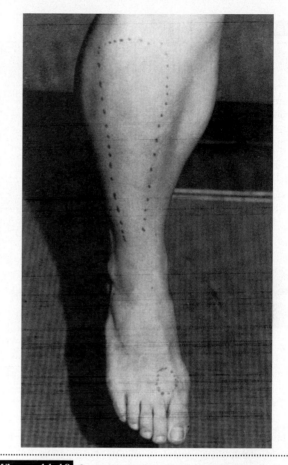

Figure 11-10 Acute traumatic anterior compartment syndrome with swelling and tenderness in anterior compartment and decreased sensation in first web space of foot as outlined.

(From Nicholas JA, Hershman EB, editors: *The lower extremity and spine in sports medicine*, ed 2, vol 1, St Louis, 1995, Mosby.)

Among the symptoms of peroneal tendon subluxation are swelling, ecchymosis, pain over the affected tendons, subluxation with eversion, and crepitus. The clinician should rule out a lateral ankle sprain.[36] Observation of the peroneal tendons during active eversion of the foot is often helpful.

Treatment for acute conditions may be conservative (i.e., immobilization), or it may involve surgery. Chronic subluxation, if disabling, warrants surgical reconstruction of the retinaculum. If the subluxation occurs concomitant with lateral ankle instability, the surgeon may split the peroneus tertius tendon and wrap it around the calcaneus, thus reconstructing the fibular ligaments.

Table 11-2 Traumatic Injuries to Lower Leg

	Acute Traumatic Anterior Compartment Syndrome	Fibula Head Subluxation	Peroneal Tendon Subluxation
Physical examination findings	Pain in anterior compartment of lower leg Possible swelling and inflammation at front of shin Painful passive stretch Need to rule out foot drop, pulselessness, and skin pallor	Painful proximal fibula "Click" or "pop" at fibula head Paresthesia or pain into distal lateral leg Swelling over lateral knee inferior to joint line Possible peroneal neurapraxia Presence of Tinel's sign	Lateral lower leg pain over proximal tendons Crepitus or deformity at distal leg over retinaculum Subluxed tendon over lateral malleolus
X-ray findings	Normal	No evidence of abnormalities Possible fibula in lateral or posterior position on standard anteroposterior film	Normal
Treatment plan	Application of ice, avoidance of compression, activity modification, electrotherapy Possibly, surgical referral, catheterization, emergency fasciotomy	Chiropractic manipulative therapy Application of ice, modified activity, soft-tissue work Need to rule out peroneal neurapraxia, foot drop	Reduction Orthopedic surgical referral

Continued

Rupture of the Achilles' Tendon

A sudden, explosive plantar flexion force, such as a quick sprint or jumping motion, is usually responsible for the rupture of the Achilles' tendon. Men between the ages of 35 and 55 years account for most cases[36]; out-of-shape, weekend athletes are the most vulnerable because of their generally poor year-round conditioning and their lack of heel-cord flexibility.

The person with a ruptured Achilles' tendon cannot walk normally; bearing weight is very painful. The calf is swollen from hemorrhage, and the musculotendinous junction is deformed. As a result of the loss in tendon continuity, squeezing the muscular bulk of the posterior lower leg does not produce the typical plantar response of the foot (i.e., positive Thompson test).

In the past, clinicians who have suspected that a patient has torn or ruptured the Achilles' tendon have used computed tomography and ultrasonography as diagnostic tools. Magnetic resonance imaging (MRI) has enhanced the imaging capability of Achilles' ruptures (Figure 11-13).[41] It has been particularly beneficial in the diagnosis of partial ruptures, which have been quite difficult to diagnose previously.[76]

Although many patients with an Achilles' tendon rupture undergo immediate surgery, it is often prefer-able to adopt a conservative, nonoperative approach. The use of a short leg cast *with the foot in equinus* allows healing to take place without the risks of anesthesia and infection associated with surgical repair. Even with alternative techniques, such as percutaneous approaches, infection at the surgical repair site of an Achilles' tendon is common. The relative thinness of the surface reduces the strength of the epidermis and can interfere with the healing process, producing a high skin slough rate with oozing and wound complications. Surgical procedures also have a longer immobilization period—approximately 11 weeks for patients undergoing surgery versus 8 weeks for those receiving conservative treatment.

On the other hand, some authorities advocate surgical repair to restore normal tendon length, which may result in better dynamic function than can be obtained nonoperatively.[58] Furthermore, evidence of rerupture is also generally lower in surgical patients. *Thus highly competitive athletes who participate in ballistic athletic events may be candidates for a surgical consult.*

Gentle gains of heel-cord flexibility and push-off strength are goals for follow-up physical therapy.[55] Activity must be modified for up to 1 year after the injury with both conservative and surgical treatment.

Table 11-2 Traumatic Injuries to Lower Leg—continued				
	Achilles' Tendon Rupture	**Gastrocnemius Muscle Strain**	**Plantaris Tendon Rupture**	**Lower Leg Fracture**
Physical examination findings	Pain and tenderness at muscle-tendon interface Deformity and sulcus 2.5-5 cm from os calcis Inability to ambulate Presence of Thompson sign Ecchymosis and swelling	Tendonitis over medial or lateral head of gastrocnemius Swelling and ecchymosis over calf Pain during passive dorsiflexion or active heel raising in a weight-bearing mode No Thompson sign	Sensation of being "shot in the calf" Plantar flexion response Pain along course of plantaris tendon No Thompson sign	History of acute trauma Deformity, bony displacement of lower leg Point tenderness or crepitus at fracture site Swelling, ecchymosis Inability to bear weight
X-ray findings	Normal	Normal, if applicable	Not applicable	Confirmation of tibial or fibular fracture Need to rule out knee or ankle injury, osseous displacement, unstable fracture
Treatment plan	RICE Cast immobilization Orthopedic surgical referral	Application of ice, rest, use of heel pad Use of crutches, if weight bearing is painful	Application of ice, rest Use of crutches for 3-4 days Electrotherapy	Immobilization Orthopedic surgical referral

RICE, Rest, ice, compression, and elevation.

Gastrocnemius Muscle Strain

Injuries to the fleshy gastrocnemius muscle may be mild, moderate, or severe. Overexertion during walking or stair climbing may lead to mild strains. More serious injuries result from ballistic events (e.g., falling from a step or curb) or sports events (e.g., running or jumping). Weekend athletes, fitness fanatics, and individuals with inflexible calf muscles are prone to gastrocnemius strains.

The mechanism of a severe gastrocnemius injury is similar to that of an Achilles' tendon rupture, but the pain that originates in a strain or tear of the gastrocnemius muscle is over the medial or lateral head of the muscle rather than at the tendinous surface or muscle-tendon junction. The Thompson test can be helpful in differentiating between the two injuries. The practitioner should also check the plantar response to rule out a rupture of the plantaris tendon. Passive stretching into dorsiflexion and ambulation are quite painful for the patient with a gastrocnemius strain. An active heel raise is impossible for those with moderate-to-severe tears. Swelling and ecchymosis are common, and there may be a deformity at the site of injury in severe cases.

Appropriate treatment consists of the application of ice, rest, the wearing of a heel pad to take the strain off the calf, and the use of crutches for 7 to 10 days (if

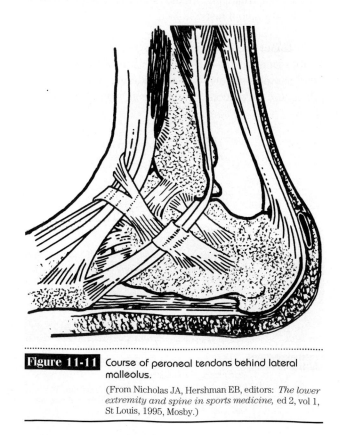

Figure 11-11 Course of peroneal tendons behind lateral malleolus.

(From Nicholas JA, Hershman EB, editors: *The lower extremity and spine in sports medicine,* ed 2, vol 1, St Louis, 1995, Mosby.)

the injury is severe enough to make weight bearing painful). Electrotherapy can relieve pain and swelling, and ultrasound can promote healing and make the scar tissue more pliable. Stretching with a towel or slant board and heel raises lead to heel-cord flexibility and proprioception during the rehabilitation stage.

Rupture of the Plantaris Tendon

In general, a rupture of the plantaris tendon in the calf occurs during an activity such as jumping or running. The patient reports a sensation like "being shot in the leg." Sometimes, a patient reports hearing or feeling a "pop" as well. Initially, walking is difficult, because of the pain rather than the lack of plantar flexion. Pain develops from medial to lateral along the course of the plantaris tendon, which helps the clinician in making the diagnosis. Some swelling and ecchymosis may become apparent within 1 to 2 days. The Thompson maneuver can rule out a ruptured Achilles' tendon.

Tears of the plantaris tendon differ from those of the gastrocnemius muscle in that the recuperation time is shorter. An individual who has a plantaris tendon rupture may need crutches for only 3 or 4 days. As with other calf injuries, treatment should include the application of ice, elevation, and rest.

Lower Leg Fractures

Acute trauma can result in a fracture of the lower leg. For example, motor vehicle accidents, motorcycle injuries, and recreational trauma (e.g., skiing) are all potential causes of acute fibular and tibial fractures. The severity of the trauma and the velocity of the external forces determine the degree of disability in most cases.

Fractures can be classified as simple (i.e., nondisplaced) or compound. Those that involve the long bones of the lower leg can be spiral, transverse, hairline, or oblique fractures. The site of the injury varies according to the mechanical lines of osseous stress, such as the proximal shaft, midshaft, or distal lower leg. Careful evaluation for deformity and neurovascular compromise is essential. Radiographic examination focuses on the possibility of bony displacement, syndesmotic shifts (i.e., Dupuytren's fracture), concomitant osseous injury, and gross ligamentous rupture. Thus it is necessary to order x-ray films not only of the entire lower leg, but also of the ankle and knee.

Because the tibia is a weight-bearing structure, a tibial fracture usually requires cast immobilization for

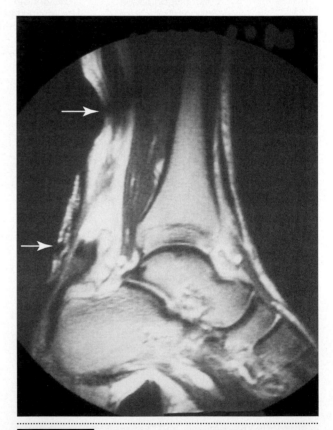

Figure 11-13 Complete tear of the Achilles' tendon as seen on a magnetic resonance image.

(From Nicholas JA, Hershman EB, editors: *The lower extremity and spine in sports medicine*, ed 2, vol 1, St Louis, 1995, Mosby.)

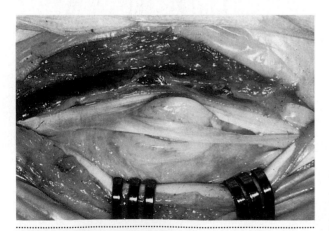

Figure 11-12 Protrusion of the malleolus through a split in a subluxed peroneal tendon.

(Courtesy of William Grana, MD. From Grana W: Chronic pain persisting after ankle sprain, *J Musculoskeletal Med*, 7(6):36, 1990.)

a minimum of 6 to 8 weeks, followed by approximately 4 weeks of bracing (Figure 11-14 *A, B*). Injuries to the fibula may be treated more conservatively, since the fibula is not critical in weight bearing. The selection of conservative or aggressive care depends on case presentation and the philosophy of the treating orthopedic surgeon.

Anatomic Factors: Tibia-Fibula Dissociation

Usually noted as an incidental finding in patients with mechanical knee pain, a tibia-fibula dissociation is only rarely the result of a traumatic event. The synovial membrane that envelops the proximal tibiofibular joint is inherently lax, which allows the mobile fibula head to slide laterally and posteriorly. The clinician notes that the fibular head is prominent and that its motion is excessive. The patient is generally hypermobile at the knee joint as well, which is a risk factor for patellofemoral dislocation. These two sites of inherent laxity accompany cases of tibia-fibula dissociations.

Lateral or posterior displacement of the fibula may appear on a plain x-ray film; otherwise, there is no other osseous abnormality. Dissociation rarely requires treatment because it is not generally painful (Table 11-3). Repetitive popping or subluxing of the fibular is certainly not advisable, however.

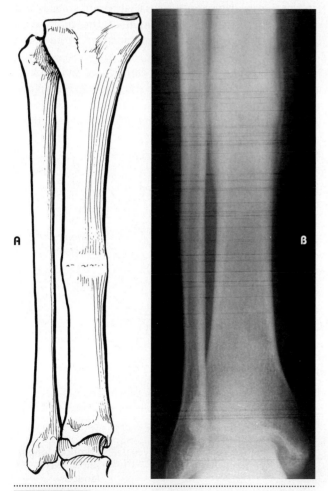

Figure 11-14 **A,** Complete union of a fracture of the tibial diaphysis. Note the negligible deformity of the contour, denoting an optimal fracture site union. **B,** Fracture of the tibial shaft demonstrating near-complete healing. A mild convexity of the cortex is visualized at the site of union and is a result of callus.

(From Deltoff MN, Kogan PL: *The portable skeletal x-ray library,* St Louis, 1998, Mosby.)

PART TWO: ANKLE

Applied Anatomy and Biomechanics of the Ankle

Talocrural Joint

The union of the fibula, tibia, and talus forms the talocrural joint, otherwise known as the ankle joint proper. The long bones of the leg form a mortise into which the dome of the talus fits. Because the medial and lateral malleoli project downward over the sides of the trochlea (i.e., talus), they improve the bony stability of the ankle joint.[57] This osseous restraint is not symmetric in nature, however. The lateral malleolus of the fibula

Table 11-3	Anatomic Factors
	Tibia-Fibular Dissociation
Physical examination findings	Hypermobility of fibula head
	Inherent laxity of proximal tibiofibular joint
	Concomitant mechanical problems of knee joint
X-ray findings	No evidence of abnormality
	Possibly, fibula in lateral or posterior position on standard anteroposterior film
Treatment plan	Knee symptomatology is the focus of treatment

projects distally further than the medial malleolus of the tibia; therefore the lateral side of the ankle has greater inherent bony stability.

Flexion and extension are the major movements of the ankle joint, although the obliquity of the axis of motion permits other minor movements.[57] The tibial plafond is wider anteriorly than posteriorly, which allows for dorsiflexion. During plantar flexion, the narrow posterior portion of the talus approximates the anterior tibia. This unique bony arrangement provides anterior ankle stability and a functioning stable position in dorsiflexion. Thus the mortise acts as a hinged joint.

The distal tibia and fibula form a syndesmosis bound by the interosseous membrane. The anterior and posterior tibiofibular ligaments contribute to stability. The syndesmosis, with the deltoid and lateral collateral ligaments of the ankle, maintains the relationship of the tibia, fibula, and talus (Figure 11-15 *A, B*). Approximately 10% of the population possess a true synovial joint at the distal tibiofibular articulation.[80]

Subtalar Joint

Inferior to the level of the mortise joint lies the articulation between the talus and the calcaneus. The subtalar joint is solely responsible for inversion and eversion movement, partly because of the peculiarities of the anatomic arrangement at the ankle. For example, the fact that the ankle's bony stability is greater laterally than medially has two biomechanical consequences. First, the deltoid ligament on the medial aspect of the ankle is strong to compensate for weak bony stability; second, inversion movement is more likely than eversion movement in pathomechanical situations. As the subtalar joint moves toward inversion, it loses its inherent stability in a neutral position. Plantar flexion of the mortise in common movements further compounds the inversion instability of the subtalar joint.

The lateral ligamentous complex of the ankle is commonly injured or torn when it is under stress. Three major ligaments make up the complex: the anterior talofibular ligament, the calcaneofibular ligament, and the

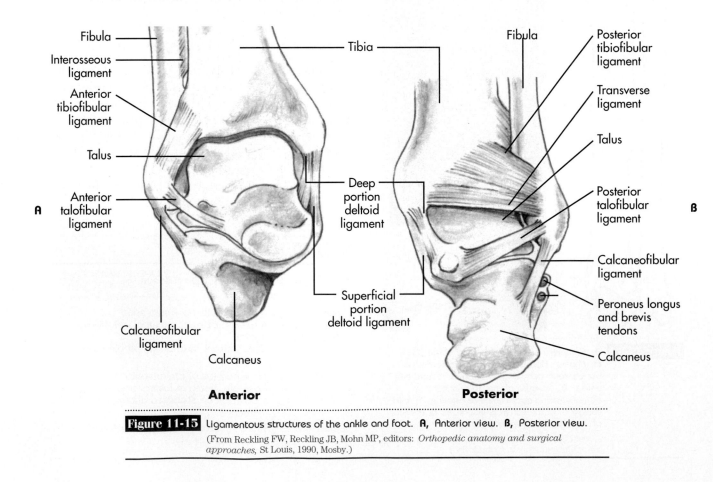

A | **B**

Anterior **Posterior**

Figure 11-15 Ligamentous structures of the ankle and foot. **A,** Anterior view. **B,** Posterior view.
(From Reckling FW, Reckling JB, Mohn MP, editors: *Orthopedic anatomy and surgical approaches*, St Louis, 1990, Mosby.)

posterior talofibular ligament (Figure 11-16). The anterior talofibular ligament is the weakest of these; it is the most commonly injured and the first to be damaged during the strain of inversion and plantar flexion. The structural integrity of the anterior talofibular ligament prevents forward talar draw under normal conditions. The calcaneofibular ligament, the largest of the three, is approximately two and one-half times stronger than the anterior talofibular ligament,[5] and it is the second most likely to be damaged in lateral ankle sprains. Finally, the posterior talofibular ligament—the strongest—is injured only in severe lateral ankle sprains and ankle dislocations.[46]

Although excessive inversion is a common mechanism for ankle sprains, the same vector of force may produce varied injury patterns according to the position of the ankle joint at the time of the force or the history of the individual involved. A plantar flexion mode increases the vulnerability of the anterior talofibular ligament to the stress of inversion. In contrast, dorsiflexion

places the calcaneofibular ligament under stress during inversion.[16] Injuries to the anterior and posterior talofibular ligaments are likely to tear the joint capsule because of the continuity of the ligaments and capsule. However, the calcaneofibular ligament is not contiguous with the joint capsule; therefore the rare isolated injury to the calcaneofibular ligament spares the joint capsule.

Excessive pronation and supination of the subtalar joint not only provides the clinician with a dynamic visual deformity of the rearfoot gait, but these may give the clinician clues to the cause and effect of distant syndromes in the lower leg, patellofemoral joint, and lumbopelvic spine.

Pathologic Conditions of the Ankle

Injuries to the ankle are so common that they sometimes seem to dominate the practice of the sports medicine specialist. Because the posterior musculature of the lower leg is strong and a primary factor in both inversion and

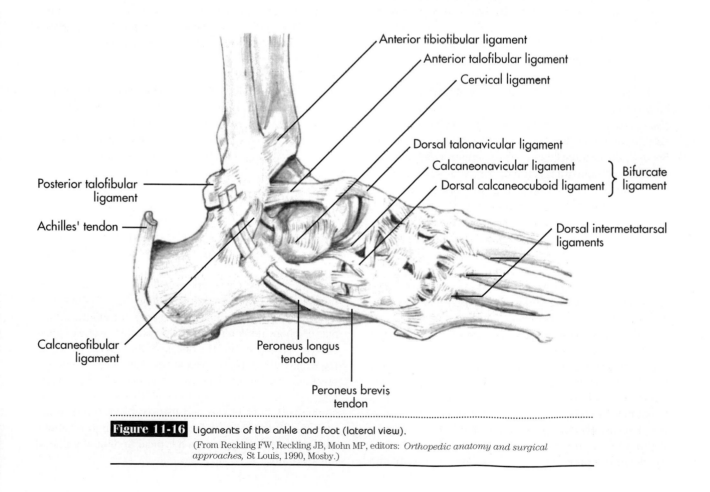

Figure 11-16 Ligaments of the ankle and foot (lateral view).

(From Reckling FW, Reckling JB, Mohn MP, editors: *Orthopedic anatomy and surgical approaches,* St Louis, 1990, Mosby.)

Labels in figure:
Anterior tibiotibular ligament
Anterior talofibular ligament
Cervical ligament
Dorsal talonavicular ligament
Calcaneonavicular ligament
Dorsal calcaneocuboid ligament
Bifurcate ligament
Dorsal intermetatarsal ligaments
Posterior talofibular ligament
Achilles' tendon
Calcaneofibular ligament
Peroneus longus tendon
Peroneus brevis tendon

plantar flexion, lateral ankle sprains are by far the most common of such injuries.

Ankle Sprains

Several researchers have noted that ankle sprains are the most frequent injuries in athletics and the most often treated condition in some hospital emergency rooms.[24,34,45] Theoretically, standards of care should be routine, and there should be little controversy concerning treatment parameters. This is not always the case, however, since many injuries are undertreated, especially if the radiographic studies are normal. Severe sprains, on the other hand, often provoke debate regarding the efficacy of surgical treatment versus conservative care.

As stated previously, the ankle mortise is less stable in plantar flexion, such as during the end of the swing phase in walking. Repetitive sprains to either or both talofibular ligaments can easily contribute to chronic ankle laxity and subtalar joint instability. The primary reason many individuals sustain recurrent sprains, however, is the lack of a properly designed, thorough rehabilitation program.

Lateral Ankle Sprains

For anatomic, biomechanical, and practical reasons, an ankle sprain involves the lateral ligaments approximately 85% to 95% of the time.[25,43] First, because the lateral malleolus is larger than the medial malleolus, there is a natural tendency for the foot to ease into inversion. Second, the plantar flexors are much stronger than the dorsiflexors; hence, it is common for the foot to be placed into equinus, which is fairly unstable under stress because of the poor bony congruence of the talus at this angle in the ankle mortise. Finally, the plantar flexion of the foot when it hits the ground during normal activity, as well as in some sports activities, leaves the ankle in a fairly unstable position. For example, activities such as jogging, running, and walking on uneven surfaces may cause a lateral ankle sprain from a plantar flexion, inversion stress force.

When the lateral ligaments are under stress, the peroneal muscles attempt to absorb some of the strain. Any weakness in these muscles allows undue strain to fall on the lateral collateral ligament complex, however. This scenario grows even worse for those individuals with a tight heel cord (i.e., Achilles' tendon) and tight calf muscles, because the foot is already in slight plantar flexion. Without proper rehabilitation to regain ankle and lower leg flexibility, aberrant mechanics become one of the

primary reasons for the high rate of recurrent ankle sprains.[39]

The danger in treating this common injury as "just a sprain" is the delay in making an accurate diagnosis and in initiating proper treatment measures, such as cryotherapy to control the sometimes enormous swelling. The reduction of inflammation early in treatment is a crucial element in reducing pain, disability, and future morbidity. It is vital to use immobilization and to avoid bearing weight on the injured limb. The use of crutches, an Unna boot (i.e., a soft-compressive cast), or an air splint brace helps reduce the length of the patient's disability.

Physical Examination for Lateral Ankle Sprains. There are two separate and distinct evaluations in the examination of the sprained ankle: under non–weight-bearing conditions and under weight-bearing conditions. Palpation of the acutely sprained ankle usually reveals swelling or ecchymosis over the sinus tarsi below the level of the lateral malleolus. Tenderness is evident directly over the anterior talofibular ligament and, depending on the grade of injury, may involve the calcaneofibular ligament. Most posterior discomfort originates in a tightened Achilles' tendon. The peroneal muscles may be strained at the distal fibula.

Grade I sprains usually involve a stretch of the ligament fibers with little functional loss and mild swelling. Most often these sprains involve the anterior talofibular ligament, and there is no gross instability at the ankle joint. Moderate injuries involving partial tears of one or more ligaments with accompanying pain, swelling, difficulty in ambulating, and ligamentous laxity with a definite end point are grade II sprains. The anterior talofibular ligament and calcaneofibular ligament are commonly involved in grade II sprains. Grade III sprains are severe; most often the anterior talofibular and the calcaneofibular ligaments are completely torn, and stability testing shows no definitive end point.[10]

It is necessary to order radiographic films to rule out a fracture. Orthopedic procedures used to screen for a possible fracture include placing pressure along the long axis of a bone, looking for pain away from the site of pressure, and compressing the tibia and fibula at the proximal leg while evaluating for pain at the distal leg. Of course, any point tenderness over the fibula and any obvious deformity warrant close scrutiny. With the patient lying supine with both ankles and feet exposed, the clinician observes the degrees of dorsiflexion in the injured ankle; the lack of a few degrees is a typical finding of a lateral ankle sprain.

The anterior draw test remains a standard procedure for the evaluation of the status of the anterior talofibular ligament. This test is most accurate when performed with the patient sitting and dangling the legs over the edge of the table. The examiner cups the patient's heel in one hand, stabilizes the distal tibiofibular syndesmosis in the other, and attempts to "draw" the calcaneus forward. (The examiner may need to remind the patient to let the leg relax completely.) Another option is to grab the mortise from the dorsal aspect of the foot and draw the articulation forward.

It is essential to test the patient's comfort in a weight-bearing mode. If weight bearing on the involved side is painful, the patient needs crutches. If not, the patient should take the unaffected foot off the floor and balance on the injured side. The ankle may need some support, such as an air splint or crutches, if the patient cannot balance on the injured foot. No support is necessary for normal ambulation if the patient can bear weight satisfactorily on the injured leg.

Diagnostic Imaging of Lateral Ankle Sprains. A physical examination alone cannot rule out a fracture.

For example, radiographic studies are necessary to differentiate a lateral ankle sprain from the following:

- Peroneal tendon dislocation
- Talar dome fracture
- Distal fibula fracture
- Jones fracture (i.e., fifth metatarsal)
- Midfoot sprain

A minimal radiographic evaluation that includes anteroposterior, lateral, and internal oblique (mortise) views is mandatory after a traumatic ankle sprain (Table 11-4). It is necessary not only to evaluate the fibula and talus for possible fracture, but also to view the fifth metatarsal. The clinician should check talar tilt and assess the stability of the mortise. In some cases, radiographic examination reveals degenerative changes from prior or cumulative trauma, congenital anomalies, and accessory bony structures (Figure 11-17).

Some patients eventually need advanced radiographic studies (Figure 11-18). Although an MRI or arthrography can confirm a tear of the anterior talofibular ligament, the clinician should be able to gather enough information from the physical examination to detect this

Table 11-4 Radiographic Studies of Ankle Trauma

X-Ray View	Position	Clinical Notes
Anteroposterior	Patient supine, heel on cassette; ankle slightly dorsiflexed so that plantar surface of foot is perpendicular to film; lower leg internally rotated so that line through malleoli is parallel to film surface; central ray through mortise	Distal tibia, distal fibula, talus, and ankle joint are visualized; if foot is not dorsiflexed, tibiotalar joint is not clearly visualized; in subtle fractures of talar dome, plantar flexion may depict fracture site
Lateral	Lateral surface of ankle in contact with film; foot slightly dorsiflexed to prevent lateral rotation of ankle; opposite leg crossed over affected leg with support for opposite knee	Distal tibia, distal fibula, ankle joint, talus, and calcaneus are visualized; posterior lip of tibia is frequently involved in fractures and can best be seen in off-lateral projection with slight external rotation of foot
Medial (internal) oblique	Ankle slightly dorsiflexed so that plantar surface of foot is perpendicular to film; leg rotated 15°-20° internally at mortise; to ensure open ankle joint, ankle rotated internally until malleoli are parallel to film surface	Invaluable for detecting subtle fractures of distal fibula, posterior tibia, and base of fifth metatarsal; width of joint space should be constant throughout entire ankle mortise—otherwise, presence of talar tilt or shift in mortise indicates ankle instability
Inversion stress	Hindfoot inverted; subtalar joint placed into inversion	Integrity of lateral collateral ligament complex is tested; comparison views of both ankles are valuable because amount of talar tilt on one side is normally within 5°-10° of that on the other; complete tear of anterior talofibular ligament results in abnormal talar tilt seen; gap is greater, if calcaneofibular ligament is also torn

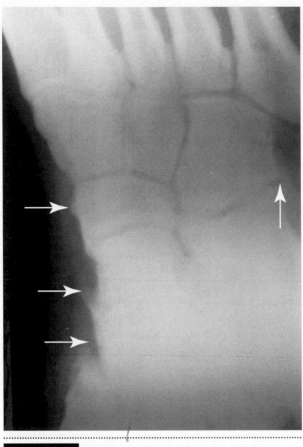

Figure 11-17 Spurring at the talar dome and capsular attachment to the midtarsal region after recurrent ankle sprains.

swelling is the application of ice with compression and electrotherapy (Table 11-5, page 385). Ice should be applied generously for as long as the injury requires treatment and rehabilitation. The use of an Unna boot is also helpful to control and reduce the edema. In addition, electrotherapy on a low pulse can be used either on the skin directly or over the Unna boot to reduce the swelling.

The patient should use crutches to avoid placing any weight on the injured ankle and should elevate the leg as much as possible; pillows under the foot of the patient's mattress facilitate lymphatic drainage. After 2 or 3 days, the practitioner should remove the Unna boot and reexamine the ankle. If the swelling has diminished, an air splint may provide sufficient support for the next stage of recovery, and the patient may begin to place weight on the involved leg—with the assistance of crutches.

Once pain and swelling have begun to subside, the patient can start gentle "gas pedal" exercise (i.e., pumping the foot up and down as if it were on a gas pedal) and towel stretching to regain heel-cord flexibility. Writing the alphabet in the air with the great toe of the affected leg (sometimes called the alphabet exercise) can also be helpful; the knee should be straight, and the motion should come from the foot and ankle only.

When the patient is ready to progress to weight-bearing exercise, performing heel raises on a stair stretches the ankle joint and Achilles' tendon, thus increasing strength and proprioception. A wobble board device is an excellent way to improve balance, proprioception, and functional movements. Isokinetic training helps restore normal muscle function at the lower leg and ankle, which is especially important for the dorsiflexor muscles.

The practitioner may recommend various types of ankle supports for follow-up treatment and rehabilitation. Active patients and those individuals involved in recreational and competitive sports may wish to have extra ankle support after rehabilitation, especially if they have a history of ankle injuries. Pneumatic braces, lace-up stirrup supports, and athletic tape all may help improve ligamentous function and ankle support in isolated instances.[4] There is no substitute, however, for sound joint rehabilitation that includes strengthening of the everter muscles,[14] heel-cord flexibility, and proprioception training of the foot and ankle.

Because chronic ankle sprains may lead to scar tissue formation at the talocalcaneal joint, contributing to the cycle of lost motion and heel-cord inflexibility, patients

condition. Inversion stress films, usually taken bilaterally, may be helpful in evaluating talar tilt on an anteroposterior view, however (Figure 11-19). There is some disagreement about the point at which the talar tilt becomes pathologically unstable. Some authors have stated than any tilt of more than 5 degrees or a difference of more than 3 mm between the two sides may be unstable.[18,40] Recently the consensus has been that it is more realistic to consider a difference of 5 to 10 degrees on comparison projections of the two sides to be within the normal range.[52]

Treatment of Lateral Ankle Sprains. As noted earlier, it is crucial to control the inflammatory process associated with a lateral ankle sprain to reduce rehabilitation time and morbidity. The initial step in the treatment of lateral ankle sprains with moderate-to-severe

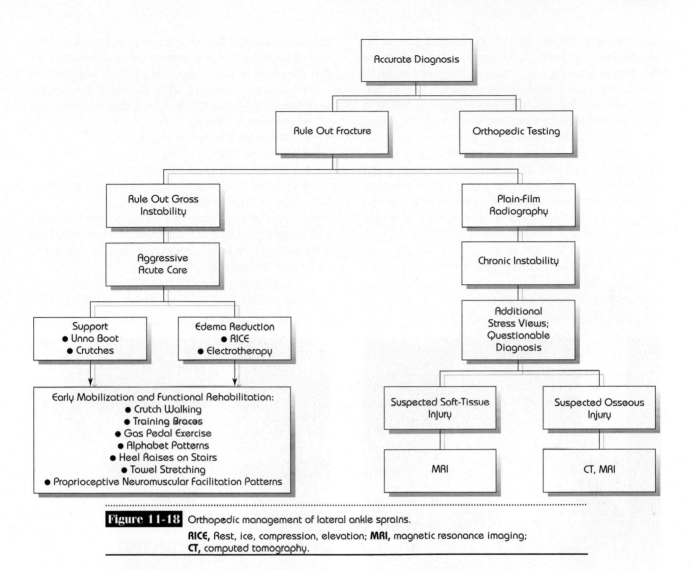

Figure 11-18 Orthopedic management of lateral ankle sprains.
RICE, Rest, ice, compression, elevation; **MRI,** magnetic resonance imaging;
CT, computed tomography.

with such a history can benefit from manipulation of the ankle mortise and supportive exercises. Distraction and anteroposterior glide should be used to check for hypomobility at the ankle. Manipulation with the patient in the supine or seated position is best (Figure 11-20 *A, B*).

There has been debate regarding the appropriate treatment of severe ankle sprains, but immobilization for 6 to 8 weeks generally provides satisfactory results. Certain conditions, such as a dislocated ankle, subluxed peroneal tendon with a torn retinaculum, and severe mortise instability, may require surgical care. Competitive athletes with a history of multiple sprains and chronic lateral instability may elect to undergo a surgical procedure that involves splitting the tendon of the peroneus tertius and drilling a hole through the fibula to po-

sition the tendon around the calcaneus. This procedure reconstructs the anterior talofibular and calcaneofibular ligaments, thus adding stability to the ankle mortise and subtalar joint.

Medial Ankle Sprains

Although relatively rare (5%) among ankle sprains, the medial sprain poses hidden dangers. Medial support comes from the strong triangular deltoid ligament, also known as the medial collateral ligament (Figure 11-21, page 387). Both superficial and deep fibers originate from the medial malleolus of the tibia. The superficial fibers split into three portions that attach onto the navicular, talus, and sustentaculum tali. Both the flexor digitorum longus and posterior tibialis tendons overlie the ligament.

Generally an eversion of the subtalar joint is the mechanism of a medial ankle sprain. Most sprains of the deltoid ligament evoke pain in the eversion mode, and the clinician notes bogginess over the deltoid ligament and capsule. Although the swelling may not be as great as that associated with lateral ankle sprains, the injury may be equally severe.

It is necessary to obtain a standard x-ray film series of the ankle, including the anteroposterior, lateral, and mortise views. A space greater than 4 mm between the talus and medial malleolus on the mortise view suggests a tear of the deltoid ligament. The mortise view also makes it possible to rule out ankle instability at the talocalcaneal joint.[65] The practitioner should carefully scrutinize the areas adjacent to the injured area on these films.

The deltoid ligament is much stronger than its lateral counterpart, so it is less likely to rupture under stress.

Even if the ballistic force is not sufficient to tear the deltoid ligament itself, it may damage other structures near the site, such as the talus, tibial plafond, interosseous membrane, and calcaneus. Thus trauma in the area requires the practitioner to rule out a variety of conditions:

- Syndesmosis sprain
- Talar dome fracture
- Medial malleolus fracture
- Tibiofibular ligament rupture
- Proximal fibula fracture (i.e., Maisonneuve's fracture), if the syndesmosis is disrupted

Severe associated injuries such as a tear of the anterior and posterior tibiofibular ligaments[82] or a rupture of the interosseous membrane should be promptly referred to an orthopedic surgeon.

Imaging techniques such as MRI are helpful in differentially diagnosing conditions that do not improve with

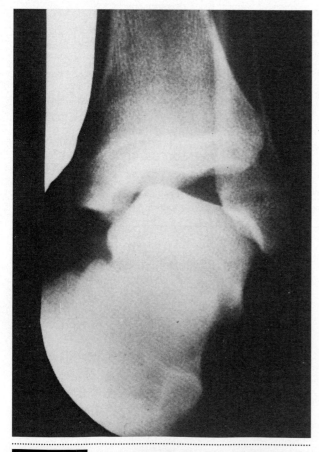

Figure 11-19 Inversion stress film showing significant talar tilt.
(From Nicholas JA, Hershman EB, editors: *The lower extremity and spine in sports medicine,* ed 2, vol 1, St Louis, 1995, Mosby.)

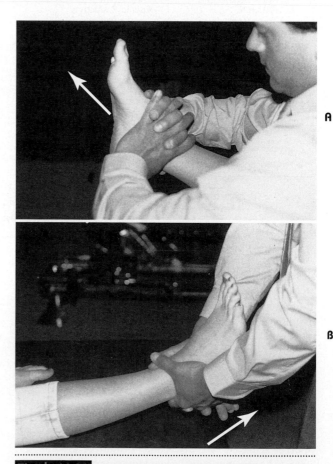

Figure 11-20 Manipulation of the talocrural joint. **A,** Position for axial distraction. **B,** Alternate position for long axis adjustment of the talocrural joint.

treatment.[68] *The period of morbidity associated with injuries to the deltoid and tibiofibular ligaments is much longer than that associated with lateral sprains of the ankle.*

Tibiofibular Syndesmosis Sprains

Also known as the *high ankle sprain*, a syndesmotic sprain is an injury to the anterior and posterior inferior tibiofibular ligaments.[74] If these structures are ruptured, there is a complete diastasis of the interosseous membrane. Tenderness and swelling occur over the distal anterior lower leg, and there is palpable pain over the fibula. These injuries are more common than previously reported, and they occur most often in association with other injuries such as ankle fractures.[48]

The clinical examination provides a tentative diagnosis. The patient usually has pain in eversion over the deltoid ligament, anteromedial ankle pain, ecchymosis, and effusion on both sides of the ankle. Squeezing the proximal tibiofibular joint and looking for pain distally over the syndesmosis should be part of the examination to detect injury in this area.

Table 11-5 Ankle Sprains

| | Lateral Ankle Sprains | | | | |
	Grade 1	Grade 1+	Grade 2	Grade 2+	Grade 3
Physical examination findings	Bogginess Ability to bear weight on one or both legs Normal result on anterior draw test Palpable tenderness over anterior talofibular ligament Full dorsiflexion, plantar flexion	Mild swelling Ability to bear weight only with both feet on ground Slightly abnormal result on anterior draw test Palpable tenderness over anterior talofibular ligament Mild loss of dorsiflexion	Moderate effusion Medial and lateral capsular tenderness Palpable pain over anterior talofibular ligament and calcaneofibular ligament Positive result on anterior draw test, talar tilt Distinct loss of dorsiflexion Inability to bear weight	Large effusion and midfoot swelling Medial and lateral capsular tenderness Palpable pain over anterior talofibular ligament and calcaneofibular ligament Achilles' tendon contracture Loss of all range of motion Inability to bear weight	Large effusion and midfoot swelling Palpable pain over anterior talofibular, calcaneofibular, and posterior talofibular ligaments Achilles' tendon contracture Positive result on anterior draw test Gross anatomic instability
X-ray findings	Normal	Normal	No gross instability	Gross instability, subluxation of talus Need to rule out fracture; examine mortise for stability	Anterior talar subluxation Need to rule out fracture
Treatment plan	Application of ice Electrotherapy Towel stretching RICE at home	Application of ice Electrotherapy Use of crutches for 2-5 days Air splint or Unna boot Dorsiflexion stretches RICE at home	Application of ice Electrotherapy Use of crutches, Unna boot for 7-10 days RICE at home Follow-up evaluation in 2-3 days with replacement of boot, if necessary	Application of ice Electrotherapy Immobilization by Unna boot for 1-2 weeks with crutches, followed by use of air splint or crutches for 1-2 more weeks (i.e., no weight bearing for 3-4 weeks total) RICE at home	No weight bearing Cast immobilization or surgical referral

RICE, Rest, ice, compression, and elevation.

Continued

Table 11-5 Ankle Sprains—continued

	Medial Ankle Sprains	Tibiofibular Syndesmosis Sprain
Physical examination findings	History of eversion, pronation mechanism of injury Palpable tenderness over deltoid ligament Medial capsule tenderness possible Tenderness over navicular Mild-to-moderate effusion	Tenderness and swelling at distal anterior lower leg Palpable pain over fibula Concomitant deltoid ligament sprain common Effusion at both sides of injured ankle Anteromedial pain on ankle palpation Need to rule out associated injuries
X-ray findings	Need to rule out avulsion fracture of medial malleolus, mortise, or syndesmotic instability	Careful scrutiny required Need to rule out separation of bony bodies between distal tibia and fibula Need to rule out associated fracture
Treatment plan	Application of ice Electrotherapy Immobilization and non–weight-bearing activity, if necessary Repeated x-ray studies on follow-up, if condition is refractory to care	Orthopedic surgical referral Immobilization and non–weight-bearing activities

---

Keys to Successful Rehabilitation of Ankle Sprains

1. Carefully make an accurate diagnosis based on history, mechanism of injury, stability testing, and radiologic evaluation.
2. Rule out concomitant fracture or other advanced pathologic conditions.
3. Use aggressive edema reduction techniques. If the swelling is not controlled or if the edema extravasates into the dorsum of the midfoot, treatment and rehabilitation time will be prolonged.
4. Do not hesitate to prescribe crutches and compression immobilization for immediate care.
5. Instruct the patient to begin non–weight-bearing flexibility exercises as soon as tolerated.
6. Make full dorsiflexion of the ankle mortise and a relaxed Achilles' tendon the primary goals of motion and flexibility rehabilitation.
7. Prevent swelling in the forefoot or dorsum of the midfoot by advising the patient to use rest, ice, compression, elevation (RICE technique) to immobilize the involved leg, and to mobilize the toes when the leg is elevated.
8. Place an Unna boot (i.e., soft compressive cast) for an initial period of 2 to 3 days; this device can control and aid in the dissipation of an effusion, thus decreasing the "downtime" from an ankle injury by as much as 50%.

Stability films may be normal initially, but standard films may show a separation between the medial fibular cortex and posterior edge of the peroneal grooves.[77] Radiographic evidence of tibiofibular diastasis includes greater than a 10-mm overlap of distal tibia and fibula on anteroposterior film, greater than a 1-mm overlap of distal tibia and fibula on mortise film, and a medial clear space of greater than 3 mm on the anteroposterior film.[68] Chronic degenerative changes are often evident in patients with prior, sometimes undetected trauma (Figure 11-22). It is critical to rule out a fibular fracture, because the presence of such a fracture and the level of the break determine the integrity of the tibiofibular ligaments. Fibular fractures at or proximal to 3 inches above the ankle joint can indicate a tear of the anterior inferior tibiofibular ligament.[77] Fractures that are distal to the ligamentous insertion 2 to 3 cm proximal to the ankle joint indicate that the syndesmosis is intact.

Because of the prolonged morbidity resulting from their injury, patients with a syndesmotic sprain should see an orthopedic surgeon. Depending on any concomitant injuries, such as fracture or joint instability, surgical intervention may be necessary. Complete syndesmotic ruptures with clinical or radiographic evidence of lateral talar subluxation require operative care with transverse screw fixation.[53]

Ankle Fractures

Avulsion or compression forces, or a combination of the two, are responsible for fractures of the ankle.[28] Trau-

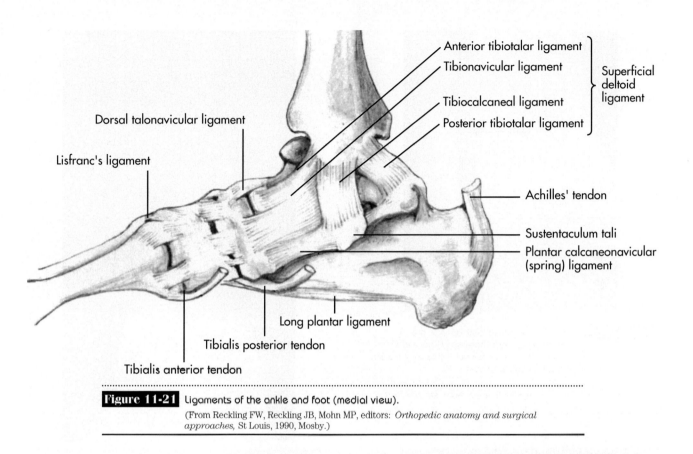

Dorsal talonavicular ligament

Lisfranc's ligament

Anterior tibiotalar ligament
Tibionavicular ligament
Tibiocalcaneal ligament
Posterior tibiotalar ligament
} Superficial deltoid ligament

Achilles' tendon

Sustentaculum tali

Plantar calcaneonavicular (spring) ligament

Long plantar ligament

Tibialis posterior tendon

Tibialis anterior tendon

Figure 11-21 Ligaments of the ankle and foot (medial view).

(From Reckling FW, Reckling JB, Mohn MP, editors: *Orthopedic anatomy and surgical approaches*, St Louis, 1990, Mosby.)

matic fractures can be divided into eversion, inversion, and compression injuries. Knowing the exact mechanism of injury can help both the primary care practitioner and the orthopedic surgeon determine which ligaments are likely to be involved.

Some ankle fractures occur concomitantly with ligamentous injuries; others are isolated injuries that are a result of blunt external trauma. If the event that prompted a ligamentous injury contained sufficient ballistic force, it may dislocate or fracture the ankle. For example, excessive forces on an everted foot in plantar flexion from a jumping position can produce an ankle dislocation with a fracture. Many severe injuries of the ankle can fracture both malleoli (bimalleolar fracture) or fracture the fibula with a deltoid ligament rupture (Figure 11-23).

Persistent swelling, pinpoint tenderness, or deformity should be treated as a fracture until imaging or radiographic techniques prove otherwise. The bony geometry of the ankle is so complex that the use of imaging techniques is mandatory. To screen for fracture, a minimum of three views is initially necessary: standard anteroposterior and lateral films, as well as one projection of the mortise (preferably an ankle mortise view). Diagnostic studies that help evaluate osseous ankle injuries include

plain radiography, computed tomography (CT), technetium bone scans, and conventional tomography. Follow-up arthrography or MRI may be helpful if the diagnosis remains in doubt after the initial studies.

Although conservative treatment with cast immobilization is successful for many fractures, some cases require open reduction and internal fixation. Ensuring proper alignment at the time of injury decreases the risk of malfunction or malunion at some later point.

Guidelines for the Clinical Evaluation of Ankle Fractures

There are several key guidelines that the primary care practitioner must always keep in mind when examining a patient with a possible fracture of the ankle:

- Evaluate the extent of trauma and, in particular, any concomitant ligament or capsular disruption around the ankle.
- Rule out any occult fracture via systematic examination and diagnostic imaging, if warranted.
- Examine the ankle for any gross deformity and malfunction of the ankle mortise.
- Assign a high priority to the restoration of prefracture anatomy.

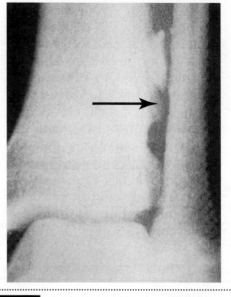

Figure 11-22 Formation of heterotopic bone in the interosseous space between tibia and fibula (arrow) indicating previous injury to the distal tibiofibular syndesmosis.

(Courtesy of William Grana, MD. From Grana W: Chronic pain persisting after ankle sprain, *J Musculoskeletal Med*, 7(6):36, 1990.)

- Pay careful attention to the status of the ankle mortise; be certain to rule out any talar shift or gross instability.
- Examine the position of the fibular as it relates to the possibility of a fracture.
- Rule out the displacement of a fracture segment, as well as any angular deformity.
- Do not hesitate to order plain radiographic films of the ankle and possibly of the knee joint and lower leg, if both presentation and mechanism of injury warrant these studies.
- Evaluate the distal epiphyses of the lower leg in skeletally immature patients.

The experienced primary care practitioner may be able to manage simple ankle fractures, but many cases require prompt referral to an orthopedic surgeon. Thus experience, any evidence of gross instability on plain films, or any indications of neurovascular compromise determine the appropriate course of primary care and referral.

Types of Ankle Fractures

The most common type of ankle injury involves supination, adduction, and internal rotation. The velocity and

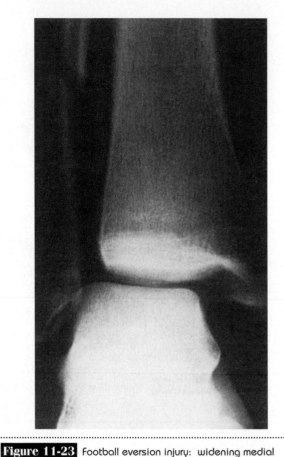

Figure 11-23 Football eversion injury: widening medial mortise with associated deltoid tear, widening distal tibiofibular syndesmosis, high fibular fracture, and small posterior malleolus fracture (not seen here).

(From Nicholas JA, Hershman EB, editors: *The lower extremity and spine in sports medicine*, ed 2, vol 1, St Louis, 1995, Mosby.)

degrees of force, along with the direction of trauma, determine the severity of injury and the fracture pattern. There are a variety of ankle fractures (Table 11-6).

Talar Fractures. The mechanisms of injury that cause ankle sprains may also cause talar fractures. Hyperextension that forces the neck of the talus against the tibia is one common mechanism of injury.

Transchondral talar fractures involve the articular surface of the joint, resulting in damage to the articular cartilage. Talar dome fractures involve either the lateral or medial aspect of the dome, depending on the position of the ankle joint at the time of injury (i.e., dorsiflexion or plantar flexion, respectively).[67] Inversion is a factor in both scenarios. Abnormal radiographic films warrant further imaging studies. If initial films are un-

Table 11-6 Types of Ankle Fractures

Fracture	Definition of Injury	Mechanism of Injury	X-Ray Views Recommended	Treatment
Wagstaffe's	Vertical fracture of anterior margin of fibular malleolus due to stressed anterior tibiofibular or talofibular ligament; subsyndesmotic fracture	Inversion or abduction force	Anteroposterior ankle, lateral ankle, oblique ankle	1
High Dupuytren's	Fracture of suprasyndesmotic shaft of fibula with rupture of tibiofibular ligaments and supra-adjacent fibers of crural interosseous membrane extending up to level of fractured fibula; there is a lateral shifting of talus and avulsion of medial malleolus or tear of deltoid ligament(s)	Violent abduction	Proximal fibula, anteroposterior ankle, lateral ankle, possibly oblique ankle stress	1
Low Dupuytren's	Fracture of fibula through inferior tibiofibular syndesmosis with tear of anterior tibiofibular ligament or avulsion of anterior tubercle of fibula; medial side of ankle displays avulsed tibial malleolus or torn deltoid ligament	Violent external rotation	Anteroposterior ankle, lateral ankle, oblique ankle	2
Maisonneuve's	Spiral fracture of proximal end of fibula or anatomic neck of fibula associated with tear of anterior-inferior tibiofibular ligament; usually an avulsion fracture of tibial malleolus or tear of deltoid ligaments accompanies this injury	External rotation (supination and eversion)	Knee and ankle, anteroposterior ankle, lateral ankle, possibly oblique ankle stress	2
Pott's	Fracture of distal fibula within 2-3 inches of lateral malleolus, usually with disruption of deltoid ligaments and medial subluxation of inferior tibia; suprasyndesmotic fracture; foot is drawn under distal fragment of fractured fibula and proximal end, which falls in toward tibia.*	Eversion injury	Anteroposterior ankle, lateral ankle, oblique ankle	3
Tillaux's	Rupture of deltoid ligaments or avulsion of tibial malleolus with fracture of distal fibula 5-6 cm above lateral malleolus; avulsion of one or both tibial tubercles may occur; detached piece of bone from tibial lateral margin is called a Tillaux's third or intermediate fracture	External rotation	Anteroposterior ankle, lateral ankle, oblique ankle, mortise view	2
Shepherd's	Fracture of trigonal process of lateral tubercle of talus, commonly of little process of bone external to groove for tendon of flexor hallucis longus muscle; fracture occurs when stretching of ligament in twisting action of foot tears off process of the bone	External rotation (twisting)	Anteroposterior ankle, lateral ankle, oblique ankle	2
Volkmann's	Fracture of anterior margin of distal weight-bearing plate of tibia; associated with fractures of tibial malleolus and fibular shaft with tibiofibular diastasis	Eversion and external rotation	Anteroposterior ankle, lateral ankle, oblique ankle	4
Bosworth	Fracture of distal fibula with upper fragment locked behind posterolateral tibia; trans-syndesmotic or low suprasyndesmotic fracture	Supination and eversion (external rotation)	Anteroposterior ankle, lateral ankle, oblique ankle	5
Cotton's	Partial dislocation of tibia forward (tibiotalar) with fracture of posterior tibial lip or medial and lateral malleoli	Planting of significant forefoot with body continuing forward over it	Anteroposterior ankle, lateral ankle, oblique ankle	4

1, Short-leg walking cast for 4-6 weeks (weight bearing permitted after 2 days); **2,** long-leg cast for 4 weeks; replace with a well-molded short-leg walking cast for 4 weeks; **3,** short-leg cast for 4-8 weeks; **4,** closed reduction with aid of redresser apparatus, and immobilization in short-leg cast for 8 weeks; **5,** open reduction with internal fixation, because of resistance to closed reduction.

*There is controversy concerning the way in which the distal segment falls. The way described by Pott requires a complete tear of the inferior tibiofibular syndesmosis and terminal tibiofibular diastasis. It is possible that this type of diastasis existed in the fractures described by Pott, but was spontaneously reduced as sometimes occurs.

(Adapted from Kelikian H, Kelikian A: *Disorders of the ankle*, Philadelphia, 1985, WB Saunders. Courtesy of Douglas Obetz, D.C.)

remarkable, follow-up tomography may be necessary and high-resolution CT may reveal subtle changes in bone density. If the initial radiographic studies are unremarkable, but the results of a bone scan are abnormal, MRI may be helpful.

Persistent pain after treatment for an ankle sprain may suggest that the original diagnosis was incorrect and the injury is actually a talar fracture rather than a sprain. Any talar fracture requires close scrutiny to determine whether it has a detrimental effect on the mortise. Displacement with ligamentous injury usually mandates surgical treatment.

Malleolar Fractures. An oblique fracture of the lateral malleolus is the most common ankle fracture. The mechanism of injury is often an eversion injury to the deltoid ligament (medial ankle sprain) or blunt trauma.

Nondisplaced malleolar fractures usually require only cast immobilization (Figure 11-24 *A, B*). If the fracture involves the fibula, which is non–weight bearing, the period of immobilization may be short (e.g., 2 to 3 weeks). Displaced fractures, on the other hand, often mandate open reduction and internal fixation, although there is a fine line and great debate over borderline cases of fibula fractures.

Bimalleolar fractures may require surgical treatment. Skin complications such as infection are common, and fractures of both the lateral and medial malleoli render the mortise unstable. In trimalleolar fractures, not only are both malleoli fractured, but the posterior lip of the tibia is fractured as well. Forces large enough to cause trimalleolar fractures result in great swelling and deformity.

Epiphyseal Fractures. Often missed on clinical examination, epiphyseal fractures produce pain and tenderness over the growth plate in youngsters. Initial radiographic studies may be normal. Follow-up x-ray films or bone scans may reveal the epiphyseal fracture; in some cases, however, tomography is necessary to confirm the diagnosis. If immobilized for 4 to 6 weeks, nondisplaced epiphyseal fractures are unlikely to interfere with the youngster's growth.[49]

Tibial Plafond Fractures. Although fractures of the tibial plafond are usually not displaced, the practitioner should evaluate the stability of the talus in the mortise. Cast immobilization allows healing at the fracture site and at the distal tibiofibular joint.

Os Trigonum Fractures. A supernumerary (accessory) bone in the posterior part of the talus, the os trigonum may be involved in an excessive plantar flexion injury. Plain films are seldom helpful in the diagnosis; bone scintigraphy is usually necessary to confirm os trigonum fracture.[37]

Osteochondritis Dissecans

Although more common in the knee joint, osteochondritis dissecans can involve the ankle joint. There is not always a history of trauma, but lateral lesions have a stronger association with antecedent trauma than do medial lesions.[3] Young athletes may sustain an injury presumed to be an ankle sprain, only to find an osteochondral defect later. Microtrauma or overuse injuries may also predispose the child athlete to osteochondritis dissecans. Variations in ossification centers may play a role as well.

The patient may describe intermittent swelling, clicking, or popping of the ankle joint.[19] Joint line tenderness may accompany limitations in motion. In some cases, radiographic films may reveal subtle findings; in others, they may be completely normal. A mortise projection will likely provide useful findings. An area of radiolucency surrounds an area of detached bone at the medial or lateral talar dome on the x-ray film (Figure 11-25).

For patients whose initial films were inconclusive and whose conditions have not responded to care as quickly as anticipated, follow-up plain films may be helpful; however, it may be advisable in questionable cases to obtain a CT scan or an MRI to evaluate the subchondral region and to determine the status of the articular cartilage (Table 11-7). MRI accurately documents

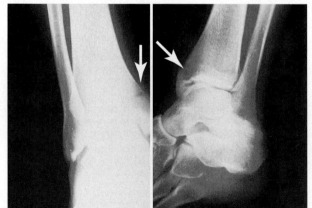

A

B

Figure 11-24 **A,** Anteroposterior projection of fractured medial malleolus of the tibia. **B,** Oblique (mortise) view showing stability of the ankle mortise and no displacement of the fractured fragment.

articular cartilage disease and osteochondral fracture.[21] The high resolution and contrast between the black cortical base and the white bone marrow make this procedure extremely useful when the diagnosis is in doubt (Figure 11-26 *A, B*).[38]

Berndt and Harty classified osteochondral lesions into four categories[54]:

Stage I: Focal region of compressed subchondral bone
Stage II: Osteochondral fragment attached to an underlying bed of trabecular bone
Stage III: Detached, nondisplaced fragment
Stage IV: Displaced fragment

Completely displaced osteochondral fragments that lie freely in the joint (i.e., stage IV lesions) are the most likely candidates for surgical treatment.[44] Several authors recommend drilling, curettage of the defect, or osteotomy for either displaced or nondisplaced fragments.[3,23] Patients with stage I or stage II lesions are candidates for conservative treatment with immobilization.

For symptomatic youngsters, however, the level of expected activity during treatment must be a major consideration in the choice of therapy. The growing child generally does well with conservative care that includes the application of ice and activity modification, with immobilization only if absolutely necessary.

As in the knee joint, osteochondritis dissecans in the ankle joint often heals with rest. An air splint provides support and allows the patient to bear weight on the involved leg. Most cases, particularly in adolescents,[59] are self-limiting, and it is far more beneficial to take a wait-and-see approach. Of course, if the condition is refractory to primary conservative care, a reevaluation and consultation with an orthopedic surgeon are the next steps in case management.

PART THREE: FOOT

Described as a fairly complex array of articulations, ligamentous restraints, musculofascial structures, and bones, the human foot is central to weight bearing and to the dynamics of locomotion. The foot is flexible enough to allow diversity in movement, yet sturdy enough to dissipate forces during ambulation.

The foot can be considered as three separate sections: the hindfoot, midfoot, and forefoot. Each serves a specific purpose and contributes to the synchronous act of stabilization. A problem that originates in the foot

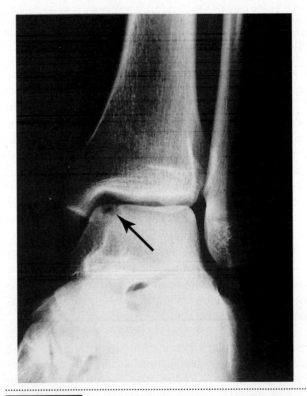

Figure 11-25 Osteochondritis dissecans of the ankle. Note the in situ osseous fragment at the superomedial aspect of the talar dome (arrow).

(From Deltoff MN, Kogan PL: *The portable skeletal x-ray library*, St Louis, 1998, Mosby.)

Table 11-7	Osteochondritis Dissecans (Talus)
Physical examination findings	Joint line tenderness Limited range of motion Intermittent swelling "Clicking" or "popping" possible
X-ray findings	Area of fragmentation or radiolucency at medial or lateral talar dome Need to rule out displacement, loose bodies
Treatment plan	Application of ice Electrotherapy Mild form of immobilization, if necessary (aircast) Activity modification Follow-up computed tomography or magnetic resonance imaging, if diagnosis is in question Orthopedic surgical consult, if necessary

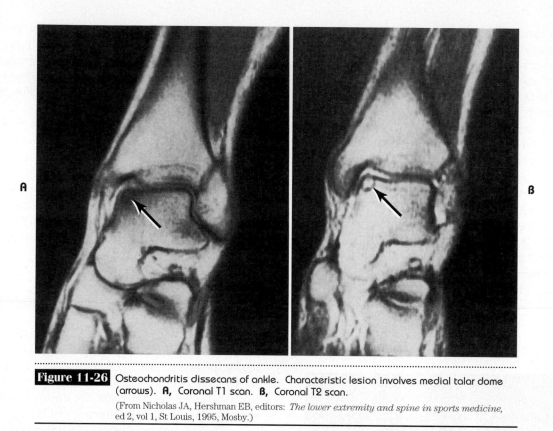

Figure 11-26 Osteochondritis dissecans of ankle. Characteristic lesion involves medial talar dome (arrows). **A,** Coronal T1 scan. **B,** Coronal T2 scan.

(From Nicholas JA, Hershman EB, editors: *The lower extremity and spine in sports medicine,* ed 2, vol 1, St Louis, 1995, Mosby.)

often causes dysfunction in the articulation and soft-tissue structures adjacent to it. Likewise, dysfunction or malalignment of the axial or appendicular skeleton can adversely affect the foot.

Applied Anatomy and Biomechanics of the Foot

As discussed earlier in this chapter, the talocrural joint is made up of the tibia, talus, and fibula. The talocalcaneal, talonavicular, and calcaneocuboid articulations all contribute to the movement of the subtalar joint.

Subtalar joint flexibility leads to limb and articular freedom of motion in dynamic movement phases. Subtalar joint motion contributes to approximately two thirds of the movement in supination and one third of the movement in pronation (Figure 11-27). Between these motions is the neutral point. If the arch of the foot in question is normal and the hindfoot is perpendicular to the floor surface, then the foot is in the neutral position. Proper dorsiflexion of the mortise with a healthy arch and normal hindfoot mechanism helps prevent shin pain, arch strain, and metatarsal problems.

Supination combines the movements of inversion, adduction, and plantar flexion. Inversion takes place around the subtalar joint; adduction occurs around the forefoot-midfoot axis; plantar flexion takes place at the talocrural articulation. Pronation combines the movements of eversion, abduction, and dorsiflexion. Eversion takes place around the subtalar joint; abduction occurs around the forefoot-midfoot axis; dorsiflexion takes place at the talocrural articulation.[33]

Twenty-six bones make up the osseous skeleton of the foot. The joints of the midfoot, which include the navicular-cuneiform and cuneiform-metatarsal joints, do not provide much movement. These midtarsal articulations provide ground stability of the foot, however.

In contrast, the joints of the forefoot provide more movement and play a dynamic function in push-off during ambulation. These articulations include the metatarsophalangeal joints. Although the interphalangeal joints play an important mechanical role in that they permit intricate movements, their position makes them quite vulnerable to trauma.

Ligamentous restraints provide anterior support for these articulations. Extrinsic muscles of the lower

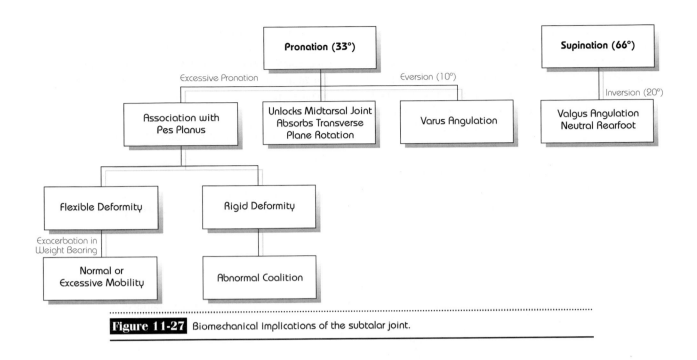

Figure 11-27 Biomechanical implications of the subtalar joint.

leg, along with the plantar fascia that aids in the distribution of weight-bearing loads, provide most of the dynamic support for the foot. The posterior, anterior, and lateral compartment musculature of the lower leg all attach at the foot and thus control its actions (Figure 11-28). The intrinsic muscles of the foot are responsible only for toe function.

Arches of the Foot

There are three arches in the foot: the medial longitudinal arch, lateral longitudinal arch, and transverse arch. The underlying osseous infrastructure of the foot is arranged to aid in the formation of the arches.

The longitudinal arches begin in the area of the plantar fascial insertion into the weight-bearing surface of the calcaneus. This arch extends distal to the metatarsal heads, where it completes its course. The longitudinal arch of the midtarsal articulation averages 15 degrees from the transverse plane and 9 degrees from the sagittal plane. Intrinsically, the longitudinal arch has the support of the spring ligament, which spans the plantar surface of the calcaneonavicular joint. The posterior tibialis tendon also helps form the floor of the arch, while the muscles of the plantar surface, along with the plantar fascia and plantar calcaneonavicular ligament, support the foot.

The transverse arch spans the metatarsal heads in a domelike fashion. During weight bearing, the arch flattens and plays no major role; each of the metatarsal heads bears the brunt of the load. In fact, because the hallux is the largest joint, the first metatarsal head bears twice the load of the other metatarsal heads.[2]

Gait Analysis

An examination of the human locomotor system is incomplete without a thorough analysis of gait, which is the summation of the individual movements of the pelvis, hip, knee, and lower leg coordinated through the spine and coming together at the foot. The fascia of the foot's arch efficiently absorbs the forces imposed by the dynamic weight of the body, thus sparing the joints.

The two phases of gait are the stance phase, when the body is in a weight-bearing mode, and the swing phase, when the limb follows through to the next heel strike.[57] In the stance phase the following events generally occur:

1. Heel strike on the involved side (i.e., contact)
2. Flattening of the foot, as the body weight is transferred
3. Beginning of heel lift-off from the surface
4. Toe-off phase, which particularly involves the metatarsal heads

Table 11-10 Conditions Associated with Heel Pain

	Calcaneal Heel Spur	Calcaneal Fracture	Calcaneal Periostitis	Plantar Fasciitis	Traction Apophysitis of Os Calcis
Physical examination findings	Subcalcaneal pain Common in obese or highly active individuals Need to rule out concomitant mechanical syndromes (e.g., subtalar dysfunction, arthritides, systemic illness)	Pain over the heel Swelling at hindfoot Difficulty in weight bearing History of axial loading	Extreme tenderness at os calcis Only mild swelling over heel pad, if present at all Difficulty in weight bearing	Palpable pain at medial tubercle of calcaneus Hindfoot, heelcord inflexibility Painful weight bearing, especially on wakening Need to rule out pes planus, hyperpronation	Palpable tenderness at os calcis Pain at Achilles' tendon–apophysis interface Painful running or jumping Reproduction of discomfort on dorsiflexion of ankle
X-ray findings	Axial projection Lateral projection best for visualizing horizontal orientation of spur	Anteroposterior, lateral, axial mortise views Need to rule out various possible fracture sites	Normal	Possible concomitant heel spur	Need to rule out fragmentation and irregularity of calcaneal apophysis
Treatment plan	Ice massage Proper footwear, heel cup or pads Underwater ultrasound Injection of corticosteroid with anesthetic, if condition is refractory to conservative therapy	Referral to orthopedic surgeon Possibly, computed tomography for further evaluation	Use of crutches for 5-7 days Elevation Follow-up radiologic examination, if pain does not subside within 1 week	Ice massage Ultrasound therapy Arch exercises Stretching of heel-cord and plantar fascia Use of heel cups, pads Active rest	Application of ice Activity modification Gentle restoration of Achilles' tendon flexibility

Swelling of the hindfoot is common in the patient with a calcaneal fracture, as well as the inability to bear weight on the involved foot. Calcaneal fractures can occur in a variety of sites and forms:

- Sustentaculum tali
- Anterior process of the calcaneus
- Calcaneal tuberosity
- Calcaneal beak
- Achilles' tendon insertion on the os calcis
- Oblique fracture that spares the subtalar joint
- Depression fracture with or without comminution

In addition, there may be a concomitant fracture of the lower extremity or lumbopelvic spine, and the practitioner must take this into consideration.

The complex anatomy of the calcaneus makes the treatment of these injuries problematic, and there is widespread disagreement over treatment protocols.[77] Most practitioners immobilize the foot with a cast or splint the foot with a bulky dressing. Patients should generally keep weight off the foot for 8 to 12 weeks. Early referral to an orthopedic surgeon is appropriate for all calcaneal fractures to reduce the risk of complications, such as widening of the heel, long-term heel pain, and subtalar arthritis.[56] Follow-up CT studies are often necessary for the evaluation of the fracture, a possible widening of the calcaneus, and the condition of the subtalar joint.

Calcaneal Periostitis (Heel [Stone] Bruise). Although painful, calcaneal periostitis is a simple injury involving a contusion to the periosteum of the heel. The cause is generally a strong external force or fall from a significant height, since the thick fascial heel pad protects the periosteum in most cases. The injury falls short of a fracture, but the heel bruise makes weight bearing difficult for a minimum period of 5 to 7 days.

X-ray films are normal. The patient should use crutches to avoid bearing any weight on the involved foot, apply ice, and elevate the foot. Within 1 or 2 weeks, the pain will decrease and the patient can begin to place some weight on the foot. There are no further complications to the injury.

Plantar Fascitis. In the primary care setting, plantar fascitis is common in adults, and it may have a preceding exertional event. The pain frequently occurs at the medial tubercle of the os calcis at the insertion of the plantar fascia. Some authorities who have reported a high incidence of plantar fascitis in athletes involved in running and jumping sports have termed this condition the "painful heel" syndrome.[11,78]

The cause of plantar fascitis is not well understood. It may start as a strain to the plantar fascia. Inflexibility, especially of the hindfoot and Achilles' tendon complex, may lead to scarring of the fascial attachments as the windlass mechanism attempts to maintain the longitudinal integrity of the foot. Pain may arise from the subcalcaneal bursa, fat pad, tendinous origins of the intrinsic muscles, or medial branch of the calcaneal nerve. As chronic tendon stress increases at the bony-tendinous interface, spurs may begin to form.

The patient usually complains of difficulty in walking when getting out of bed in the morning. Because the heel strike hurts as it stretches the plantar fascia, the individual may attempt to walk on the ball of the foot. Unfortunately, this simply perpetuates heel cord shortening and muscle tightness in the foot flexors. Hyperpronation may further aggravate the condition because it stretches the fascia as well.

Treatment begins with the correction of any biomechanical faults at the foot or ankle, such as pes planus, excessive pronation, or loss of ankle dorsiflexion. Ice massage and stretching of the plantar fascia are also components of the initial treatment. The use of a soft orthosis with a cutout heel cup can alleviate pressure on the painful area. Underwater ultrasound therapy (4- to 8-minute sessions up to four or five times each week for several weeks) can reduce pain as well. Exercises to strengthen the intrinsic foot muscles, especially the tibialis posterior muscle, help improve the integrity of the arch. The patient should wear sneakers or shoes with a good arch support.

Traction Apophysitis of the Os Calcis. The differential diagnosis for heel or Achilles' tendon pain in a growing child must include traction apophysitis of the os calcis (i.e., calcaneal apophysitis, Sever's disease). The child usually has pain from running or jumping and often participates in an organized athletic endeavor. Tenderness is palpable over the insertion of the Achilles' tendon

at the apophysis on the os calcis. Occasionally, there is bogginess over the calcaneus.

Because dorsiflexion stretches the attachment of the tendon, this maneuver reproduces the pain. Radiographic studies should include an axial projection, which frequently shows an irregular or fragmented apophysis, depending on the length and intensity of the pain (Figure 11-33 *A, B*).

Treatment includes the application of ice, the cessation of ballistic movements (e.g., jumping), the stretching of the Achilles' tendon, and a gradual resumption of normal activities. A good sneaker is usually all that the youngster needs, because a heel pad may alter the gait or the dynamics of the lower extremity of a growing child. The key to rehabilitation is the restoration of ankle and heel-cord flexibility to reduce the traction pull on the tendinous apophyseal attachment.

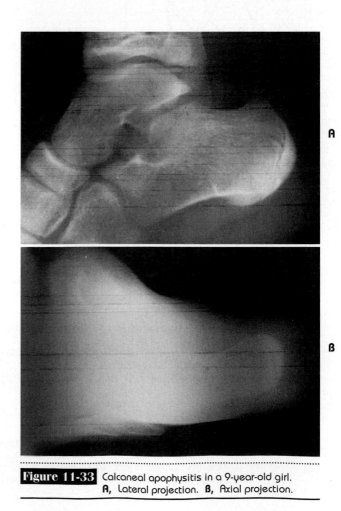

A

B

Figure 11-33 Calcaneal apophysitis in a 9-year-old girl. **A,** Lateral projection. **B,** Axial projection.

Tarsal Tunnel Syndrome

The flexor retinaculum, medial calcaneal wall, postero-medial talus, and posteromedial portion of the distal tibia make up the tarsal tunnel.[66] The condition, known as tarsal tunnel syndrome, involves entrapment of the tibial nerve and its branches in the lower leg, medial ankle, and medial heel. By the time foot pain has prompted the patient to seek care, a significant amount of degeneration and nerve entrapment may have taken place.

The patient may describe numbness and tingling in the toes via the lateral or medial plantar nerves, with or without concomitant heel pain. The plantar nerves branch off from the posterior tibial nerve (Figure 11-34).

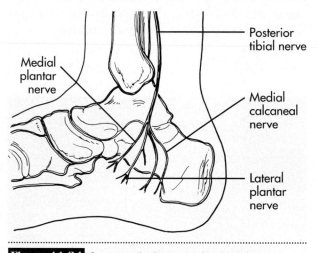

Medial plantar nerve

Posterior tibial nerve

Medial calcaneal nerve

Lateral plantar nerve

Figure 11-34 Posterior tibial nerve and its branches.
(From Post M, editor: *Physical examination of the musculoskeletal system,* St Louis, 1987, Mosby.)

The deep nerve to the abductor digiti minimi branches off from the lateral plantar nerve, passes through the fascial compartment of the tarsal tunnel, and then wraps around the inferior aspect of the calcaneus. At this point a heel spur or arthritic changes of the subcalcaneal region can entrap the nerve. The plantar nerve becomes entrapped just distal to the tarsal tunnel, causing foot and toe pain on the plantar aspect. Electrodiagnostic studies confirm the diagnosis.

In addition to the heel spur commonly seen with the disorder, a planus and pronated foot may be associated with tarsal tunnel syndrome.[75] Night and early morning pain are common. Thus plantar fascitis, gouty arthritis, and systemic illness (e.g., diabetes mellitus) are included in the differential diagnosis.

It can be quite difficult to treat tarsal tunnel syndrome conservatively. Nevertheless, a trial of nonsurgical treatment may be appropriate (Table 11-11). It centers on any arch or rearfoot injury that may have led to mechanical insult.[50] Heel pads or cups, good footwear, and underwater ultrasound therapy may be helpful in alleviating pain. Oral antiinflammatory medication can be used, if necessary; however, a surgical procedure (e.g., decompression of the tarsal tunnel and lysis of the painful nerve) may be required, if the condition interferes with the patient's activities of daily living.

Pes Planus

There are three classes of pes planus, with the first two categories prevailing (Table 11-12). The first, the flexible type of flatfoot, is usually caused by excessive joint mobility at the rearfoot and midfoot articulation, although it is possible to have both normal joint mobility

Table 11-11 Conditions of the Hindfoot

	Tarsal Tunnel Syndrome	Pes Planus
Physical examination findings	Pain emanating to plantar surface of toes, with or without heel pain Often, concomitant heel spurs, arch problems or other rearfoot abnormalities Possible numbness or tingling at night or early morning Need to rule out systemic illness (e.g., diabetes mellitus)	Hyperpronation Dropped navicular Fallen arch on weight bearing Either flexible or rigid foot possible
X-ray findings	Possible calcaneal spur Possible degenerative arthritis in talocrural region	Need to rule out tarsal coalition or accessory navicular bone
Treatment plan	Underwater ultrasound Footwear correction, heel pads, or cups to resolve mechanical faults in arch and rearfoot Electrodiagnostic studies to confirm diagnosis Possible referral to podiatrist or orthopedic surgeon	Arch exercises Footwear modification with arch supports Orthotics

and pes planus. It is common in flexible pes planus to see the foot "roll over" into excessive pronation during walking, however.

In flexible pes planus, the patient does not have a rigid deformity, and the weight-bearing posture exacerbates the flatfoot. The navicular drop test shows pes planus during the examination of the foot. The practitioner places a mark on the tarsal navicular while the foot is in the non–weight-bearing mode. Then, when the patient bears weight on the foot, the practitioner again marks the height of the tarsal navicular from the same reference point to determine whether there has been a drop in its height; the presence of such a drop may indicate a fallen arch. Exercises and orthotics are the usual course of treatment.

Not as common as the first, the second type of pes planus involves a fixed foot. It is the result of an abnormal osseous condition. If the patient is debilitated, surgical recourse may be necessary.

The presence of a planus foot, in itself, does not mandate the use of an orthotic to correct the foot posture. Furthermore, flatfootedness can be the result of a racial or ethnic factor; for example, it is a common condition in African and Native Americans.[71] Many runners and other athletes with pes planus have had great success in competition. Flat feet in children should not cause concern, *especially if the condition is asymptomatic.* In painful cases of pes planus, it is necessary to rule out a tarsal coalition or accessory navicular.[30]

Table 11-12 Classification of Pes Planus

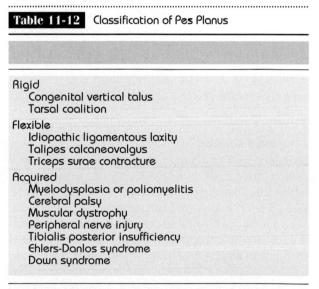

Rigid
  Congenital vertical talus
  Tarsal coalition
Flexible
  Idiopathic ligamentous laxity
  Talipes calcaneovalgus
  Triceps surae contracture
Acquired
  Myelodysplasia or poliomyelitis
  Cerebral palsy
  Muscular dystrophy
  Peripheral nerve injury
  Tibialis posterior insufficiency
  Ehlers-Danlos syndrome
  Down syndrome

From: Post M: *Physical examination of the musculoskeletal system,* St Louis, 1987, Mosby.

What About Orthotics?

It is a mistake to believe that only a foot specialist can alleviate the problem of disabling foot pain. Sometimes, a simple approach is effective. To identify those patients most likely to be helped by an uncomplicated technique, the primary care provider's first task must be to distinguish a flexible from a rigid foot deformity, a manipulative lesion from an advanced malalignment, and a serious deformity from a biomechanical dysfunction.

As strange as it may seem, commercially available or generic orthotics may reduce a mechanical fault and ease the pain of foot dysfunction. Simple arch supports, heel cushions or doughnuts with a cutout for the painful region, and other similar inserts for shoes are all less expensive than most office-prepared orthotics and are worth a trial in treatment. For example, a simple arch support purchased in a drugstore can dramatically alleviate the heel pain of a patient with a planus foot or heel spur.

Placing a soft material or insert beneath the first metatarsal head or transverse arch of the forefoot may encourage dorsiflexion during push-off of the great toe. The resultant shortening at the plantar aponeurosis lifts the arch and encourages supination. Thus this approach may benefit the patient with rearfoot pronation or pes planus.

The patient whose condition is refractory to the use of purchased or generic orthotics and those who have a severe deformity or advanced dysfunction may need an office-prepared orthotic and a podiatric evaluation. Flexible, custom-made orthotics may improve the capacity of a rigid cavus foot to absorb shock and help distribute weight more equally along the plantar surface.

Whether purchased or custom-made, orthotics have several functions designed to improve the working capability of the foot. The following is a list of their uses:

- Compensation for foot deformity
- Reduction of impact forces on the foot
- Increased ability of subtalar joint to function in the neutral position
- Treatment of overuse problems, such as tendonitis or fasciitis
- Alteration of malalignment problems
- Improvement in overall foot function

Midfoot

Although infrequently reported and poorly understood, joint dysfunction of the midfoot can be the cause of nagging discomfort and gait abnormality. The midfoot links the subtalar joint to the forefoot. Because the tarsals provide a conduit for movement generated at the hindfoot and culminated at the forefoot, tarsal fixation or hypomobility can alter gait, propulsion, and foot flexibility.

The articulation at the calcaneocuboidal and talocrural interface generates movement in a plane perpendicular to the joint surfaces. Although the former is a saddle joint and the latter is a condyloid joint, the midfoot acts as a communicator with the foot in the "locked" position as the forefoot moves in direct relationship with the hindfoot.[57] Pronation and supination begin with the hindfoot, for example, but take place via the subtalar articulation through the midtarsal joint.[79]

As in the evaluation of the hindfoot and subtalar joints, the clinician examines the midfoot with the patient in both the non–weight-bearing and upright positions. To assess the status of the arch, the clinician pays careful attention to the navicular bone during the navicular drop test. Inspection for anatomic deformity, malalignment, or joint abnormality during walking focuses not only on the midfoot, but also on the lower extremity. Finally, the practitioner checks the movement of the midtarsal articulation and makes bilateral comparisons for end feel and congruency of motion.

The midtarsal complex consists of two main joints: the talonavicular and calcaneocuboidal. The manual evaluation of both should be part of any midfoot examination. For the talonavicular joint, the examiner checks the anteroposterior (dorsal-plantar) glide with the patient in the supine position. Stabilizing the talus with the proximal hand, the examiner grasps the tarsal navicular with the thumb and forefinger of the inferior or active hand.[81] This technique restores joint mobility to the medial aspect of the midtarsal complex.

Under normal conditions, the calcaneocuboidal joint also provides for anteroposterior (dorsal-plantar) glide. With the patient in either the supine or standing position, the practitioner may perform a manipulative procedure called the "cuboid snap" to restore joint motion. The patient bends the knee to approximately 60 degrees while the clinician grasps the calcaneocuboidal articulation between the thumb and forefinger of both hands. The "snap" move is similar to the carpal snap in manipulating the lunate bone.

Most midfoot injuries seen in primary care are the result of overuse or of a sudden change in exertional activities. Extensor tendonitis and tarsal (midtarsal) dysfunction are directly related to overuse. Metatarsal fractures and tubercle deformities are usually the result of macrotraumatic events, such as violent supination of the foot in sports (e.g., basketball, baseball). Some tarsal conditions can remain dormant and asymptomatic, only to become a problem when the individual begins to participate strenuously in an athletic activity.

Extensor Tendonitis

Pain over the extensor tendon sheath on the proximal aspect of the dorsum of the foot is characteristic of extensor tendonitis. Swelling and erythema localized over the extensor tendons are evident, and stretching of the tendons is painful. Inflammation usually involves the inferior extensor retinaculum, because it contains the tendons of the three major muscles for dorsiflexion of the foot: the anterior tibialis, extensor digitorum longus, and extensor hallucis longus. The pain may branch out more distally over the individual tendon affected from the midtarsal joint to the region of the metatarsal heads. In acute cases of inflammation, pinpoint palpation can elicit a painful response. Heel walking can provoke pain if the injury is acute.

Although the cause of extensor tendonitis is generally overuse, certain activities can precipitate the condition. Jumping or running on hills, especially running downhill, can lead to inflammation of the foot extensors. Ski boots or tight running shoes can cause a local irritation over the extensor retinaculum.

Treatment includes rest, the application of ice, electrotherapy (in cool water if the pain is distal to the extensor retinaculum and more aggressive treatment is necessary to overcome the effects of gravity), and a well-padded, properly fitted shoe (Figure 11-35). Most patients do well with a relatively short course of conservative treatment and activity modification (Table 11-13).

Tarsal Coalition

Described as a structural abnormality in the midtarsal joint, a tarsal coalition involves a fibrous or an osseous bridge that spans the talocalcaneal or calcaneonavicular joint. A bony bar or a cartilaginous defect may be present.

Patients with a tarsal coalition may have unremitting foot and ankle pain or an extended period of pain and dysfunction after a mild ankle sprain.[7] It is common to find a concomitant inflexible case of pes planus. (Thus the plain x-ray films of anyone with a painful, rigid flatfoot, particularly children and active adolescents, require

Table 11-13 Problems of the Midfoot

	Extensor Tendonitis	Tarsal Coalition	Accessory Navicular	Proximal Fifth Metatarsal Fracture
Physical examination findings	Palpable tenderness over dorsum of foot Pain over extensor retinaculum Passive stretching painful Point tenderness over involved tendon Bogginess or swelling over extensor tendons of foot and ankle	Loss of hindfoot motion Peroneal shortening, subtalar hypomobility Possible rigid flatfoot	Bony prominence over navicular bone Palpable tenderness over os, if symptomatic Possible pes planus	Palpable tenderness over proximal aspect of fifth metatarsal History of violent inversion or forced supination of foot Difficulty inverting or supinating foot Swelling at base of fifth metatarsal
X-ray findings	Normal	Cartilaginous, fibrous, or osseous bridge at talonavicular joint	Difficulty in identifying accessory bone	Need to rule out Jones fracture of diaphysis and tuberosity
Treatment plan	Application of ice Electrotherapy Use of proper footwear Activity modification	CT or MRI to outline congenital deformity Symptoms as the focus of treatment CMT for lumbopelvic or lower extremity dysfunction Flexibility program for rearfoot–Achilles' tendon junction	Application of ice Massage Use of proper footwear Use of arch support or flexible orthotic device, if required	Referral to orthopedic surgeon

CMT, Chiropractic manipulative therapy; **CT,** computed tomography; **MRI,** magnetic resonance imaging.

careful inspection for a tarsal coalition.) The combination of a rigid flatfoot with a subsequent loss of rearfoot movement markedly decreases subtalar motion (i.e., inversion, eversion) and leads to peroneal contracture. Many of these individuals are asymptomatic unless a traumatic event brings the problem to the attention of a practitioner, however.

A talocalcaneal coalition is difficult to detect radiographically, and a calcaneonavicular coalition may need axial or oblique films to reveal a beak of the talus. Preferable routes for inquiry include CT and MRI scans in coalition cases (Figure 11-36 *A, B*). Similar to CT, MRI aids in the diagnosis when plain films are inconclusive. Furthermore, fibrous coalition is more difficult to visualize on CT than on MRI.[64]

Treatment centers around symptoms such as stiffness and contracture. The prescription of flexibility exercises for a shortened Achilles' tendon, as well as arch support for pes planus, is appropriate. Chiropractic manipulative therapy to the lumbopelvic spine may be necessary for chronic joint fixation secondary to faulty ambulation.

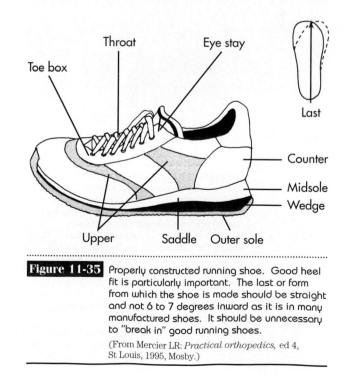

Figure 11-35 Properly constructed running shoe. Good heel fit is particularly important. The last or form from which the shoe is made should be straight and not 6 to 7 degrees inward as it is in many manufactured shoes. It should be unnecessary to "break in" good running shoes.

(From Mercier LR: *Practical orthopedics*, ed 4, St Louis, 1995, Mosby.)

Accessory Navicular Bone

There are many sesamoid and accessory bones in the foot (Figure 11-37). One of the most common is the accessory navicular bone (sometimes called the os navicular

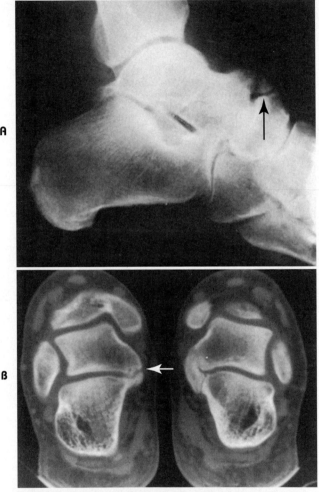

A

B

Figure 11-36 Talocalcaneal coalition. **A,** Secondary signs are evident, including talar breaking and talonavicular degenerative changes. Anterior navicular osteophyte with cartilaginous or fibrous component is present (arrow). This should not be confused with a fracture. **B,** Coronal computed tomography scan of both ankles shows bilateral coalitions at middle facets. In the right ankle (arrow) fusion is cartilaginous or fibrous as evidenced by irregularity and narrowing of middle facet and cortical hyperostosis. Left ankle is also fused at middle facet by what was once a solid osseous bar.

(From Nicholas JA, Hershman EB, editors: *The lower extremity and spine in sports medicine,* ed 2, vol 1, St Louis, 1995, Mosby.)

or the os tibiale externum), which lies near the navicular tuberosity. Although these structures are usually asymptomatic, mechanical pressures in the active adolescent years may cause symptoms. For example, a large accessory bone or the pressure of ill-fitting shoes may irritate local areas. Symptoms are more likely to develop in female than in male adolescents.[31] Pes planus may be associated with the presence of an accessory navicular bone.

Physical examination reveals a bony prominence over the navicular bone on the medial aspect of the midtarsal region. This scenario differs from that of Köhler's disease, which is usually found in the young child (i.e., 4 to 8 years of age)and involves osteochondritis of the navicular bone.[61] It can be difficult to isolate the accessory bone in radiographic analysis, because it may appear to be an apophysis; however, the tarsal navicular bone *does not have an apophysis.* The basis for diagnosis is the history, a careful examination, and radiographic evidence of bone. A minimum of three projections is necessary for a diagnostic evaluation.

Treatment is usually conservative and palliative. An arch support is often helpful in cases of exaggerated pes planus. Orthotic prescription is beneficial if the material is flexible. It is necessary to avoid rigid orthotics, however, because they add to the pressure over the bony prominence of the accessory navicular and thus increase the patient's symptoms.[17] Massage therapy may also be useful.

Fracture of the Proximal Fifth Metatarsal

Although fairly common in athletes, osseous injury to the proximal aspect of the fifth metatarsal can pose a diagnostic challenge to the primary care practitioner. All injuries are not the same in this region, especially those involving bony defects. The plethora of anatomic structures that attach to the proximal fifth metatarsal makes this area dynamic in nature. The peroneus brevis and tertius, abductor digiti minimi and flexor minimi, interosseous muscle, joint capsule, and lateral cord of the plantar aponeurosis all insert in this area.[12]

Among the structures at the proximal fifth metatarsal that can be fractured are the tuberosity and proximal diaphysis (i.e., Jones fracture). The mechanism of injury for the fracture of the tuberosity is often similar to that of a lateral ankle sprain, since the individual "rolls over" the ankle in a plantar flexion-inversion stress mode. Avulsion forces play a major role in this mechanism of injury. This particular injury is common in both baseball and basketball players, who forcibly supinate the foot, sometimes landing on an object (e.g., first base) or the foot of another player. A fracture to the tuberosity usually heals completely and uneventfully with conservative treatment, including cast immobilization.

The cause of a Jones fracture may be repetitive stress from overuse or blunt trauma. If detected with scintigraphy in the acute stage—before changes are visible on x-ray films—a Jones fracture heals well with conservative care. Chronic injury accompanied by radiographic evidence of sclerosis, however, may require surgical bone grafting.

In youngsters and adolescent athletes with a history of fifth metatarsal trauma, the apophysis of the fifth metatarsal is usually apparent on a radiographic film (Figure 11-38 *A, B*). Its presentation changes with age, because it appears first at the age of 7 to 10 years and closes by the age of 16 years.[12] On the lateral x-ray film, a small fleck of bone longitudinally positioned from the lateral aspect of the fifth metatarsal represents the apophysis. In all cases of suspected or confirmed radiographic osseous injury in this region, it is wise to consult an orthopedic surgeon.

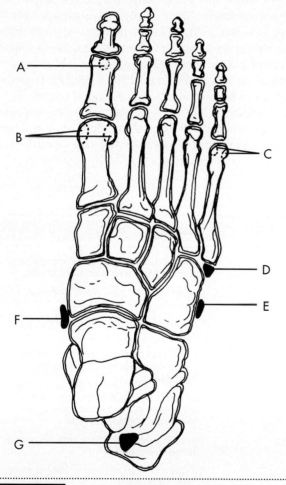

Figure 11-37 Common accessory bones of the foot. **A,** Interphalangeal accessory. **B,** Sesamoids of great toe. **C,** Sesamoids under fifth metatarsal head. **D,** Os vesalianum. **E,** Os peroneum in peroneus longus tendon. **F,** Os tibiale externum or accessory navicular, and **G,** os trigonum.

(From Post M, editor: *Physical examination of the musculoskeletal system,* St Louis, 1987, Mosby.)

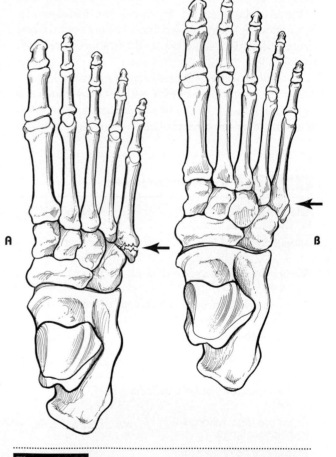

Figure 11-38 Jones fracture. **A,** The horizontal orientation of the fracture line is perpendicular to the long axis of the fifth metatarsal (arrow). **B,** The Jones fracture must be differentiated from the normal secondary growth center (arrow) of the styloid process of the fifth metatarsal base. The vertical orientation of the physis is parallel to the metatarsal shaft.

(From Deltoff MN, Kogan PL: *The portable skeletal x-ray library,* St Louis, 1998, Mosby.)

Forefoot

A combination of trauma and soft-tissue deformity is the most likely cause of an abnormality of the forefoot (Table 11-14). Clinical findings in each diagnosis determine whether conservative care is appropriate. Excessive pain, deformity, or dysfunction may warrant a referral to a podiatric or orthopedic surgeon, however.

The Hallux

Any osseous or soft-tissue pathologic condition around the hallux, often called the great toe, can potentially cause severe foot dysfunction. For example, the hallux serves as an anchor in medial foot stabilization because of the attachment of the plantar aponeurosis on the base of the proximal phalanx.[47] Pathologic joint malalignment (hallux valgus), joint hypomobility (hallux rigidus), and other dysfunctions can seriously alter the mechanical role of the hallux.

Hallux Valgus. Described as a subluxation of the first metatarsophalangeal joint, hallux valgus culminates in medial deviation of the first metatarsal and in lateral deviation of the proximal phalanx.[15] Bony and soft-tissue enlargement at the metatarsophalangeal joint is the primary feature of a bunion (Figure 11-39). This deformity occurs primarily in women, and it runs in families. Wearing improper footwear, such as ill-fitting shoes, also plays a role in the development of this condition.

As the soft tissues around the hallux become inflamed and tender, a compensatory deformity in hyperextension causes calluses to form at the second toe. Osseous deviations and deformities at the great toe become visible on radiographic films, and there is a possibility of a bony extensor of the metatarsophalangeal joint.

The use of sneakers and the avoidance of rigid dress shoes, which have a notoriously narrow toe box, are the keys to treatment (Table 11-15). The application of cold and underwater ultrasound therapy can aid in alleviating the pain and swelling of a flare-up. Consistent impairment of gait, frequent painful episodes, and general interference with the patient's ability to lead a satisfactory and active life are indications for surgical correction.

Hallux Rigidus. Appearing primarily in people who are in late middle age, hallux rigidus is a dorsal compression of the metatarsophalangeal joint. It can be a di-

---

Table 11-14 Causes of Distal Foot Pain

Site of Pain	Diagnosis	Cause(s)
Lateral dorsum of foot into toes	Sural neuritis	Contusion, compression of lateral sural cutaneous nerve from tight shoes
Medial or lateral plantar surface of foot and toes	Tarsal tunnel syndrome, medial or lateral plantar neuritis	Osteoarthritis, heel spur, diabetes, trauma
Between third and fourth or between fourth and fifth toes	Morton's neuroma	Growth of benign tumor on interdigital nerve
Metatarsal head	Metatarsalgia	Mechanical overuse, anatomic status (e.g., cavus foot), inflammatory conditions
Plantar aspect of first metatarsophalangeal joint at flexor hallucis tendon	Sesamoiditis	Traumatic episode of violent hyperextension of metatarsophalangeal joint, mechanical overuse
Great toe, first metatarsophalangeal joint	Hallux valgus, hallux rigidus	Heredity, degenerative arthritis, poorly fitted footwear
Metatarsophalangeal joint (extension deformity), proximal interphalangeal joint (flexor deformity)	Hammer toes	Congenital factors, hallux valgus, poorly fitted footwear
Metatarsophalangeal joint (volar displacement), interphalangeal joint (flexor deformity)	Claw toes	Congenital factors, cavus foot
Distal interphalangeal joint (flexor contracture)	Mallet toes	Trauma

rect result of degenerative arthritis of the metatarsophalangeal articulation, although runners and ballet dancers may develop the condition through overuse. It may be associated with a bunion.[8] The telltale signs are pain (frequently on passive extension of the great toe) and a lack of dorsiflexion at the first metatarsophalangeal joint. The toe is not always swollen. Many individuals with hallux rigidus have experienced previous discomfort and injury, and they may find forefoot propulsion and heel raises difficult to perform.

Radiographic findings are consistent with osteoarthritis; they include the typical narrowing, eburnation, and spurring at the joint. Gentle manipulation of the first metatarsophalangeal joint, cold therapy, or therapeutic ultrasound performed underwater may provide temporary relief. For resistant cases, it may be necessary to prescribe antiinflammatory medication and to recommend the use of a metatarsal bar. Wearing footwear with a wide toe box and a proper cushion (e.g., a good pair of walking shoes or sneakers) is advisable.

Phalangeal Deformities

Deformation of the toes can be congenital (e.g., webbing of the toes, an absent digit, an extra digit) or acquired (e.g., the result of blunt trauma). Plain x-ray films are always initially necessary to determine whether there is a fracture. Deformation of the lesser toes, such as Morton's foot (longer second toe), may accompany deformities of the hallux and congenital forefoot malformations.[69] An overlapping fifth toe is a fairly common deformity that warrants evaluation during examination.

When examining a patient with a phalangeal complaint, the clinician puts each joint of the toes through active motion and, if there is a deformity, determines how rigid it is. In addition, the practitioner generally checks the dorsum and plantar surfaces for abnormal skin response to pressure. Internal pressure from a bony outgrowth, combined with external mechanical pressure (from a tight shoe, for example), often produces corns and skin calluses. These findings are consistent with underlying pathologic deformities. A podiatrist can alleviate pressure by applying a pad or shaving these skin lesions. Treatment of the specific phalangeal deformity should be prompt, particularly if there is a risk of progression and disability.

Hammer Toe. A flexor deformity at the proximal interphalangeal joint with a hyperextended metatarsophalangeal articulation is a hammer toe. Because the

Table 11-15	Conditions of the Hallux	
	Hallux Valgus	**Hallux Rigidus**
Physical examination findings	Lateral deviation of great toe Bony enlargement, soft-tissue deformity at metatarsophalangeal joint Callus formation at forefoot	Tenderness at first metatarsophalangeal joint Limited, painful dorsiflexion of great toe
X-ray findings	Bony deformity at great toe Subluxation of metatarsophalangeal joint	Evidence of degenerative arthritis at first metatarsophalangeal joint
Treatment plan	Use of proper footwear Application of ice Therapeutic ultrasound Referral to orthopedic or podiatric surgeon in resistant cases	Use of proper footwear Gentle manipulation Application of ice Underwater ultrasound

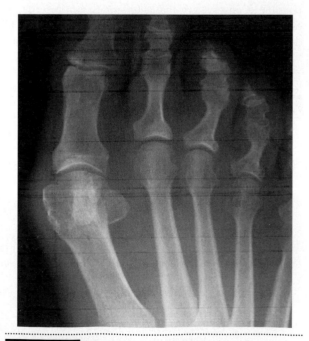

Figure 11-39 Hallux valgus with bunion exostosis.

(From Mercier LR: *Practical orthopedics*, ed 4, St Louis, 1995, Mosby.)

proximal phalanx extends up, a callus or corn usually develops on the dorsum of the foot at the proximal segment. In cases of severe deformity, the metatarsal head is subluxed toward the sole of the foot; as a result of the abnormal position of the toe, the shoe can irritate the skin and lead to a painful skin lesion in this location as well.

Tight, poorly fitted shoes can once again be contributing factors, along with hallux valgus. If the patient has a hallux valgus deformity, it frequently occurs at the second toe.

Mobilization or manipulation that straightens the proximal phalanx may resolve mild cases of hammer toes (Table 11-16). Rigid, advanced cases may require surgical correction, however, so referral to a podiatric surgeon is advisable.

Claw Toe. Often associated with a cavus foot, the claw toe is an extension deformity at the metatarsophalangeal joint with a concomitant flexing or "clawing" of the toe at both the proximal and distal interphalangeal joints. The claw toe deformity indicates a weakness of the intrinsic muscles of the foot and warrants screening for a neurologic disorder. The condition occurs in more than one toe at a time, and bilateral involvement is common.

As with other toe malalignments, the clinician first determines whether passive correction of the problem is possible. Conservative management (e.g., prescription of stretching exercises) is often successful with flexible deformities, although the foot position may make it diffi-cult to fit footwear properly. In fact, some patients may need an orthosis to ensure a proper fit. Advanced cases of claw toes may require consultation with an orthopedic or podiatric surgeon.

Mallet Toe. Most commonly seen in a single toe, a mallet toe involves a flexion deformity at the distal interphalangeal joint; it is the result of a flexor contraction of the end joint. On physical examination and gait assessment, the problem is obvious. Furthermore, there is usually a corn on the top of the involved toe because the position of the toe causes it to dig into the shoe.

Frequent visits to the podiatrist, who can shave the skin or callus down, alleviates the pressure. Because the difficulty usually involves the fourth toe, it is possible to treat the condition by taping the distal portions of the fourth and fifth digits to each other in the neutral position.

Sesamoiditis

The function of the great toe and first metatarsal head is crucial in weight bearing and dynamic propulsion; it is easy to see how active individuals can develop a problem in the region of the two small sesamoid bones, which lie in the tendon of the flexor hallucis brevis muscle beneath the first metatarsophalangeal joint. Athletes such as those who run long distances and those who use cleated shoes or spikes are extremely vulnerable to injury of the sesamoids. Moreover, the close proximity of the medial digital nerve to the medial sesamoid can complicate an injury in this area.

Table 11-16 Phalangeal Deformities

	Hammer Toe	Claw Toe	Mallet Toe
Physical examination findings	Flexor deformity in proximal interphalangeal joint Commonly seen with hallux valgus Second toe often affected Volar displacement of metatarsal head or affected toe	Passive correction possible, if deformity is flexible Commonly seen with cavus foot Intrinsic muscle weakness Volar displacement of metatarsophalangeal articulation with interphalangeal flexor deformity	Flexor contraction at distal interphalangeal joint Typically, corn on top of involved toe
X-ray findings	Usually seen, if flexor deformity is large	Visible on lateral film	Not usually significant
Treatment plan	Use of proper footwear Concomitant treatment of hallux valgus, if present Manipulation to reduce deformity Referral to podiatric surgeon in severe cases	Need to rule out neurologic disease Stretching exercises in flexible cases Referral to orthotist for footwear Referral to orthopedist or podiatrist for severe deformity	Use of soft footwear to relieve callus buildup Buddy taping Referral to podiatrist to relieve pressure

Athletes with intermittent pain at the first metatarsal head over a long period of time may have a fractured or "cracked" sesamoid bone. Violent hyperextension of the great toe can also fracture the sesamoid bone. Such a fracture appears as either a fracture line or fragmentation on an anteroposterior foot projection (Figure 11-40). Fractures of the medial sesamoid may often appear to be sesamoiditis, metatarsalgia, or, in some cases, a stress fracture. The medial sesamoid is often bipartite, which contributes to the clinical confusion. A nuclear bone scan will aid in the diagnosis.[28]

Because the sesamoid bones are so essential in weight bearing, the individual with an injured or inflamed sesamoid bone finds it quite painful to ambulate. Rest, the application of ice, taping or strapping the toe, and a limited use of crutches are the usual components of treatment. The importance of the function of these bones eliminates surgical intervention as an option; they should be left in place and treated conservatively (Table 11-17).

Metatarsalgia

The term *metatarsalgia* refers to an acute or chronic pain syndrome involving the metatarsal heads. Such pain may prevent the extension of the metatarsophalangeal joints that is necessary to negotiate the dynamics of gait.

It has a variety of possible causes, including overuse, anatomic malalignment, foot deformity, or degenerative processes in the forefoot (Table 11-18). Any condition that drastically changes the forces of normal weight bearing, such as weight gain and a fallen arch, can cause this problem.

Tenderness under the lesser metatarsal heads generally is the result of pathomechanical compensation for an adjacent injury, such as sesamoiditis or hallux valgus. The hyperextension associated with hammer or claw toes can also cause metatarsalgia.[29] Callus formation in the plantar aspect of the head of the affected metatarsal is common. Freiberg's disease of the second metatarsophalangeal joint may also be a contributing factor.

Metatarsalgia at the great toe usually is the result of a traumatic episode or degenerative arthritis. Patients with metatarsalgia should undergo screening for hallux valgus or rigidus, as well as for sesamoiditis. In addition, these patients may have a cavus foot.

Treatment for metatarsalgia consists of soaks for callus formation, modification of footwear with foot pads or inserts, and a referral to an orthopedist or orthotist for a metatarsal bar in cases of advanced disease and disability. Cryotherapy can help to control initial pain and swelling, if any.

Table 11-17   Sesamoiditis, Metatarsalgia, and Morton's Neuroma

	Sesamoiditis	Metatarsalgia	Morton's Neuroma
Physical examination findings	Palpable tenderness at first metatarsophalangeal joint Swelling at head of first metatarsal Pain on extension of great toe	Palpable tenderness over plantar aspect of metatarsophalangeal joint Pain at metatarsal head reproduced by extension of metatarsophalangeal joint Cavus foot commonly associated	Tenderness to pressure at affected interspace between heads of metatarsals Usually 3-4 interspace affected Limited, painful extension of metatarsophalangeal joint
X-ray findings	Possibly, normal Fracture of sesamoid possible, usually medial sesamoid Need to rule out bipartite medial sesamoid	Degenerative changes sometimes seen in metatarsophalangeal joint Need to rule out concomitant, adjacent deformities or degenerative conditions	Need to rule out concomitant degeneration or arthritic conditions
Treatment plan	Rest Application of ice Taping or strapping Crutches to avoid weight bearing for a limited time, if injury is from acute trauma	Cryotherapy Shoe modification Restoration of normal gait Metatarsal pads, inserts, or bars	Underwater ultrasound Metatarsal pads Use of proper footwear Referral for steroid injection, if necessary Neurectomy as last resort

The High Price of Fashion

A majority of the foot problems seen in women are the direct result of dress shoes. Many women insist on wearing high-fashion shoes with high heels and narrow, rigid toe boxes because they believe that these shoes create a longer leg line and a more "feminine" appearance. These women often pay a price in the form of pain, however. High heels place the foot into an equinus position, which transmits an enormous amount of stress onto the metatarsal heads during weight-bearing activities and causes a shortening of the Achilles' tendon that, in turn, leads to hindfoot inflexibility.[70] In addition, the narrow, pointy toe box causes deformities of the phalanges and can lead to hammer toes, claw toes, bunions, corns, and calluses. Walking in a "moderate" 3-inch heel can also cause lower back pain.

Most foot conditions resulting from dress shoes respond to conservative care, including the purchase of shoes that are properly fitted (Table 11-19). Women should wear their high-fashion shoes only on special occasions and their sneakers during leisure time. The practitioner should ask those who resist this change in footwear to remove their shoes and stand next to them. When they observe that their feet are clearly bigger than the narrow shoe, it will become "painfully" apparent to them that they must make the recommended concessions to eliminate foot pain. Above all, these patients should remember the general rule: the lower the heel, the better.

Morton's Neuroma

Fibrosis in the perineural region of the intermetatarsal plantar digital nerve is the pathologic condition that underlies Morton's neuroma. The patient may have a chief complaint of metatarsalgia, and the pain may extend, with paresthesia, into the toe. Motion at the metatarsophalangeal joint, especially extension, aggravates the symptoms. The patient may experience a burning or deep aching pain from the neuroma. It is more common at the interspace between the third and fourth toes (i.e., 3-4 interspace), but it can occur in the intermetatarsal region (i.e., the 2-3 interspace).[29]

With the thumb, the practitioner places pressure at the interspace between the heads of the metatarsals in the region affected to find any immobility that suggests a degenerative condition at the metatarsophalangeal joint. A bunion, which is often seen with a neuroma, can contribute to an increased pressure on the lateral metatarsals. The use of narrow footwear aggravates interdigital neuromas because of inadequate toe room.[1]

Treatment centers on the use of underwater ultrasound in cool water, metatarsal pads, good footwear, and possibly a referral for a steroid injection. Only cases recalcitrant to these interventions require referral for surgical neurectomy.

Table 11-18 Causes of Metatarsalgia

Primary metatarsalgia
  Statis disorders of forefoot
  Iatrogenic after forefoot surgery
  Hallux valgus or rigidus
  Freiberg's disease
Secondary metatarsalgia
  Stress fracture of metatarsal bone
  Sesamoid abnormality
  Rheumatoid arthritis
  Neurogenic disorders
Other forefoot pain
  Morton's metatarsalgia
  Tarsal tunnel syndrome
  Plantar warts
  Plantar fibromatosis

From: Post M: *Physical examination of the musculoskeletal system*, St Louis, 1987, Mosby.

Table 11-19 Shoe Prescription for Foot Problems

Condition	Shoe Prescription
Foot pronation	Shoes with control features, such as strong heel counters
Pes cavus	Well-cushioned and padded shoes
Pes planus	Shoes with sufficient internal arch support
Osteoarthritic foot	Shoes with a strong and rigid midsole
Phalangeal deformities	Flexible shoes with a wide and ample toe box

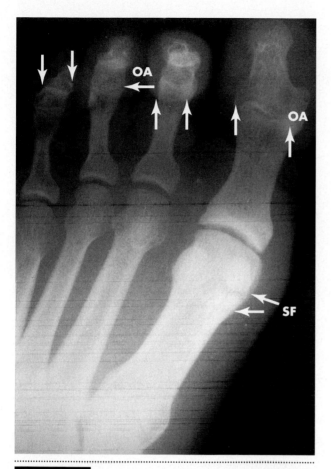

Figure 11-40 Fracture line and separation through the medial sesamoid in the flexor hallucis brevis tendon (SF) of a 53-year-old tennis player with a history of intermittent and chronic pain in the forefoot and metatarsals. Note the typical osteoarthritic changes (OA) at the distal interphalangeal joints.

Review Questions

1. Name the three compartments of the lower leg and the anatomic structures in each compartment.
2. Rear foot pronation has been associated with several musculoskeletal conditions. State which articulation is involved in pronation and the conditions that may arise with this pathomechanical situation.
3. (a) Name the broad, strong ligament that resists eversion at the medial aspect of the ankle joint. (b) What conditions are associated with eversion trauma? (c) Standard x-ray films for this injury include which projections?
4. What are the keys to a successful outcome in treating lateral ankle sprains?
5. Your female patient exhibits faulty gait mechanics, including insufficient heel strike with a pronounced toe-off phase. (a) What conditions may become evident on examination of the lower leg and foot? (b) What pathomechanical condition may exist as a result of high-fashion footwear?
6. (a) What is the most common cause of tarsal tunnel syndrome? (b) What other conditions must be considered in the differential diagnosis?

References

1. Alexander IJ: *The foot: examination and diagnosis,* New York, 1980, Churchill Livingstone.
2. American Academy of Orthopaedic Surgeons: *Athletic training and sports medicine,* Chicago, 1984, AAOS.
3. Anderson IF, Crichton KJ, Grattan-Smith T et al: Osteochondral fractures of the dome of the talus, *J Bone Joint Surg [Br]* 71(8):1143, 1989.
4. Ashton-Miller JA, Ottaviani RA, Hutchinson C et al: What best protects the inverted weightbearing ankle against further inversion? *Am J Sports Med* 24:800, 1996.
5. Attarian DE, McCracken HS, DeVito DP et al: Biomechanical characteristics of human ankle ligaments, *Foot Ankle* 6(2):54, 1985.
6. Balduini FC: Compartment syndromes, *Postgraduate Adv Sports Med,* vol 2, Berryville, Vir, 1987, Forum Medicum.
7. Bassewitz HL, Shapiro MS: Persistent pain after ankle sprain: targeting the cause, *Phys Sports Med* 25(12), 1997.
8. Baxter DE: Treatment of bunion deformity in the athlete, *Orthop Clin North Am* 25(1):37, 1994.
9. Bogden R: Biomechanical principles of running injuries. In Valmassy RL, editor: *The lower extremities,* St Louis, 1996, Mosby.
10. Buschbacher RM: Ankle sprain evaluation and bracing. In Buschbacher RM, Braddom RL, editors: *Sports medicine and rehabilitation: a sport-specific approach,* St Louis, 1994, Mosby.
11. Busseuil C, Freychat P, Guedj EB, Lacour JR: Rearfoot-forefoot orientation and traumatic risk for runners, *Foot Ankle Int* 19:32, 1998.
12. Carlsen TJ: The proximal fifth metatarsal fracture: is it a "Jones fracture?" *Postgraduate Adv Sports Med,* Pennington, NJ, 1986, Forum Medicum.
13. Cave EF: Fracture of the calcis: the problem in general, *Clin Orthop* 30:64, 1963.
14. Chandler TJ: Muscle strength and ankle sprains, strength and conditioning, *Strength and Conditioning* 19(4):39, 1997.
15. Churchill RS, Donley BG: Managing injuries of the great toe, *Phys Sports Med* 26(9), 1998.
16. Clanton TO: Instability of the subtalar joint, *Orthop Clin North Am* 20(4):583, 1989.
17. Conti SF: Posterior tibial tendon problems in athletes, *Orthop Clin North Am* 25(1):118, 1994.

18. Cox TS: Surgical and non-surgical treatment of acute ankle sprains, *Clin Orthop* 198:118, 1988.

19. Davis AW, Alexander IJ: Problematic fracture and dislocations in the foot and ankle of athletes, *Clin Sports Med* 9(1):163, 1990.

20. Deltoff MN, Kogan PL: *The portable skeletal x-ray library,* St Louis, 1998, Mosby.

21. De Smet AA, Fisher DR, Burnstein MI et al: Value of MR imaging in staging osteochondral lesions of the talus: results in 14 patients, *Am J Roentgenol* 154:555, 1990.

22. Engsberg JR: A new method for quantifying pronation in over-pronating and normal runners, *Med Sci Sports Exercise* 28(3):299, 1996.

23. Flick AB, Gould N: Osteochondritis dissecans of the talus: review of the literature and new surgical approach for medial dome lesions, *Foot Ankle* 5:165,1985.

24. Garrick JG: The frequency of injury, mechanism of injury, and epidemiology of ankle sprains, *Am J Sports Med* 5:241, 1977.

25. Gehlsen GM, Pearson D, Bahamarde R: Ankle joint strength, total work, and ROM: comparison between prophylactic devices, *Athletic Training* 26:62, 1991.

26. Gerber L: Foot and ankle problems in the arthritides, *J Musculoskeletal Med* 6(12):13, 1989.

27. Giladi M, Milgrom C, Simkin A et al: Stress fractures: identifiable risk factors, *Am J Sports Med* 19(6):647, 1991.

28. Glick JM, Sampson TG: Ankle and foot fractures in athletes. In Nicholas JA, Hershman EB, editors: *The lower extremity and spine in sports medicine,* ed 2, vol 1, St Louis, 1995, Mosby.

29. Gould JS: Metatarsalgia, *Orthop Clin North Am* 20(4):553, 1989.

30. Griffin LY: Common sports injuries of the foot and ankle seen in children and adolescents, *Orthop Clin North Am* 25(1):85, 1994.

31. Grogan DP, Gasser SI, Ogden JA: The painful accessory navicular: a clinical and histopathological study, *Foot Ankle* 10:164, 1989.

32. Hicks JH: The mechanisms of the foot, *J Anat* 88:25, 1954.

33. Hossler P, Maffei P: Podiatric examination techniques for in-the-field assessments, *Athletic Training* 25(4):311, 1990.

34. Jackson DW, Ashley RL, Powell JW: Ankle sprains in young athletes: relation of severity and disability, *Clin Orthop* 101:201, 1984.

35. Jones D, James SL: Overuse injury of the lower extremity, *Clin Sports Med* 6(2):275, 1987.

36. Jones DC, Singer KM: Soft-tissue conditions of the ankle and foot. In Nicholas JA, Hershman EB, editors: *The lower extremity and the spine in sports medicine,* ed 2, vol 1, St Louis, 1995, Mosby.

37. Keene J, Lange RH: Diagnostic dilemmas in foot and ankle injuries, *JAMA* 256(2):247, 1986.

38. Kingston S: Magnetic resonance imaging of the ankle and foot, *Clin Sports Med* 7(1):21, 1988.

39. Konradsen L, Olesen S, Hansen HM: Ankle sensorimotor control and eversion after acute ankle inversion injuries, *Am J Sports Med* 26:72, 1998.

40. Lassiter TE, Malone TR, Garrett WE: Injury to the lateral ligaments of the ankle, *Orthop Clin North Am* 20(4):629, 1989.

41. Lazzarini KM, Troiano RN, Smith RC: Can running cause the appearance of marrow edema on MR images of the foot and ankle? *Radiology* 202:540, 1997.

42. Lutte LD: Pronation biomechanisms in runners, *Contemp Orthop* 2:579, 1980.

43. Mack RP: Ankle injuries in athletes, *Clin Sports Med* 1:75, 1982.

44. McManama GB Jr: Ankle injuries in the young athlete, *Clin Sports Med* 7(3):556, 1988.

45. Maehlums Dalijord OA: Acute sports injuries in Oslo—a one year study, *Br J Sports Med* 18:181, 1984.

46. Marder RA: Current methods for the evaluation of ankle ligament injuries, *J Bone Joint Surg (Am)* 76(7):1103, 1994.

47. Mann RA: The great toe, *Orthop Clin North Am* 20(4):519, 1989.

48. Marderson EL: The uncommon sprain: ligamentous diastasis of the ankle without fracture or bony deformity, *Orthop Rev* 15:664, 1986.

49. Mercier LR: *Practical orthopedics,* ed 2, Chicago, 1987, Year Book Medical Publishers.

50. Mercier LR: *Practical orthopedics,* ed 3, St Louis, 1991, Mosby.

51. Michaud T: *Foot orthoses and other forms of conservative foot care,* Baltimore, 1993, Williams & Wilkins.

52. Milbauer DL, Patel SA: Radiographic techniques. In Nicholas JA, Hershman EB, editors: *The lower extremity and spine in sports medicine,* ed 2, vol 1, St Louis, 1995, Mosby.

53. Miller CD, Shelton WR, Barrett GR et al: Deltoid and syndesmosis ligament injury of the ankle without fracture, *Am J Sports Med* 23(6):746, 1995.

54. Miller TT, Ghelman B, Potter HG: Imaging of the foot and ankle. In Nicholas JA, Hershman EB, editors: *The lower extremity and spine in sports medicine,* ed 2, vol 2, St Louis, 1995, Mosby.

55. Neumann D, Vogt L, Banzer W, Schreiber U: Kinematic and neuromuscular changes of the gait pattern after Achilles tendon rupture, *Foot Ankle Int* 18:339, 1997.

56. Neviaser RJ, Eisenfeld LS, Wiesel SW, Lewis RJ: *Emergency orthopedic radiology,* New York, 1988, Churchill Livingstone.

57. Nuber GW: Biomechanics of the foot and ankle during gait, *Clin Sports Med* 7(1):1, 1988.

58. O'Donnell CS, Good RP, Snedden HE: Closed rupture of the Achilles' tendon, *Orthop Consultation* 8(1):8, 1987.

59. Pappas AM: Osteochondrosis: disease of growth centers, *The Physician and Sportsmedicine* 17(3):21, 1988.

60. Perry J: *Gait analysis: normal and pathological function,* New York, 1992, McGraw-Hill.

61. Post M: *Physical examination of the musculoskeletal system,* Chicago, 1987, Year Book Medical Publishers.

62. Prentice WE, Arnheim DP: *Modern principles of athletic training,* ed 5, St Louis, 1993, Mosby.

63. Reckling FW, Mohn MP: The leg. In Reckling FW, Reckling JB, Mohn MP, editors: *Orthopedic anatomy and surgical approaches,* St Louis, 1990, Mosby.

64. Roberts AK, Pomeranz SJ: Current status of magnetic resonance in radiologic diagnosis of foot and ankle injuries, *Orthop Clin North Am* 25(1):64, 1994.

65. Ryan JB, Hopkinson WJ. Wheeler JH, Arciero RA, Swain JH: Management of the acute ankle sprain, *Clin Sports Med* 8(3):477, 1989.

66. Schon LC: Nerve entrapment, neuropathy, and nerve dysfunction in athletes, *Orthop Clin North Am* 25(1):47,1994.

67. Shea MP, Maroli A II: Recognizing talar dome lesions, *The Physician and Sportsmedicine* 21(3):109, 1993.

68. Singer KM, Jones DC, Taillon MR: Ligament injuries of the ankle and foot. In Nicholas JA, Hershman EB, editors: *The lower extremity and spine in sports medicine,* ed 2, vol 1, St Louis, 1995, Mosby.

69. Singh M, Johnson KA: Physical diagnosis of the foot and ankle. In Post M, editor: *Physical examination of the musculoskeletal system,* Chicago, 1987, Year Book Medical Publishers.

70. Snow RE, Williams KR: High heeled shoes: their effect on center of mass position, posture, three dimensional kinematics, rearfoot motion, and ground reaction forces, *Arch Phys Med Rehabil* 75(5):568, 1994.

71. Stewart S: Human gait and the human foot: an ethnological study of flatfoot: I, *Clin Orthop* 70-111, 1970.

72. Subotnick SI: *Podiatric sports medicine,* Mt Kisco, NY, 1975, Futura Publishing.

73. Subotnick S: *Sports medicine of the lower extremity,* New York, 1989, Churchill Livingstone.

74. Taylor DC, Bassett FH III: Syndesmosis ankle sprains, *The Physician and Sportsmedicine* 21(12):39, 1993.

75. Valmassy RL: Pathomechanics of lower extremity function. In Valmassy RL, editor: *Clinical biomechanics of the lower extremities,* St Louis, 1996, Mosby.

76. Weinstabl R, Stiskel M, Neuhold B et al: Classifying calcaneal tendon injury according to MRI findings, *J Bone Joint Surg* 73B:683, 1991.

77. Weissman BN, Sledge CB: *Orthopedic radiology,* Philadelphia, 1986, WB Saunders.

78. Welsh RP, Huffer BR: Disorders affecting tendon structures about the ankle. In Welsch RP, Shephard RJ, editors: *Current therapies in sports medicine,* St Louis, 1985, Mosby.

79. Wernick J, Volpe RG: Lower extremity function and normal mechanics. In Valmassy RL, editor: *Clinical biomechanics of the lower extremities,* St Louis, 1996, Mosby.

80. Williams PL, Warwick R: *Gray's anatomy,* Edinburgh, Churchill Livingstone, 1980.

81. Wooden MJ: Mobilization of the lower extremity. In Donnatelli R, Wooden MR, editors: *Orthopedic physical therapy,* New York, 1989, Churchill Livingstone.

82. Xenos JS, Hopkinson WJ, Mulligan ME et al: The tibiofibular syndesmosis: evaluation of the ligamentous structure, methods of fixation, and radiographic assessment, *J Bone Joint Surg* (Am) 77(6):847, 1995.

Musculoskeletal Challenges 2000

Primary care practitioners are seeing a surge of musculoskeletal complaints that in the past have not fallen into any clear-cut clinical entity. Generalized and vague flu-like complaints such as fatigue and myalgias were once thought to be stress-related diseases or somatoform disorders. Only in recent years have the academic and orthodox medical communities begun to devote research grants and funding to nonrheumatic diseases of the neuromusculoskeletal system.

Three conditions that are being diagnosed with increasing frequency present a formidable challenge to the clinician as the 21st century approaches. It has in the past been difficult to diagnose Lyme disease, fibromyalgia, and chronic fatigue immune dysfunction syndrome (CFIDS), and the effective treatment of these conditions continues to be problematic for the clinician. The signs and symptoms of these three entities often overlap one another, thereby adding to the confusion.

Lyme disease is bacterial in origin, with the pathogen known since the 1970s. Diagnosis and treatment remain a major challenge for clinicians, however, and the number of cases reported in endemic regions continues to rise. Practitioners have recognized fibromyalgia as a separate, distinct condition only since the 1980s; there are several theories on the cause of the condition, but there is no known cause and thus no cure. The Centers for Disease Control and Prevention (CDC) did not rec-ognize CFIDS until recent years, and research efforts to find a causative agent and cure have been increasing in the 1990s. It is thought that a retrovirus may be the culprit, but none has been isolated to date.

All students and providers of primary care–musculoskeletal health care are seeing these conditions with increasing frequency, and a clear understanding of the differential diagnosis and various treatment options is essential to improve the likelihood of a successful outcome. As a result of their conditions, many of these patients have chronic problems that have drastically changed their once active lives. Noninvasive and conservative care to enhance the patients' quality of life remains the common goal for all clinicians.

Lyme Disease

The bacterial agent that causes Lyme disease is *Borrelia burgdorferi*. This poorly understood spirochete is transmitted through a painless deer tick bite. The tick vectors include *Ixodes dammini* and *Ixodes scapularis,* which are commonly present in the northeastern United States; *Amblyomma americanum* (lone star tick); and *Ixodes pacificus,* which is found in the Pacific Northwest. Depending on the location, infection rates of ticks can be extremely low (1%) or extremely high (90%).

The deer tick has a 2-year life cycle and feeds three times in this period. In the larval stage, the tick feeds on rodents (e.g., mice), which may be infected with the spiral-shaped bacterium. During the nymph stage, it is the size of a pinhead and feeds on larger animals (e.g., dogs, cats, and humans). Ticks are active in the spring and early summer, which is prime time for infectious transmission to human beings.

A person who has been bitten by a tick should carefully remove the tick with a pair of tweezers in a way that does not disengage the body, place the tick in a glass vial or a Ziploc bag, and preserve it for testing. Treatment should begin if

1. Tests show that the tick is infected with spirochetes;
2. The person who has been bitten develops signs and symptoms consistent with a diagnosis of Lyme disease;
3. The person is symptomatic and pregnant; and,
4. The incident has occurred in a hyperendemic area and involves a tick that is engorged, indicating that a bite and, possibly, transmission may have taken place.

The incidence of Lyme disease is rapidly increasing in the United States. Although cases of the disease have been reported in virtually every state, endemic areas include the Northeast, the Great Lakes region, and the Pacific Northwest. Most cases occur in the Northeast, especially in New York, New Jersey, and Connecticut.[5] More specifically, the majority of diagnosed cases in the United States originate in the suburbs of New York City.

Diagnosis of Lyme Disease

Referred to as the "great imitator," Lyme disease may mimic many other illnesses, making diagnosis particularly difficult. Early signs and symptoms include generalized viral complaints, such as aches and pains in the muscles and joints, low-grade fevers, and fatigue.[6] A rash may appear several days after infection or not at all. A bull's-eye rash (i.e., erythema migrans) is the disease's prototypical dermatologic manifestation, but not all patients with Lyme disease develop a rash. Multiple rash sites are possible in disseminated disease, and atypical rashes have also been reported, further adding to the difficulty of early diagnosis.

Patients with late disease have more musculoskeletal impairment, higher rates of morbidity, and a higher prevalence of memory and cognitive impairment.[32] They may experience polyarthralgia, joint effusions, crepitus, polymyalgia, cephalalgia, profuse fatigue, radiculopathy, peripheral neuropathies, and stiffness. Cervical lymphadenopathy, stiff neck, Bell's palsy, and severe headaches are also common in Lyme encephalopathy.

The diagnosis of Lyme disease is based on history, clinical symptoms, epidemiology, and serologic studies. Laboratory tests, such as the enzyme-linked immunosorbent assay (ELISA) and Western Blot, which produce both false-positive and false-negative results, are often inconclusive. Specific IgG and IgM antibody titers to *B. burgdorferi* are the focus of serologic tests. Medications and preexisting conditions can all alter test results, however.

The condition of children with symptoms, including joint pain, needs careful assessment. Again, the diagnosis must be made on historical and clinical grounds. Lyme disease in children is difficult to diagnose if there is no rash or if the parents fail to notice one.[22] In addition, a significant number of children with erythema migrans have no antibodies on serologic testing.[17]

It may be difficult to diagnose new or acute cases of Lyme disease by conventional assays, especially in patients who have antibodies to *B. burgdorferi* proteins.[31] Furthermore, early disease, which usually takes approximately 6 weeks to become seropositive, and late (chronic) disease that is resistant to drug therapy, may be seronegative.[29] Plasmid polymerase chain reaction (PCR) studies for *B. burgdorferi* have been evaluated for serum, cerebrospinal fluid, synovial fluid, urine, and ethylenediaminetetraacetic acid (EDTA) whole blood specimens, but their accuracy has yet to be proved. Although there is a report of *B. burgdorferi* isolated from the arthritic joint of patients with Lyme disease,[28] several recent studies show laboratory findings that conflict with the clinical symptomatology.[2,19]

Differential Diagnosis for Lyme Disease

As noted earlier, patients with Lyme disease have many of the symptoms associated with fibromyalgia and CFIDS. In many cases, however, the patient with Lyme disease can provide the clinician with a history compatible with an infectious disease process, including tick bites, exposure to a hyperendemic area, and a prodrome of viral-type symptoms. Conversely, the history of patients with fibromyalgia and CFIDS may not be nearly as clear-cut. In addition, patients with fibromyalgia and CFIDS are usually women, 20 to 50 years of age.

In fibromyalgia, the chief complaint is pain; in CFIDS, the complaint is progressive, profound fatigue. Patients with either disease may experience primary or secondary depression, along with sleep disturbances. Constitutional symptoms (e.g., memory loss) commonly seen in these patients may also occur in those with late Lyme disease. For all three disorders, the diagnosis is based on clinical findings.

The practitioner caring for a patient who has active symptoms and a history consistent with Lyme disease should also consider the possibility that the patient has one of the other emerging tick-borne diseases, such as babesiosis (i.e., infection with *Babesia microti*) and ehrlichiosis (i.e., infection with *Rickettsia*), including human monocytic and human granulocytic ehrlichiosis. Finally, the clinician should be aware that because of the recognized ability of *B. burgdorferi* to evade host defenses, even in the presence of antibiotics,[7,12,25] definitive diagnosis may be elusive.

Treatment of Lyme Disease

Confusion and ambiguity have created great controversy in the treatment of patients with Lyme disease (Table 12-1). Clinicians approach Lyme disease in a variety of ways, but those who practice in endemic regions tend to advocate more aggressive treatment.[13] As the incidence has increased, these field practitioners have been quick to discover that Lyme disease has more serious sequelae than previously understood. Therefore modern approaches based on clinical experiences are replacing simplistic techniques. In some cases, treatment requires longer trials of medication and more complex combinations of antibiotics. The controversy has become quite political as insurance companies, alarmed by the high cost of treatment, have attempted to deny care to some patients.[15,30]

If untreated, Lyme disease may cause irreparable damage to the nervous, immune, musculoskeletal, and cardiac systems. The treatment for patients with Lyme disease is the oral or intravenous administration of antibiotics, usually for a period of at least 4 to 6 weeks. Patients whose disease is at a later stage when diagnosed may require the parenteral administration of antibiotics, and they may need drug therapy over a longer period.[8] Treatment is more likely to be successful if it begins early, however. Therefore if erythema migrans appears, treatment should begin immediately.

For adults, acute treatment with antibiotics frequently includes the oral administration of doxycycline

---

Table 12-1 Management of Lyme Disease, Fibromyalgia, and Chronic Fatigue Immune Dysfunction Syndrome (CFIDS)

	Lyme Disease	Fibromyalgia	CFIDS
Physical examination findings	History of tick bite, exposure, or rash Generalized viral or flulike complaints in early disease (e.g., muscle or joint aches, headaches, fatigue, low-grade fever) Arthritis, cognitive or memory impairment, cardiac and neurologic disease, debilitating fatigue, joint effusions in late disease Variable findings on serologic tests	Multiple tender points, especially the scalene, trapezius, levator scapula, and suboccipital muscles Hypomobility of cervical spine Headaches, anxiety, depression, and sleep disturbance	Profound progressive fatigue of at least 6 months' duration Headaches, sore throat, cervical lymphadenopathy Allergy, anxiety, depression; co-existing psychiatric diagnosis possible Cognitive impairment, poor short-term memory
X-ray findings	Applicable only to rule out arthritis	Usually unremarkable, which contributes to diagnosis	Not applicable
Treatment plan	Antibiotic therapy (oral or parenteral) Physical therapy, graded exercise for debilitated patients CMT for joint stiffness, immobility Acidophilus, vitamin supplementation Massage therapy	CMT, particularly soft-tissue techniques Regular graded aerobic exercise, physical therapy for debilitated patients Stress management and psychologic counseling Massage therapy Multidisciplinary support, including medication for sleep disturbances or depression, if clinically indicated	Modification of activities of daily living Gentle, graded therapeutic exercise, physical therapy for debilitated patients Stress reduction, control CMT, massage therapy possibly beneficial Medication and counseling, if indicated

CMT, Chiropractic manipulative therapy.

(100 to 300 mg twice a day) or amoxicillin (1 g every 8 hours) plus probenecid (500 mg every 8 hours). Localized disease recognized in its early stages may require treatment for only 4 to 6 weeks. Acute disseminated infection, however, may require more aggressive treatment.[10] Early, mild disseminated disease may resolve with 1 to 4 months of oral therapy, but disseminated disease with organ involvement, chronic or resistant infection, and late diagnosis generally mandates parenteral therapy for 6 weeks to several months with ceftriaxone, cefotaxime, doxycycline, or benzathine penicillin.[7] Patients who are extremely ill may require extended intravenous therapy, especially if their infection is refractory to treatment.

Because of the administration of antimicrobial therapy and possible chronic stress to the immune system, patients should supplement their daily diet with acidophilus or daily yogurt with active cultures, multivitamins, and B complex. Physical therapy and a supervised, graded therapeutic exercise program are helpful for debilitated patients. Massage therapy is often palliative for muscle and joint pains and for headaches. Chiropractic manipulation may be beneficial to counteract joint stiffness and immobility

In some individuals, Lyme disease is a chronic infection. Seronegativity, the existence of chronic persistent infections, relapses, and treatment failures have all been documented.[9,11,21] The persistence of spirochetal nucleic acids in active Lyme arthritis has also been documented,[4] as has recurrent erythema migrans despite extended antibiotic treatment.[24]

Patients with chronic disease may respond to the reinstitution of antibiotic therapy, which can suppress, but does not eradicate, the infection. The mechanisms of bacteriostatic treatment patterns are not clearly understood. Possible scenarios include intracellular sequestration, dormant states of pathogenesis, and antigenic variation of surface proteins.[23] Seropositive test results indicate only exposure, not the current presence of the spirochete in the blood. Although peaking IgMs are common in late disease, reactivity may not distinguish early from late disease. It does suggest an active infection, however. In cases of late seronegative disease, transient seroconversion may follow completion of successful therapy.[7]

Unfortunately, Lyme disease may not be curable for all patients in a bacteriologic sense. Until laboratory science learns more about this illness, treatment of Lyme borreliosis will remain clinically difficult, politically controversial, and subject to great debate in health care.

Fibromyalgia

An often disabling condition that affects 2% to 4% of the population,[14] fibromyalgia has been described in the medical literature since the mid-1800s, but it remains poorly understood. Not until the 1970s did researchers begin to unfold the multisystem involvement of fibromyalgia. The first laboratory-based findings were the disturbances in non–rapid eye movement (non-REM) deep sleep patterns that Smythe and Moldofsky discovered.[33] There is still much to be learned about the cloudy mechanism of this disorder, which continues to be commonly encountered in orthopedic, rheumatologic, and chiropractic practices.

Fibromyalgia is characterized by diffuse myalgia, with multiple sites of tender points, chronic pain, and spinal hypomobility. The common symptoms of anxiety, headache, sleep disturbances, and depression frequently complicate the diagnostic process. It is often difficult to determine whether these patients have myofascially triggered cervicogenic headaches or tension cephalalgia derived from stress.

Tender points usually differ from myofascial trigger points in that they have no distant referral pattern in fibromyalgia. The locations of the tender points seem to have a characteristic pattern; in fact, pain or tenderness on digital palpation at 11 of 18 common tender point sites is one criterion for the diagnosis (Figure 12-1). Common anatomic sites of tenderness include the inferior lateral epicondylar region, greater trochanter of the hips, and second costochondral junctions. The paracervical region is often affected at multiple sites. The most common tender point regions, however, are the middle trapezius, the belly of the scalene muscles, the suboccipital region, the muscles of mastication, and the levator scapula at the lower cervical spine.

Women far outnumber men among patients with fibromyalgia syndromes; 5 or 10 to 1.[14] Most patients are between the ages of 30 to 50 years, and there is seldom any clinical evidence of organic disease or antecedent trauma.[3] The fact that so many of the symptoms are related to stress disorders (e.g., bowel disturbances, nonrefreshing sleep, fatigue, depression, headaches) causes further confusion in diagnosis. In addition, systemic disease (e.g., hypothyroidism, rheumatologic disease, viral illnesses) have similar presentations (Table 12-2).

It is often thought that depression and fatigue in these patients are the results of chronic pain, not the causes of the pain. Many patients with chronic neck and

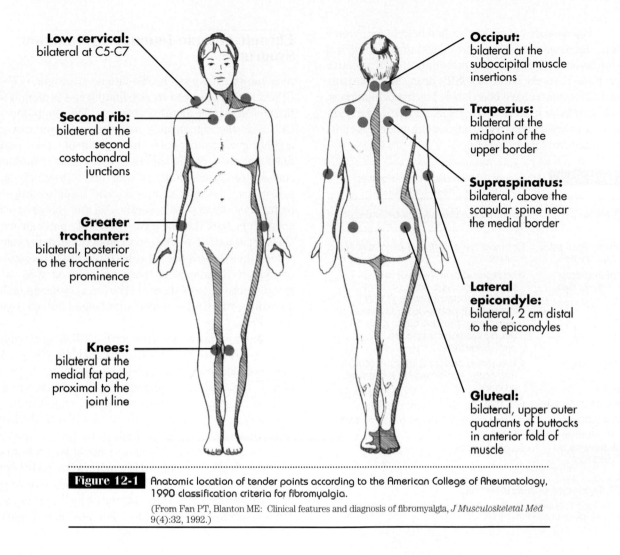

Low cervical: bilateral at C5-C7

Second rib: bilateral at the second costochondral junctions

Greater trochanter: bilateral, posterior to the trochanteric prominence

Knees: bilateral at the medial fat pad, proximal to the joint line

Occiput: bilateral at the suboccipital muscle insertions

Trapezius: bilateral at the midpoint of the upper border

Supraspinatus: bilateral, above the scapular spine near the medial border

Lateral epicondyle: bilateral, 2 cm distal to the epicondyles

Gluteal: bilateral, upper outer quadrants of buttocks in anterior fold of muscle

Figure 12-1 Anatomic location of tender points according to the American College of Rheumatology, 1990 classification criteria for fibromyalgia.

(From Fan PT, Blanton ME: Clinical features and diagnosis of fibromyalgia, *J Musculoskeletal Med* 9(4):32, 1992.)

back pain suffer psychosomatic overlays in their clinical presentation. The difficulty of distinguishing fibromyalgia from chronic fatigue syndrome has been the subject of many reports.[18,34] The primary complaint in fibromyalgia, however, is pain—not fatigue. This is the key factor in differentiating the two conditions.

A multidisciplinary approach may be necessary to treat the patient with fibromyalgia (Figure 12-2). Chiropractic management is beneficial because of the practitioner-patient rapport established in the hands-on orientation of the treatment. Cervical manipulation, soft-tissue techniques, massage therapy, and alleviating patient fears are helpful in reducing anxiety, headaches, and spinal pain.

Although patients with chronic pain should not receive narcotics, antidepressant medication may be help-ful. Medication to improve sleep not only may assist in controlling pain, but it also may enhance concentration and memory. Many clinicians prescribe amitriptyline (Elavil) as treatment for sleep disturbance, headaches, and depression. Cyclobenzaprine (Flexeril), diphenhydramine (Benadryl), zolpidem tartrate (Ambien), and alprazolam (Xanax) are also used as sleep aids.[20] Patients with fibromyalgia should also go to bed at the same time each night to maintain a regular schedule of sleep.

Stress management is an integral component of case management. Recreational activities and exercise can reduce stress and promote feelings of well-being and self-esteem. For example, daily graded aerobic exercise improves muscle function and reduces constitutional symptoms. Supervised physical therapy is necessary for debilitated patients.

Psychologic counseling is often helpful for chronic pain. Some patients with severe debilitation from clinical depression may require the prescription of a selective serotonin reuptake inhibitor (SSRI) drug. Many patients with fibromyalgia have been labeled as hypochondriacs, malingerers, or hysterics. Therefore it is particularly important to treat them with compassion, understanding, and long-term follow-up care.

Table 12-2 Fibromyalgia Mimickers and Features that Distinguish These Conditions

Disorder	Features not shared by fibromyalgia
Myofascial pain syndrome	Regional pain, referred pain, sudden onset
Polymyalgia rheumatica	Widespread pain in neck and shoulder girdles, back and hip girdles; moderate-to-high ESR; absence of pathologic weakness or myopathy; patient older than 60 years; dramatic response to corticosteroids
Polymyositis	Objective weakness; inflammatory myopathy confirmed by laboratory studies
Hypothyroidism	Positive thyroid function tests
Metastatic carcinoma	History of local malignancy; positive bone scan
Rheumatoid arthritis	Swollen joints

ESR, Erythrocyte sedimentation rate.

(From Fan PT, Blanton ME: Clinical features and diagnosis of fibromyalgia, *J Musculoskeletal Med* 9(4):32, 1992.)

Chronic Fatigue Immune Dysfunction Syndrome

Also known simply as chronic fatigue syndrome (CFS), CFIDS is characterized by debilitating and profound fatigue of at least 6 months' duration. The symptoms of CFIDS overlap significantly with those of Lyme disease and fibromyalgia; patients with any one of these conditions may demonstrate multiple nonspecific symptoms such as headaches, recurrent sore throats, tender lymph nodes, myalgias and arthralgias, and cognitive impairment. In addition to musculoskeletal and constitutional complaints that do not ease with rest, patients with chronic fatigue commonly report anxiety and depression. Some studies have reported a high incidence of coexisting psychiatric diagnoses in these patients, as well as a greater prevalence of allergy.[1] The chief complaint of the individual with CFIDS remains prolonged fatigue, however (Table 12-3).

Most individuals who have CFIDS are white, women, and between their mid-20s and late 40s in age. The condition seldom occurs in children under 12 years of age. Postviral syndrome after an infectious disease such as mononucleosis is possible, and exposure to *B. burgdorferi* can trigger CFIDS in some patients who have received adequate antibiotic therapy for Lyme disease.[26]

Patients with CFIDS require an initial work-up of laboratory tests, including a minimum of a complete blood cell count with leukocyte differential; a urinalysis; the erythrocyte sedimentation rate, as well as the levels of total protein, alkaline phosphatase, glucose, and thyroid-

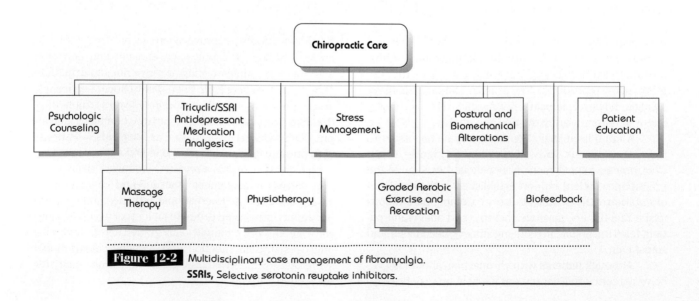

Figure 12-2 Multidisciplinary case management of fibromyalgia.
SSRIs, Selective serotonin reuptake inhibitors.

Table 12-3 Clinical Comparison of Lyme Disease, Fibromyalgia, and Chronic Fatigue Immune Dysfunction Syndrome

	Lyme Disease	Fibromyalgia	CFIDS
Sex of typical patient	M/F	F	F
Age of typical patient	Any age	30-50 yrs	25-50 yrs
Joint pain	Yes	Yes	Possibly
Headaches	Yes	Yes	Yes
General viral and influenza complaints	Yes	Yes	Yes
Sore throat, lymphadenopathy	Possibly	Rare	Yes
Bowel disturbances	Possibly	Yes	Yes
Characteristic tender points	No	Yes	No
Skin rash	Possibly	No	No
Fevers	Possibly	Rare	Low grade
Sleep disturbances	Possibly	Yes	Yes
Pain as chief complaint	Possibly	Yes	No
Fatigue as chief complaint	Possibly	No	Yes
Peripheral neurologic complaints	Possibly	Possibly	Rare
Depression and anxiety	Possibly	Possibly	Usually
Cognitive and memory impairment	Possibly	Possibly	Yes
Abnormal laboratory test results	Possibly	No	No
Rehabilitation, exercise indicated	Yes	Yes	Yes
Antibiotic therapy indicated	Yes	No	No
SSRIs and tricyclic medications helpful	No	Usually	Yes
Causative agent	Spirochete	Unknown	Unknown
ADLs modification necessary	Yes	Usually	Yes

SSRIs, Selective serotonin reuptake inhibitors; **ADLs,** activities of daily living.

stimulating hormone (TSH).[16] These tests are helpful in ruling out certain causes of chronic fatigue, such as hypothyroidism, obesity, sleep apnea, substance abuse, multiple sclerosis, primary depression and bipolar disorder, and infectious disease (e.g., hepatitis).

Although the National Institutes of Health, particularly the National Institute of Allergy and Infectious Disease (NIAID), have provided research grants since 1986, investigators have not yet isolated a causative agent for CFIDS. The condition does not seem to be easily transmissible, but there may be multiple contributory factors, including neuroendocrine or other systemic dysfunction. Studies of single viral agents as the cause of the condition, such as the Epstein-Barr virus, herpesvirus 6, retroviruses, and enteroviruses have not been fruitful.[27]

Because of the variety of problems associated with CFIDS, treatment requires a multidisciplinary approach. Total care involves both symptomatic treatment and emotional support. Modification of the person's daily activities seems to be paramount to the success of treatment. Balancing activity and rest; gentle, graduated exercise to limit deconditioning; counseling, if appropriate; and possibly the administration of medication with tricyclic antidepressants or selective serotonin reuptake inhibitors are often helpful. Physical therapy, chiropractic treatment, and massage therapy may also be beneficial.

Review Questions

1. (a) In what tissue systems does the Lyme organism commonly manifest itself? (b) From what methodology is the diagnosis of Lyme disease made?
2. Name the differences in medical treatment seen in the late stage of Lyme disease versus the early stage.
3. What are the clinical differences between chronic fatigue immune dysfunction syndrome and fibromyalgia?
4. How would you differentiate myofascial pain syndrome and fibromyalgia?
5. (a) What do Lyme disease, chronic fatigue immune dysfunction syndrome, and fibromyalgia have in common? (b) What similarity is present in the treatments for these conditions?

References

1. American Association for Chronic Fatigue Syndrome: *Disease overview*, Albany, NY, 1997, The Association.
2. Barkley M, Harris N, Szantyr B: *The Lyme Urine Antigen Test (LUAT) during antibiotic therapy in women with recurrent menstrual cycles.* 10th Annual International Conference on Lyme Borreliosis, 1997, Bethesda, MD, National Institutes of Health (NIH).
3. Bennett RM, Smythe HA, Wolfe F: Recognizing fibromyalgia, *Patient Care,* 8(3):211, 1992.
4. Bradley JF, Johnson RD, Goodman JL: The persistence of spirochetal nucleic acids in active Lyme arthritis, *Ann Intern Med* 120(6):487, 1994.
5. Brier SR: Lyme disease: a case report, *J Manipulative Physiol Ther* 13(6):24, 1990.
6. Brier SR: Lyme disease and joint pain in children (correspondence), *Dynamic Chiropractic* 15(23):37, 1997.
7. Burrascano JJ: *Managing Lyme disease—diagnostic hints and treatment guidelines for Lyme borreliosis,* ed 11, East Hampton, NY, 1996, Author.
8. Cimmino MA, Accardo S: Long-term treatment of chronic Lyme arthritis with benzathine penicillin, *Ann Rheum Dis* 51(8):1007, 1992.
9. Coyle PK, Deng Z, Schutzer SE et al: Detection of *B. burgdorferi* antigens in cerebrospinal fluid, *Neurology* 43(6):1093, 1993.
10. Dattwyler R, Luft BJ, Kunkel MR et al: Ceftriaxone compared with doxycycline for the treatment of acute disseminated Lyme disease, *N Engl J Med* 337(5):289, 1997.
11. Dorward DW, Fischer ER, Brooks DM: Basic and clinical approaches to Lyme disease: a Lyme disease foundation symposium, *Clin Infect Dis* 25:S2, 1997.
12. Duffy J: Cardiac manifestations of Lyme disease, *J Musculoskeletal Med* 9(9):17, 1992.
13. Eppes SC, Klein JD, Caputo CM, Rose CD: Physician beliefs, attitudes, and approaches toward Lyme disease in an endemic area, *Clin Pediatr (Phila)* 33(3):130, 1994.
14. Fan PT, Blanton ME: Clinical features and diagnosis of fibromyalgia, *J Musculoskeletal Med* 9(4):24, 1992.
15. France D: Reality bites—Lyme disease is proving hard to lick, *New York Magazine* 4:24, 1997.
16. Fukuda K, Straus SE, Hickie I et al: The chronic fatigue syndrome: a comprehensive approach to its definition and study, *Ann Intern Med* 121:953, 1994.
17. Gerber MA, Shapiro ED, Burke GS, Parcells VJ, Bell GL: Lyme disease in children in southeastern Connecticut, *N Engl J Med* 335(17):1270, 1996.
18. Goldenberg DL: Fibromyalgia and other chronic fatigue syndromes: is there evidence for chronic viral disease? *Semin Arthritis Rheum* 18:111, 1988.
19. Harris NS, Stephens BG: Antigenuria detected in 30% of patients with active Lyme symptoms without treatment and confirmed rash, *J Spirochete Tick-Borne Diseases* 2:37, 1995.
20. Kroha K: *Syndromes associated with fibromyalgia,* Portland, OR, 1996, Conference on Fibromyalgia Syndrome.
21. Lawrence C, Lipton RD, Lowry FD, Coyle PK: Chronic neuroborreliosis, *Eur Neurol* 35(2):113, 1995.
22. Leib-Feldman B, Wormser GP, McKenna D, Nadelman RB et al: Lyme disease in children [correspondence], *N Engl J Med* 336(15):1107, 1997.
23. Liegner KB: *Chronic persistent infection in Lyme disease,* Atlantic City, NJ, 1993, Sixth Annual Lyme Disease Scientific Symposium.
24. Liegner KB, Shapiro JR, Ramsay D et al: Documentation of recurrent EM despite extended antibiotic therapy, *J Am Acad Dermat* 28(2):312, 1993.
25. Luft BJ, Steinman CR, Neimark HC et al: Invasion of the central nervous system by *Borrelia burgdorferi* in acute disseminated infection, *JAMA* 267:1364, 1992.
26. Mawle AC, Reyes M, Schmid DS: Is chronic fatigue syndrome an infectious disease? *Infectious Agents and Disease* 2:333, 1994.
27. National Institute of Allergy and Infectious Disease, National Institutes of Health: *Overview of the chronic fatigue syndrome research program,* Bethesda, MD, 1997, The Institute.
28. Noctum J, Dressler F, Rutledge B, Rys P, Persing D, Steere A: Detection of *B. burgdorferi* by PCR in synovial fluid for a patient with Lyme arthritis, *N Engl J Med* 330(4):229, 1994.
29. Preac-Mursic V, Weber K, Pfister HW et al: Survival of *Borrelia burgdorferi* in antibiotically treated patient with Lyme disease, *Infection* 17(6):355, 1989.
30. Schemo DJ: Prolonged Lyme treatments, *The New York Times* 1:1, 1994.
31. Schutzer SE, Luan J: Detection of Lyme disease after OspA vaccine, *N Engl J Med* 337(11):794, 1997.
32. Shadick NA, Phillips CB, Logigian EL et al: The long-term clinical outcomes of Lyme disease: a population-based retrospective cohort study, *Ann Intern Med* 121(8):560, 1994.
33. Smythe HA, Moldofsky H: Two contributions for understanding of the "fibrositis" syndrome, *Bull Rheum Dis* 28:928, 1977.
34. Wolfe F, Smythe HA, Yanus MB et al: The American College of Rheumatology 1990 criteria for the classification of fibromyalgia: report of the Multicenter Criteria Committee, *Arthritis Rheum* 33:160, 1990.

Glossary

acetabuli protrusio (ch 9) Abnormal protrusion of the femoral head into the pelvis, which usually occurs secondary to arthritis; also called Otto's pelvis.

acromioplasty (ch 3) Surgical technique performed via arthroscopy or an arthrotomy in which the surgeon reduces the acromion so that the greater tuberosity of the humerus can clear and achieve overhead motion and a free arc of abduction.

active rest (ch 7) Continuation of an injured person's normal everyday activities that provide healthy movement, but avoidance of the activity that caused the injury.

Adam's test (ch 7) Determines whether a scoliosis curve disappears when the patient flexes forward at the waist with the hands in the prayer position and the arms hanging to the floor. Its disappearance suggests a mild-to-moderate deformity that is not structural in nature. The examiner may take a position anterior or posterior to the patient.

adhesive capsulitis (ch 3) Formation of scar tissue at the glenoid labrum that leads to restricted, painful loss of glenohumeral movement.

adolescent scoliosis (ch 7) Spinal curvature presenting at or about the onset of puberty and before maturity.

adult scoliosis (ch 7) Spinal curvature existing after skeletal maturity.

air splint (ch 11) Brace designed for the ankle or lower leg that features pneumatic support. If used on ankle sprains, it can help maintain the subtalar joint in a neutral position and allow for early weight-bearing and active rehabilitation.

anal wink (ch 8) Reflex contraction of the anal sphincter after perianal sensation.

ankle mortise (ch 11) Articulation between the talus and tibia; also known as the talocrural joint.

anterior capsulolabral repair (ACLR) (ch 3) The preferred surgical procedure when chronic anterior instability is present with significant labral and capsular damage.

anterior cruciate ligament–deficient knee (ch 10) Pathologic state of knee kinematics that includes at least excessive anterior translation of the tibia, possibly as a result of a prior tear or sprain of the ligament.

apprehension sign (ch 3) Pain or alarm when the examiner slowly abducts the patient's arm, rotates it externally, and palpates the glenohumeral joint with the other hand. This maneuver can mimic the feeling of a prior anterior dislocation.

arcuate complex (ch 10) Ligamentous arrangement of the lateral knee joint that aids the lateral collateral ligament in stabilizing the joint. It is located deep to the lateral collateral ligament and popliteus muscle.

arthrography (chs 2, 10) Use of air and a contrast agent to outline anatomic structures, such as joint capsules and cartilage. Arthrograms are used to diagnose capsular injuries, rotator cuff tears, and torn menisci in the knee joint.

arthroscopy (chs 3, 10) Microsurgical technique that enables quick and efficient diagnostic and reconstructive procedures (e.g., for tears of the glenoid labrum or meniscus). It may be carried out via two or three portals.

atlantoaxial instability (ch 6) Ligamentous disruption caused by trauma or disease that results in a dissociation at the interodontoid space or posterior interspinous space and is visible radiographically.

attenuation (chs 2 and 3) Reduction in radiation intensity that is the result of absorption and scattering. It is a thinning or weakening of a structure, perhaps the result of disease, aging, or trauma.

axial compression (ch 6) Vertical loading of a segmented cervical spinal column through the crown or vertex of the head.

axonotmesis (ch 6) Nerve injury that interrupts the axon's connection with intact surrounding tissues.

Babinski sign (ch 8) Extension of the great toe as the other toes splay when the examiner runs a sharp instrument across the plantar surface of the foot and along the calcaneus and lateral border of the forefoot. The presence of this sign suggests an upper motor lesion involving the corticospinal tract.

Bankart lesion (ch 3) Area of calcification secondary to trauma of the anterior glenohumeral ligament, indicative of a sclerotic reaction to chronic glenohumeral instability.

barroom fracture (ch 5) Fracture to the neck of the fifth metacarpal; also called boxer's fracture.

Bechterew's test (ch 8) Determines whether the extension of the patient's legs, one at a time, increases backache or sciatic nerve pain. The examiner may add downward resistance to the extended leg to aggravate symptoms while he or she is sitting.

Bennett's fracture (ch 5) Fracture or dislocation of the thumb metacarpal.

Bertilotti's syndrome (ch 2) Condition in which the individual has multiple congenital variants at the lumbosacral joint, including a transitional vertebra and a unilateral pseudoarthrosis.

biplanar instability (ch 10) Pathologic laxity in the knees from injury in two planes, typically involving a torn anterior cruciate ligament and a damaged collateral ligament.

Böhler's angle (ch 11) Measured on a lateral x-ray film of the foot. The angle is created by connecting the highest points of the anterior process of the calcaneus, posterior facet, and calcaneal tuberosity. The normal angle is approximately 25 to 40 degrees.

bone scan (scintigraphy) (ch 2) Imaging technique that uses a radioactive isotope and x-ray films to measure the physiologic component of bone and confirm the presence of occult pathologic conditions (e.g., metastatic disease and stress fractures). This procedure is used when plain films are negative or equivocal.

Boston brace (ch 7) Thoracolumbosacral orthosis (TLSO) made from an impression of the area extending from the xiphoid to the greater trochanter of the femur for the patient with scoliosis.

Bouchard's nodes (ch 5) Abnormal fusiform enlargement of the proximal interphalangeal joints of the hand that is indicative of synovitis secondary to rheumatoid arthritis.

boutonniere deformity (ch 5) Flexion deformity of the proximal interphalangeal joint and the resultant hyperextended position of the distal interphalangeal joint. The central extensor slip is ruptured proximally, and the profundus tendon is lax distally.

bowstring sign test (ch 8) Exertion of pressure on the popliteal fossa with the patient in the supine position with both legs extended and the affected leg on the examiner's shoulder. Pain in the lumbar spine or along the course of the sciatic nerve suggests lumbosacral nerve root compression.

brachial plexopathy (ch 6) Diffuse weakness of the upper extremity ("dead arm") from a contusion or stretching of the brachial plexus.

buddy system taping (ch 5) Method of immobilizing an injured finger by taping it to an adjacent digit.

capsulorrhaphy (ch 3) Surgical procedure performed to alleviate excessive capsular laxity in unstable shoulders that do not have Hill-Sachs or Bankart lesions.

carpal tunnel syndrome (ch 5) Peripheral entrapment neuropathy at the carpal tunnel of the wrist, involving compression of the median nerve.

carpus (ch 5) Complex arrangement of joints that encompass eight small bones at the wrist distributed into two rows.

carrying angle (ch 4) Normal anatomic angle of the humeral-ulnar joint, which is approximately 10 to 15 degrees of valgus angulation.

cavus foot (ch 11) Foot with an accentuated high arch, which usually places undue stress on the metatarsal heads.

cervical acceleration-deceleration (CAD) (ch 6) Cervical whiplash injury to the cervical spine, sometimes called a hyperextension-hyperflexion injury; often the result of a motor vehicle accident.

cervical whiplash syndrome (ch 6) Traumatic cervical acceleration-deceleration (CAD) injury that usually involves hyperextension and hyperflexion of the spinal column.

chiropractic manipulative therapy (CMT) (chs 6, 7, 8, 9) Spinal manipulation that usually involves high-velocity, low-amplitude adjusting of specific hypomobile vertebral articulations.

chondromalacia patellae (ch 10) Histopathologic condition of the patellofemoral joint that entails softening of the articular cartilage at the retropatellar surface.

cinema sign (ch 10) Locking, crepitus, and pain experienced at the patellofemoral joint when the leg is straightened after a period of prolonged flexion.

claw toe (ch 11) Flexion deformity at both the metatarsophalangeal joint and proximal interphalangeal joint.

Clay Shoveler's fracture (ch 6) Avulsion fracture of the spinous process, usually at the C7 or T1 level.

closed manipulation (ch 3) Technique to regain movement in a frozen shoulder in which the practitioner places the patient under anesthesia (sometimes local anesthesia) and forcefully moves the patient's shoulder through the restricted arcs.

closed reduction (ch 5) Conservative restoration of a fracture or dislocation with traction, splinting, or casting.

Cobb angle (ch 7) Measurement of the scoliotic curve derived by drawing lines along the superior end plate of the uppermost vertebra and the inferior end plate of the lowermost vertebra and determining the angle between a line drawn perpendicular to these two lines and the lines indicating the uppermost and lowermost aspects of the curve.

Codman's drop-arm test (ch 3) Procedure to determine an individual's ability to maintain arm abduction at 90 degrees. This procedure requires an intact rotator cuff.

compensatory curve (ch 7) Spinal curve in the patient with scoliosis that is smaller and generally more flexible than the primary curve. It usually compensates for the body's changing center of gravity in relation to the primary curve.

computerized arthrotomography (chs 2, 3) Imaging procedure in which the clinician injects the patient with double contrast material (dye and air) to detect soft-tissue lesions in joints that have complex anatomy, such as the shoulder.

computed tomography (ch 2) Imaging procedure in which special films produce high-contrast resolution pictures that are superior to plain radiographic films of areas that have soft-tissue structures and complex osseous anatomy, such as the hand and foot.

congenital hip dysplasia (CDH) (ch 9) Common disorder involving displacement of the infant's femoral head, attributable to such factors as malformation of the acetabulum or breech delivery and other concomitant congenital deformities.

congenital scoliosis (ch 7) Curvature of the spine as a result of a birth abnormality (e.g., muscular disorders).

conventional tomography (ch 2) Imaging technique in which there is synchronous motion of both x-ray film and tube to isolate the focal plane and diagnose occult fractures, such as a hairline fracture.

costochondritis (Tietze's syndrome) (ch 7) Inflammation of the costal cartilage at the sternal border.

costovertebral dysfunction (ch 7) Rib subluxation or fixation together with the corresponding level of vertebral dysfunction.

countercoup mechanism (ch 6) Contact of the brain with the skull during rapid acceleration of the head and neck.

counterforce brace (ch 4) Support device that is placed just inferior to the extensor aponeurosis of the lateral elbow to decrease the working arm of the tendon and reduce the tension of the muscle in active lateral epicondylitis.

Cozen's test (ch 4) Procedure in which the patient maintains an extended, pronated, and clenched fist against resistance, thus activating the lateral elbow-forearm mass. If the procedure reproduces pain at the lateral epicondyle of the elbow, the patient has lateral epicondylitis.

cubital tunnel (ch 4) Region between the olecranon process of the ulna and medial epicondyle of the humerus that houses the ulnar nerve at its superficial course.

cubital tunnel syndrome (ch 4) Insult to the ulnar nerve at the cubital tunnel caused by adhesions, scar tissue, bony spurs, and inflammation that usually arises secondarily to chronic medial compartment changes at the elbow; also known as ulnar neuritis.

Dejerine's sign (ch 6) Reproduction of spinal pain as a result of coughing, sneezing, or any straining that increases intrathecal pressure.

De Quervain's tenosynovitis (ch 5) Tendonitis that involves the abductor pollicis longus and extensor pollicis brevis; also known as stenosing tenosynovitis or first extensor compartment tendonitis.

diagnostic ultrasound (ch 2) Use of ultrasonography to detect soft-tissue conditions, such as tendon injuries, pediatric hip lesions, or fluid-filled cysts.

diffuse idiopathic skeletal hyperostosis (DISH) (ch 6) Flowing calcifications in the anterior vertebral body region that appear radiographically along the anterior longitudinal ligament and involve several spinal segments; also known as Forestier's disease.

discography (ch 2) Controversial and invasive imaging procedure used for patients with chronic spinal pain in which a needle is moved and pain stimuli are tracked to identify various pain patterns and neurologic distributions of pain. It involves roentgenography of the spine for visualization of the intervertebral disk after injection of an absorbable contrast medium into the disk itself. Computerized tomography usually makes the technique biplanar.

double-major curves (ch 7) Left lumbar and right thoracic scoliosis. These curves have a predilection for progression.

double major scoliosis (ch 7) Scoliosis with two structural curves.

double thoracic curves (scoliosis) (ch 7) Two structural curves within the thoracic spine.

Dupuytren's contracture (ch 5) Contracture of the palmar fascia of the hand, possibly caused by alcoholism or diabetes.

electrodiagnostic testing (ch 2) Series of tests to detect abnormal physiology or function of nerve tissue, such as electromyographic analyses and nerve conduction velocity studies; also called electrophysiologic testing.

equinus (ch 11) Foot in the plantar flexed position.

Erb's palsy (ch 6) Neurologic disorder that involves the brachial plexus and places the arm in an awkward position of internal rotation and adduction.

extensor mechanism (ch 10) Quadriceps muscle and tendon that are involved in active knee extension.

extensor/supinator group (ch 4) Group of muscles at the lateral portion of the elbow and proximal forearm that extend and supinate the forearm. The group includes the extensor carpi ulnaris longus and brevis and the supinator muscle.

F wave (ch 2) Impulse resulting from the application of an external stimulus to a myelinated nerve that conducts impulses, both anterograde and retrograde. F wave tests determine the state of proximal nerve root function.

facet tropism (ch 2) Asymmetry in the angles (planes) of the facet joints of a particular spinal level.

Fajersztajn's test (ch 8) Test to determine whether a straight leg raise on the asymptomatic side while the patient is supine causes pain on the symptomatic side. Such pain may signal a medial disk lesion. The test is also known as the well–leg raise test.

fasciotomy (ch 11) Surgical procedure for compartment syndromes of the lower leg that decompresses the tightly wound fascia in the anterior compartment.

fat pad sign (ch 4) Elevation of the anterior and posterior fat pads (usually of the elbow), visible on a plain film, which is generally caused by an effusion and often signifies an osseous pathologic abnormality, most commonly a fracture.

fibromyalgia (ch 12) Soft-tissue condition that presents itself as a diffuse and achy pain at specific multiple sites in the absence of positive clinical test findings.

Finkelstein's test (ch 5) Test for De Quervain's extensor tendonitis in which, with the patient's forearm pronated, the examiner tucks the affected thumb into the palm of the patient's hand, asks the patient to make a fist over the thumb, and then moves the hand and wrist into ulnar deviation. Pain at the abductor pollicis longus or extensor pollicis brevis indicates De Quervain's tenosynovitis.

flexion loading (ch 10) Load placed on the knee joint during flexion, which makes the patella vulnerable to injury.

flexor/pronator mass (ch 4) Musculature at the medial aspect of the forearm and elbow, which is responsible for wrist flexion and forearm pronation. These muscles include the pronator teres and flexor carpi ulnaris.

frank herniation (ch 6) Uncontained prolapse of the nucleus pulposus in an intervertebral disk.

Freiberg's disease (ch 11) Osteonecrosis of the second metatarsal head with loss of extension of the metatarsophalangeal joint.

frog-lateral projection (ch 9) Plain x-ray film taken with the thigh abducted and hip flexed to visualize the hip joint without obstruction of the femoral head.

Froment's paper sign (ch 5) Patient's inability to hold a piece of paper between two digits when the clinician tries to take it away; used for documenting the intrinsic motor weakness of the interosseous muscles of the hand.

frozen shoulder (ch 3) Painful condition that consists of an exaggerated loss of glenohumeral motion in all planes.

gadolinium-diethylenetriamiane pentetic acid (gadolinium-DTPA) (ch 2) Paramagnetic contrast agent used in conjunction with standard magnetic resonance imaging scans.

Gaenslen's test (ch 8) Test for sacroiliac joint disease, which involves the patient in a supine position with the unaffected thigh flexed toward the abdomen. The examiner stresses the affected thigh by placing the leg into extension. The test is positive if hyperextension reproduces pain at the sacroiliac joint in question.

genu recurvatum (ch 10) Hyperextension of the knee joint, as seen in individuals with laxity in the posterior capsule.

glenohumeral (scapulohumeral) rhythm (ch 3) Normally a synchronous motion of abduction that encompasses 3 degrees of glenohumeral motion for every 2 degrees of scapulothoracic excursion.

golfer's elbow (ch 4) Generic term for a strain of the flexor mass or flexor tendonitis at the medial epicondylar insertion at the humerus.

gravity stress film (ch 4) X-ray film taken to screen for medial instability at the elbow; the patient is placed the supine position with the arm in abduction and the elbow in a valgus position.

Guyon's canal syndrome (ch 5) Peripheral entrapment of the ulnar nerve between the hook of the hamate and the pisiform bone.

H reflex (ch 2) Electrophysiologic analog to the ankle jerk reflex; the monosynaptic reflex arc measures afferent and efferent conduction along the S1 nerve root.

Haglund's disease (deformity) (ch 11) Combination of calcaneal spurring and chronic retrocalcaneal bursitis that occurs commonly in endurance athletes.

hallux valgus (ch 11) Lateral deviation of the great toe with an outgrowth of soft tissue and bone at the first metatarsophalangeal joint; also called a bunion.

hammer toe (ch 11) Flexion contracture at the proximal interphalangeal joint of the toe, which may be accompanied by a mild extensor malalignment of the metatarsophalangeal joint.

Heberden's nodes (ch 5) Nodules that form as a result of the cystic degeneration of the joint capsule at the dorsal aspect of the distal interphalangeal joint in osteoarthritic patients.

heel-cord flexibility (ch 11) Ability of the Achilles' tendon to be stretched, thus allowing the ankle to achieve dorsiflexion.

hemarthrosis (ch 10) Joint effusion tinged with blood, which usually signifies a serious internal derangement.

high-contrast resolution (ch 2) Ability to demonstrate small objects with clear delineation between subjects; also known as spatial resolution.

Hill-Sachs lesion (ch 3) Fracture of the posterolateral portion of the humeral head, which is the result of a subluxation or dislocation of the shoulder joint and is most readily evident on an axillary (notch) x-ray projection.

Hughston projection (ch 10) View of the patellofemoral joint taken with the patient in the prone position and in flexion to visualize the position of the patella on the trochlear groove, the facets of the patella, and the femoral condyles.

hyperkyphosis (ch 7) Sagittal alignment of the thoracic spine in which there is more than the normal amount of kyphosis.

hypokyphosis (ch 7) Sagittal alignment of the thoracic spine in which there is less than the normal amount of kyphosis, but not so severe as to be truly lordotic.

idiopathic scoliosis (ch 7) Spinal curvature of unknown etiology, as in 85% to 90% of all cases of scoliosis.

iliac apophysitis (ch 9) Traumatic avulsion of the hip flexor tendon at the attachment of the anterior superior iliac spine with inferior displacement of the apophysis.

infantile scoliosis (ch 7) Spinal curvature developing during the first 3 years of life.

inferior vertebral subluxation (ch 7) Tenderness over the supraspinous ligament with an associated inferiorly malpositioned spinous process; also called anteriority.

instability (chs 1, 10) Excessive motion or mobility in a joint, as seen in the pathologic knee joint, which always indicates a degree of abnormal laxity in the associated ligaments.

internal derangement of the knee (ch 10) Trauma-induced injury that disrupts one of the knee's internal structures: meniscus, ligaments, joint capsule, or bone.

intersegmental instability (ch 6) Translation of one vertebral body over the adjacent vertebra greater than 3.5 mm, as seen on a neutral lateral radiographic film.

joint effusion (chs 1, 2) Presence of fluid inside an articulation, often signifying an internal derangement or disease state.

Jones fracture (ch 11) Fracture to the base of the fifth metatarsal at the physis just distal to the tuberosity as a result of violent supination or inversion.

juvenile scoliosis (ch 7) Spinal curvature developing between the skeletal age of 3 years and the onset of puberty.

Kienböck's disease (ch 5) Condition of avascular necrosis at the lunate carpal bone that often, but not always, is preceded by a traumatic event.

Klippel-Feil syndrome (ch 6) Deformity in which two or more cervical vertebrae are fused, leading to significant loss of cervical range of motion.

Köhler's disease (ch 11) Poorly understood disease of the tarsal navicular bone that occurs in young children and is usually classified as osteochondrosis.

kyphoscoliosis (ch 7) Spine with scoliosis and a true hyperkyphosis. A rotatory deformity with only apparent kyphosis should not be described by this term.

kyphotic deformity (ch 7) Excessive curvature of the spine to the posterior, usually associated with senile age and advanced curvature of the dorsal spine.

Lasègue's test (ch 8) Straight leg raise test for nerve root or sciatic nerve inflammation, which has several variations (e.g., patient seated or supine) and may involve raising the leg from the bent knee position of hip flexion to a fully extended leg posture. Pain during the first 30 degrees of hip flexion suggests a nerve root abnormality, whereas pain during 30 to 60 degrees of motion may stem from mechanical conditions of the sacroiliac or lumbosacral articulation.

laser-assisted capsular shift (LACS) (ch 3) Surgical option for the chronically injured shoulder with no labral damage and with a large capsular pouch present. Heat is used to augment the procedure by shrinking the capsule.

lateral ankle instability (ch 11) Chronic laxity in the lateral collateral ligament complex at the ankle, seen as excessive talar tilt on comparison stress views.

laxity (chs 1, 10) Looseness in a joint, either as a direct function of a slack ligament or as a sequel to excessive joint motion.

Legg-Calvé-Perthes disease (ch 9) Condition of childhood involving avascular necrosis of the femoral head nucleus. The etiology is largely unknown, although hormonal factors may be involved.

Lisfranc's joint (ch 11) Fracture or dislocation at the base of a metatarsal that may be associated with trauma or the severe sensory neuropathies of diabetes.

Little League elbow (ch 4) General term that describes the adverse effects of overuse in an immature elbow, especially at the apophyses.

magnetic resonance imaging (MRI) (ch 2) Use of surface coils and electromagnetic fields together with computer software to provide multiplanar imaging of neuraxes and other soft-tissue areas without the use of ionizing radiation.

major curve (ch 7) Term used to designate the largest structural curve.

mallet finger (ch 5) Rupture of the extensor tendon at the distal interphalangeal joint, making finger extension insufficient.

mallet toe (ch 11) Lack of extension at the distal interphalangeal joint, resulting in the typical flexion deformity of the distal toe.

McKenzie extension program (ch 8) Series of exercises performed in the prone position and designed to place the low back in extension as part of a program for disk rehabilitation, which has the goal of "centralizing" the individual's pain.

mechanoreceptor (ch 6) Nerve endings in joint capsules, such as those in the spine, that measure muscle tone, mechanical pressure, or inhibit pain.

Merchant view (ch 10) X-ray tangential projection of the patellofemoral joint taken with the patient in the supine position and the knee flexed to 45 degrees; x-ray is directed in a caudal and inferior direction.

metatarsal bar (ch 11) External orthotic device placed outside the shoe to take pressure off the metatarsal heads; sometimes referred to as an anterior heel.

Mills' test (ch 4) Procedure to detect lateral epicondylitis by determining whether passive flexion of the patient's wrist and forearm, followed by passive pronation and extension of the forearm, reproduces lateral elbow pain.

Milwaukee brace (ch 7) Cervicothoraciclumbosacral orthosis (CTLSO) for a child with a moderate-to-severe curvature or progressive deformity during pubescence that is made from an impression of the child's torso.

minor curve (ch 7) Term refers to the smallest curve, which is always more flexible than the major curve.

mobilization (ch 3) Gentle technique employed to regain ranges of motion in patients with restrictive joint pathologic conditions; involves moving a joint to its end range of motion, but not into the paraphysiologic space.

Morton's neuroma (ch 11) Fibrosis of the interdigital branch of the plantar nerve, which usually causes burning in the third web space and third and fourth toes.

muscle-energy technique (ch 6) Form of soft-tissue manipulation that includes contraction, relaxation, and passive movement of body structures.

myelography (ch 2) Administration of either a water-soluble or fat-soluble contrast medium to evaluate intrinsic spinal cord lesions or nerve root defects. Myelography can be used for motion analysis (flexion or extension films) or with computerized tomography in acute spinal trauma.

myelopathy (chs 6, 8) Clinical signs of cord compression, including muscle wasting, spasticity, clonus, and lower limb sensory disturbances.

myofascitis (chs 6, 8) Pain or inflammation that emanates from the muscles or connective soft tissues.

myositis ossificans (ch 9) Calcium formation, usually in the belly of a large muscle, that is secondary to a traumatic hematoma or contusion.

needle electromyography (EMG) (ch 2) Test to determine the denervation potential, denervation of paraspinal muscles, and motor disturbances from both nerve root compression and neuromuscular disease. It is helpful in differentiating a central spinal lesion from a peripheral entrapment neuropathy.

nerve conduction velocity (NCV) (ch 2) Test to rule out peripheral nerve entrapment by determining the speeds of conduction of impulses from two separate stimuli along the course of the peripheral nerve.

neurapraxia (ch 6) Transient weakness attributable to mild demyelinization of the axon sheath of a nerve without disruption.

neurotmesis (ch 6) Injury to a nerve that causes disruption of the axon and supportive tissues. Recovery is not likely in these cases.

nonstructural curve (ch 7) Curve that has no structural component and that corrects or over corrects on recumbent side-bending roentgenograms.

open manipulation (ch 3) Surgical procedure to debride a joint of scar tissue and calcific deposits that is used primarily as a salvage procedure after a closed manipulation has failed.

Ortolani reduction test (ch 9) Test to reduce a congenitally dislocated hip by abducting the hip, which produces an audible click, if successful.

osteochondritis dissecans (chs 4, 10) Disease of adolescents that involves a breakdown of subchondral bone (e.g., in the lateral portion of the medial femoral condyle) and that may lead to vascular insult and fragmentation of bone.

osteogenic scoliosis (ch 7) Structural or "fixed" curvature associated with bony changes that do not correct with side bending and may be associated with an osseous pathologic or a degenerative process.

Panner's disease (ch 4) Disease of childhood that is actually an osteochondrosis of the capitellum and affects primarily boys between the ages of 5 and 10 years.

paraphysiologic movement (ch 1) Movement that extends beyond active and passive motion without compromising the structural integrity of the joint.

patella subluxation (ch 10) Incomplete or partial dislocation at the patellofemoral joint as a result of trauma. Retinacular tearing culminates in a joint effusion.

patellar malalignment syndrome (ch 10) Usually involves a myriad of structural problems such as excessive Q angle, lateral tracking patella, femoral anteversion, and tibial torsion.

patellar retinaculum (ch 10) Fibrous connective tissue extension of the patellar tendon that envelops the patellofemoral joint.

patellar tracking (ch 10) Ability of the patella to maintain congruity in the trochlear groove of the femur during flexion and extension of the knee joint.

Patrick's test (ch 8) Test to detect pathologic abnormalities in the hip or sacroiliac joint. With the patient lying supine, placing the foot on the affected side on the opposite knee and putting the hip in a flexed, abducted, and externally rotated position, the examiner checks for pain in the inguinal or hip region. The examiner may also press down on the bent knee to place pressure on the sacroiliac joint.

pectus carinatum (ch 7) Excessive prominence of the sternum; also known as pigeon breast.

pectus excavatum (ch 7) Excessive depression of the sternum; also known as funnel breast.

pelvic obliquity (ch 8) Tilt of the pelvis or hip region; also known as tortipelvis.

perionychium (ch 5) Superficial skin that grows over the edges of the nailbed.

peripatellar pain (ch 10) Pain adjacent to the patella or over the patellar retinaculum that usually results from a faulty tracking mechanism secondary to injury or weakness.

pes planus (ch 11) Flatfoot deformity, commonly associated with a hyperpronated foot.

Phalen's wrist flexion test (ch 5) Patient's flexing of both wrists to their maximum position and holding them in that position for 60 seconds. Pain in the distribution of the median nerve evoked by this maneuver indicates carpal tunnel syndrome.

Philadelphia collar (ch 6) Rigid cervical orthosis made from hard plastic for advanced ligamentous or osseous injury.

phonophoresis (ch 4) Therapeutic use of ultrasound and a topical pharmaceutical agent, such as hydrocortisone cream, to reduce pain and inflammation from musculoskeletal injury.

pivot shift test (ch 10) Test designed to elicit a subluxation of the tibial plateau and thus to detect a deficiency of the anterior cruciate ligament.

positron emission tomography (PET) (ch 2) Noninvasive imaging technique in which the administration of radioactive substances makes it possible to create computer images of the brain, central nervous system, and various organ systems.

posterior interosseous nerve syndrome (ch 4) Lateral elbow pain, usually of a chronic nature, resulting from peripheral entrapment of the radial nerve near the supinator muscle at the arcade of Frohse.

posttraumatic carpal instability (ch 5) Abnormal bony alignment of the carpus with concomitant ligamentous injury that follows a fall on the extended wrist.

primary curves (ch 7) Spinal curves that are large in magnitude and structural in nature.

pronator teres syndrome (ch 4) Pain caused by compression of the median nerve between the two heads of the pronator teres muscle at the forearm.

pubic symphysitis (ch 9) Inflammation of the pubic symphysis, usually diagnosed radiographically as sclerosing of the symphysis, which can be attributable to repetitive adductor strains or tendonitis or to simple overuse in endurance sports.

Q angle (ch 10) Angulation of the patella in relation to the thigh and pelvis, which reflects the alignment of the lower extremity. The angle is determined by drawing lines from the anterior superior iliac spine to the midpoint of the patella and from the tibial tubercle to the midpoint of the patella. The angle formed at the intersection of these lines is the Q angle, which is normally approximately 13 degrees in men and 18 degrees in women.

quantitative computed tomography (QCT) (ch 2) Noninvasive test that measures bone mineral density. It is often used to screen for osteoporosis of the axial skeleton in postmenopausal women.

radiculopathy (chs 6, 8) Painful or dysthetic response originating from a spinal nerve root and extending outward to the peripheral nerves.

radiofrequency (ch 2) Electromagnetic radiation with frequencies from 0.3 kHz to 300 GH. Magnetic resonance imaging employs a radiofrequency in the range of approximately 1 to 100 mHz.

reconstruction (ch 10) Surgical procedure that involves an unstable joint. Autogenous grafts, such as tendons or allografts of compatible synthetic substances, are used to reinforce damaged ligaments and the joint capsule.

repair (ch 10) Surgical procedure that usually involves the use of sutures to restore the functional capacity of joint structures. In ligament repairs (e.g., anterior cruciate tear), tendinous augmentation may also be used.

retropatellar pain (ch 10) Pain perceived as in the patellofemoral joint or underneath the knee cap.

rib hump (ch 7) Rib prominence associated with scoliosis and vertebral rotation, best seen in the forward bending position (i.e., Adam's position).

ring sign (ch 5) Radiographic evidence of an abnormal rotation of the scaphoid bone that is best visualized on the posteroanterior wrist projection; also known as the cortical ring sign.

Risser grading (ch 7) Skeletal maturity scale of 0 to 5 according to the extent of ossification at the iliac apophysis.

Risser sign (ch 2) Indication of the stage of maturity at the iliac apophyseal ring that helps the clinician determine an individual's skeletal maturity.

Rolando fracture (ch 5) Intraarticular fracture to the base of the thumb that is a precursor to basal joint arthritis.

Romberg's sign (ch 6) Body sway, loss of balance when an individual closes the eyes and stands still following head and neck injury.

Rust's sign (ch 6) Difficulty in maintaining the cervical spine in an erect position against the forces of motion and gravity, which indicates ligamentous instability.

scapholunate angle (ch 5) Angle between the scaphoid and lunate, which is a major factor in determining carpal stability, as visualized on the lateral x-ray projection of the wrist. A normal angle is 30 to 60 degrees.

scapholunate dissociation (ch 5) Interval of 4 mm or more between the scaphoid and lunate, which is definitive of ligamentous (carpal) instability.

Scheuermann's disease (ch 7) Condition of congenital weakness of the end-plate ring apophysis in adolescents, which occurs predominantly in the thoracolumbar region of the spine and may be associated with radiographic evidence of Schmorl's nodes; sometimes called juvenile kyphosis.

scleratogenous pain (ch 6) Peripheralization of spinal pain originating from the somatic structures of the vertebral column, such as the joint capsule, articular cartilage, bone, and ligaments; also termed somatic pain referral.

secondary restraint (ch 10) Structures outside the bony arrangement of a joint that contribute to joint stability.

selective serotonin reuptake inhibitors (SSRIs) Medication used to treat clinical depression to boose the brain's level of serotonin.

sesamoiditis (ch 11) Inflammation, bruise, or fracture involving one of the two small sesamoid bones in the tendon of the flexor hallucis brevis muscle under the first metatarsal head.

Sever's disease (ch 11) Inflammation at the attachment of the Achilles' tendon at the calcaneal apophysis; also called traction apophysitis of the os calcis or calcaneal apophysitis.

skeletal age (ch 2) Bony maturity, an individual's progress in the physical maturation process, as opposed to the individual's chronologic age.

skier's thumb (ch 5) Sprain or rupture of the ulnar collateral ligament as a result of a forceful fall on an abducted thumb; also called a "gamekeeper's" thumb.

slipped capital femoral epiphysis (ch 9) Childhood disorder involving a displacement of the femoral epiphyseal plate that appears radiographically as "ice cream slipping off the cone."

somatosensory evoked potentials (SSEP) (ch 2) Test to investigate spinal abnormalities (e.g., spinal cord disease, spinal trauma, demyelinating disorders, neuromuscular disease) by evaluating the condition of a peripheral nerve through its spinal cord connection up to the somatosensory region of the brain.

Soto-Hall test (ch 6) Sharp, passive flexion of the head and neck to detect any pain in the cervicothoracic spine that suggests subluxation, exostoses, disk lesion, sprain, strain, or fracture of vertebrae.

spinal stenosis (chs 6, 8) Vertebral canal compromise in size via congenital, bony, or soft-tissue means.

spondyloarthropathies (chs 6, 8) Group of arthritides (e.g., ankylosing spondylitis, Reiter's disease) that often affect the spine, although serologic tests show no sign of the rheumatoid factor.

spondylolysis (ch 8) Fatigue or stress fracture at the pars interarticularis, most often diagnosed on an oblique projection of the lumbar spine.

Sprengel's deformity (ch 6) Partially undescended (from neck to thorax) scapula.

Spurling's maneuver (ch 6) Placement of the patient into cervical compression, rotation, and extended positions toward the side of involvement to determine whether these movements cause pain.

Stenner lesion (ch 5) Injury to the ulnar collateral ligament in a grade III rupture where the ligament lies on top of the adductor pollicis muscle.

stress films (ch 2) Special projections taken when ligaments and joint capsules are stretched (i.e., stressed) to help diagnose occult instability.

structural curve (ch 7) Segment of the spine with a lateral curvature that lacks normal flexibility. Radiographically, it is identified by the complete absence of a curve on a supine film or by the failure to demonstrate complete segmental mobility on supine side-bending films.

subluxation (ch 2) Presence of joint incongruency and deviation from normal articulation of two bony surfaces or points of articulation in a joint (i.e, a partial dislocation).

superior labral repair (SLAP) (ch 3) Surgical repair from the anterior to the posterior aspect of the structure. This procedure is an option when the long head of the biceps is unstable.

supination anteroposterior projection (ch 4) Standard oblique view at the elbow that is particularly useful when an injury to the radial head is suspected.

supracondylar fracture (ch 4) Difficult-to-treat childhood fracture that usually occurs just above the humeral condyles and often results in neurovascular compression of the limb.

swan neck deformity (ch 5) Hyperextension injury at the proximal interphalangeal joint with volar plate damage. This extension deformity results in flexion of the distal interphalangeal joint.

sympathetic injury (ch 6) Trauma to the autonomic chain ganglia of the paracervical region common in whiplash injuries, causing diverse symptomatology such as dizziness, lightheadedness, visual disturbances, nausea, and headache.

synovitis of the hip (ch 9) Inflammation of the hip joint that may be caused by infection, trauma, or degenerative processes.

T1 relaxation time (ch 2) Time required for the interactions between nuclear spins and the tissue lattice to return to normal following radiofrequency excitation during magnetic resonance imaging; also called spin-lattice or longitudinal relaxation time.

T2 relaxation time (ch 2) Time required for the interaction between nuclear spins and adjacent nuclear spins to return to normal after radiofrequency excitation during magnetic resonance imaging; also called spin-spin or transverse relaxation time.

talipes equinovarus (ch 11) Rigid deformity of the foot present at birth; also called congenital clubfoot.

tarsal coalition (ch 11) Fibrous or cartilaginous bridge between two tarsal bones or at the hindfoot, which may become symptomatic or play a direct role in foot hypomobility.

tarsal tunnel syndrome (ch 11) Pain in the medial or lateral plantar nerve caused by entrapment of the tibial nerve and its branches in the region between the medial malleolus and the calcaneus.

temporomandibular joint (TMJ) syndrome (ch 6) Articular or soft-tissue dysfunction of the craniofacial muscles with mandibular pain. Often the cause of head, face, eye or ear, or neck pain, this syndrome may be the result of whiplash trauma or stress.

tennis elbow (ch 4) Generic term for lateral epicondylitis or extensor tendonitis of the elbow caused by repeated terminal extension of the elbow.

Terry Thomas sign (ch 5) Gap of more than 2 mm between the scaphoid and lunate, as measured on an anteroposterior film, which suggests ligamentous instability at the scapholunate articulation.

thermography (ch 2) Imaging procedure that measures heat emissions and temperature differentials to document soft-tissue injury. There are two types of thermographic imaging: electronic infrared and liquid crystal thermography.

Thompson test (ch 11) Test in which the examiner squeezes the involved calf and looks for plantar flexion of the foot to screen for an Achilles' tendon rupture. The test is positive when this motion is absent, suggesting rupture.

thoracic outlet syndrome (TOS) (ch 6) Condition involving neurovascular compression at the thoracic outlet with medial arm and hand pain, positional symptomatology of the shoulder and arm, night pain, and pulse changes of the upper extremity.

thumb opposition (ch 5) Motion of the thumb to the little finger of the hand.

thumb-spica immobilization (ch 5) Use of a brace to keep both the wrist and thumb-basal articulation in a neutral, immobile position.

Tinel's sign (chs 4, 5) Procedure in which the examiner taps a nerve at a superficial point to elicit a painful response or paresthesias distal to the stimulus in cases of compression and irritation. Commonly used at the cubital tunnel (ulnar nerve), the carpal tunnel (median nerve), and the fibular head (common peroneal nerve).

torque (ch 8) Load that is applied by a coupling of forces (parallel and directed opposite each other) about the long axis of a structure.

torticollis (ch 6) Muscle spasm and stiffness in the cervical region; also known as wry neck.

total hip arthroplasty (ch 9) Surgical replacement of a diseased hip joint with an artificial joint for the diseased articulation. A medullary rod or stem are cemented into the femur to reduce pain and improve function.

transient cervical quadriplegia (ch 6) Temporary paresis in both the upper and lower extremity, which may result from spinal cord shock (vertebral contusion) or from a soft-tissue injury in a patient with cervical stenosis.

tricyclic antidepressants (ch 6) Group of drugs (e.g., amitriptyline [Elavil]) that are used commonly for chronic back pain and headaches.

trigger finger (ch 5) Incongruous motion of the finger in the tendon sheath, usually caused by swelling of the flexor tendon pulley with nodular and fibrotic changes.

two-point discrimination (ch 7) Ability to differentiate between two points of stimulation on the skin surface simultaneously.

ulnar nerve transposition (ch 4) Surgical procedure in which the surgeon moves a traumatized ulnar nerve from the compromised cubital tunnel to the anterior position of the arm.

ulnar variance (ch 5) Relationship between the length of the ulna and that of the radius at the wrist, as indicated by the distance in millimeters of a line extended anteriorly from the distal radial articular surface to the distal ulna. Normally, the two bones are almost the same length. A positive ulnar variance indicates that the ulna projects farther distally than the radius.

Unna boot (ch 11) Soft, medicated compressive case used for early compression, immobilization, and protection of the ankle against further injury.

vertebral apophysitis (ch 7) Nonunion or traumatic inflammation that involves the secondary centers of ossification of the vertebrae and most commonly affects the superior-anterior aspect of the vertebral body.

vertebral end plates (chs 6, 7, 8) Superior and inferior plates of cortical bone of the vertebral body adjacent to the intervertebral disk.

vertebral growth plate (ch 7) Cartilaginous surface covering the top and bottom of a vertebral body, which is responsible for the linear growth of the vertebra.

vertebral ring apophyses (chs 7, 8) Most reliable index of vertebral immaturity, seen best in lateral roentgenograms or in the lumbar region in side-bending anteroposterior views.

vertebrogenic cephalgia (ch 6) Head pain, either neuromuscular or vascular, from a source within the cervical spine.

wallerian degeneration (ch 6) Disruption and breakdown of nerve tissue.

windlass mechanism (ch 11) Function of the plantar fascia as it forms the longitudinal arch from the metatarsal heads to the os calcis.

Yeoman's test (ch 8) Test for a sacroiliac lesion in which, with the patient lying prone and bending one knee, the examiner places one hand over the affected sacroiliac joint as a stabilizer and lifts the knee off the examination table. Increased sacroiliac pain denotes a positive test.

Answers to Review Questions

Chapter 1

1. Internal derangement, such as a torn ligament or meniscus (cartilage)
2. Arthritis (e.g., osteoarthritis, rheumatoid arthritis)
3. Scleratogenous referral, also known as somatic-referred pain
4. Effusion
5. Organic disease
6. To rule out fracture, arthritis, tumor, skeletal age assessment
7. Immature bones of the child possess strong periosteum, weak growth centers (apophysis, epiphysis) and are susceptible to load deformation. Mature bones of the adult have closed growth centers, are resistant to load deformation, and have weaker periosteum.

Chapter 2

1. (a) Plain-film radiography
   (b) Two
   (c) Hand and wrist joint and foot and ankle joint, because of the complex anatomy of each, and sometimes the knee and elbow, require three projections. An oblique projection is necessary to rule out trauma.
2. (a) Ask the woman of childbearing age if she is pregnant before obtaining x-ray films, because of the danger to the fetus.
   (b) Ask the patient if she has had significant exposure in the past few years to large numbers of imaging procedures.
   (c) Reduce the gonadal dosage by using rare-earth screens, protecting the area with a shield, and limiting the total number of films.

3. Posteroanterior view of the wrist, iliac apophyseal ring (Risser's sign), epiphyseal plate of long bones, and apophysis at the tendon-bone interface
4. (a) To screen for bone tumors in patients with an increased alkaline phosphatase level
   (b) To identify early bone and joint infection (sepsis)
   (c) To diagnose ankylosing spondylitis, diskitis, posterior element stress fracture, or metastatic disease
   (d) To diagnose a stress or fatigue fracture of the extremities
5. (a) Superior contrast resolution for bone and soft-tissue, potential for cross-sectional display, and image reconstruction in additional planes
   (b) Imaging of cortical bone, acute brain injury, fracture confirmation, lung disease, and general survey for neoplasm
6. Spinal cord abnormalities that include the intradural space, spinal disk disease, multiple sclerosis, avascular necrosis, meniscal tears, and fibrocartilage conditions
7. Needle electromyogram (EMG) to rule out denervation from cervical nerve root compression (NCV); NCV to rule out concomitant peripheral entrapment of the median nerve

Chapter 3

1. (1) Glenohumeral joint—dislocations, subluxations, and chronic instability
   (2) Acromioclavicular joint—sprains (separations), arthritis, subacromial bursitis
   (3) Sternoclavicular joint—sprains (separations), clavicle fractures

(4) Scapulothoracic joint—myofascitis, dysfunction, dyskinesia, postural faults

2. A–4; B–3; C–1; D–2

3. (a) Anterior (subcoracoid)

(b) Sudden or forced hyperabduction with external rotation

(c) Plain films to rule out fracture, including an axillary (Stryker notch) projection; and immobilization for a minimum of 3 weeks for first-time dislocators

4. (a) Point tenderness and swelling over the acromioclavicular joint and painful horizontal adduction; difficulty in abducting the arm over 90 degrees and possible instability of the acromioclavicular joint

(b) Ice hockey, downhill skiing, football, weight-training

5. Bony borders include the acromion process, acromioclavicular joint, and tuberosity of the humeral head. Structures that can be involved in pathologic abnormalities of the space include a thickened coracoacromial ligament, subacromial bursa, biceps tendon, acromioclavicular arthritis or spurring, and supraspinatus tendon.

6. (a) Adhesive capsulitis

(b) Arthrography

(c) Physical therapy, chiropractic manipulative therapy, and mobilization and therapeutic range-of-motion exercises

7. (a) Lung tumor

(b) Apical (lordotic) chest x-ray, complete blood count and chemistry, and urinalysis

Chapter 4

1. (a) Medial shear and lateral compression

(b) Valgus strain

2. (a) Medial collateral ligament, ulnar nerve, flexor and pronator muscles

(b) Extensor mass or tendon, bony fragments, osteochondral lesion, posterior interosseous-radial nerve

(c) Joint capsule, biceps tendon, median nerve

(d) Triceps tendon or muscle, arthritic bone, olecranon bursa

(e) Elbow fracture

3. (a) Lateral epicondylitis (tennis elbow)

(b) (1) Repetitive extension of the elbow (overuse in weight training)

(2) Tennis (using too heavy a racquet, improper grip, racquet strung too tight, poor technique)

(3) Excessive carrying of heavy bags or briefcase with a straight arm

(c) Rest, ice, ultrasound, therapeutic exercises, use of a counterforce brace, antiinflammatory medication, and manipulation

4. (a) Ulnar neuritis (cubital tunnel syndrome)

(b) Numbness or paresthesias in the ulnar nerve distribution of the hand, pain at the medial forearm into the fourth and fifth digits, positive Tinel's sign in elbow flexion over the ulnar nerve, weakness in pinch and grip strength; late motor changes, including positive Froment's sign, atrophy of the intrinsic muscles of the hand, and difficulty in handwriting

5. (a) Overuse syndrome that usually occurs from the repetitive valgus stress of throwing in skeletally immature persons

(b) Limiting the number of innings a pitcher throws per week and stressing proper throwing mechanics, including the avoidance of sidearm throwing

Chapter 5

1. (a) Posteroanterior, posteroanterior oblique, and lateral

(b) Posteroanterior film—examine for normal wrist arcs, the spacing of the intercarpal articulations, and the angles between the carpals to evaluate stability, especially the scapholunate space to rule out a Terry Thomas sign.
Posteroanterior oblique film—examine for the same indications and bony integrity of the scaphoid in cases of trauma.
Lateral film—examine for scapholunate angle measurement and the radiolunate interface.

(c) (1) Carpal tunnel projection evaluates the bony borders of the tunnel and is used to rule out fractures of the hamate.

(2) Posteroanterior ulnar deviation film confirms the presence of a scaphoid fracture.

2. (a) Inflammation of the first extensor compartment of the wrist involving the tendons of the abductor pollicus longus and the extensor pollicis brevis

(b) Repetitive motions of the wrist and hand that require ulnar deviation, hormonal influx of estrogen during pregnancy

(c) Finkelstein's test

3. (a) Scaphoid fracture
   (b) Posteroanterior, posteroanterior oblique, lateral, and posteroanterior ulnar deviation projection to rule out scaphoid fracture
   (c) If x-ray findings are normal or equivocal and the examination suggests scaphoid fracture, the patient's wrist should be immobilized and x-ray films should be retaken in 10-14 days.
4. (a) Numbness and tingling in the wrist, thumb, and first and second digits on the involved hand; weakness in pinch and grip strength; thenar atrophy; nocturnal pain; reduced two-point discrimination
   (b) Tinel's tap over the volar carpal ligament, Phalen's test
   (c) Immobilization, underwater ultrasound, vitamin B6 therapy, antiinflammatory medication
   (d) Cervical radiculopathy, pronator teres syndrome
5. (a) Ulnar nerve
   (b) Cervical radiculopathy, cubital tunnel entrapment, Guyon's canal syndrome, ulnar neuritis
6. (a) Ulnar collateral ligament of the thumb
   (b) Metacarpophalangeal joint of the thumb
   (c) Avulsion fracture at the base of the proximal phalanx

Chapter 6

1. (a) C0-C1: Primarily flexion and extension
       C1-C2: Primarily posteroanterior rotation
       C3-C7: Aids in considerable flexion and extension, with the greatest range at C5-C6 level
   (b) Height of the cervical disks and their relatively small diameter in both the sagittal and coronal planes
   (c) Lateral bending that produces concomitant posteroanterior rotation with spinous movement to the contralateral side of lateral bend; coupling movements that decrease gradually from C2 to C7 as the incline of the facet joints change
2. (a) Leading with the crown of the head induces initial contact at the top of the helmet in football, for example, which involves the skull rapidly decelerating on impact.
   (b) The head in flexion will segmentalize the vertebral column, leaving the vertebral end-plates vulnerable to compression forces. The end result of axial loading to the cervical spine may be disk failure, vertebral compression fracture, vertebral burst fracture, or spinal cord injury.
3. 1–b; 2–d; 3–c ; 4–a
4. (a) Restoration of synovial joint motion, altering existing myofascial tension, lengthening connective tissues through adhesion disruption, and correcting and relieving muscular hypertonicity
   (b) Causes of global hypomobility, such as fracture or dislocation, gross spinal cord impairment (e.g., quadriplegia, paraplegia), carotid artery disease, vertebrobasilar insufficiency, Wallenberg's syndrome, malignant tumors, gross ligamentous instability, and spinal infection
5. (a) Cervical sympathetic insult, recurrent headaches, vestibular dysfunction, myofascitis, altered cognitive ability, temporomandibular joint complaints
   (b) Active, manual intervention that is instituted as early as clinically possible during the course of care, avoidance of prolonged immobilization
   (c) Plain film x-rays
6. (a) Cervical disk lesion with radiculopathy
   (b) Ice, clinical modalities to reduce pain and swelling, gentle manual traction, immobilization as indicated, isometrics
7. (a) Disk disease, degenerative arthritis, and acute flexion loading injuries
   (b) Transient quadriplegia in athletes, cervical cord neuropraxia, chronic degenerative disk disease, ligamentous instability
   (c) Magnetic resonance imaging (MRI) or computed tomography (CT); MRI is superior for imaging the spinal cord. CT is the diagnostic tool of choice for assessing bony canal size.
8. (a) Thoracic outlet syndrome
   (b) C8,T1 nerve roots
   (c) Normal EMG and NCV
   (d) Shoulder depression, hyperabduction test, costoclavicular test

Chapter 7

1. (a) Primary curve
   (b) Infection, scoliosis, metabolic disorders, Scheuermann's disease
   (c) Iliocostalis thoracis, erector spinae muscles, ribs, and synovial joints
2. (a) Upper seven rib pairs
   (b) Lower five rib pairs

(c) Rib pairs 11 and 12, because of the lack of anterior attachment

3. Ankylosing spondylitis

4. (a) No radicular signs, tenderness over the neural arch, supraspinous ligament or spinous process; end-range joint block, provoking flexion-extension of the cervicodorsal spine, unilateral paraspinal hypertonicity

   (b) Repetitive trauma, postural faults, previous rib injury, somatic dysfunction possible

   (c) Over the supraspinous ligament

5. (a) Idiopathic

   (b) Loss of physiologic kyphosis, convex vertebral body rotation and lateral bending possible, loss of spine's inherent resistance to deforming loads (especially rotation), development of secondary curves or half-curve possible, asymmetry in resting muscle tone, muscle length and gross joint motion, altered postural reflexes, pelvic obliquity with or without a short leg, and lumbopelvic inflexibility

   (c) Progression factor $= \dfrac{\text{Cobb angle} \times \text{Risser's sign}}{\text{chronologic age}}$

   (d) Maintain flexibility of the spine and curve, improve paraspinal strength, use spinal movements that include transverse loads and joint distraction to normalize intervertebral segmental motion.

Chapter 8

1. (a) Direct—costs of administrating claims; provider, hospitalization, surgical, and medication costs; workers' compensation premiums; costs of rehabilitation, including occupational and physical therapy and work hardening; cost of absenteeism and sick leave

      Indirect—loss of productivity, retraining and hiring new workers, workplace morale, costs of corporate safety programs, litigation, and medical-peer review vendor costs

   (b) Excessive compressive forces on the erector spinal muscles of the back; shearing forces on the lumbar facets and posterior ligaments in lifting objects and exaggerated flexion movements; large moment forces in flexion and exaggerated rotation on the lower lumbar disks; muscular fatigue, postural alterations, and accelerated disk degeneration attributable to repetitive vibration

   (c) Shift from high-tech, surgical, and hospital-based care and passive therapies (e.g., bedrest, ongoing medication) to more low-tech, hands-on, office-based treatment systems that use active therapies (e.g., early forms of mobilization, manipulation, and rehabilitative exercise)

2. (a) Aging and degeneration of the intervertebral disk, including internal resorption, carbohydrate binding, loss of water content (dessication), and hydraulic power, that lead to failure under axial loading and compression through fissures and compression fractures. This failure, in turn, may lead to improper transfer of spinal loads at the intervertebral joint, which ultimately places excessive weight-bearing demands on the posterior facet joints of the lumbar spine, leading to arthrosis and fibrosis.

   (b) Mechanical (true nerve root compression) and biochemical (inflammatory exudates)

3. The proper transfer of loads and sequencing of forces occurs through the efficient use of the pelvic-hip extensor mass and legs in the absence of independent erector spinal recruitment. Final compensation of load occurs through the lumbodorsal fascia, which ultimately transfers force to the upper extremities.

4. (a) (1) Prior neoplasm and infection

       (2) Lack of reproducible orthopedic and neurologic findings

       (3) Full range of motion in the presence of unrelenting pain

       (4) Pain that is constant, worse at night, and consistent

       (5) Weight loss accompanied by changes in bowel or bladder habits

   (b) Patients with unexplained weight loss, significant trauma, suspicion of ankylosing spondylitis, history of drug or alcohol abuse at age 50 years or older, history of cancer or metabolic disease, prolonged use of corticosteroids, temperature higher than 100° F

5. (a) Radicular pain is often described as sharp, stabbing, or shooting in a pinpoint zone, 1 to 2 inches in width. Radicular problems may be associated with sensory distribution (paresthesia), motor changes (weakness, atrophy), or pain radiating outward from the spine (radiculopathy). Disk disease, infection, and space-occupying lesions are examples of radicular pain. Somatic-referred pain originates in vertebral structures such as disks, neural elements, and the posterior

joint, as well as in articular capsules, cartilage, and vertebrae. Sacroiliac and facet sprain can cause somatic (scleratogenous) referral, which is described as dull and achy pain that is harder to localize than radicular patterns.

(b) Myotogenous pain stems from active trigger points that radiate to a distant site from the muscle tissue and is not as well-localized as pain in the more "traditional" dermatomal pattern, which is sharp and localized via a specific dermatome or dermatomes. Dermatomal pain usually stems from nerve root irritation or compression, as seen in a herniated disk and radiculopathy.

6. (a) Mechanical effects—alters joint capsule tension, activates type I and II mechanoreceptors, influences muscle tone and spinal cord reflexes, increases spinal and articular mobility.

Neurohormonal effects—may affect beta-endorphin levels and the elevation of immune and biologic markers.

(b) McKenzie extension series, functional squatting program, spinal stabilization series, mobility training including dynamic weight-bearing exercise such as ground-reactive movements

7. (a) L4-L5 disk herniation with radiculopathy (L5)

(b) McKenzie extension series, manipulation-distraction in extension, ice, spinal stabilization exercise, clinical modalities

(c) Central disk herniation

(d) MRI

8. (a) History of repetitive flexion and extension, intermittent history of low back pain, child athletes (especially gymnastics and football), painful lumbar extension with radiation into the buttock or leg, pain over the area of defect during unilateral weight bearing

(b) Defect of the pars interarticularis without forward displacement on the lateral or oblique projection

(c) Dysplastic, isthmic, degenerative, traumatic, or pathologic defects

(d) Chiropractic manipulative therapy, antilordic exercises (i.e., Williams flexion exercises), flexibility program for hamstrings, psoas, and gluteal muscles

Chapter 9

1. (a) Range of motion impairment, most severe in flexion and internal rotation

(b) Adults with a history of systemic illness, degenerative diseases, steroid therapy, or infection; children with a history of trauma, fever and infection, or severe limitation of hip motion

2. (a) Elderly

(b) Fall secondary to visual impairment, Parkinson's disease, previous stroke, or lower limb dysfunction

(c) Greater trochanter of the femur, lesser trochanter of the femur, and femoral neck

3. (a) Thigh (quadriceps) contusion

(b) Never

(c) Myositis ossificans

4. (a) Painful limp, hip or leg pain, limited internal rotation and flexion

(b) Children, 1 to 3 years of age: congenital dislocation, transient synovitis with a recent history of upper respiratory infection, trauma
Children, 4-10 years of age: Legg-Calvé-Perthes disease, slipped capital femoral epiphysis, tumors, infection

5. (a) Iliac Apophysitis (apophyseal avulsion)

(b) Plain x-ray films, including anteroposterior and oblique projections of the affected hip to rule out a slipped apophysis

(c) Treatment is conservative and symptomatic, directed at controlling pain and swelling. Acute care includes ice, non–weight-bearing rest, the use of crutches, and electrotherapy.

Chapter 10

1. (a) Rotation (medial-lateral), translation (flexion-extension)

(b) Medial and lateral collateral ligaments prevent excessive adduction and abduction, respectively. Anterior and posterior cruciate ligaments prevent hyperextension and hyperflexion, respectively.

2. (a) (1) Aids in load transmission
   (2) Functions as a major shock absorber
   (3) Helps control excessive joint motion
   (4) Aids in joint nutrition

(b) (1) Positive joint effusion
   (2) Joint line tenderness
   (3) Painful flexion and rotation
   (4) Positive McMurray test

(c) MRI and arthrography

3. (1) Anterior knee pain and bogginess
   (2) Retropatellar (facet) and peripatellar (retinac-

ulum) discomfort
  (3) Patellar malalignment (genu valgum, tibial varum)
  (4) Excessive Q-angle
  (5) Quadriceps weakness
  (6) Atrophy
  (7) Lateral tracking patella
  (8) Hypermobility of the patellofemoral joint
  (9) Painful flexion of the knee
4. (a) Grade II medial collateral ligament sprain and mild medial capsule sprain; rule out a medial meniscus tear
   (b) Application of ice, immobilization, use of crutches, isometrics, and electrotherapy
5. (a) Anterior cruciate ligament sprain and medial meniscus tear
   (b) MRI to confirm the torn meniscus and to evaluate whether the patient is a candidate for arthroscopic meniscal repair
6. Isometrics in terminal extension (quadriceps sets), isometrics in partial flexion (wall squats), short arc isotonics without resistance, short arc isotonics with resistance, functional multijoint closed–kinetic chain movements (therapeutic squats)
7. Traction apophysitis (Osgood-Schlatter Disease)

Chapter 11

1. Posterior compartment contains the soleus and gastrocnemius muscles, along with the posterior tibial nerve; anterior compartment contains the tibia and fibula, tibialis anterior, extensor hallucis longus and extensor digitorum longus muscles, and deep peroneal nerve and tibial artery. Lateral compartment contains the peroneus longus and peroneus brevis, along with the superficial branch of the peroneal nerve.
2. Subtalar joint; pes planus, posterior tibialis strain or tendonitis, plantar fascitis, tarsal tunnel syndrome, patellofemoral pain, mechanical low back pain
3. (a) Deltoid ligament
   (b) Medial ankle sprain, mortise instability, syndesmosis (high ankle) sprain, talar dome fracture, medial malleolus fracture, rupture of the tibiofibular ligament, Maisonneuve fracture (anteroposterior)
   (c) Anteroposterior, lateral, mortise views
4. Aggressive control of acute edema and inflammation through the use of crutches, compressive Unna boot, cryotherapy, electrotherapy, and non–weight-bearing flexibility exercises will enable the clinician to institute earlier ambulation, proprioception and strengthening movements for the ankle.
5. (a) Metatarsalgia, plantar fasciitis
   (b) Shortened or tightened Achilles' tendon, and/or gastrocnemius muscle, foot in equinus position
6. (a) Peripheral entrapment of the plantar nerve just distal to the tarsal tunnel causing foot and toe pain
   (b) Diabetes mellitus, plantar fascitis, gouty arthritis, and calcaneal spurs

Chapter 12

1. (a) Musculoskeletal, nervous, dermatologic
   (b) Clinical diagnosis
2. Early stage of Lyme disease will respond to proper oral administration of antibiotics for 4 to 6 weeks with favorable results. Late stage of the disease will require intravenous antibiotic therapy, with varying results.
3. Although there is crossover in the signs and symptoms of both illnesses, the major difference between the two is fatigue in chronic fatigue syndrome and pain in fibromyalgia, the chief complaint in both.
4. Patients with myofascitis have active trigger points with distant-site referral and a lack of constitutional symptoms. Patients with fibromyalgia have multiple tender point sites with no active referral zones, and, in addition, these patients have secondary constitutional complaints, such as depression, sleep disturbances, gastrointestinal ailments, and headaches.
5. (a) Generalized viral complaints, including headache, muscle and joint pain, and fatigue
   (b) All treatments for these conditions are conservative and nonsurgical. Gentle-graded therapeutic exercise is important to improve or maintain general fitness levels in all three conditions.

Index

Page number in italics denotes an illustration; page number followed by a *t* denotes a table.

439

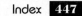

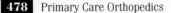